9.50

85-239-C
WM 100

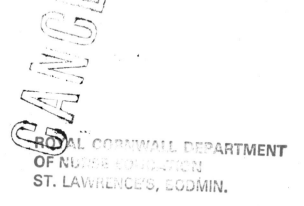

TREATMENT AND MANAGEMENT
IN ADULT PSYCHIATRY

Treatment and Management in Adult Psychiatry

Edited by

G. E. BERRIOS

MA(Oxon), MD, DPhilSci (Oxon), DPM, FRCPsych
Director of Medical Studies and Fellow of Robinson College, Cambridge;
University Lecturer in Psychiatry, and Honorary Consultant Psychiatrist
at the University of Cambridge Clinical School

J. H. DOWSON

MA, MB, BChir (Cantab), DPM (Edin), FRCPsych, PhD (Edin)
Member of Queens' College, Cambridge; University Lecturer in Psychiatry,
and Honorary Consultant Psychiatrist at the University of Cambridge
Clinical School

BAILLIÈRE TINDALL · LONDON

Published by BAILLIÈRE TINDALL,
a division of Cassell Ltd,
1 St Anne's Road,
Eastbourne, East Sussex
BN21 3UN

First published 1983

ISBN 0 7020 0927 X

Phototypeset by Scribe Design, Gillingham, Kent

**Printed and bound in Great Britain by
Robert Hartnoll Ltd. Bodmin, Cornwall**

British Library Cataloguing in Publication Data

Treatment and management in adult psychiatry.
1. Mental illness
I. Berrios, G.E.   II. Dowson, J.H.
616.89   RC 454

ISBN 0-7020-0927-x

Contents

Preface

There are many publications concerned with aspects of the wide variety of pharmacological, physical, psychological and social treatment methods, or of the management of psychiatric disorder, but a relatively concise, inclusive, integrated and up-to-date account of the practice of psychiatry was not available. This book is an attempt to meet this need, and reflects an eclectic philosophy combined with a belief that the value of our discipline must be judged, ultimately, on the basis of scientific enquiry.

Part One provides a detailed account of the range of treatment methods which are available to the psychiatrist, while Part Two considers the selection of the appropriate interventions for the various psychiatric syndromes. Although this book is not designed as a comprehensive textbook of psychiatry, descriptive and other aspects are included where necessary. Certain contributions cover relatively neglected aspects of psychiatric practice. These include the chapters on: 'Treatments for Chronic Cognitive Impairment'; 'Group Psychotherapies', in which the focus is on the group activities in a routine psychiatric service; 'Management of Disorders of Sexual Function'; and 'Management of Sleep Disorders'.

Treatment and Management in Adult Psychiatry is principally written for trainee and practising psychiatrists, but we hope that it will also be of value to medical students, general practitioners, and other professions working in the psychiatric services. Most of the contributions are derived from the teaching programmes at the University of Cambridge Clinical School.

We would like to express our gratitude to our contributors; also to Mrs E. Barry, Mrs E. Broad, Mrs M. Coburn, Miss R. Hammond and Mrs M. Lockwood for their help with the preparation of the typescripts; and to the people at Baillière Tindall for their encouragement and patience.

November, 1982

G.E. Berrios
J.H. Dowson

Contributors

Dr. F. Arroyave, LMS (Salamanca), MRCPsych, Consultant Psychiatrist in Alcoholism, Ley Clinic, Littlemore Hospital, Oxford.

Dr. T.R.E. Barnes, MB, BS, MRCPsych, Wellcome Research Fellow, Department of Psychiatry, University of Cambridge Clinical School, Addenbrooke's Hospital, Hills Road, Cambridge, CB2 2QQ.

Dr. G.E. Berrios, MA, MD, DPhilSci, DPM, FRCPsych, Honorary Consultant Psychiatrist, University Lecturer in Psychiatry, Department of Psychiatry, University of Cambridge Clinical School, Addenbrooke's Hospital, Hills Road, Cambridge, CB2 2QQ.

Dr. W.M. Braude, BA, MB, ChB, MRCPsych, Wellcome Research Fellow, Department of Psychiatry, University of Cambridge Clinical School, Addenbrooke's Hospital, Hills Road, Cambridge, CB2 2QQ.

Dr. C.P.B. Brook, MA, MD, DPM, FRCPsych, Consultant Psychogeriatrician, Associate Lecturer in Psychiatry, University of Cambridge, Fulbourn Hospital, Cambridge, CB1 5EF.

Dr. J.H. Dowson, MA, MB, BChir, DPM, FRCPsych, PhD, Honorary Consultant Psychiatrist, University Lecturer in Psychiatry, Department of Psychiatry, University of Cambridge Clinical School, Addenbrooke's Hospital, Hills Road, Cambridge, CB2 2QQ.

H.M. Evans, BSc, (Lately MRC Research Psychologist, Research Associate, Department of Psychiatry, University of Cambridge Clinical School, Addenbrooke's Hospital, Hills Road, Cambridge, CB2 2QQ.) The Wellcome Research Laboratories, Langley Court, Beckenham, Kent, BR3 3BS.

Dr N.J.R. Evans, MA, BM, BCh, MRCPsych, (Lately Research Associate, Department of Psychiatry, University of Cambridge Clinical School, Addenbrooke's Hospital, Hills Road, Cambridge, CB2 2QQ.) Consultant Psychiatrist, Coney Hill Hospital, Coney Hill, Gloucester, GL4 7QJ.

Dr. A.V.P. Mackay, MA, BSc, PhD, MB, ChB, DPM, MRCPsych, Physician Superintendent, Argyll and Bute Hospital, Lochgilphead, Argyll, PA31 8LD. (Formerly Deputy Director, MRC Neurochemical Pharmacology Unit, Cambridge.)

Dr. S. Morley, BSc, PhD, MPhil, Senior Psychologist, Cambridge District Health Authority, Senior Clinical Psychologist, Fulbourn Hospital, Cambridge, CB1 5EF.

Dr. C.Q. Mountjoy, MB, BS, DPM, MRCPsych, Honorary Consultant Psychiatrist, Wellcome Research Fellow, Department of Psychiatry, University of Cambridge Clinical School, Addenbrooke's Hospital, Hills Road, Cambridge, CB2 2QQ.

Professor Sir Martin Roth, MD, FRCP, FRCPsych, ScD, Professor of Psychiatry, University of Cambridge Clinical School, Addenbrooke's Hospital, Hills Road, Cambridge, CB2 2QQ.

Professor D.J. West, MD, DPM, MRCPsych, PhD, LittD, Professor of Clinical Criminology, Institute of Criminology, 7 West Road, Cambridge, CB3 9DT.

Dr. C. de B. White, MB, BS, MRCP, MRCPsych, MD, Wellcome Research Fellow, Department of Psychiatry, University of Cambridge Clinical School, Addenbrooke's Hospital, Hills Road, Cambridge, CB2 2QQ.

PART ONE

Treatment

1

Anxiolytic Drugs

G.E. Berrios

BENZODIAZEPINES

Introduction

When the search for tranquillizers superior to barbiturates or meprobamates started in the 1950s, Sternbach (1979) chose the benzheptodiazines because they were 'relatively unexplored, readily accessible, easily modifiable and looked as if they could lead to biologically active products'.

Over 1000 derivatives were tested by three screening tests and in 1957 a compound which had been synthesized 2 years earlier was rediscovered. Screening showed it to be superior to meprobamate, chlorpromazine and phenobarbitone. The drug 7-chloro-2 methylamino-5-phenyl-3H-1, 4-benzodiazepine 4-oxide (chlordiazepoxide) was patented in July 1959. The relevant nucleus was identified as 2-amino-1, 4 benzodiazepine 4-oxide, which has three crucial positions for manipulation.

More than 4000 compounds have since been reported in over 12 000 publications. Latterly, modifications in the structure have produced the 1-5 benzodiazepines (such as clobazam), and an additional ring has given rise to the triazolobenzodiazepines (e.g. triazolam, alprozam), which have been claimed to be ideal hypnotics on the basis of their short half-life and absence of active metabolites.

The benzodiazepines (BZDs), when taken on their own, carry a relatively small risk of serious effects from self-poisoning, have only a minor teratogenic effect (i.e. involving cleft lip), produce less cognitive impairment than other sedating compounds (such as barbiturates), and interact to a lesser extent with other drugs. However, BZDs can lead to dependence (Bard 1979; Tyrer 1980; Petursson and Lader 1981), and alarm at the 'benzodiazepine bonanza' (Tyrer 1974) has been fuelled by occasional reporting of side effects that include release of aggressive behaviour (Gaind and Jacoby 1978), amnesia (Frumin et al. 1976; Clark et al. 1979), withdrawal states (Marks 1978; Bard 1979; Winokur et al. 1980) and psychotic episodes (Dukes 1980). BZDs have also been found to be

3

significantly associated with traffic accidents (Honkannen et al. 1980). Claims that BZDs may produce cerebral atrophy or cancer remain unsubstantiated. Marks (1980) has concluded that 'in general, benzodiazepines are used conservatively by doctors (in the UK) rather than overused, and their current consumption is not excessive relative to the level of emotional morbidity in the community'.

The simplistic view is frequently taken that predictions about differential indications for BZDs can be made on the basis of half-life alone, but psychiatrists should be aware of other factors such as absorption, distribution, half-life of active metabolites, interactions with other drugs, and possible relationships between nuclear structure and clinical effect (Curry and Whelpton 1979). Also, the clinical effect may be related to the rate of increase in plasma concentration as well as to specific levels (Greenblatt and Shader 1978a; Allen et al. 1980; Amrein and Leishman 1980).

In spite of advances in pharmacokinetics and pharmacodynamics, clinical trials are still essential to determine the value and indication of BZDs (Rickels 1978), and although estimations of the plasma (or saliva) concentration of these drugs are increasingly available (Rosenblatt et al. 1979), the weak correlations found between plasma or saliva concentration and clinical effect are discouraging (Lader 1979; Bittencourt and Dhillon 1981).

The discovery of high affinity binding sites for BZDs in the mammalian central nervous system (Fulton and Burrows 1980; Robertson 1980) has widened the area of enquiry and also suggested new hypotheses as to the nature of anxiety (Gray 1979). The possible role of γ-*aminobutyric acid* (*GABA*), *glycine*, and *carbolin*-like compounds as endogenous ligands (Baastrup and Nielsen 1980), is currently a major concern of clinical psychopharmacologists. The anxiety disorders seem to constitute at least two separate groups; BZDs are indicated only in states of high arousal, muscular tension, autonomic symptoms and subjective anxiety (Hoehn-Saric 1982).

Pharmacokinetics

General points.   BZDs are not well absorbed by the intramuscular route, and intravenous administration is only slightly more efficient than oral doses. Antacids, anticholinergic compounds and achlorhydria delay absorption (Greenblatt and Shader 1980), while clorazepate is hydrolized in the stomach to its active metabolite desmethyldiazepam.

The major site for the metabolism of BZDs is the liver. It is believed that most of these compounds do not significantly induce the synthesis of microsomal liver enzymes, but some, such as flurazepam (Hasegawa and Matsubara 1975), nitrazepam, and diazepam (Linnoila et al. 1975), appear to do so. Protein-binding capacity is high for the BZDs, and is affected by a number of factors including hypoproteinemia, drug competition for binding sites, age and disease-induced changes in alpha-1 acid glycoprotein (Perucca and Richens 1979). BZDs are lipid soluble and are rapidly absorbed from the intestine, which explains their prompt bioavailability after using the oral route. The blood–brain barrier is easily crossed, leading to an early onset of action if an adequate plasma level (i.e. 'minimum effective concentration', MEC) is achieved. This rapid action is advantageous in certain clinical situations that require urgent control, such as panic attacks. However, persisting anxiety, convulsions and muscle spasticity require relatively steady plasma levels.

Distribution. Most BZDs (with the exception of nordiazepam) initially distribute into both blood and extracellular fluid, and then show a fast distribution stage in which cerebral cortex levels peak in a matter of minutes. This is followed by a more prolonged and slower distribution phase, which can take several hours. The latter is particularly relevant when BZDs are used as hypnotics (Breimer 1979a). Not all BZDs, however, behave in the same way; for example, a significant part of an oral dose of diazepam, nitrazepam and probably bromazepam, becomes trapped in the enterohepatic circulation and is therefore secreted unchanged in the bile, to be reabsorbed from the gut. The intake of food leads to still less of the drug reaching the plasma, while distribution may be delayed in pathological states such as congestive cardiac failure.

Metabolism. BZDs are complex organic molecules which are broken down by hepatic microsomal enzymes at a rate proportional to the concentration of the compound. However, genetic and various exogenous factors also affect metabolic rate. There are three metabolic pathways for the 1-4 benzodiazepines and certain metabolites are eliminated in the urine. Factors relevant to the rate of metabolism are diet, drug interactions, liver disease and age (Greenblatt and Shader 1980). Induction of microsomal enzymes may, with a minority of BZDs, influence the breakdown rate of both parent drug and active metabolites.

Consideration of absorption, protein binding, distribution, metabolism, age, sex, physical state, other medication and smoking is important to the prediction of clinical effects. Even then, as a recent review concludes, 'the clinical consequences of alterations in benzodiazepine kinetics due either to the ageing process or to drug interaction are not readily predictable' (Greenblatt and Shader 1980).

General Systemic Physiological Effects

The respiratory and cardiovascular systems are more affected than the gastrointestinal or urinary tracts. For example, diazepam in moderate doses slightly depresses alveolar ventilation and may cause respiratory acidosis by attenuating hypoxic drive. Lorazepam has a similar depressing effect but the mechanism involved in this case seems to be a reduction in hypercapnic drive (i.e. the response to increased PCO_2). This makes lorazepam contraindicated in the sleep apnoea syndromes which may involve a hyposensitivity of the repiratory centre to CO_2. In spite of these effects on respiration, overdosage of

BZDs is not usually lethal (Greenblatt and Shader 1978a) provided that they are not mixed with barbiturates, alcohol or tricyclic antidepressants. However, the relatively 'harmless' nature of poisoning by BZDs has recently been called into question (Meredith and Vale 1981).

Moderate anaesthetic doses of diazepam (>20 mg) reduce systolic blood pressure. Chlordiazepoxide has been described as having an antiarrhythmic effect in mammalian cardiac tissue (Lasagna 1977; Wang and James 1978), but this effect has not yet been investigated in humans.

The Major Benzodiazepines

Chlordiazepoxide (CDX). CDX exhibits the four main pharmacological effects of benzodiazepines, i.e. sedative, muscle relaxant, 'taming' and anticonvulsant activity. In man and other species CDX is metabolized into the active compounds *N*-desmethylchlordiazepoxide (the major metabolite), desoxyde-moxepam and demoxepam. The elimination half-life ranges from 9–18 h for the parent drug, to 34–44 h for its metabolites. Regular oral doses, such as three times daily, can lead to a steady state (i.e. when the daily dose is equivalent to the rate of metabolism into inactive products) in about 3 days, after which a single daily dose regimen can be established without causing fluctuations of clinical effect. Oral CDX is absorbed at a faster rate than from the intramuscular route, so that intramuscular administration (as is sometimes used in alcoholic withdrawal syndromes) may result in a delayed onset of activity.

After a single 25-mg dose in the adult, plasma levels of CDX range from about 0.26 to 1.63 μg/ml. The correlation between plasma level and time interval since intake is not high, and there is much interindividual variability (Lader 1979). No clear correlation seems to exist between plasma level of CDX and clinical response, but recently a correlation has been identified between two of its metabolites (desethylchlordiazepoxide and demoxepam) and anxiety reduction (Lin and Friedel 1979). Active metabolites can be detected in plasma 84 h after discontinuation of the parent drug. An overdose with CDX is not usually dangerous (Gjerris 1966).

Diazepam (DZP). Diazepam is the active metabolite of medazepam, and has an elimination half-life of about 32 h. Its three main active metabolites are *N*-desmethyldiazepam, 3-hydroxydiazepam (temazepam) and exazepam (Hillstad et al. 1974), and a steady state may be reached after about 5–7 days. The elimination half-life of the parent drug and metabolites can be up to 100 h. Advancing age increases these times.

Diazepam used as a hypnotic may lead to accumulation with side effects (Kleinknecht and Donaldson 1975). Peak plasma levels can be reached about 30 min after oral intake, and about 60 min after i.m. injection. In normal volunteers a correlation can be found between plasma levels and self-reported side effects such as drowsiness, slowness and clumsiness. Plasma levels of active metabolites correlate better with subjective reports of side effects than do those of the parent drug. Genetic factors may be important determinants of plasma levels, and it has been suggested that those who metabolize the drug relatively quickly may be better responders to diazepam. Liver enzyme induction occurs after chronic therapy (Linnoila et al. 1975) but, even then, routine doses of diazepam remain effective (Ladewig and Schwarz 1980). Accumulation of active metabolites in white matter, thalamus, hypothalamus and hypophysis may be responsible for some of the long-term side effects (Placidi et al. 1976). Plasma levels of N-desmethyldiazepam below 287 μg/ml do not appear to correlate with autonomic symptoms (Dasberg et al. 1974). Ageing leads to a three- to six-fold increase in elimination half-life and so does liver disease, principally cirrhosis (Greenblatt and Shader 1980). Because of the accumulation of its active metabolites, DZP is not a suitable hypnotic unless the insomnia to be treated is of the 'hyperarousal' type (see Chapter 25), which is often accompanied by marked diurnal anxiety. A withdrawal reaction has been described in patients taking low doses of diazepam (15–25 mg daily) for 6 years (Winokur et al. 1980).

Diazepam is the most widely prescribed benzodiazepine, and a survey in the Oxford region showed that it comprised 4.1% of all prescriptions in general practice (Skegg et al. 1977). Intravenous injection of diazepam carries a risk of vein thrombosis (as a result of damage to the endothelium), which has been reported to occur with about 6% of injections if a large antecubital vein is used, and with about 23% when a vein in the hand or wrist is chosen (Hegarty and Dundee 1977). This risk is even higher in the elderly, smokers, women taking an oral contraceptive and after repeated injections of diazepam. These figures are high, and steps must be taken to reduce the risk, such as dilution of the ampoule in 20 ml of 5% dextrose + Ringer's lactate, or the use of the patient's own blood as a diluent. It is recommended that diazepam (and lorazepam) should not be mixed with another drug in the same syringe (Anon 1981). Diazepam, when taken during the first trimester of pregnancy, has been associated with a two- or three-fold increase in the occurrence of cleft lip (Safra and Oakley 1975). A slow-release preparation of DZP has recently become available (Müller-Lissner 1981); it seems to possess some clinical advantage (Saletu et al. 1981).

Lorazepam (LZP). Lorazepam is excreted in urine as a glucuronide metabolite (Schillings et al. 1975). Despite its designation as a 'short-acting' compound (C.R.M. 1980) its elimination half-life ranges from about 13 h (Greenblatt et al. 1977) to 22 h (Kraus et al. 1978). Lorazepam glucuronide reaches peak plasma levels within 6 h of the dose and, with regular administration, a steady state is reached in about 3 days. Oral, intramuscular and intravenous routes are equally effective, and peak plasma levels are reached 2 h after oral intake. Anterograde amnesia has been described after parenteral use (Pandit et al. 1976; Greenblatt and Shader 1978a; Korttila 1979). Overdose with LZP does not appear to produce serious effects; in three reported cases, the patients were alert and symptom-free despite high plasma levels (Allen et al. 1980).

Nitrazepam (NZP). This is a widely used hypnotic in spite of the fact that its elimination half-life of about 28 h (De Boer et al. 1978) leads to accumulation, which itself may lead to a reduction in the half-life in some patients due to hepatic enzyme induction (Reider and Wendt 1973; Breimer 1979). In the elderly the rate of accumulation is more marked, as the elimination half-life is relatively longer (Kangas et al. 1979).

Following oral administration, about 80% of NZP is absorbed and reaches peak plasma concentration within 2 h. Only one of its five unconjugated metabolites seems to be biologically active. Headache, dizziness and motor clumsiness are not uncommon in patients on chronic NZP therapy (Mendelson 1980).

Oxazepam (OXP). Oxazepam is a metabolite common to chlordiazepoxide, chlorazepate, diazepam, temazepam, medazepam and desmethyldiazepam, and is used clinically in its own right (Garattini 1978). It has a half-life within the range of 7–25 h, does not accumulate or break down into active metabolites, and is conjugated with glucuronic acid prior to excretion in the bile. It is less soluble than DZP, so that no parenteral preparation of OXP is available (Alvan and Odar-Cederlöf 1978). Peak plasma concentration occurs in humans between 1 and 4 h after oral intake. Although its pharmacological characteristics should recommend OXP as a good hypnotic (Lehmann 1978), clinical experience has not shown this conclusively, and it has been suggested that the degree of penetration to the brain is low (Breimer 1979b).

Flurazepam (FZP). Flurazepam has two main metabolites: a hydroxyethyl compound and an N-1-desalkyl derivative. The former does not accumulate, has a half-life of about 2 h, and is barely detectable in the urine after 12 h. The N-1-desalkyl derivative is, however, the major metabolite, and its accumulation, due to its half-life of about 100 h, may be responsible for the reported diurnal side effects (Bond and Lader 1972). FZP is quickly absorbed, and forms relatively weak bonds with proteins; this may explain its relative success as a sleeping pill (Paula 1980).

Temazepam (3-hydroxydiazepam). This is an active metabolite resulting from the breakdown of diazepam. Most is metabolized to a glucuronide which is excreted in urine, but about 5% is transformed to oxazepam. Only about 8% is metabolized in the first 'pass' through the liver. It has a short half-life of between 5 and 8 h (Fuccella et al. 1977), is lipid soluble and hence highly bound to plasma proteins. It is rapidly absorbed, and peak plasma levels occur in about 30 min. It may be a useful hypnotic (Breimer 1979a).

Triazolam. This belongs to the new group of triazole BZDs and has a short elimination half-life of around 3 h. No appreciable accumulation seems to take place. Its main effect is due to the activity of its main metabolite, α-hydroxytriazolam, which also has a very short half-life. Triazolam is claimed to be a good hypnotic, carrying a particular indication in patients who have delayed onset of sleep or who show a marked 'hangover' to other BZDs (DTB 1979). However, a report that triazolam can induce an acute psychotic state has raised doubts as to the safety of this compound but more evidence is needed (Lasagna 1980). Triazolam is an expensive benzodiazepine when compared to oxazepam or diazepam (DTB 1979).

Alprazolam. Information on the pharmacokinetics of this triazolobenzodiazepine is scanty, and it is being tried as an anxiolytic and antidepressant. So far there is no evidence that it is any better than other BZDs (Aden and Thein 1980).

Clobazam. This is the first 1-5 benzodiazepine to be marketed. Its half-life is about 18 h and that of its main active metabolite, desmethylclobazam, up to 46 h (Rupp et al. 1978). It is claimed that it has a good anxiolytic action but with relatively less sedative, depressant and muscle relaxant effects (Fielding and Hoffman 1978). There do not seem to be major toxic effects, and the fact that it produces less psychomotor changes than other BZDs may particularly recommend it as an anxiolytic in the elderly.

Behavioural Pharmacology of the Benzodiazepines

Animal models of anxiety are useful for the identification of new tranquillizing agents, and a popular model since 1960 has been an operant conditioning method for studying 'conflict behaviour' (Geller and Seifter 1960). The animal is trained on an operant schedule of intermittent food reinforcement, which is alternated with another schedule that combines punishment with food reward (Sepinwall and Cook 1978). Punishment (usually footshock) produces a characteristic suppression of response which is called 'conflict behaviour'. Drugs can then be administered to the animal to determine their effect upon this response suppression (Iversen 1980). Characteristically, BZDs, and barbiturates to a lesser extent (McMillan and Leander 1976), increase response during the 'conflict' period, so that these compounds have been called 'anticonflict', 'conflict-attenuating' or 'antipunishment' drugs, whose effect has been considered to indicate an 'antianxiety' property. There is some correlation between therapeutic doses in humans and the minimum effective doses which increase conflict response in animals (Cook and Sepinwall 1975). However, some other properties of BZDs, such as the anticonvulsive effect, do not correlate well with clinical efficacy in anxiety (Sepinwall and Cook 1978).

By means of the Geller and Seifter task, behavioural pharmacologists can separate the effect of BZDs from other substances which may produce general tranquillization, such as neuroleptics or chloral hydrate; the essential difference is that the latter drugs reduce response during the conflict stage. The Geller and Seifter task does not differentiate BZDs from barbiturates, ethanol or meprobamate. Thus it has been claimed that experimental evidence for the superiority of BZDs over other anxiolytic agents is not yet adequate (Iversen 1980).

It has been suggested that the 'anticonflict' Geller and Seifter effect is mediated by serotonergic pathways, and that the effects of BZDs may be partially due to a reduction of serotonergic activity (Stein 1980).

Biological Basis for the Action of Benzodiazepines

Advances in the neurochemistry of γ-aminobutyric acid (GABA) and the discovery of 'benzodiazepine receptors' in the mammalian brain (Tallman et al. 1980) have led to new hypotheses for the action of BZDs (Stein 1980). Traditional views on anxiety have undergone revision (Horvath 1980) and its homogeneous nature has been questioned (Hoehn-Saric 1982); the relevance of the septohippocampal system has also been highlighted (Gray 1981).

Schmidt et al. (1967) reported that diazepam potentiated presynaptic inhibition in the cat spinal cord, and the possibility that this potentiation might be mediated by GABA became clear once it was demonstrated that this effect of diazepam was reduced by GABA antagonists (e.g. picrotoxin and bicuculline) and abolished by GABA depletion (produced by synthesis inhibitors such as thiosemicarbazide) (Haefely 1978).

Similar interactions were soon reported as occurring in the central nervous system, (i.e. in the cuneate nucleus and cerebellum), and the question arose as to what were the mechanisms responsible for this BZD-related facilitation of GABA-ergic transmission. It became clear that this effect did not require a change in the rate of synthesis or utilization of GABA (Tallman et al. 1980), and that BZDs might be affecting the GABA receptor itself. The idea that these drugs might actually bind to specific receptors emerged from a number of sources, including the discovery that BZDs can bind to specific sites (Baastrup and Nielsen 1980; Paul et al. 1980); the fact that BZDs increase inhibition only if sufficient GABA is present in the synapse; and the finding that GABA receptors and BZD receptors tend to be found together in certain location sites (Enna 1979).

It seems that BZD receptors are bound to cell membranes and are only present in brain tissue (Baastrup and Nielsen 1980; Costa 1980). They are not evenly distributed in the brain, and the highest concentrations (in the human) are found in the cortical areas and limbic system.

The belief in the existence of BZD receptors in the brain started the search for an endogenous ligand, and ethyl β-carboline-3 carboxylate has been suggested for this role (Baastrup and Nielsen 1980). However, there may be more than one type of BZD receptor in the brain, and it has been postulated that one group of 'type I' receptors may mediate the anxiolytic effect of BZDs while the 'type II' receptors (functionally linked with GABA receptors) would mediate other effects such as ataxia and the anticonvulsive effect (Antoniadis et al. 1979; Phillis and Wu 1980).

The identification and location of BZD receptors has also led to the development of new theories of anxiety. Gray (1979, 1981) has suggested that there is a substantial overlap between the behavioural changes observed after septal and hippocampal lesions, and those resulting from the administration of antianxiety drugs. This similarity may indicate that antianxiety drugs may act on the septal–hippocampal system.

Conclusion

The BZDs are a relatively new group of compounds whose neurochemistry, behavioural pharmacology and clinical usefulness are still in the process of clarification. They are widely prescribed as anxiolytics, hypnotics, muscle relaxants and antiepileptics. Probably too many are now available, and only three or four are required for routine clinical purposes. The prescribing of BZDs has probably been abused, in terms of dose, variety of compounds and duration of treatment, because of their margin of safety. Indications, therefore, must be clearly defined, and periods of treatment should be specified. As with other psychotropic drugs the early hopes that plasma level determinations could lead to a scientific control of therapy have not been fulfilled, as there is much intra- and interpersonal variability. Further, the final effect of a BZD often depends upon the summation of the effect of the parent drug and of its active metabolites. A combination of a BZD and a β-adrenergic receptor blocking compound is probably useful in cases when subjective and somatic symptoms of anxiety are combined.

Herrington and Lader (1981) have summarized the way in which BZDs are clinically superior to the barbiturates as anxiolytics: they are more effective, with less steep dose–effect curves and a lower incidence of dose-related side effects; they are several orders of magnitude safer in overdosage; and they are less likely to produce physical dependence. Also, as these compounds do not materially induce hepatic microsomal oxidizing enzymes, they are much less likely to interact with other drugs.

β-BLOCKERS

Introduction

Drugs which antagonize β-adrenergic receptor activity have acquired a limited but distinct place in psychiatric pharmacotherapy. β-Blockers are primarily used in the treatment of the somatic concomitants of anxiety and in the control of certain drug-induced tremors, while they have also been used, controversially, in the treatment of acute schizophrenia (see Chapter 2).

The Adrenergic Receptor (Bacq 1975)

Ahlquist (1948) proposed the existence of two types of adrenergic receptors to explain the dissimilar effects of adrenaline, noradrenaline and other sympatho-mimetic amines. It was suggested that α-receptors show the strongest response to adrenaline, less to noradrenaline and the weakest to isoprenaline, while β-receptors show the strongest response to isoprenaline, less to adrenaline and weakest to noradrenaline. Based on this distinction, Powell and Slater (1958) reported the β-blocking effect of dichloroisoprenaline, and Black and Stephenson (1962) described 'a new adrenergic beta-receptor-blocking compound', i.e. pronethalol. Soon, however, the carcinogenic effect of this agent led to its withdrawal from the market (Paget 1963), and its replacement by propranolol in 1964 (Prichard and Gillam 1964).

Clinical Use

A number of β-blockers have been developed and are available in the UK. They have a chemical structure similar to isoprenaline, the central agonist of the β-receptor, and include acebutolol, oxprenolol, practolol and propranolol. Some of these are used in cardiovascular medicine for the management of certain forms of hypertension, arrhythmias, coronary heart disease and cardiomyopathies. Also they are occasionally used in other disorders such as hyperthyroidism, glaucoma, migraine and tremor.

The early β-blockers affected all populations of β-receptors whether in the cardiovascular system, bronchial muscle or gastrointestinal tract. Lands et al. (1967) postulated the existence of two types of β-receptor: β_1-receptors, consisting principally of the cardiac β-receptors (and also of populations in the gastrointestinal tract and in fatty tissue) and β_2-receptors which include the receptor populations in vascular and bronchial muscle. On the basis of this receptor differentiation, β-blockers can be classified as β_1-selective (atenolol, metoprolol, practolol and acebutolol) and non-selective (pindolol, exprenolol, timolol, propranolol, sotalol and nadolol).

This two-fold classification, however, is still an oversimplification. There is some evidence that the ratio of β_1- to β_2-receptors is a dynamic one in that the numbers of receptors change under the influence of various factors (Lydtin and Lohmöller 1980).

Pharmacokinetics of β-Blockers

The basic structure of the β-blockers is similar to that of isoprenaline, the β-receptor agonist, and consists of an *N*-alkylated phenoxypropanolamine. β-Blocking activity is confined to the L-isomers.

β-Blockers are rapidly absorbed from the gastrointestinal tract and neither pH nor presence of food in the stomach are of significance. About 90% of the administered dose will be absorbed, although this may be reduced in the elderly or during renal failure. However, bioavailability is poor, as much is metabolized by the liver before entering the circulation. The extent of this effect varies both intra- and interindividually, and, as the dose increases, a form of 'saturation' of the hepatic extraction mechanism takes place (Evans et al. 1973). Some metabolites (such as 1-hydroxy-propranolol) also show β-blocking activity.

In plasma, about 90% of the drug is protein bound. The lipid solubility of the various compounds varies considerably and those which are lipophilic, such as metoprolol, oxprenolol, pindolol and propranolol, enter the brain rapidly. The elimination half-life varies between 2 and 13 h, and knowledge of the individual half-life of β-blockers is useful for determining the optimal dose frequency. For example, oxprenolol, metoprolol, pindolol, propranolol and timolol have short half-lives (2–6 h) and therefore must be prescribed on a three or four times daily basis, while sotalol and atenolol have longer half-lives (up to 24 h) and therefore can be prescribed once a day. Correlation between half-life and clinical effect is not good, perhaps because plasma levels may be affected by transfer to and from the storage 'compartments' of the body.

Renal excretion is the major route of elimination, especially for atenolol, acebutolol, sotalol and nadolol. Hence patients with impaired renal function may need smaller doses. There is no evidence that β-blockers induce liver microsomal enzymes.

General Physiological Effects

The β-blocking action can be described as competitive and reversible, and occurs because the compound does not usually elicit any specific response in the effector organ, although some β-blockers (for example, practolol, pindolol and exprenolol) can, at certain doses, stimulate β-receptors (Prichard 1978).

Effects on the Cardiovascular System

The cardiovascular system possesses both β_1- and β_2-receptor populations, and β-blockers may affect the heart rate, contractility and output. They may also affect blood vessel contractility. In general, β-blockers have little influence on the function of the normal heart at rest but may have profound effects when the heart is under sympathetic stimulation (e.g. as a response to anxiety or during exercise). Selective blockers acting on β_1-receptors attenuate sympathetic drive by reducing the rate of impulse formation in the sinoatrial node and the degree of myocardial contractility.

Cardiac output also drops in response to β-blockade, but this effect seems to be partially independent from heart rate, as pacemaker-induced increases of heart rate during β-blockade are not accompanied by increases in cardiac output. However, this reduction in cardiac output may not be sustained during chronic treatment, especially in hypertensives. The generalized depression of myocardial function may lead to heart failure, but it is believed that β-blockers without membrane-stabilizing properties (such as sotalol, timolol and atenolol) are less likely to induce failure than propranolol.

The effect of β-blockers on blood vessels results from blockade of β_2-adrenergic receptors which have an inhibitory (i.e. dilatating) effect upon peripheral vessels. β-Blockers therefore increase arteriolar muscle tone and lead to a rise in total peripheral vascular resistance. However, no major change in mean arterial pressure takes place, as the reduction in cardiac output is 'balanced' by the increase in peripheral resistance. Pulmonary arterial pressure increases under the influence of β-blockade, which also decreases venous tone, but flow in coronary and cerebral vessels does not seem to be significantly affected (Nies et al. 1973).

Effects upon the Respiratory System

Adrenergic bronchodilatation is mediated by β_2-receptor populations, so that β-blockers increase airway resistance. This effect is probably without clinical significance in normal individuals, but bronchospasm can be precipitated in asthmatics, in whom a selective β_1 agent should be prescribed. It is claimed that the use of β-blockers with partial agonistic activity (e.g. labetalol) may reduce the incidence of bronchospasm (Fleisch et al. 1970), but this has not been confirmed (Connolly et al. 1976).

Metabolic Effects and Effects upon the Gastrointestinal Tract

β_2-Receptors exert an inhibitory role upon gastrointestinal tract motility, so that β-blockers can produce an increase in motility with diarrhoea and occasional spasm. Also, carbohydrate and fat metabolism are influenced by β-receptor activity and β-blockers must be used with caution in diabetic patients. Fat tissue contains both β_1- and β_2-receptor populations, and it has been shown experimentally in animals that β-blockers can prevent the development of fatty degeneration of the liver resulting from chronic alcoholic intake (Lydtin and Lohmöller 1980).

Effects upon the Central Nervous System

The ability of β-blockers to cross the blood–brain barrier varies, but propranolol readily enters the brain. However, the distribution and function of β-receptor populations in the brain are unclear. β_2-Receptors seem to be distributed relatively homogeneously, while β_1-receptors are subject to regional and experimentally induced variation (Minneman et al. 1979a,b). Some recent evidence suggests that β_1-receptor populations play an important neuronal role (Chang et al. 1980). β-Adrenergic activity has been associated with a disturbance of eating behaviour (finickiness); this so-called 'β-adrenergic satiety' may be reversed by propranolol (Hoebel 1977).

β-Blockers and Psychiatric Disorders

The psychiatric use of β-blockers has been reviewed by Jefferson (1974), Atsmon and Blum (1978), Tyrer (1976) and Lydtin and Lohmöller (1980), and these drugs have been used in anxiety states, schizophrenia, mania, alcoholism, heroin abuse, amphetamine abuse, tremor and tricyclic antidepressant toxicity.

β-Blockers and Anxiety

Granville-Grossman and Turner (1966) showed, in 15 anxious patients, that somatic symptoms (but not subjective anxiety) improved significantly after 80 mg propranolol. Wheatley (1969) compared propranolol and chlordiazepoxide in 105 patients and found no significant difference, but a placebo was not used. Bonn et al. (1972) compared practolol (a β-blocker with low lipid solubility which does not readily enter the brain) and placebo in 15 patients; on doses of 400 mg daily, the β-blocker was significantly better for anxiety relief. Tyrer and Lader (1973) compared sotalol with placebo in 14 patients with chronic anxiety, and found no significant difference in overall motor performance or subjective assessment, but there was an improvement in cardiovascular symptoms of anxiety, tremor and diarrhoea. More recently, Kathol et al. (1980) reported results from a double-blind crossover study of propranolol in 26 patients with chronic anxiety, 17 of whom were improved both in their subjective and somatic symptoms. Side effects such as dizziness, fatigue and insomnia were mild and difficult to separate from the anxiety symptoms; the authors concluded that the pattern of side effects and therapeutic response suggest a central effect.

Most studies seem to show the β-blockade is beneficial in the control of the somatic symptoms of anxiety, and this conclusion is supported by studies on patients suffering from episodic bouts of anxiety characterized by cardiovascular symptomatology. Frohlich et al. (1966) described the so-called hyperdynamic β-adrenergic circulatory state in 14 patients whose main complaint was a sensation of cardiac awareness, palpitations, chest discomfort and tachycardia, and who experienced a worsening of their symptoms when challenged by isoproterenol, a β-receptor agonist; their symptoms were reversed by propranolol but not placebo. A similar symptomatology, often accompanied by feelings of panic, can be elicited by the infusion of lactic acid and it has been suggested that β-blockade may achieve its anxiolytic effect by inhibiting lactic acid production (Lydtin and Lohmöller 1980).

Heiser and De Francisco (1976) have reported propranolol to be of benefit in the treatment of ten patients with acute panic attacks, but to be less successful in the control of chronic anxiety associated with agoraphobia. Bernadt et al. (1980) reported that tolanolol abolished stress-induced tachycardia but not subjective distress in a group of 22 females suffering from animal phobias. Easton and Sherman (1976) described six patients with cardiac hyperactivity, diagnosed as 'β-adrenergic hyperactivity' who, when challenged by isoprotere-nol, produced an exacerbation of their disorder and who responded to treatment with propranolol.

It can be concluded that there is prima facie evidence that β-blockade may be of some use in the control of somatic anxiety of the cardiovascular type. The author has successfully treated four patients with cardiovascular symptomatology associated with the hyperventilatory state. Further research is needed to identify the diagnostic subgroups most likely to benefit.

β-Blockers and Schizophrenia

The use of β-blockade in the treatment of schizophrenia was suggested after Atsmon and Blum (1970) described the chance observation of a patient suffering from porphyria with tachycardia and hypertension who had developed an organic psychosis. Improvement followed the administration of propranolol. The same authors then reported a series of 44 patients suffering from various forms of psychoses who had been treated with propranolol, and it was claimed that seven out of 11 acute schizophrenic patients showed marked improvement. A number of trials have been carried out since (Auriol et al. 1972; Rackensper-ger et al. 1974; Gardos et al. 1973; Maurice et al. 1974; Yorkston et al. 1974; Sheppard 1979) but, because of methodological defects in the studies, no firm conclusions can be drawn. Concerning interaction between phenodiazines and β-blockers, it has recently been shown that this may give rise to higher plasma levels of chlorpromazine and its active metabolites (Peet et al. 1980, 1981b).

Recent controlled studies cast doubt on the usefulness of propranolol in chronic schizophrenia (King et al. 1980; Lindström and Persson 1980; Peet et al. 1981a), and it can be concluded that, so far, the evidence for the clinical usefulness of β-blockade in the treatment of either acute or chronic schizophrenia is unconvincing. Furthermore, the severity of side effects usually precludes its use in the high dose levels which have been recommended.

β-Blockers and Mania

The occasional reports of successful treatment by β-blockers of excited psychotic states of organic (Atsmon and Blum 1970; Voltina et al. 1971) or puerperal (Steiner et al. 1973) origin led to the view that manic excitement may also respond to β-blockade. This was reinforced by the experimental finding that propranolol could control excited and abnormal behaviour in rats (produced by prolonged isolation) which has been considered as an animal model for mania. Six patients with acute mania were treated with propranolol (up to 2320 mg daily) by Rackensperger et al. (1976) and two of the patients became symptom free only to relapse after the discontinuation of the drug. Side effects, such as insomnia, precordial pain, hypotension and bradycardia were described. However, the number of patients in this study is small, and replication is required.

Other Psychiatric Applications of β-Blockers

The finding that tremor induced by isoprenaline can be controlled by propranolol led to the belief that tremor caused by other factors might also respond to β-blockade. Parkinsonian tremor has been found to be reduced by propranolol (Owen and Marsden 1965), although other studies found this effect to be marginal (Vas 1966). Essential tremor also has responded favourably to propranolol (Winckler and Young 1974), especially in younger subjects (Murray 1976), but the initial benefit seems to be lost after months of treatment. This may result from the development of β-receptor hypersensitivity. In addition, lithium-induced tremor has been found to respond to propranolol (Floru et al. 1974; Kirk et al. 1973; Lapierre 1976). The patient should be started on 20–40 mg daily in divided doses, and this can be increased up to 80 mg. It should not be prescribed in patients with asthma or cardiovascular disorder. Finally, the 'restless leg syndrome' which may follow treatment with neuroleptics may occasionally respond to small doses of propranolol (Strong 1967).

BARBITURATES

Introduction

Barbiturates are the oldest group of hypnotic–sedative drugs. They result from the condensation of malonic acid and urea, and mostly have a depressant action upon the central nervous system. The first commercially viable barbiturate, Veronal (diethylbarbituric acid), was introduced by Fisher in 1903, and variations in the molecular structure of the barbiturates led to changes in sedative, hypnotic and antiepileptic effects.

Between 1970 and 1975 the number of barbiturate prescriptions in the UK declined by about 40% (Williams 1980) and this downward trend probably still continues (Bennett 1981). The reasons for this are clear: evidence has accumulated on the high poisoning risk and physical dependence associated with these drugs. For example, about 50% of all deaths due to drug addiction in the Greater London Coroners' area in the years 1970–74 were due to barbiturates and, in children under 10 years, barbiturates were the fourth commonest cause of death from poisoning in a sample of 1300 (1968–78) (Vale and Meredith 1981*b*). Since the early 1960s barbiturate abuse (Brandon 1975) and the phenomena of physical dependence, such as withdrawal fits (Gardner 1967), have been well known.

The Advisory Council on the Misuse of Drugs set up a working party in 1974 'to establish and consider the facts relevant to the use of barbiturates and similar drugs in medical use'. This led to the organization of the Campaign on the Use and Restriction of Barbiturates (CURB) which had two objectives: to help doctors reduce the prescribing of barbiturates as hypnotics or sedatives (although it was recognized that phenobarbitone had a place for the treatment of epilepsy), and educate the public on the hazards of unnecessary consumption of hypnotics and sedatives (Bennett 1981). Furthermore, a recommendation by the Committee on the Review of Medicines (1979) emphasized that although the prescription of barbiturates might be justified in rare cases of 'severe intractable insomnia', they had high addiction potential, they interacted dangerously with other drugs, and they had no confirmed antianxiety effect (Hunt 1981).

Pharmacology

The route of administration for barbiturates is determined by the main indication. This should be oral when the drug is used as a maintenance antiepileptic, and intravenous when used as a general anaesthetic, as an 'abreactive' drug, or in the management of convulsive emergencies. The intramuscular route is not appropriate, as barbiturates may cause pain and necrosis at the injection site. A barbiturate which is well diluted in water and taken on an empty stomach will be rapidly absorbed in the intestine, but food in the stomach will decrease the rate of this process.

Intravenously administered lipid-soluble barbiturates (e.g. thiopentone, methohexitone) can rapidly induce sleep, while in 30 min only about 10% of the peak amount will remain in the grey matter. Protein binding of the various barbiturates varies considerably, and the highly bound barbiturates have a relatively low rate of renal excretion, while the rate of hepatic metabolism is relatively slow in the poorly bound compounds (Curry 1980). The concentration in fetal blood is similar to that in maternal plasma.

Barbiturates are eliminated by kidney and liver. Renal filtration depends upon the concentration of the plasma free (i.e. unbound) fraction, and can be enhanced by making the urine alkaline with bicarbonate. Barbiturates are metabolized by the hepatic microsomal enzymes into compounds which are less lipophilic and which are then filtered by the kidneys. Hepatic enzymes can be 'induced' (i.e. their synthesis can be accelerated) by the barbiturates, which may partially explain the development of tolerance. Barbiturates may also accelerate the metabolism of other drugs such as coumarin-type anticoagulants, steroids, oral contraceptives, chlorpromazine and amitriptyline. This is of practical importance, as concomitant intake of barbiturates can drastically reduce plasma levels of tricyclic antidepressants and phenothiazines, and thus impair their pharmacological actions. This may be of relevance in the treatment of depressive or schizophrenia-like episodes in epileptics maintained on pheno-barbitone. Barbiturates may also produce deficiencies in the coagulation factors II and VIII, which may have been responsible for the reported cases of coagulation defects in infants born to mothers taking phenobarbitone. Barbitu-rates also enhance porphyrin synthesis, and this explains the fact that they can precipitate attacks of acute intermittent porphyria which may be accompanied by abdominal pain, clouding of consciousness, perceptual disorders, severe insomnia and excitement. The prescription of barbiturates may be wrongly contemplated for the control of the disorder or in the course of anaesthesia for an exploratory laparotomy.

The old classification of long-, intermediate- and short-acting barbiturates is not substantiated. Their elimination half-lives show considerable intra- and interpatient variation and, amongst the commonly used barbiturates, only hexobarbitone seems to have an elimination half-life of less than 24 h. Thus, all other barbiturates accumulate during repetitive administration to an extent which is partly determined by the degree of hepatic enzyme induction, which leads to the development of increased tolerance. Half-life is influenced by a number of factors; it is shortened by hepatic enzyme induction, and lengthened by liver disease (Richter et al. 1972), pregnancy (due to increased protein binding) and old age.

Metabolism to inactive compounds occurs in the liver. Oxybarbiturates, such as amobarbitone or phenobarbitone, are exclusively degraded in the liver, whilst thiobarbiturates, such as thiopentone, may also be transformed in other tissues such as kidney and brain. The metabolites are easily filtered by the kidneys, although a small portion is excreted in the faeces via the bile.

It has been found that pentobarbitone can potentiate neurotransmission (Nicoll 1978), and this effect of barbiturates on both excitatory and inhibitory synapses may be mediated by a number of mechanisms that include neuro-transmitter release, or the enhancement of postysnaptic sensitivity. It has been suggested that enhancement of inhibition may be mediated by a prolongation of the action of GABA, and high concentrations of barbiturates seem to activate GABA receptors. Barbiturates also affect noradrenergic and cholinergic trans-mission and release calcium from neuronal mitochondria, resulting in an increased membrane permeability to sodium.

Behavioural Effects

The anticonvulsant action of barbiturates can be dissociated from the hypnotic effect, as these activities depend on different parts of the molecule. While the former can be achieved without producing a degree of central nervous system depression, the latter is always associated with a degree of drowsiness. Another interesting feature of the barbiturates is that, even at small doses, they produce an awareness of pain, which can cancel out their sedating or hypnotic effect. Barbiturates may occasionally produce overexcitement, and this may be associated with depression of inhibitory centres.

Effects on the Central Nervous System

Barbiturates are central nervous system depressants which produce sedation, an hypnotic effect and coma (after an overdosage), although there may be an initial excitatory phase of behaviour which follows cortical release from inhibitory control. Complex psychological functions, such as judgement, become disorganized first, although the subject may believe himself to be unimpaired. The effects of barbiturates on the awake EEG are dose dependent, and small doses tend to decrease low-frequency electrical activity and to increase low-voltage, fast (β-) activity. Although there may be a feeling of euphoria, a degree of clouding (i.e. drowsiness and disorientation) tends to accompany the so-called barbiturate activation of the EEG, and widespread β-activity in a patient suffering from a confusional state of unknown aetiology should raise the suspicion of a barbiturate intoxication. The same EEG findings are present in barbiturate withdrawal. At higher doses, barbiturates produce a different EEG appearance, which involves large-amplitude, random, slow waves (5–10 Hz). As the patient loses consciousness, bursts of spindles can be seen in the tracing. A further increase in dosage leads to behavioural unresponsiveness and to slower activity (1–3 Hz), which is often interrupted by brief periods of electrical silence.

The sleep EEG is also altered, mainly by the oxybarbiturates. Behaviourally, barbiturates accelerate sleep onset, increase total sleep time (by increasing the duration of light sleep states) and decrease the duration of REM periods (Kay et al. 1972). With chronic administration, the REM suppression is eventually reversed, when a subsequent 'rebound' period with increased REM duration seems to take place (Kales et al. 1970).

Barbiturates also depress transmission in the peripheral nervous system, which may contribute to hypotension after intravenous oxybarbiturates, or after self-poisoning episodes.

Effects on Respiration

Respiration is maintained by three mechanisms: the neurogenic drive (originating in the reticular activating system), the response to $P\text{CO}_2$ and to arterial and to CSF pH, and the hypoxic drive. The neurogenic drive is diminished even by hypnotic doses of barbiturates, while higher doses also impair both the chemoreceptor and hypoxic drives. The majority of deaths resulting from barbiturate poisoning are due to respiratory complications (Cochrane 1981).

Effects on the Cardiovascular System

Hypotension is the commonest cardiovascular response to barbiturate injection or to barbiturate poisoning. This fall in blood pressure results from a number of factors such as partial inhibition of ganglionic transmission with peripheral venous pooling, direct myocardial depression, and medullary depression in cases of severe poisoning. Hypotension seems to be more frequent amongst hypertensives. There is also a decrease in cardiac output, cerebral blood flow, CSF pressure and renal plasma flow. Myocardial depression may also take place. Arrhythmias are uncommon.

Effects on the Gastrointestinal Tract

Oxybarbiturates reduce gastric secretion and motility, although colonic hypermotility may occasionally be seen after barbiturate-induced sleep. The induction effect on hepatic enzymes may be caused by even a few days of barbiturate use and may explain the development of tolerance and a number of drug interactions.

Effects on the Kidney and Genitourinary Tract

Barbiturates reduce urine flow and this may be partly due to a stimulation of antidiuretic hormone production and to systemic hypotension. In cases of poisoning, this effect may lead to oliguria or anuria.

The Better Known Barbiturates

Thiopentone. This is commonly used to induce anaesthesia for ECT and occasionally for 'abreactive' techniques. Thiopentone is highly lipid-soluble and its duration of action is short (c. 15 min) as it is rapidly taken up into fat stores. Cerebral blood flow is reduced by this barbiturate. Acute intermittent porphyria may be precipitated by thiopentone, and laryngospasm is occasionally induced.

Amylobarbitone. This oxybarbiturate is available in oral and injectable form, and 250 mg intravenously can occasionally be helpful in the differential diagnosis of stupor (Perry and Jacobs 1982). It has also been recommended as an adjuvant for the clinical interview in patients who are too inhibited to talk freely (Sargant and Slater 1963); however, this is based on anecdotal evidence and controlled research seems to show that there is no difference between the effects of the active drug and a saline control (Dysken et al. 1979). This barbiturate has also been recommended as a means to differentiate functional and organic confusion (see Chapter 13) (Ward et al. 1978).

Phenobarbitone. The only indication for this drug is as an antiepileptic. It has low lipid solubility and crosses the blood–brain barrier slowly. Between 20% and 40% is excreted unchanged in the urine. It reaches peak concentration after oral intake in about 6 h (Jalling 1974). It is degraded (parahydroxylated) in the liver and, in plasma, about 50% is bound to protein. Primidone is metabolized to phenobarbitone and phenylmalonamide (PEMA), so that patients taking this drug may have significant plasma levels of phenobarbitone (PEMA accumulates to a smaller extent). The therapeutic range of phenobarbitone in the treatment of epilepsy is between 60 and 120 mmol/litre. This is, however, not a very reliable index of efficacy. Since tolerance occurs to the effects of barbiturates, a plasma level of 20 mmol/litre which is rapidly produced may have a greater antiepileptic effect than a level of 200 mmol/litre which has been maintained chronically. Phenobarbitone may produce irritability, belligerence and hyperactivity in children, and drowsiness, cognitive impairment and psychomotor slowing in the adult. It has been suggested that a deficiency of folates may be responsible for some of these symptoms (Reynold 1971; Smith and Obbens 1979).

Barbiturate Poisoning

Poisoning by barbiturates is almost always the result of a deliberate attempt at self-injury. Death occurs in 0.5%–10% of overdoses, and this risk varies in relation to factors such as proximity to intensive care units (Herrington and Lader 1981; Bates and Cartlidge 1981). If coma is reached, the mortality can be as high as 32% (Arieff and Friedman 1973), and the concomitant intake of alcohol worsens the prognosis of barbiturate self-poisoning. It has been claimed that barbiturate poisoning can result from 'drug automatism', when the patient takes an overdose as a result of confusion induced by the first two or three tablets; however, there is no clear evidence that this can occur (Aitken and Proudfoot 1969; Dorpat 1974).

The symptoms of barbiturate poisoning are impairment of the level of consciousness, respiratory depression, hypotension and hypothermia (Meredith and Vale 1981). Death is often due to respiratory complications. Bowel sounds may be absent, renal failure is an infrequent complication and the EEG is of the 'burst suppression' type interspersed with electrical silences. The coma induced by barbiturate poisoning is often accompanied by extensor plantaris and the degree of impairment of consciousness is proportional to the amount taken. The pupils are small and reactive, while corneal reflexes are preserved and symmetrical, except in profound coma. The eyes are fixed and divergent (due to involvement of upper brain stem centres associated with spontaneous and reflex eye movements) and there are no roving eye movements which are characteristic of a 'metabolic' coma. Also, when the head is moved, the eyes fail to retain their position in relation to the eye sockets. Caloric responses are absent or depressed. These findings are so consistent that, if the above eye signs are present in any comatose patient, it can be assumed that a drug overdosage is probably responsible (Cartlidge 1981).

Treatment consists of gastric aspiration and lavage, with appropriate and intensive supportive measures. The lethal dose of phenobarbitone is 6–10 g, and that of amylobarbitone 2–3 g. Forced alkaline diuresis is only effective in cases of phenobarbitone poisoning and it is not indicated in other cases (Linton et al. 1967). Plasma levels must be estimated and efforts made to calculate the total dose taken. In cases of severe poisoning haemoperfusion can be tried (Vale and Meredith 1981a), although others claim that conservative therapy produces similar results (Davis and Benvenuto 1975).

Conclusions

Barbiturates are potentially dangerous compounds and, in routine psychiatric practice, should be restricted to the management of epilepsy (i.e. by phenobarbitone), the induction of anaesthesia for ECT (i.e. by thiopentone and methohexitone), and the occasional abreaction of diagnostic procedure (i.e. with amylobarbitone). Although there is pharmacological evidence that barbiturates may have an antianxiety effect, the clinical evidence for this is poor in humans (Lader et al. 1974), and any reduction in anxiety may be secondary to drowsiness.

The hypnotic effect of barbiturates is well documented but it is probably no better than that achieved by adequately prescribed benzodiazepines. There is, therefore, no reason for barbiturates to be commenced either as a treatment for anxiety or as a hypnotic.

However, there are a number of patients (usually elderly) who have been on a stable dose of a barbiturate hypnotic for many years. Opinion varies as to what should be the correct ethical and clinical procedure in these cases. Some argue that these patients must be suffering from a covert form of dependence and hence must be weaned off their drugs as they are at risk of escalating the dose or of being unwittingly withdrawn (e.g. during a hospital admission) (Herrington and Lader 1981). In such cases it has been claimed that substitution of the barbiturate by a benzodiazepine must always be attempted (Wells 1973). Despite the theoretical attraction for such a policy, clinical experience has shown that, in a number of these patients, the discontinuation of the barbiturate or its replacement by benzodiazepines destabilizes the patient, and results in severe insomnia, restlessness and protestations.

References

ADEN, G.C. & THEIN, S.G. (1980) Alprazolam compared to diazepam and placebo in the treatment of anxiety. *J. clin. Psychiat.*, **41**, 245.

AHLQUIST, R.P. (1948) A study of the adrenotropic receptors. *Am. J. Physiol.*, **153**, 586.

AITKEN, R.C.B. & PROUDFOOT, A.T. (1969) Barbiturate automatism—myth or malady. *Postgrad. med. J.*, **45**, 612.

ALLEN, M.D. et al. (1980) Pharmacokinetic study of Lorazepam overdosage. *Am. J. Psychiat.*, **137**, 1414.

ALVAN, G. & ODAR-CEDERLÖF, I. (1978) The pharmacokinetic profile of oxazepam. *Acta psychiat. scand.* (Suppl. 274), 47–55.

AMREIN, R. & LEISHMAN, B. (1980) Importance of pharmacokinetic data for clinical practice. In: *Benzodiazepines Today and Tomorrow*, ed. Priest, R.C. et al. pp. 61–75. Lancaster: MTP.

ANON. (1981) Local problems of injecting some benzodiazepines. *Drug Therap. Bull.*, **19**, 11.

ANTONIADIS, A. et al (1979) Benzodiazepine receptor interactions may be involved in the neurotoxicity of various penicillin derivatives. *Ann. Neurol.*, **8**, 71.

ARIEFF, A.I. & FRIEDMAN, E.A. (1973) Coma following non-narcotic drug over-dosage: management of 208 adult patients. *Am. J. med. Sci.*, **266**, 405.

ATSMON, A. & BLUM, I. (1970) Treatment of acute porphyria variegata with propranolol. *Lancet*, **i**, 196.

ATSMON, A. & BLUM, I. (1978) Beta-adrenergic blocking drugs in psychiatry: present status, future approach and research. *l'Encéphale*, **IV**, 173.

AURIOL, B., PALANDJIAN, N., BORD, M. & VALS, A. (1972) Les beta-bloquants en psychiatrie. *Nouv. Presse méd.*, **1**, 1439.

BAASTRUP, C. & NIELSEN, M. (1980) Benzodiazepine receptors. In: *New Perspectives in Benzodiazepine Therapy, Arzneimittel-Forsch.*, **30**, 852.

BACQ, Z.M. (1975) *Chemical Transmission of Nerve Impulses: A Historical Sketch.* Oxford: Pergamon Press.

BARD, M.L. de (1979) Diazepam withdrawal syndrome: A case with psychosis, seizure and coma. *Am. J. Psychiat.*, **136**, 104.

BATES, D. & CARTLIDGE, N.E.F. (1981) Self-poisoning. In: *Advanced Medicine*, ed. Tunbridge, W.M.G. London: Pitman Books.

BENNETT, J.R. (1981) Campaign on the use and restriction of barbiturates. In: *The Misuse of Psychotropic Drugs*, ed. Murray, R., Ghodse, H., Harris, C. et al. London: Royal College of Psychiatrists Publication.

BERNADT, M.W., SILVERSTONE, T. & SINGLETON, W. (1980) Behavioural and subjective effects of beta adrenergic blockade in phobic subjects. *Br. J. Psychiat.*, **137**, 452.

BLACK, J.W. & STEPHENSON, J.S. (1962) Pharmacology of a new adrenergic beta-receptor-blocking compound (nethalide). *Lancet*, **ii**, 311.

BITTENCOURT, P.R.M. & DHILLON, S. (1981) Benzodiazepines: clinical aspects. In: *Therapeutic Drug Monitoring*, ed. Richens, A. and Marks, V., pp. 255–71. Edinburgh: Churchill-Livingstone.

BOND, A.J. & LADER, M.H. (1972) Residual effects of hypnotics. *Psychopharmacologia*, **25**, 117.

BONN, J.A., TURNER, P. & HICKS, D.C. (1972) Beta adrenergic receptor blockade with practolol in treatment of anxiety. *Lancet*, **i**, 814.

BRANDON, S. (1975) Barbiturate abuse and the withdrawal syndrome. In: *Sleep Disturbance and Hypnotic Drug Dependence*, ed. Clift, A.D. Amsterdam: Excerpta Medica, American Elsevier, p.207.

BREIMER, D.D. (1979a) Clinical pharmacokinetics and biopharmaceutical aspects of hypnotic drug therapy. In: *Sleep Research*, ed. Priest, R.G. et al. Lancaster: MTP.

BREIMER, D.D. (1979b) Pharmacokinetics and metabolism of various benzodiazepines used as hypnotics. *Br. J. clin. Pharmac.*, **8**, 75.

CARTLIDGE, N.E.F. (1981) Drug-induced coma. *Adverse Drug Reaction Bull.*, **88**, 320.

CHANG, R.S.L., TRAN, V.T. & SNYDER, S.H. (1980) Neurotransmitter receptor localization. *Brain Res.*, **190**, 95.

CLARK, E.O. et al. (1979) The pattern of memory loss resulting from I.V. diazepam. *Arch Neurol. (Chicago)*, **36**, 296.

COCHRANE, G.M. (1981) Respiratory complications and their management in self poisoned patients. In: *Poisoning, Diagnoses and Treatment*, ed. Vale, J.A. & Meredith, T.J., pp. 52–58. London: Update Books.

COMMITTEE ON THE REVIEW OF MEDICINES (1979) Recommendations on barbiturate preparations. *Br. med. J.* **2**, 719.

CONNOLLY, M.E., KERSTING, F. & DOLLERY, C.T. (1976) The clinical pharmacology of beta adrenoreceptor-blocking drugs. *Prog. cardiovas. Dis.*, **19**, 203.

COOK, L. & SEPINWALL, J. (1975) Behavioural analysis of the effects and mechanisms of action of benzodiazepines. In: *Mechanisms of Action of Benzodiazepines*, ed. Costa, E. & Greengard, P., pp. 1–28. New York: Raven Press.

COSTA, E. (1980) Benzodiazepines and neurotransmitters. In: *New Perspectives in Benzodiazepine Therapy. Arzneimittel-Forsch.*, **30**, 852.

CRM (Committee on the Review of Medicines) (1980) Systematic review of the benzodiazepines. *Br. med. J.*, **i**, 910.

CURRY, S.H. (1980) *Drug Disposition and Pharmacokinetics*. Oxford: Blackwells Scientific Publication.

CURRY, S.H. & WHELPTON, R. (1979) Pharmacokinetics of closely related benzodiazepines. *Brit. J. clin. Pharmacol.*, **8**, 515.

DASBERG, H.H., VAN DER KLEIJN, E., GUELEN, P.J.R. et al. (1974) Plasma concentration of diazepam and of its metabolite N-desmethyl-diazepam in relation to anxiolytic effect. *Clin. Pharmac. Ther.*, **15**, 473.

DAVIS, J.M. & BENVENUTO, J.A. (1975) Acute reactions from drug abuse problems. In: *Emergency Psychiatric Care*, ed. Resnik & Ruben, pp. 81–101. Bethesda: NIMH Publication.

DE BOER, A.G., RÖST-KAISER, J., BRACHT, H. & BREIMER, D.D. (1978) Assay of underivatized nitrazepam and clonazepam in plasma by capillary glass chromatography applied to pharma-cokinetics and bioavailability studies in humans. *J. Chromatograph. Biomed. Appl.*, **145**, 105.

DORPAT, T.L. (1974) Drug automatism, barbiturate poisoning, and suicide behaviour. *Arch. gen. Psychiat.*, **31**, 216.

DTB (1979) Two more benzodiazepines. *Drug Ther. Bull.*, **17**, 65.

DUKES, M.N.G. (1980) The Van der Kroef syndrome. In: *Side Effects of Drugs Annual* 4, ed. Dukes, M.N.G, pp. v–ix. Amsterdam: Excerpta Medica.

DYSKEN, M.W., KOOSER, J.A., HARASZTI, J.S. & DAVIS, J.M. (1979) Clinical usefulness of sodium amobarbital interviewing. *Arch. gen. Psychiat.*, **36**, 789.

EASTON, J.D. & SHERMAN, D.G. (1976) Somatic anxiety attacks and propranolol. *Arch Neurol. (Chicago)*, **33**, 689.

ENNA, S.J. (1979) Regional variation and characteristics of GABA receptors in the mammalian CNS. In: *GABA-Biochemistry and CNS Functions*, ed. Mandel, P. & De Feudis, F.V., pp. 326–337. New York: Plenum Press.

EVANS, G.H., WILKINSON, G.R. & SHAND, D.G. (1973) The disposition of propranolol IV. A dominant role for tissue uptake in the dose dependent extraction of propranolol by the perfused rat liver. *J. Pharmac. exp. Ther.*, **186**, 447.

FIELDING, S. & HOFFMAN, I. (1978) Pharmacology of antianxiety drugs with special reference to clobazam. *Br. J. clin. Pharmacol.*, **7**, (Suppl. 1), 7.

FLEISCH, J.H., MALING, H.M. & BRODIE, B.B. (1970) Evidence for existence of alpha-adrenergic receptors in the mammalian trachea. *Am. J. Physiol.*, **218**, 596.

FLORU, L., FLORU, L. & TEGELER, J. (1974) Therapeutische Bedeutung der β-Rezeptorenblockade bei Lithium bedingtem Tremor. *Med. Welt*, **25**, 450.

FROHLICH, E.D., DUNSTAN, H.P. & PAGE, I.H. (1966) Hyperdynamic beta adrenergic circulatory state. *Archs intern. Med.*, **117**, 614.

FRUMIN, M.J., HERCKAR, V.R. & JARVIK, M.E. (1976) Amnestic action of diazepam and scopolamine in man. *Anaesthesiology*, **45**, 406.

FUCCELLA, L.M., BOLCIONI, G., TAMASSIA, V. et al. (1977) Human pharmacokinetics and bioavailability of temazepam administered in soft gelatine capsules. *Europ. J. clin. Pharmac.*, **12**, 383.

FULTON, A. & BURROWS, G.D. (1980) Benzodiazepine receptors in the central nervous system. In: *Handbook of Studies of Anxiety*, ed. Burrows, G.D. & Davies, B., p.316. North Holland: Elsevier.

GAIND, R. & JACOBY, R. (1978) Benzodiazepines causing aggression. In: *Current Themes in Psychiatry 1*, ed. Gaind, R.N. & Hudson, B.L., pp. 371–379. London: Macmillan.

GARATTINI, S. (1978) Biochemical and pharmacological properties of Diazepam. *Acta psychiat. scand.* (Suppl. 274), 9–18.

GARDOS, G., COLE, J.O., VOLICER, L. et al. (1973) A dose–response study of propranolol in chronic schizophrenics. *Curr. ther. Res.*, **15**, 314.

GARDNER, A.J. (1967) Withdrawal fits in barbiturate addicts. *Lancet*, **ii**, 337.

GELLER, I. & SEIFTER, J. (1960) The effect of meprobamate, barbiturates, *d*-amphetamine and promazine on experimentally induced conflict in the rat. *Psychopharmacologia*, **I**, 482.

GJERRIS, F. (1966) Poisoning with chlordiazepoxide (Librium). *Dan. med. Bull.* **13**, 170.

GRANVILLE-GROSSMAN, K.L. & TURNER, P. (1966) The effect of propranolol on anxiety. *Lancet*, **i**, 788.

GRAY, J.A. (1979) Anxiety and the brain; not by neurochemistry alone. *Psychol. Med.*, **9**, 605.

GRAY, J.A. (1981) Anxiety as a paradigm case of emotion. *Br. med. Bull.*, **37**, 193.

GREENBLATT, D.J., COMER, W.H., ELLIOTT, H.W. et al. (1977) Clinical pharmacokinetics of Lorazepam III: Intravenous injections. *J. clin. Pharmacol.*, **17**, 490.

GREENBLATT, D.J. & SHADER, R.I. (1978a) Prazepam and Lorazepam, two new benzodiazepines. *New Engl. J. Med.*, **299**, 1342.

GREENBLATT, D.J. & SHADER, R.I. (1978b) Effects of age and other drugs on benzodiazepine kinetics. *Arzneimittel-Forsch.*, **30**, 886.

GREENBLATT, D.J. & SHADER, R.I. (1980) Pharmacokinetic aspects of anxiolytic drug therapy. *J. Canad. Sci. Neurolog.*, **7**, 269.

HAEFELY, W.E. (1978) Central actions of benzodiazepines. *Br. J. Psychiat.*, **133**, 231.

HASEGAWA, M. & MATSUBARA, I. (1975) Metabolic fates of flurazepam. *Chem. pharm. Bull. (Tokyo)*, **23**, 1826.

HEGARTY, J.E. & DUNDEE, J.W. (1977) Sequelae after intravenous injection of three benzodiazepines. *Br. med. J.*, **ii**, 1384.

HEISER, J.F. & DE FRANCISCO, D. (1976) The treatment of pathological panic attacks with propranolol. *Am. J. Psychiat.*, **133**, 1389.

HERRINGTON, R.H. & LADER, M.H. (1981) Drug Treatment in Psychiatry—Psychotropic Drugs. In: *Handbook of Biological Psychiatry*, Part V, ed. Van Praag. New York: Marcel Dekker.

HILLESTAD, L., HANSEN, T., MELSOM, H. & DRIVENESO, A. (1974) Diazepam metabolism in normal man. *Clin. Pharmac. Ther.*, **16**, 479.

HOEBEL, B.G., (1977) The psychopharmacology of feeding. In: *Handbook of Psychopharmacology, Vol. 8*, ed. Iversen, L.L., Iversen, S.D. & Snyder, S.H., pp. 55–129. New York: Plenum Press.

HOEHN-SARIC, R. (1982) Neurotransmitters in anxiety. *Arch. gen. Psychiat.* **39**, 735.

HONKANNEN, R., ERTAMA, L., LINNOILA, M. et al (1980) Role of drugs in traffic accidents. *Br. med. J.*, **281**, 1309.

HORVATH, T. (1980) Arousal and anxiety. In: *Handbook of Studies on Anxiety*, ed. Burrow, G.D. & Davies, B., pp. 89–116. North Holland: Elsevier.

HUNT, B. (1981) The British Government's review of psychotropic drugs. In: *The Misuse of Psychotropic Drugs*, ed. Murray, R., Ghodse, H., Harris, C. et al., pp. 99–102. London: Royal College of Psychiatrists Publication.

IVERSEN, S.D. (1980) Animal models of anxiety and benzodiazepine action. In: *New Perspectives in Benzodiazepine Therapy. Arzneimittel Forschung*, **30**, 862.

JALLING, B. (1974) Plasma and CSF concentrations of phenobarbital in infants given single doses. *Dev. Med. and Child Neurol.*, **16**, 781.

JEFFERSON, J.W. (1974) Beta-adrenergic receptor blocking drugs in psychiatry. *Arch. gen. Psychiat.*, **31**, 681.

KALES, A., ALLEN, C., SCHARF, M.B. & KALES, J.D. (1970) Hypnotic drugs and their effectiveness. All night studies of insomniac subjects. *Arch. gen. Psychiat.*, **23**, 226.

KANGAS, L., LISALO, E., KANTO, J. et al (1979) Human pharmacokinetics of nitrazepam: effect of age and diseases. *Eur. J. clin. Pharmac.*, **15**, 163.

KATHOL, R.G., NOYES, R., SLYMEN, D.J. et al (1980) Propranolol in chronic anxiety disorders. *Arch. gen. Psychiat.*, **37**, 1361.

KAY, D.C., JASINSKI, D.R., EISENSTEIN, R.B. & KELLY, O.A. (1972) Quantified human sleep after pentobarbital. *Clin. Pharmac. Ther.*, **13**, 221.

KING, D.J., TURKSON, S.N.A., LIDDLE, J. & KINNEY, C.D. (1980) Some clinical and metabolic aspects of propranolol in chronic schizophrenic. *Br. J. Psychiat.*, **137**, 458.

KIRK, L., BAASTRUP, P.C. & SCHOU, M. (1973) Propranolol treatment of Lithium-induced tremor. *Lancet*, **ii**, 1086.

KLEINKNECHT, R.A. & DONALDSON, D. (1975) A review of the effects of diazepam on cognitive and psychomotor performance. *J. neur. ment. Dis.*, **161**, 399.

KORTTILA, K. (1979) Amnesic action and residual effects of benzodiazepines used for intravenous sedation. In: *Sleep Research*, ed. Priest, R.G. et al., pp. 123–133. Lancaster: MTP Press.

KRAUS, J.W., DESMOND, P.V., MARSHALL, J.P. et al. (1978) Effects of ageing and liver disease on disposition of lorazepam. *Clin. Pharmac. Ther.*, **24**, 411.

LADER, M. (1979) Correlation of plasma concentrations of benzodiazepines with clinical effects. In *Sleep Research*, ed. Priest, R.G. et al. pp. 99–108. Lancaster: MTP Press.

LADER, M.H., BOND, A.J. & JAMES, D.C. (1974) Clinical comparison of anxiolytic drug therapy. *Psychol. Med.*, **4**, 381.

LADEWIG, D. & SCHWARZ, E. (1980) Long term treatment with diazepam: Clinical and electroencephalographic variables. In: *Benzodiazepines, Today and Tomorrow*, ed. Priest, R.G. et al. Lancaster: MTP Press.

LANDS, A.M., ARNOLD, A., MCAULIFF, J.P. et al. (1967) Differentiation of receptor systems activated by sympathomimetic amines. *Nature*, **214**, 597.

LAPIERRE, Y.D. (1976) Control of Lithium tremor with propranolol. *Cand. med. Ass. J.*, **114**, 619.

LASAGNA, L. (1977) The role of benzodiazpines in non-psychiatric medical practice. *Am. J. Psychiat.*, **134**, 657.

LASAGNA, L. (1980) The Halcion story: trial by the media. *Lancet*, **i**, 815.

LEHMANN, W. (1978) The effect of oxazepam on sleep in normal healthy volunteers. *Acta psychiat. scand.* (Suppl. 274), 33.

LIN, K.M. & FRIEDEL, R.O. (1979) Relationship of plasma levels of Chlordiazepoxide and metabolites to clinical response. *Am. J. Psychiat.*, **136**, 18.

LINDSTRÖM, L.H. & PERSSON, E. (1980) Propranolol in chronic schizophrenia: A controlled study in neuroleptic treated patients. *Br. J. Psychiat.*, **137**, 126.

LINNOILA, M., KORTTILA, M. & MATTILA, M.J. (1975) Effect of food and repeated injections on serum diazepam levels. *Acta Pharmacol. Toxicol.*, **36**, 181.

LINTON, A.L. LUKE, R.G. & BRIGGS, J.D. (1967) Method of forced diuresis and its applications in barbiturate poisoning. *Lancet*, **ii**, 377.

LYDTIN, H. & LOHMÖLLER, G. (1980) *Beta Blockers*. Bern: Hans Huber Publishers.

MARKS, J. (1978) *The Benzodiazepines*. Lancaster: MTP Press.

MARKS, J. (1980) The benzodiazepines: use and abuse. In: New Perspectives in Benzodiazepine Therapy. *Arzneimittel-Forsch.*, **30**, 898.

MAURICE, E., REMY-SCHMETZ, J., DENYS, W.J. & SPRUYT, L. (1974) Essai préliminaire d'un béta bloqueur (pindolol) chez trois schizophrènes et trois malades psychiatriques non psychotiques. *Acta psychiat. belg.*, **74**, 294.

MCMILLAN, D.E. & LEANDER, J.D. (1976) Changes in the effect of pentobarbital and chlordiazepoxide on punished and unpunished behaviour as a function of chronic pentobarbital drinking. *Pharmacologist*, **18**, 235.

MENDELSON, W.B. (1980) *The use and misuse of sleeping pills*. New York: Plenum Press.

MEREDITH, T.J. & VALE, J.A. (1981) Poisoning due to hypnotics, sedatives, tranquillizers and anticonvulsants. In: *Poisoning, Diagnosis and Treatment*, ed. Vale, J.A. & Meredith, T.J., pp. 84–89. London: Update Books.

MINNEMAN, K.P., DIBUER, M.D., WOLFE, B.B. & MOLINOFF, P.B. (1979a) B_1 and B_2 adrenergic receptors in rat cerebral cortex are independently regulated. *Science*, **204**, 866.

MINNEMAN, K.P., HEGSTRAND, L.R. & MOLINOFF, P.B. (1979b) Simultaneous determination of B_1 and B_2 adrenergic receptors in tissues containing both receptor types. *Mol. Pharmacol.*, **16**, 21.

MÜLLER-LISSNER, S.A., WILL, N., MÜLLER-DUYSING, W. et al. (1981) Schwimmkapseln mit langsamer Wirkstoffabgabe. *Dtsch. med. Wschr.* **106**, 1143.

MURRAY, T.J. (1976) Long-term therapy of essential tremor with propranolol. *Cand. med. Ass. J.*, **115**, 892.

NICOLL, R. (1978) Selective actions of barbiturates on synaptic transmission. In: *Psychopharmacology: A generation of progress*, ed. Lipton, M.A., DiMascio, A., & Killam, K.F., pp. 1337–1348. New York: Raven Press.

NIES, A.S., EVANS, G.H. & SHAND, D.G. (1973) Regional haemodynamic effects of beta-adrenergic blockade with propranolol in the unanaesthetised primate. *Am. Heart J.*, **85**, 97.

OWEN, D.A.C. & MARSDEN, C.D. (1965) Effect of adrenergic β-blockade on parkinsonian tremor. *Lancet*, **ii**, 1259.

PAGET, G.E. (1963) Carcinogenic action of pronethalol. *Br. med. J.*, **ii**, 1266.

PANDIT, S.K., HEISTERKAMP, D.V. & COHEN, P.J. (1976) Further studies of the antirecall effect of Lorazepam. *Anaesthesiology*, **45**, 495.

PAUL, S.M., MARANGOS, P.J., GOODWIN, F.K. & SKOLNICK, P. (1980) Brain-specific benzodiazepine receptors and putative endogenous benzodiazepine-like compounds. *Biol. Psychiat.*, **15**, 407.

PAULA, A.J.M. de (1980) Flurazepam in insomnia. In *Benzodiazepines, today and tomorrow*, ed. Priest, R.G. et al., pp. 241–250. Lancaster: MTP Press.

PEET, M., BOTHELL, M.S., COATES et al. (1981*a*) Propranolol in schizophrenia I: Comparison of propranolol, chlorpromazine and placebo. *Br. J. Psychiat.*, **139**, 105.

PEET, M., MIDDLEMISS, D.N. & YATES, R.A. (1980) Pharmacokinetic interaction between propranolol and chlorpromazine in schizophrenic patients. *Lancet*, **ii**, 978.

PEET, M., MIDDLEMISS, D.N. & YATES, R.A. (1981*b*) Propranolol in schizophrenia II. Clinical and biochemical aspects of combining propranolol with chlorpromazine. *Br. J. Psychiat.*, **138**, 112.

PERRY, J.C. & JACOBS, D. (1982) Overview: clinical applications of the Amytal Interview in psychiatric emergency settings. *Amer. J. Psychiat.* **139**, 552.

PERUCCA, E. & RICHENS, A. (1979) Interpretation of drug levels; relevance of plasma protein binding. In: *Drug Contentrations in Neuropsychiatry*. Ciba Foundation Symposium 74 (New Series). Amsterdam: Excerpta Medica.

PETURSSON, H. & LADER, M.H. (1981) Benzodiazepine dependance. *Br. J. Addiction*, **76**, 133.

PHILLIS, J.W. & WU, P.H. (1980) Interactions between the benzodiazepines, methylxantines and adenosine. *J. canad. Sci. Neurol.*, **7**, 247.

PLACIDI, G.F., TOGNONI, G. & PACIFICA, G.M. (1976) Regional distribution of Diazepam and its metabolites in the brain of cat after chronic treatment. *Psychopharmacology*, **48**, 133.

POWELL, C.E. & SLATER, I.H. (1958) Blocking of inhibitory adrenergic receptors by a dichloroanalogue of isoproterenol. *J. Pharmac. exp. Ther.*, **122**, 480.

PRICHARD, B.N.C. (1978) β-Receptor adrenergic blockade in hypertension, past, present and future. *Br. J. clin. Pharmacol.*, **5**, 379.

PRICHARD, B.N.C. & GILLAM, P.M.S. (1964) Use of propranolol (Inderal) in treatment of hypertension. *Br. Med. J.*, **ii**, 725.

RACKENSPERGER, W., FRITSCH, W., SCHWARZ, D. et al. (1976) Wirkung des Beta-Rezeptoren-Blockers Propranolol auf Manien. *Arch. Psychiat. Nervenkr.*, **222**, 223.

RACKENSPERGER, W., GAUPP, R., MATTKE, D.J. et al. (1974) Behandlung von akuten schizophrenen Psychosen mit Beta-Rezeptoren-Blockern. *Archs Psychiat. Nervenkr.*, **219**, 29.

REIDER, J. & WENDT, G. (1973) Pharmacokinetics and metabolism of the hypnotic nitrazepam. In: *The Benzodiazepines*, ed. Garattini, S., Mussini, E. & Randall, L.O., pp. 99–127. New York: Raven Press.

REYNOLDS, E.H. (1971) Anticonvulsant drugs, folic acid, metabolism, fit frequency and psychiatric illness. *Psychiat. Neurol. Neurosurg.*, **74**, 167.

RICHTER, E., ZILLY, W., BRACHTEL, D. (1972) Zur Frage der Barbiturattoleranz bei Patienten mit akuter Hepatitis. *Dt. med. Wschr.*, **97**, 254.

RICKELS, K. (1978) Use of antianxiety agents in anxious patients. *Psychopharmacologia*, **58**, 1.

ROBERTSON, H.A. (1980) The benzodiazepine receptor: the pharmacology of emotion. *J. Can. Sci. Neurol.*, **7**, 243.

ROSENBLATT, J.E. et al. (1979) A novel method for measuring benzodiazepines in saliva. *Communs Psychopharmacol.*, **3**, 49.

RUPP, W., BADIAN, M., CHRIST, O. et al. (1978) Pharmacokinetics of single and multiple doses of clobazam in humans. *Br. J. clin. Pharmacol.*, **7** (Suppl. 1), 51.

SAFRA, M.J. & OAKLEY, G.P. (1975) Association between cleft lip with or without cleft palate and prenatal exposure to diazepam. *Lancet*, **ii**, 478.

SALETU, B., GRÜNBERGER, J., AMREIN, R. & SKRETA, M. (1981) Assessment of pharmacodynamics of a new "controlled release" form of DZP by quantitative EEG and psychometric analysis in neurotic subjects. *J. int. med. Res.*, **9**, 408.

SARGANT, W. & SLATER, E. (1963) *Physical methods of treatment in psychiatry*. Edinburgh: Churchill Livingstone.

SCHILLINGS, R.T., SISENWINE, S.F., SCHWARTZ, M.H. et al. (1975) Lorazepam glucuronide formation in the cat. *Drug Metab. Dispos.*, **3**, 85.

SCHMIDT, R.F., VOGEL, E. & ZIMMERMANN, K. (1967) Die Wirkung von Diazepam auf die präsynaptische Hemmung und andere Rückenmarksreflexe. *Naunyn-Schmiedebergs Arch. exp. Path. Pharmak.*, **258**, 69.

SEPINWALL, J. & COOK, L. (1978) Behavioural pharmacology of antianxiety drugs. In: *Handbook of Psychopharmacology*, Vol. 13, ed. Iversen, L.L., Iversen, S.D. & Snyder, S.H., pp. 345–393. New York: Plenum Press.

SHEPPARD, G. (1979) High dose propranolol in schizophrenia. *Br. J. Psychiat.*, **134**, 470.

SKEGG, D.C.G., DOLL, R. & PERRY, J. (1977) Use of medicines in medical practice. *Br. med. J.*, **i**, 1561.

SMITH, D.B. & OBBENS, E.A.M.T. (1979) Antifolate-antiepileptic relationships. In: *Folic Acid in Neurology, Psychiatry and Internal Medicine*, ed. Botez, I. & Reynolds, E.H. New York: Raven Press.

STEIN, L. (1980) Behavioural neurochemistry of benzodiazepines. In: *New Perspectives in Benzodiazepine Therapy. Arzneimittel-Forsch.*, **30**, 868.

STEINER, M., LATZ, A., BLUM, J. et al. (1973). Propranolol versus chlorpromazine in the treatment of psychoses associated with childbearing. *Psychiat. Neurol. Neurochir. (Amst.)*, **76**, 421.

STERNBACH, L.H. (1979) The benzodiazepine story. *J. med. Chem.*, **22**, 1.

STRONG, R.R. (1967) The symptom of restless legs. *Med. J. Aust.*, **i**, 1211.

TALLMAN, J.F., PAUL, S.M., SKOLNICK, P. & GALLAGER, D.W. (1980) Receptors for the age of anxiety: Pharmacology of the benzodiazepines. *Science*, **207**, 274.

TYRER, P. (1974) The benzodiazepine bonanza. *Lancet*, **ii**, 709.

TYRER, P. (1976) *The Role of Bodily Feelings in Anxiety.* Maudsley Monograph No. 23, pp. 10–23. Oxford: Oxford University Press.

TYRER, P. (1980) Dependence on benzodiazepines. *Br. J. Psychiat.*, **137**, 576.

TYRER, P.F. & LADER, M.H. (1973) Effects of beta adrenergic blockade with sotalol in chronic anxiety. *Clin. Pharmac. Ther.*, **14**, 418.

VALE, J.A. & MEREDITH, T.J. (1981a) Forced diuresis, dialysis and haemoperfusion. In: *Poisoning, Diagnosis and Treatment*, ed. Vale, J.A. & Meredith, T.J, pp. 59–68. London: Update Books.

VALE, J.A. & MEREDITH, T.J. (1981b) 'Epidemiology of poisoning in the UK.' In: *Poisoning*, ed. Vale, J.A. & Meredith, T.J., pp. 1–8. London: Update Books.

VAS, C.J. (1966) Propranolol in parkinsonian tremor. *Am. J. Cardiol.*, **18**, 484.

VOLTINA, E.J., THOMPSON, S.I. & TISUE, J. (1971) Treatment of acute organic brain syndrome with propranolol. *Clin. Toxicol.*, **4**, 357.

WANG, C.M. & JAMES, C.A. (1978) An analysis of the direct effect of chlordiazepoxide on mammalian cardiac tissues and crayfish and squid giant axons: possible bases of antiarrhythmic activity. *Life Sci.*, **24**, 1357.

WARD, N.G., ROWLETT, D.B. & BURKE, P. (1978) Sodium Amylobarbitone in the differential diagnosis of confusion. *Am. J. Psychiat.*, **135**, 75.

WELLS, F.O. (1973) Prescribing barbiturates: drug substitution in general practice. *J. Roy. Coll. gen. Prac.*, **23**, 164.

WHEATLEY, D. (1969) Comparative effects of propranolol and chlordiazepoxide in anxiety states. *Br. J. Psychiat.*, **115**, 1411.

WILLIAMS, P. (1980) Recent trends in the prescribing of psychotropic drugs. *Health Trends*, **12**, 6.

WINCKLER, G.F. & YOUNG, R.R. (1974) Efficacy of chronic propranolol therapy in the action tremors of the familial, senile or essential varieties. *New Engl. J. Med.*, **290**, 984.

WINOKUR, A., RICKELS, K., GREENBLATT, D.J. et al. (1980) Withdrawal reaction from long-term low dosage administration of diazepam. *Arch. gen. Psychiat.*, **37**, 101.

YORKSTON, N.J., ZAKI, S.A., MALIK, M.K.U. et al. (1974) Propranolol in the control of schizophrenic symptoms. *Br. med. J.*, **4**, 633.

2

Antischizophrenic Drugs

A.V.P. MacKay

INTRODUCTION

Historical Perspectives

Diagnosis must precede treatment and it was during the late nineteenth and early twentieth centuries that the classification of mental disorder matured to a state compatible with specific remedies. The description and delineation of the major functional psychoses illuminated clear targets for chemotherapy in the form of manic-depressive psychosis and the schizophrenias. During the first half of the twentieth century schizophrenic patients were liable to receive several heroic physical remedies, including the barbiturates (to induce prolonged sleep), insulin (to induce coma) and metrazol (to induce epileptiform fits). Psychiatrists could not have been accused of nihilism in matters therapeutic; nevertheless, wards remained 'disturbed' and overcrowded. The impact of the introduction of chlorpromazine was clear and indisputable; the time was 1952 and the place the Val-de-Grâce military hospital in Paris (Caldwell 1970; Hollister 1977).

The French surgeon Laborit had decided in 1947 that, in order to control the physical reaction to surgical stress, the autonomic nervous system had to be inhibited. In 1949 he began to use the antihistaminic drug promethazine for this purpose. He was struck by its central actions, observing that patients became calm and relaxed without being heavily sedated, and appeared to suffer less pain. Laborit was not satisfied, however, and in collaboration with the Parisian anaesthetist Huguenard, tested a whole range of drugs active on the autonomic nervous system, the majority of them belonging to the phenothiazine family. Vital support in this quest came from the French drug house Specia, through their Rhône-Poulenc laboratories. They initiated a systematic programme of drug synthesis and in December 1950 one of the chemists, Charpentier, produced a phenothiazine (code number RP 4560) which was weakly antihistaminic but also adrenolytic and parasympatholytic. This was chlorpromazine, and in May of the following year Laborit was delighted to find that this new drug produced tranquillity without lowering consciousness.

The first psychiatrists persuaded by Laborit to use the new drug were his own colleagues at the Val-de-Grâce; Hamon, Paraire and Velluz. The first psychotic patient to be treated showed dramatic improvement and the word quickly spread. It was now January 1952 and four weeks later chlorpromazine was introduced to the nearby St Anne's psychiatric hospital where Delay, Deniker and their colleagues correctly evaluated the therapeutic importance of the drug. Results were reported at the Centennial of the Société Médico-Psychologique; the occasion was dramatic and of profound international importance. During 1952 chlorpromazine raced through the mental hospitals of France and entered Italy. A symposium in Basle in 1953 was devoted entirely to the therapeutic use of chlorpromazine and between 1953 and 1954 it had crossed the channel to the United Kingdom and the Atlantic Ocean to North America.

The discovery of the antipsychotic activity of a quite unrelated plant alkaloid, reserpine, was made at about the time chlorpromazine became available. Although this drug is seldom used in the treatment of schizophrenic illness, it must be acknowledged as probably the first effective antipsychotic drug to be documented in modern times (Hollister 1977). The parent plant from which the pure alkaloid is derived is Rauwolfia Serpentinia, a climbing shrub found in India, extracts of which were described in ancient Hindu writings as a remedy for snakebites, hypertension, insomnia and insanity. In 1931 Sen and Bose published a claim that Rauwolfia was useful in the management of severely disturbed patients and over the following twenty years this claim was supported by several reports. Reserpine, the active principle, was isolated in 1952, and Kline was soon thereafter to report on its antischizophrenic activity. Guilty of producing a high incidence of depressive side effects, reserpine was soon to be abandoned as a treatment for schizophrenic illness in favour of chlorpromazine and its relatives. Curiously, its place in the history of psychopharmacology is assured on account of this unwanted side effect of depression (a crucial component of the biogenic amine hypothesis for depressive illness) and also in view of its usefulness as a reliable pharmacological tool which can be used to deplete neuronal stores of monoamines.

In the years following the discovery of chlorpromazine there was intense activity by groups of synthetic chemists exploring the pharmacological properties of structural variants of the tricyclic phenothiazine prototype. This activity produced two families of 'second generation' antipsychotic agents—the thioxanthenes and butyrophenones which, together with the phenothiazines, were to provide the main pharmacological repertoire for the treatment of schizophrenic illness for a period of over twenty years.

The thioxanthene family is structurally related to the phenothiazines. In the course of systematic work, Petersen and colleagues succeeded in synthesizing a series of tricyclic compounds with preserved antipsychotic efficacy but reduced toxicity by replacing the phenothiazine nucleus with a thioxanthene nucleus. Chlorprothixene, clopenthixol, thiothixene and flupenthixol are the thioxanthene analogues of chlorpromazine, perphenazine, thioproperazine and fluphenazine, respectively.

The butyrophenones are the most potent and among the most selective antipsychotic agents, developed almost single-handedly through the brilliant efforts of Paul Janssen at Beerse in Belgium. They were the progeny of a methodical 'production line' approach to drug development. The starting point was a bicyclic chemical (4-phenyl-4-piperidinol) from which compounds with both chlorpromazine-like and morphine-like activity evolved, and eventually haloperidol emerged with relatively pure and very potent activity. Chemically quite unrelated to the phenothiazines, the haloperidol molecule is structurally reminiscent of γ-aminobutyric acid (GABA). Successful clinical trials of haloperidol were first reported in 1958 and by 1960 the drug was in common use in Europe.

While sporadic developments occurred in the 1960s and early 1970s, the third and most recent generation of antipsychotic drugs is still in the throes of proper clinical evaluation. Pimozide, fluspirilene and penfluridol represent a completely new class of potent and long-acting drugs; derivatives of diphenylbutylpiperidine. Clozapine is a tricyclic drug of the dibenzodiazepine family, but the drug has been withdrawn from clinical use due to haemopoetic toxicity. Sulpiride and tiapride are examples of yet another new class, the benzamide derivatives, which are in many ways atypical and the first to claim relative specificity at one subtype of dopamine receptor.

It is perhaps fitting that one of the most recent developments in the general field of antischizophrenic chemotherapy brings this historical account back full circle to the Specia drug house, and to Professor Paul Deniker. and his colleagues at St Anne's Hospital in Paris. Specia have produced an agent, carpipramine, which contains a tricyclic moiety reminiscent of imipramine but with a butyrophenone-like side chain. The drug has a most unusual pharmacological profile and in limited preliminary studies by Deniker, carpipramine is reported to have particularly beneficial effects on certain intractable aspects of schizophrenic psychopathology (Deniker 1978).

Nomenclature

The term 'neuroleptic' has been used to refer to the group, alternatively referred to as 'major tranquillizers' or 'ataractics', which made their debut in Europe with the introduction of chlorpromazine. Neuroleptic was the term proposed by Delay and Deniker in 1955 to the French Academy of Medicine and was derived from the term 'psycholepsis' coined by Janet for his concept of reduced psychological tension. Neuroleptic was meant to designate substances which reduced extrapyramidal function while having effects on mental state. This is a rather odd and unsatisfactory definition, depending as it does on the occurrence of neurological side effects in conjunction with psychotropic actions.

In the fourth edition of Goodman and Gilman, neuroleptics are described as drugs which 'cause general quiescence and a state of psychic indifference to environmental stimuli but do not produce sleep'. As Shepherd et al. (1968) have pointed out, such behavioural definition also lacks precision and scarcely covers the wide use of this group of drugs in the treatment of schizophrenias, where environmental indifference may already be a feature of the illness. The drugs were first used to reduce psychomotor excitement, and were then established as a symptomatic treatment for acute, and later chronic, schizophrenia. Thus terms such as 'antipsychotic' and 'antischizophrenic' agent have tended to coincide with the term neuroleptic, implying some specific remedial action. However, the relationship between the manifestations of schizophrenia and its pathology remains so obscure that symptomatic improvement cannot be regarded as radical treatment, and clinical evidence barely warrants the assumption of a specific antipsychotic or antischizophrenic action. While it is true that the majority of patients suffering from the acute symptoms of schizophrenic illness and paranoid psychosis will benefit from treatment with this class of drugs, so will patients suffering from psychomotor agitation associated with affective psychoses and organic psychoses.

Thus none of the currently used terms appears to be satisfactory for the definition of agents commonly used in the treatment of schizophrenic illness; 'neuroleptic' requires associated neurological impairment and 'antischizophrenic' perhaps misleadingly implies total specificity. In the absence of anything better, however, the terms 'anti-schizophrenic agent' and 'antipsychotic agent' will be used here, and will be used interchangeably. They are to be preferred to the term neuroleptic since some of the drugs referred to are virtually devoid of extrapyramidal side effects. Specificity is not claimed; the terms will be used merely in a pragmatic sense in that the drugs to which they refer have been found useful in the treatment of psychotic illness in general, and schizophrenic illnesses in particular.

Unconventional Chemotherapy

The vast majority of drugs included in this chapter can be thought of as conventional to the extent that their historical development has followed some sort of natural progression based upon the essential pharmacological ingredients of chlorpromazine. There are, however, other agents whose use in the treatment of schizophrenia could not have been predicted by accepted animal screening methods and whose pharmacology differs in fundamental respects from chlorpromazine and its many descendants. Their history is relatively short and their proper clinical evaluation at an early stage:

β-*Blockers.* Following an anecdotal report in 1971, interest has grown in the use of high doses of propranolol in the treatment of schizophrenic illness. Recent reports cast doubt on the efficacy of propranolol (Peet et al. 1981*a, b*) and no studies to date have been carried out with other β-receptor antagonists. As a departure from conventional antischizophrenic chemotherapy this remains an area of theoretical interest, particularly in the context of arousal mechanisms, but clinical application may be premature.

Endorphin-related chemotherapy. One of the most significant developments in neurobiology of the past decade has been the demonstration that the mammalian brain, the human included, contains morphine-like chemicals in the form of small proteins, or peptides, which interact with central opiate receptors. The generic name 'endorphin' has been used to describe this family of peptides and particular interest has been directed towards *met-* and *leu-*enkephalin (5 amino acid chain) and β-endorphin (31 amino acid chain). The endorphins exist in discrete neuronal systems in the brain and probably perform physiological functions as neurotransmitters and neuromodulators. There is no primary clinical evidence for a disturbance of central endorphin systems in the major psychoses, apart from scattered reports of diminished pain perception in chronic schizophrenic patients (Marchand 1955; Watson et al. 1981; Buchsbaum et al. 1981). Behavioural experiments with rats have demonstrated that direct injection of endorphin material into the brain can induce motor abnormalities which have been variously interpreted as schizophrenia-like, or like the extrapyramidal impairment induced by antischizophrenic drugs. Based upon these rather crude and diametrically opposed inferences, two broad therapeutic strategies have been assessed in schizophrenic patients. One is based upon the assumption that schizophrenic illness is associated with excessive release of endorphins, suggesting treatment with the opiate receptor antagonist naloxone. The other is based upon the assumption that schizophrenic illness is associated with reduced endorphin activity, suggesting treatment with natural endorphins or their more stable synthetic analogues. Neither therapeutic approach has so far proved to be of general clinical use but this remains an area of intense research activity (Mackay 1980).

The endorphin era has seen the revival of haemodialysis as a treatment for schizophrenic illness, stimulated by claims that a psychotogenic, atypical endorphin (β-*leu*⁵-endorphin) was present in excess in the blood of schizophrenic patients and that this psychotogen was dialysable (Palmour et al. 1977). Attempts to replicate the detection of this abnormal peptide in body fluids of schizophrenic patients have failed (Berger 1981) and a double-blind evaluation of haemodialysis in the treatment of schizophrenia has likewise failed to reveal any therapeutic effect (Diaz-Buxo et al. 1980).

PHARMACOLOGY OF ANTISCHIZOPHRENIC DRUGS

The Dopamine (DA) Hypothesis

The dopamine (DA) hypothesis states that the therapeutic action of antischizophrenic drugs depends upon their ability to block central DA receptors. The formulation of this, the most coherent hypothesis for the therapeutic action of conventional antischizophrenic drugs, represents one of the most intriguing pieces of clinical pharmacological detective work in recent years. Origins of the hypothesis can be traced in two main directions. In the early 1950s the clinicians originally responsible for the therapeutic evaluation of chlorpromazine noted that parkinsonism was a common accompaniment of the antipsychotic action of the drug. This observation preceded by more than a decade the pioneering work of Honykiewicz and his colleagues, which was to demonstrate that idiopathic and postencephalitic parkinsonism were associated with substantial degeneration of DA-releasing neurons in the nigrostriatal tract, leading to loss of dopaminergic transmission in the caudate-putamen. The other major source of the DA hypothesis arose out of clinical and behavioural observations of the effects of amphetamine.

Amphetamine psychosis. Connell (1958) was the first to suggest that a psychosis 'indistinguishable from acute or chronic paranoid schizophrenia' was a not uncommon phenomenon in habitual abusers of large doses of amphetamine. Although the facsimile may not be exact, there is general agreement that amphetamine psychosis provides the best available pharmacological model of schizophrenia (Snyder 1973; Angrist et al. 1974) and that the psychotogenic effect is due to a direct action of the drug and is neither mediated through sleep deprivation nor requires a previous history of, or predisposition to schizophrenia. Similar psychotogenic actions are observed with the DA precursor L-DOPA. The model psychoses induced by amphetamine and L-DOPA are readily reversed by antischizophrenic drugs.

Amphetamine in animals. Amphetamine has numerous behavioural actions in animals; suppressing eating, stimulating locomotor activity and, in high doses, causing striking forms of stereotyped behaviour in which the animal constantly repeats selected items from its behavioural repertoire in a meaningless fashion. Randrup and his colleagues in Denmark (for review see Randrup and Munkvad 1974) first suggested that stereotyped behaviour in response to amphetamine might represent an animal model for amphetamine psychosis and schizophrenia. They also suggested that these effects of amphetamine depended critically upon an interaction of the drug with dopaminegic mechanisms in the brain.

Brain DA systems and behaviour. DA-containing neurones are localized mainly in the mid-brain. The zona compacta of the substantia nigra contains dopaminergic neurons (A-9 cell group) whose axons form the nigrostriatal tract projecting to the caudate nucleus and putamen. The globus pallidus also receives a small, but diffuse, DA innervation and the functions of these various elements of the basal ganglia appear to include involuntary sensormotor coordination and the maintenance of a balanced motor output. Medial to the substantia nigra lies another group of DA-containing cells, designated A-10, which surrounds the interpeduncular nucleus, and these cells (with their axonal projections) form the so-called mesolimbic and mesocortical DA systems. The former includes axonal projections to the nucleus accumbens, the olfactory area, septal nuclei and amygdala, and the latter includes projections to the frontal, cingulate and entorhinal cortex (Iversen 1980). The functions of the mesolimbic DA system may be intimately involved in processes of behavioural arousal and motivation and the mesocortical systems appear to react to environmental stress (Iversen 1980).

A series of careful studies, involving pharmacological and neurosurgical manipulations, has shown quite clearly that the behavioural effects of amphetamine in animals are mediated through DA. Amphetamine is known to release DA from dopaminergic neurons and the stereotyped behaviour is mediated through increased DA release in the nigrostriatal tract, whereas increased locomotor responses are mediated largely through a similar action on mesolimbic systems. These behaviours induced by amphetamine are DA dependent and independent of any important contribution by brain noradrenaline systems (Kelly et al. 1975). The behaviours are selectively blocked by small doses of antischizophrenic drugs—indeed the ability of a drug to block amphetamine-induced stereotypy in animals has become a standard screening test of proven predictive value in the commercial development of antischizophrenic drugs.

Neurochemical studies. More direct support for the DA hypothesis for the mode of action of antischizophrenic drugs has come from in vitro biochemical and pharmacological investigations of DA receptors. This approach was launched in 1972 by Greengard and Kebabian and their colleagues at Yale University with the demonstration that adenylate cyclase (the enzyme which converts ATP into cyclic AMP), which is enriched in brain areas receiving DA innervation, can be stimulated in vitro by the addition of DA. This proved to be a receptor-mediated stimulation, and the DA-stimulated adenylate cyclase thus became the first in vitro model in which DA receptor pharmacology could be investigated directly. Results from this system showed that most conventional antischizophrenic drugs were potent DA receptor antagonists, with an order of antagonist potency roughly equal to clinical therapeutic potency. There were however, some discrepancies; namely the butyrophenones, whose apparent antagonist potency in the adenylate cyclase system was far less than clinical potency would have predicted.

An even more direct assessment of DA receptor interaction with antischizophrenic drugs came from the work of Snyder and Creese and their colleagues at Johns Hopkins Medical School. With the advent of radioactively labelled DA antagonists and agonists of high specific activity, it became possible to quantify precisely the affinity of antischizophrenic drugs for the DA receptor. When crude membrane preparations of DA-innervated areas, such as the caudate nucleus, are incubated with a radioactively labelled DA receptor ligand (i.e. which combines with the receptor) such as ^{3}H-haloperidol, the potency with which an unlabelled antischizophrenic drug can compete with the labelled ligand for binding to the tissue is proportional to the affinity of the unlabelled drug for the DA receptor. Through the application of ligand binding studies such as these it became clear that the clinical potency of a drug as an antischizophrenic agent was very closely related to its ability to bind to DA receptors (Figure 2.1). There was an equally close relationship between receptor binding data and potency in the earlier animal behavioural models such as antagonism of amphetamine-induced stereotypy.

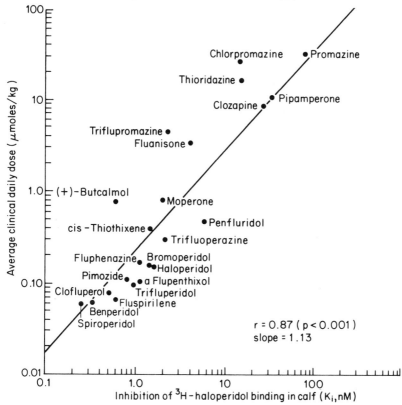

Figure 2.1. Antischizophrenic drugs: correlation between affinities for (^{3}H)haloperidol binding and clinical potencies. Clinical data were derived from the published results. Mean of each daily dose range listed for each drug was meaned and converted to moles/kg assuming a human body weight of 70 kg. The correlation coefficient $r = 0.87$ is significant at the $P < 0.001$ level. (From Creese et al. 1976.)

Although the strength of the association between DA receptor antagonism and clinical effect was persuasive support for the DA hypothesis, a compelling observation was that for no other transmitter receptor model is there a correlation at a level even approaching that seen for DA; ability to bind to receptors for noradrenaline, serotonin and histamine has been shown to have little relationship to clinical potency. The possibility of putting the DA blockade hypothesis to a stringent test in a clinical setting arose from the availability of geometrical isomers (*cis*: α and *trans*: β) of the thioxanthene flupenthixol. The isomers are chemically similar and differ only in their three-dimensional configuration, a property governing receptor interaction. Only the α isomer possesses DA-receptor antagonist properties and therefore a comparison of the antischizophrenic activity of α- and β-flupenthixol provides an interesting direct test of the relationship between DA receptor blockade and antipsychotic activity. In a clinical trial of the two isomers against placebo in the treatment of acute schizophrenic illness, only the α-isomer was found to possess pharmacotherapeutic activity (Johnstone et al. 1978). This result rules out many alternative mechanisms of therapeutic action, including non-receptor-mediated membrane effects. While this observation on its own does not rule out an action at serotonin receptors (the α-isomer being more active than the β-isomer as·a serotonin receptor antagonist), this mechanism seems highly unlikely in view of the complete lack of correlation between serotonin receptor affinity and antipsychotic activity in a wide range of psychotropic drugs.

So, in summary, the ability to act as an antagonist at central DA receptors is at present the single best predictor of antischizophrenic activity of a drug.

DA receptor subtypes. It has become clear that DA, in keeping with the majority of its fellow neurotransmitters, interacts with more than one type of receptor in brain and two have been designated as D1 and D2. The D1 receptor appears to be linked to adenylate cyclase activation (and is therefore analogous to the β-adrenergic receptor) whereas the D2 is not. Established antischizophrenic drugs (such as chlorpromazine) show little selectivity between D1 and D2 receptors and, although not completely selective, the butyrophenones show preferential affinity for the D2 receptor. A new family of antipsychotic drugs, the substituted benzamide derivatives (such as sulpiride), appear to be highly selective antagonists at D2 receptors.

D1 and D2 receptors appear to coexist in most DA-innervated areas of the brain. The only site so far shown to possess exclusively one sort is the pituitary gland, where only D2 receptors exist on mammotroph cells which react to DA released from the hypothalamus by reducing their output of prolactin. While the relative significance of D1 and D2 receptors for the antischizophrenic activity of DA antagonists can only be fully evaluated once a specific D1 antagonist is made available, it can be said at present that all of the known clinical effects of DA antagonists (including antipsychotic activity, extrapyramidal side effects and hyperprolactinaemia) can be sufficiently explained through an interaction with D2 receptors.

Non-DA-Related Pharmacology

With the advent of techniques to label neurotransmitter receptors in the brain by the use of radioactive ligands it has become possible to investigate directly the interaction of antischizophrenic drugs with several discrete types of receptor. In addition to a potent interaction with DA receptors, antischizophrenic drugs are also active at muscarinic acetylcholine (ACh), α-noradrenergic

(NA), serotonergic and histamine (H) receptors. In several instances these drugs are just as potent or even more potent at neurotransmitter receptor sites other than DA. While non-DA-related receptor interactions do not appear to be related to general antischizophrenic activity, they undoubtedly contribute to the total clinical profile of the drug and in particular to the various side effects, both desirable and undesirable.

Anticholinergic activity. The majority of conventional antischizophrenic drugs possess the ability to block muscarinic ACh receptors in the mammalian brain, but their potency in this respect varies very widely (Table 2.1). Anticholinergic

Table 2.1. Relative affinities of antischizophrenic agents for muscarinic cholinergic receptor sites in brain

Drug	Affinity for muscarinic receptor	Parkinsonian side effects
Phenothiazines		
a) Alkylamino : chlorpromazine	10	+
b) Piperidine : thioridazine	119	±
c) Piperazine : fluphenazine	1.25	++++
Thioxanthenes		
α-Flupenthixol	2.56	+++
Butyrophenones		
Haloperidol	1.16	++++
Spiroperidol	0.6	++++
Diphenylbutylpiperidines		
Pimozide	4	++
Dibenzodiazeprines		
Clozapine	204	±
Substituted Benzamides		
Sulpiride	0.06	
(Benztropine)	(4347)	

Affinity for the muscarinic receptor defined as the reciprocal $\times$ 10^{-5} of the IC_{50} value (the molar concentration of drug capable of inhibiting the specific binding of ^{3}H-PrBCM to rat brain homogenates by 50%). Figures calculated from the data of Fjalland et al. (1977).

activity bears importantly on two aspects of the clinical use of this group of drugs: peripheral autonomic side effects and extrapyramidal side effects.

Blockade of ACh receptors in the iris will produce blurring of vision and increased intraocular pressure through pupillary dilatation, and similar actions in the gastrointestinal tract and genitourinary system will produce dry mouth, constipation, urinary retention, etc. (see below).

On the other hand, anticholinergic activity in the extrapyramidal motor system may be clinically beneficial, in the short term at least. In the basal ganglia there appears to exist a reciprocal interaction between DA and ACh transmission such that a functional balance between the two is necessary for normal extrapyramidal function (Figure 2.2). In parkinsonism there is effectively a reduction in the ratio of DA:ACh transmission due to an absolute drop in DA output. Redress of the functional balance by administration of an ACh blocker such as benztropine (Cogentin) or procyclidine (Kemadrin) will tend to restore extrapyramidal performance. All conventional antischizophrenic drugs are DA receptor blockers and at therapeutic doses will tend to induce a pharmacological facsimile of Parkinson's disease. However, with some, this

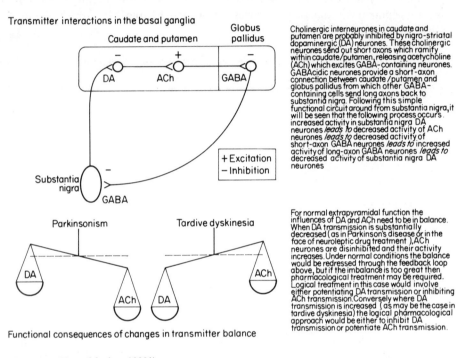

Figure 2.2. (From Mackay 1980*b*).

parkinsonogenic action is offset by a propensity to block ACh receptors, thus minimizing the net effect upon the ratio of DA:ACh transmission. This principle is well illustrated within the phenothiazine family in which piperidinyl compounds (such as thioridazine) rarely produce parkinsonism whereas piperizinyl compounds (such as fluphenazine and trifluoperazine) frequently produce moderate to severe extrapyramidal impairment, with the aliphatic alkylamino compounds such as chlorpromazine occupying a middle position (Table 2.1). As far as extrapyramidal function is concerned, therefore, giving thioridazine is crudely equivalent to giving fluphenazine plus an anti-ACh anti-Parkinson drug. This intriguing pharmacological bonus explains the apparently puzzling

Table 2.2. Relative affinities of antischizophrenic agents for α-noradrenergic (NA) and dopaminergic (DA) receptor sites in brain

Drug	Affinity for NA receptor	Affinity for DA receptor	Ratio of affinity for NA:DA receptors	Sedation and hypotension
Phenothiazines				
a) Alkylamino : chlorpromazine	192	98	1.96	+++
b) Piperidine : thioridazine	185	67	2.76	+++
c) Piperazine : fluphenazine	101	1111	0.09	±
Thioxanthenes				
α-Flupenthixol	100	1000	0.1	±
Butyrophenones				
Haloperidol	83	714	0.12	±
Spiroperidol	55	4000	0.01	
Droperidol	1429	1000	1.43	++
Diphenylbutylpiperidines				
Pimozide	55	1250	0.04	
Dibenzodiazepines				
Clozapine	58	8	7.25	
(Phentolamine)	(277)	(0.5)	(554)	

Receptor affinity defined as reciprocal $\times 10^{-6}$ of K_i (inhibitory constant) for drugs competing for ^{3}H-WB-4101 (for NA receptors) or ^{3}H-haloperidol (for DA receptors) in binding to rat brain homogenates. Figures calculated from the data of Peroutka et al. (1977)

anomaly of why, if anti-DA activity is important for treating schizophrenic illness, all antischizophrenic agents at antischizophrenic doses do not induce similar intensities of extrapyramidal side effects. This explanation linking anticholinergic activity and extrapyramidal side effects requires that the relative affinities of the drugs for the DA and ACh receptors do not follow each other in parallel. For example, regardless of absolute affinities, if fluphenazine had only one-hundredth the affinity of thioridazine for DA receptors as well as for ACh receptors, the two drugs should elicit extrapyramidal side effects to the same extent at effective antipsychotic doses. In fact, this is not the case; affinities at the two receptors show no correlation, the affinity of fluphenazine for the DA receptor being at least ten times greater than thioridazine (Table 2.2). This suggests that therapeutic antischizophrenic DA receptor blockade requires approximately ten times higher brain concentrations of thioridazine than of fluphenazine. At these much higher brain concentrations, thioridazine will block cholinergic receptors and hence minimize extrapyramidal impairment (Snyder et al. 1974).

Antinoradrenergic activity. Among the most prominent side effects of conventional antischizophrenic drugs are sympatholytic effects such as orthostatic hypotension and sedation. Both sedation and hypotension can be attributed to blockade of central and peripheral α-noradrenergic (α-NA) receptors. In a series of antipsychotic drugs, the tendency to produce autonomic and sedative side effects is roughly related to their affinity for the α-NA receptor. The absolute affinity of some antipsychotic agents for the NA receptor is even greater than that of a classic α-antagonist such as phentolamine (Table 2.2). It must be remembered that the therapeutic antischizophrenic brain concentrations of these drugs will be determined by satisfactory blockade of DA receptors. The extent to which an antipsychotic agent would block α-receptors at therapeutic dose levels would then be not purely related to absolute potency as an α-blocker, but to the *ratio* of its potency as an α-blocker to potency as a DA blocker (Peroutka et al. 1977; Table 2.2). Drugs with high ratios would be expected to exert substantial α-blockade. This prediction appears to be borne out in practice; drugs such as fluphenazine, α-flupenthixol and haloperidol have low ratios and are not usually sedative or hypotensive at therapeutic doses, whereas chlorpromazine, thioridazine, droperidol and clozapine have high ratios and show the greatest tendency to sedation and orthostatic hypotension. Therefore the ratio of α-NA to DA affinity may represent a useful predictor of sedation and the incidence of autonomic sympatholytic side effects.

Antihistamine activity. Ability to block central H_1 histamine receptors is yet another pharmacological property of most antischizophrenic drugs. Most potent H_1-antihistamines possess prominent sedative properties and drugs such as chlorpromazine, thioridazine and droperidol have antihistaminic potencies equivalent to the classic antihistamines such as chlorpheniramine (Quach et al.

1979). Antihistamine activity would be expected to enhance any sedative action arising out of the coincidental ability to block central α-NA receptors.

Antiserotonin activity. Many antischizophrenic drugs have high affinity for central serotonin (5-HT) receptors, but no statistically significant correlation exists between this pharmacological property and clinical therapeutic potency. The clinical effects of central 5-HT antagonism are less clear than those associated with blockade of central DA, ACh, NA or histamine receptors. The drugs fluspirilene, droperidol, benperidol, spiroperidol and pipamperon are particularly potent antagonists at 5-HT receptors (Peroutka and Snyder 1980). Both fluspirilene and pipamperone have been reported to be particularly effective in relieving schizophrenic hallucinations. While these drugs differ by more than 100-fold in their clinical antischizophrenic potencies and in vitro activity at DA receptors, they have equally high potency at 5-HT receptors. Since the 5-HT system has been implicated in hallucinogenesis it is interesting to speculate that at least some of their antihallucinatory action may derive from blockade of central 5-HT receptors.

Pharmacokinetics

Phenothiazines. While the characteristics of individual phenothiazines vary somewhat, certain main pharmacokinetic characteristics are common:

(1) Wide tissue distribution resulting from high lipid solubility.

(2) High degree of tissue binding—for example over 95% of chlorpromazine in plasma is bound to plasma protein, leaving only a small percentage in bioavailable form.

(3) Efficient and rapid elimination by hepatic metabolism.

(4) Autoinduction of hepatic and intestinal mucosal enzymes.

(5) Very wide individual range of plasma concentrations within any group of patients taking the same oral dose.

Over 80% of an oral dose of chlorpromazine is metabolized by the liver and by enzymes present in the intestinal mucosa (collectively termed 'first-pass metabolism'). Intramuscular chlorpromazine will avoid first-pass metabolism and it is important to appreciate that, on average, an intramuscular dose of chlorpromazine will be equivalent to about *five times* the oral dose. The overall plasma elimination half-life of chlorpromazine has been estimated at between 10 and 20 h. There exist over 150 theoretical metabolites of chlorpromazine, but only 7-hydroxy-chlorpromazine (7-OH-CPZ) and chlorpromazine-sulphoxide (CPZ-SO) occur in plasma at approximately the same concentrations as the parent molecule (Mackay et al. 1974). CPZ-SO is biologically inactive but 7-OH-CPZ is of potential importance for the clinical effects of chlorpromazine since its DA receptor blocking potency is roughly equivalent to the parent molecule. The proportion of 7-OH-CPZ which exists in unbound form in plasma is about ten times higher than chlorpromazine. It is therefore arguable that the therapeutic effects of chlorpromazine are mediated to an appreciable extent by its 7-OH metabolite (Snyder 1981).

The pharmacokinetics of thioridazine are similar to those of chlorpromazine but its strong anticholinergic actions on the gut can modify its own absorption. Major metabolites include mesoridazine, and free levels of this metabolite in plasma are 50 times higher than thioridazine. Mesoridazine is roughly equipotent with thioridazine as a DA receptor antagonist and thus most of the therapeutic activity of the parent drug may be accounted for by the metabolite (Snyder 1981).

Butyrophenones. Haloperidol is metabolized in liver and no biologically active metabolite has so far been demonstrated. Approximately 60% of the drug is bioavailable after oral administration and the plasma elimination curve is multiphasic with a plasma half-life of 12–38 h (Forsman et al. 1977). There is no evidence of enzyme autoinduction and a closer relationship between oral dose and plasma level has been observed than for the phenothiazines.

Thioxanthenes.   These are absorbed and metabolized in ways essentially similar to phenothiazines, except that metabolism to ring-hydroxylated metabolites is uncommon.

Relationship of Plasma Drug Concentration to Clinical Effect

While clinical pharmacological activity in this area has been sustained for well over a decade, it still remains to be established for any antischizophrenic agent that a clear and useful relationship exists between plasma levels and clinical result. For only one phenothiazine, butaperazine, has a crude relationship been demonstrated between plasma concentration and therapeutic outcome in a small number of schizophrenic patients. There appears to be an optimal plasma level or 'therapeutic window' and this relationship is much clearer for the concentration of drug in red blood cells than in plasma (Garver et al. 1977). It may be that the physicochemical factors regulating drug entry into erythrocytes are similar to those governing entry into strategic sites in the brain.

Long-Acting Antischizophrenic Agents

In order to facilitate drug administration over long periods, two ways of reducing the required frequency of administration have been developed. Firstly, by increasing the elimination time of an orally administered drug and, secondly by dispensing the drug in an oily vehicle which can be injected intramuscularly to form an absorption depot.

The diphenylbutylpiperidines such as pimozide, fluspirilene and penfluridol provide examples of potent antischizophrenic drugs with remarkably long biological half-lives after oral administration. Pimozide has an elimination half-life in man of 53 h (McCreadie et al. 1979) and perfluridol and fluspirilene remain biologically active for between 1 and 2 weeks following a single dose. Fluspirilene is an injectable drug and is dispensed in an aqueous solution of microcrystals from which the drug is released quite rapidly.

A widely employed mechanism for achieving sustained action is that of slow release of an ester of the active drug from an oily vehicle. Fluphenazine hydrochloride possesses an alkyl-piperazine side chain that allows it to be esterified with long-chain fatty acids. Among the commonly used phenothiazines only fluphenazine and perphenazine have this property. On a molar equivalent basis, fluphenazine is about ten times more active than chlorpromazine as a DA receptor antagonist and the effective duration of oral fluphenazine is 24 h. However, when fluphenazine hydrochloride is esterified with a long-chain fatty acid (such as decanoic acid) and dissolved in sesame oil, the duration of effect following a single intramuscular injection can be from 1 to 4 weeks. The rate of liberation of the ester from the oily depot is inversely proportional to the length of the fatty acid chain—fluphenazine enanthate persists for approximately 1 week and fluphenazine decanoate (Modecate) for 2–4 weeks. Once injected, the drug ester, still in the oil, is fairly rapidly redistributed about the body in 'secondary depots' in fat. The ester cannot penetrate the brain but must first diffuse out of the oily vehicle into the aqueous phase of tissue fluids where hydrolysis will cleave the fatty acid from the active drug. Hydrolysis occurs in the liver, at the primary injection site, and at secondary depots (Groves and Mandel 1975). In most important respects the pharmacokinetics of α-flupenthixol decanoate (Depixol) are similar to fluphenazine decanoate.

The most popular injection sites for depot drugs are the deltoid, thigh or buttock musculature, but it should be appreciated that regional blood flow can vary significantly between sites and according to local muscular activity. This may affect the rate of release of the ester from the oily depot and its removal from the injection site. Blood flow is usually greatest in deltoid, followed by thigh and buttock. The volume of injection will also bear upon the speed of absorption; assuming a crudely spherical injection depot, the absorption rate will be proportionately higher for small injection volumes.

Work by Wiles and his colleagues in Oxford, using a sensitive radioimmunoassay for fluphenazine, has shown that after a fleeting initial peak of fluphenazine immediately following injection, plasma concentrations of drug are roughly constant over a 2-week injection cycle in patients established on fluphenazine decanoate. Plasma levels of fluphenazine decline remarkably slowly after discontinuation of chronic treatment. In many patients drug is still detectable in plasma for up to *6 months* after the last injection and hyperprolactinaemia (a reflection of biological activity) persists for similar periods (Wistedt et al. 1981). This strikingly long elimination time should be taken into account when interpreting results from any study involving the withdrawal of patients from depot drugs.

Neuroendocrine Markers

The fact that the release of certain anterior pituitary hormones is directly affected by DA transmission in the tuberoinfundibular system offers the possibility of monitoring the presence in plasma of DA antagonist drugs by monitoring circulating hormone levels. Dopaminergic cell bodies lying in the median eminence of the hypothalamus send short axons to the arcuate nucleus whence DA is released into the hypothalamo-hypophyseal portal system to reach DA receptors on endocrine cells of the anterior pituitary. DA normally inhibits the release of prolactin and stimulates the secretion of growth hormone; thus pharmacologically active concentrations of antischizophrenic drugs will produce hyperprolactinaemia and reduced circulating levels of growth hormone.

The hyperprolactinaemic response to antischizophrenic agents has been extensively studied. Administration of drug is associated with marked, prompt and sustained rises in plasma prolactin concentrations. During withdrawal from medication prolactin levels drop back to normal. While hyperprolactinaemia may offer a biological marker for DA receptor-active concentrations of drug in plasma, it may not reflect accurately the situation at DA receptors in the brain. For example, it is now clear that whereas brain DA receptors show tolerance to the effects of chronic blockade, pituitary receptors show no such tolerance. Furthermore, it appears that prolactin estimations are of limited usefulness in predicting or monitoring clinical response because the prolactin system is too sensitive. That is, maximal prolactin rises are attained at drug doses insufficient for clinical response. In practical terms, the absence of a prolactin response would indicate the unlikelihood of clinical response, but the presence of a prolactin response has no predictive value (Lader 1980).

Non-Dopamine-Regulated Drugs

Propranolol. This drug was established on the basis of its peripheral neuropharmacology as an antagonist at adrenergic β-receptors. Noradrenergic β-receptors have been demonstrated in the mammalian CNS in areas such as frontal cerebral cortex, basal ganglia, hypothalamus and medulla. Evidence has accumulated that β-receptor antagonists such as propranolol have the ability to antagonize certain biochemical and behavioural actions in which 5-HT is involved (Green and Grahame-Smith 1976; Middlemiss et al. 1977). At the high doses of propranolol claimed to be of some benefit in the treatment of schizophrenic illness, it is impossible to say with certainty whether any effect is being mediated centrally and/or peripherally, and whether β-adrenergic or 5-HT receptor interactions are operative. Insofar as arousal may exert potent effects on the likelihood of schizophrenic breakdown it may be that an arousal-reducing action of propranolol is fundamental to any therapeutic action. Recent summaries of the role of NA in stress-induced arousal indicate an NA–DA interaction (Iversen 1980) and it may be at that point that NA blockers such as propranolol and DA blockers such as the conventional antischizophrenic drugs converge on a final common therapeutic pathway.

The pharmacokinetic properties of propranolol in humans are complicated (Greenblatt et al. 1976). There is a very high rate of first-pass clearance by the liver and a variety of metabolites. The drug is widely distributed with ready access into the brain. Propranolol is removed rapidly from the body, with an elimination half-life from plasma of 2–5 h.

Oxypertine. This is an indole derivative with a phenylpiperazine side chain whose main pharmacological effects are qualitatively similar to reserpine. It depletes neuronal stores of monoamines by inhibiting uptake and storage by intraneuronal vesicles. Unlike reserpine, it has an amine-selective action, depleting NA vesicles predominantly, with less potent effects on DA stores and only weak effects on 5-HT stores. It is generally less potent than reserpine, is more readily reversible and is claimed to be free of depressive side effects— perhaps by virtue of its sparing effect on 5-HT transmission. Rarely used in the West, most clinical experience with oxypertine in the treatment of schizophrenic illness has been derived in Japan.

Endorphin-Related Drugs

Drugs acting to inhibit or potentiate central endorphin transmission can interact with at least two species of endorphin receptor (Chang et al. 1980) (Table 2.3). One sort, the μ or morphine receptor, has highest affinity for morphine-like compounds and is found in the dorsal horn of the spinal cord, periaqueductal grey matter, thalamus and raphe nucleus. These areas are

Table 2.3. Opioid receptor subtypes (modified from Chang et al. 1980)

	μ *(Morphine)*	δ *(Encephalin)*
Morphine	+++	+
β-Endorphin	+++	+++
met-Enkephalin	+	++++
Naloxone	+++	+
Main responses	Analgesia	Behavioural effects

concerned with the processing of sensory information and it is likely that morphine exerts its analgesic actions through interaction with opiate receptors in mid-brain and spinal cord. The other opioid receptor type, the δ or enkephalin receptor, has preferential affinity for the enkephalins and their stable synthetic analogues, and is enriched in forebrain structures such as hippocampus, frontal cerebral cortex, amygdala and corpus striatum. While stimulation of the morphine receptor produces mainly analgesia, stimulation of enkephalin receptors produces complex behavioural responses in animals which hold more significance for psychiatry.

Of the agents investigated clinically, the opiate antagonist naloxone has been most widely tested. The drug is a classic opiate receptor blocker. It is very poorly absorbed after oral administration and must be given systemically. Naltrexone, a closely related opiate antagonist, can be given orally but has recently been withdrawn from clinical use due to toxicity. Naloxone has preferential affinity for the morphine receptor (Table 2.3).

Synthetic β-endorphin must be administered systemically, and after i.v. administration, the elimination from plasma is very rapid (biphasic elimination curve shows half-lives of 15 and 39 min) although CSF β-endorphin concentrations remain raised by approximately 50% 6 h after i.v. injection (Berger 1981). Stable synthetic enkephalin analogues are now available for clinical experimentation but they too must be given systemically.

The endorphin fragment des-tyrosynyl-γ-endorphin (DTγE) possesses behavioural activity in rats reminiscent of chlorpromazine but lacks typical morphine-like activity (de Wied et al. 1978). Like most other agents used to influence central endorphin systems, it cannot be given orally.

CLINICAL EFFICACY

The Phenothiazines

Of all the drugs used in psychiatric practice none have been evaluated so widely as the phenothiazines in the treatment of schizophrenic illness. The decade following the introduction of chlorpromazine saw the emergence of an impressive American phenomenon, the Multi-Centre Veterans Administration Collaborative Projects. These and similar trials undertook the careful evaluation of a range of phenothiazines in huge samples of patients (numbered in the high hundreds) and employing standardized clinical rating instruments. The first large VA collaborative study of this sort was mounted by Casey et al. (1960a). Eight hundred and five male schizophrenic patients (in 37 VA Hospitals) under the age of 51 years were randomly allocated to receive either chlorpromazine, promazine, phenobarbital or placebo in a double-blind crossover design. Chlorpromazine emerged with flying colours and phenobarbital emerged no better than placebo. Promazine (a relatively weak DA receptor blocker) occupied an intermediate position. Two additional monolithic studies were soon to follow (Casey et al. 1960b; Lasky et al. 1962) and with a collective patient sample of 1152 they addressed the important question of relative efficacy of various antipsychotic agents. The accumulated evidence of many such trials has been usefully reviewed (Davis 1965; Davis and Cole 1975; Davis and Garver 1978) and the evidence in support of the therapeutic action of the phenothiazines in the management of schizophrenic illness is indisputable. In general, roughly two-thirds of patients are seen to improve significantly under phenothiazine treatment, only one-tenth fail to improve to some degree, and virtually none get worse. On average, most of the therapeutic gain occurs within the first 6 weeks of treatment, although individual variation is wide (Davis and Garver 1978).

The crucial question of whether chlorpromazine and its relatives were merely a new class of sedatives or 'chemical straightjackets' was specifically explored by Goldberg et al., (1965). Re-analysis of the results of an earlier collaborative trial (NIMH-PSC 1964) confirmed that the clinical effects of phenothiazine treatment went far beyond simple sedation.

It is also quite clear that, on average, there is nothing to choose between the phenothiazines of the three chemical subgroups (aliphatic, piperidine, piperazine) in terms of overall efficacy or therapeutic profile; the only distinctions lie in side effects (see below). The notion that certain of the piperazine phenothiazines possess 'activating' rather than sedating properties has entered clinical mythology, but this is based on the most slender evidence. The myth holds that chlorpromazine is the treatment of choice for excited patients because of its sedative action, and that fluphenazine or trifluoperazine are best for withdrawn patients because of alerting properties. These beliefs have never been demonstrated to be true (Davis and Cole 1975).

Despite the absence of any clear indication that any phenothiazine is a more effective antipsychotic agent than the prototype chlorpromazine, psychiatrists continue to observe clinically that patients who fail to respond to one drug will occasionally show a good response to another. Given an adequate trial of one agent it would seem sensible to change to another in the face of therapeutic failure. The reasons for differential individual response are probably numerous, including the straightforward one of bioavailability.

The Butyrophenones

Haloperidol, the prototype and main representative of this group of antipsychotic agents, was synthesized and clinically tested in the late 1950s. Its main therapeutic place in psychiatric disorder is undoubtedly in the management of manic illness, but efficacy against acute schizophrenic illness has also been shown. Motor hyperactivity appears particularly amenable to this drug and one of the earliest demonstrations of clinical efficacy was in the treatment of the syndrome of Gilles de la Tourette.

The quantity of published experience with haloperidol in the management of schizophrenic illness is much less than for the phenothiazines and is confined mostly to European trials (Davis 1965). In general, properly controlled trials have consistently shown haloperidol to be superior to placebo and to be as effective as chlorpromazine. For reasons that are not altogether clear, haloperidol has never achieved the clinical popularity of the phenothiazines as the first treatment of choice in schizophrenic illness. Haloperidol is more commonly used as a second-line agent in patients who show an inadequate response to phenothiazines. A depot injection of haloperidol is a recent development.

The administration of very high doses of antipsychotic drugs to abort a psychosis ('rapid neuroleptisation') was first reported by Mountain in 1963. This megadose strategy was later adopted by Oldham and Bott (1971) with haloperidol. It has been reported that high dosage haloperidol (100 mg daily) might evoke improvement in the mental state of chronic drug-resistant schizophrenic patients, albeit at the expense of some deterioration in ward behaviour (McCreadie and MacDonald 1977). Recent trials in which low- and high-dose regimens of haloperidol have been compared in the management of acute schizophrenic psychoses have, however, failed to show any advantage of high over routine dose levels (Donlon et al. 1980; Neborsky et al. 1981). A curious phenomenon reported with high-dose haloperidol was a threshold effect of increasing doses on extrapyramidal impairment. A potent DA receptor blocker with weak anticholinergic activity like haloperidol is naturally prone to producing parkinsonian side effects. It was observed that as doses were increased, a threshold was reached above which extrapyramidal side effects not only levelled off in intensity but actually lessened (Sangiovanni et al. 1973; McCreadie and MacDonald 1977). It has been suggested that this is due to a ceiling effect of maximal DA receptor blockade, over which increasing doses of haloperidol start to exert significant anticholinergic activity. However, the occurrence of this extrapyramidal phenomenon appears to be in some doubt (Neborsky et al. 1981). There seems to be no clear support for the efficacy of high-dose regimens in the routine management of acute schizophrenic illness, and such a practice is best avoided for fear of increasing the likelihood of long-term neurotoxicity.

The Thioxanthenes

Chlorprothixene and thiothixene are marketed in the US and there is ample evidence that they are effective antischizophrenic agents (Davis and Garver 1978). Flupenthixol, the thioxanthene analogue of fluphenazine, is the one most used in the UK. A recent clinical trial in the UK not only demonstrated the antischizophrenic efficacy of α-flupenthixol but also highlighted two issues of

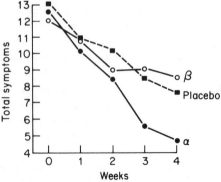

Figure 2.3. The clinical effects of α- and β-fluphenthixol compared to placebo in recently admitted patients with acute schizophrenia. (From Johnstone et al. 1978.)

general importance; the significant early placebo component in recovery from acute schizophrenic illness in hospital (patients tend to improve somewhat merely by removal to a nonstressful hospital environment), and the fact that the pharmacological influence on recovery takes at least 2–3 weeks to become apparent (Johnstone et al. 1978) (Figure 2.3). The time-course of the pharmacotherapeutic action of α-flupenthixol suggests that although the antipsychotic effect may depend upon DA receptor blockade, such blockade may be necessary only to allow other, longer term, restorative processes to take place. An interesting extension to this study was the observation that patients whose arousal in response to an auditory stimulus did not habituate tended to show a poorer antipsychotic response to medication than those who did habituate (Frith et al. 1979).

The Diphenylbutylpiperidines

This is a relatively new class of potent and long-acting antipsychotic agents and includes pimozide, fluspirilene and penfluridol. While their clinical efficacy has been established reasonably but not rigorously, the use of pimozide continues to increase in the UK. Although pimozide was clinically available in Europe in 1970, systematic evaluation has occurred slowly. Pimozide has now been shown to be effective in acutely ill schizophrenic patients (Freeman 1979) and to be effective in reducing the rate of relapse in schizophrenic patients discharged from hospital (Falloon et al. 1978). Penfluridol is used as a long-acting oral medication which can be taken once weekly and its efficacy as a prophylactic antischizophrenic agent has been demonstrated (Davis and Garver 1978). Fluspirilene is given intramuscularly in aqueous solution. The drug has not yet been evaluated in a sufficient number of double-blind placebo-controlled studies to allow definite conclusions, but the available evidence suggests that fluspirilene may also be an effective maintenance drug when given once weekly.

The Substituted Benzamides

This new class of compounds, which includes metoclopramide, sulpiride, sultopride and tiapride was introduced into clinical use in the 1960s by Justin-Besancon and colleagues in France. Most of the relevant clinical literature is French and there is a dearth of published reports from blind placebo-controlled studies. Open studies have shown that sulpiride has antipsychotic properties in chronic and withdrawn schizophrenic patients and that it produces parkinsonian side effects (Davis and Garver 1978). Evidence for the antipsychotic efficacy of metoclopramide is conflicting and requires clarification (Borenstein and Bles 1965; Stanley and Wilks 1979). As yet there is no conclusive information on the two clinically most important questions relating to these D-2 DA receptor blockers; does their clinical profile offer advantages over the older and less specific DA receptor antagonists, and are they less prone to extrapyramidal side effects? The answer to the latter question is at present the clearer and it seems to be no.

Others

Propranolol. It is always useful to have at one's disposal a drug, or group of drugs, which act in a way quite different from the therapeutic mainstays and which might offer some advantages in terms of side effects or prospect of response in the drug-resistant case. Propranolol might be considered in this category although thorough evaluation in treatment-resistant schizophrenic patients remains to be done. Claims that propranolol is effective either alone or in combination with conventional agents in both acute and chronic schizophrenic illness (Atsmon et al. 1971; Yorkston et al. 1977, 1981) have not been substantiated by some (Peet et al. 1981*a*; Myers et al. 1981). While the question of the place, if any, of propranolol in the management of schizophrenic illness must remain open, it seems likely that the interpretation of any beneficial effect observed when the drug is used in combination with a phenothiazine is complicated by the fact that propranolol increases the bioavailability of the phenothiazine (Peet et al. 1981*b*; Yorkston et al. 1981).

It has been a matter for concern that large oral doses of propranolol have been recommended as necessary for any antipsychotic effect, although recent studies claim encouraging results and little toxicity at daily doses under 1 g. Nonetheless, caution needs to be exercised (Tyrer 1980); hallucinations have been a reported side effect at relatively modest doses of β-blockers. Several other side effects are attributed to propranolol, the most important being fatigue, depressed affect, bradycardia, hypotension (and occasionally paradoxical hypertension), congestive cardiac failure, dizziness and sleep disturbance. Unlike conventional DA-blocking antipsychotic agents, propranolol causes neither hyperprolactinaemia nor extrapyramidal impairment.

Oxypertine. This unconventional drug may also fall into the category of an adjunct to established antischizophrenic medication. Two early controlled trials in the West were encouraging (Davis 1965) and the drug has recently been used quite widely in Japan. A monoamine depletor (see above), it appears to avoid the depressive side effects typical of reserpine and may therefore turn out to have useful synergistic actions with the DA receptor blockers in the treatment of refractory cases. Early reports of a selective beneficial effect on variables such as poverty of speech and motor retardation have not so far been substantiated.

Endorphin-related agents. The manipulation of central endorphin systems in the treatment of schizophrenic psychoses is at an early experimental stage and the agents available for this purpose are few. Clinical strategies have so far crudely aimed at either inhibiting or stimulating endorphin transmission.

Of the agents investigated clinically, the opiate antagonist naloxone has been most widely tested. Conflicting reports exist concerning its efficacy in the treatment of schizophrenic illness (Mackay 1980) but the results of a World Health Organization Multi-Centre Collaborative Study suggest that it may be of benefit in some patients suffering from intractable auditory hallucinations (Pickar and Bunney 1981).

The opposite strategy has most commonly involved the systemic administration of β-endorphin or one of its stable analogues. Administration of synthetic β-endorphin to schizophrenic patients has been variously reported to evoke either deterioration or improvement which is statistically significant but clinically unimportant (Gerner et al. 1980; Berger et al. 1980). Double-blind evaluation of a *met*-enkephalin analogue (FK-33-824) has failed to reveal any significant therapeutic effect in schizophrenic illness (Ruther et al. 1981). Early clinical trials of the endorphin fragment DTγE were encouraging, but subsequent work has shown this peptide to be at best of limited efficacy in a small subgroup of schizophrenic patients (Manchanda and Hirsch 1981).

Clinical results so far are, therefore, not very encouraging but it must be remembered that apart from the obvious limitations imposed by the need to give all these agents systemically, the proper clinical evaluation of endorphin-active agents in schizophrenic illness must await the availability of a wider range of receptor-specific drugs.

Target Symptomatology—What Changes?

From the very first, it was clear to clinicians using chlorpromazine and its descendants that here was a group of drugs which were not simply sedative or tranquillizing. They facilitated a restitution of the cognitive and perceptual abnormalities which are the hallmarks of schizophrenic illness. The early efficacy trials employed diagnostic criteria and indices of improvement which relied heavily upon the views of Eugen Bleuler. Bleuler's 'fundamental' symptoms (thought disorder, affective blunting, ambivalence and autistic behaviour) were all found to be responsive to the phenothiazines. In recent years, diagnostic habits and foci for therapeutic improvement have moved from Bleuler's list of fundamental phenomena to a list of symptoms which are more readily defined, and therefore more readily rated. These are embodied in the Wing Present State Examination (PSE), a highly reliable diagnostic instrument of proven operational value (Wing et al. 1972). It has been shown that the nuclear schizophrenic syndrome of the PSE (thought insertion, thought broadcast, thought commentary, thought withdrawal, auditory hallucinations of voices speaking about the patient, delusions of control and delusions of alien penetration) resolves steadily over the first few weeks of treatment of acute schizophrenic psychosis with chlorpromazine (Phillipson et al. 1977). It thus appears that even when viewed through a different and more rigorous experimental instrument, there is clear evidence of general improvement in the clinical features which distinguish schizophrenic illness. This is not to say that the therapeutic extent of these drugs is confined to the symptoms of schizophrenia—it must be emphasized that they appear to be antipsychotic in general and antischizophrenic in particular.

Positive versus negative phenomena. An important issue which has not been satisfactorily resolved is whether this group of drugs is effective in ameliorating the so-called negative (as opposed to the positive or productive) phenomena such as flattened affect, poverty of speech, slowness, underactivity, withdrawal and lack of motivation which tend to be relatively refractory to medication. There is no doubt that positive phenomena such as delusions and hallucinations, which are typical of the acute psychosis, respond well to medication, but it is the negative features (or defect state) which contribute most to the crippling stigmata of chronic schizophrenic illness. The early multicentre trials of the phenothiazines seemed to show that, indeed, these negative features responded just as well as the positive. However, a recent drug trial suggested otherwise and tends to confirm the clinical impression to the contrary (Johnstone et al. 1978). It has been suggested that this apparent discrepancy may arise out of differences in what was actually measured. The early trials made behavioural ratings of negative *features* of the disease (such as social withdrawal and lack of self-care) which are not uncommon in the acute stages of the illness, whereas negative *symptoms* are only rateable through clinical interview. When symptoms are elicited, it seems that conventional antischizophrenic medication is relatively ineffective against the defect state typical of chronic schizophrenic illness (Mackay and Crow 1980).

Chronicity and failure of functional restoration are often common features of schizophrenia, and while many patterns of individual morbidity exist, chronic schizophrenic illness carries a poor prognosis. While there is little doubt that medication reduces the probability of relapse into florid psychosis, there is absolutely no evidence that suppression of florid psychotic episodes affects the long-term course and eventual outcome of the schizophrenias (Ciompi 1980).

Social Environment, Arousal and Drugs

In research on chronic schizophrenic patients there have been many indications that drug treatments and social treatments are not alternatives but must be used to complement each other. The better the environmental conditions, the less the need for medication; the poorer the social milieu, the greater the need for drugs. If the phenothiazines and their descendants work, at least in part, by reducing a high level of physiological arousal (Venables and Wing 1962; Goldberg et al. 1965) then they should be most effective in conditions of social overstimulation. The elegant studies of the MRC Social Psychiatry Unit have shown that the emotional climate generated between the patient and the

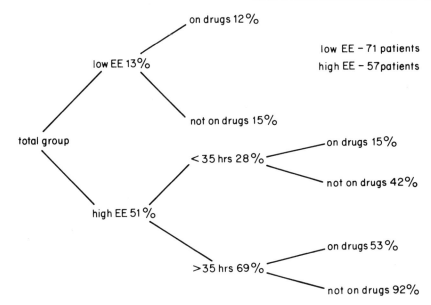

on drugs 12%

low EE – 71 patients
high EE – 57 patients

low EE 13%

not on drugs 15%

total group

< 35 hrs 28%

on drugs 15%

not on drugs 42%

high EE 51%

on drugs 53%

>35 hrs 69%

not on drugs 92%

Figure 2.4. Nine-month relapse rates in a group of 128 schizophrenic patients according to expressed emotion (EE) rated in a relative and time per week in contact with that relative. (From Vaughn and Leff 1976)

relative with whom he lives, in particular, the intensity of 'expressed emotion' (EE) and the time spent in enforced face-to-face contact with the relative, has a direct influence on the likelihood of relapse. It appears that maintenance antischizophrenic medication exerts a protective action against the damaging effects of high EE, reducing the risk of psychotic relapse to a level similar to that for patients in an ideal nonthreatening environment (Figure 2.4). It has further been shown that patients in high EE environment have a particular pattern of hyperarousal (Tarrier et al. 1979) which might represent a target for therapeutic drug action (Sturgeon et al. 1981).

Maintenance Medication: How Long to Treat?

There is abundant evidence that once an optimal level of remission from the acute stage of schizophrenic illness has been achieved, the risk of relapse into florid psychosis is substantially reduced if patients continue to take medication (Davis 1975). It appears that while the majority of patients derive some benefit from continued medication, there is a small group (some 15%) who will remain well for long periods without medication (Hogarty and Ulrich 1977). Two important questions arise; firstly, who to treat chronically with drugs, and secondly, for how long should drug therapy be maintained? The answer to the first is, unfortunately, quickly dealt with—the characteristics of this group are unclear. The only prediction that can be made on present evidence is that patients being discharged to low EE environments will have a relatively good prognosis even in the absence of medication.

The duration of drug administration must be guided by knowledge of the extent of any protective effect of medication in the patient who remains well, and by knowledge of the risks of long-term toxicity (see below). Sophisticated long-term prospective follow-up studies have shown that relapse rates in drug-maintained patients are at least half those of patients maintained on placebo. While risk of relapse does decline the longer a patient remains well, at the 2½ year stage the risk in drug-free patients is still nearly three times higher than in drug treated patients (Hogarty and Ulrich 1977). There is evidence from one study that even in patients who have remained well for 3–5 years on medication, replacement of antischizophrenic medication by a benzodiazepine results in a four-fold higher rate of relapse in the subsequent 18 months (Cheung 1981). It is thus a dangerous clinical intuition that if a patient does well after a period of successful maintenance chemotherapy then the risk of relapse is so reduced as to render continued medication unnecessary.

The majority of relapses occur within 3 months of stopping medication and it has been proposed that rather than being a natural expression of the underlying disease process, such a relapse is a drug-induced supersensitivity psychosis; a mesolimbic dopaminergic rebound following prolonged DA receptor blockade (Chouinard and Jones 1980). This possibility makes the interpretation of most studies of maintenance medication rather difficult (Mackay 1981b).

The choice of maintenance medication is governed by ease of administration, toxicity, and avoidance of non-compliance. For the phenothiazines, such as fluphenazine, there is equivalent efficacy in both the oral and depot intramuscular preparations, but maintenance therapy using multiple daily dosage of oral preparations is accompanied by a high rate of default. While they do not eliminate overt default (open refusal), injected preparations undoubtedly eliminate covert default since administration is always professionally supervised. It has been shown that, provided patients are seen regularly at a systematic follow-up clinic, daily oral pimozide is as effective as fortnightly injections of fluphenazine decanoate (Falloon et al. 1978). Johnson and Freeman (1973) found that 15–20% of patients receiving intramuscular medication dropped out of treatment, mostly within the first 6 months. The reasons for default are largely attributable to unwanted side effects, in particular an awareness of extrapyramidal symptoms such as akathisia, akinesia, tremor and dystonia (Van Putten 1974).

There is nothing to choose between the two most popular depot intramuscular preparations used in the UK, fluphenazine decanoate and α-flupenthixol decanoate. Clinical efficacy and prevalence of a variety of side effects are essentially equal at dose equivalents of 25 mg fluphenazine to 40 mg α-flupenthixol (Knights et al. 1979).

UNWANTED EFFECTS

The price paid by patients for treatment with antischizophrenic drugs is quite high in the form of unwanted side effects. A good working knowledge of the full range of unwanted effects is essential if the clinician is to react quickly and appropriately to relieve unnecessary distress, to prepare the patient against emergence of these side effects, and to weigh the benefits of medication against the cost, particularly when embarking upon chronic therapy.

Antipsychotic drugs have a high therapeutic index in terms of life threat. Most phenothiazines have a rather flat dose–response curve and can therefore be used over a wide dose range. Death from overdose is extremely rare. However, short of threat to life, this group of drugs is guilty of a long list of unwanted effects and should be treated with great respect.

Most commonly encountered side effects are *dose related* and understandable in the light of the known pharmacological actions of this group of agents. These can be classified into effects on the extrapyramidal system, other CNS effects, autonomic effects, endocrine effects, skin and eye effects. Other, less common, side effects are not clearly dose related and probably reflect an idiosyncratic or allergic response by the patient and are therefore largely unpredictable.

Extrapyramidal Side Effects

Dysfunction of the extrapyramidal motor system is the commonest of the unwanted side effects of antischizophrenic chemotherapy. While it is now generally agreed that overt extrapyramidal side effects are not a *conditio sine qua non* for therapeutic effectiveness, any antipsychotic agent which substantially inhibits central DA transmission will carry the risk of such disorders, acute and chronic. The nature, prevalence and management of drug-induced extrapyramidal side effects have recently been extensively reviewed (Marsden et al. 1981).

Overall at least 30% of all patients receiving antischizophrenic medication will suffer extrapyramidal dysfunction. There is a wide interdrug variation, the most troublesome in this respect being the newer, more selective and potent DA antagonists which are devoid of anticholinergic activity (see above). With them, the prevalence of extrapyramidal disorder is over 50%, and, in the case of the depot intramuscular preparations, can be as high as 80% (Knights et al. 1979). Many of these untoward reactions occur early in the course of drug treatment, particularly after systemic administration, and it is important to appreciate that this may represent the patient's earliest experience of this form of treatment.

Acute Toxicity

Acute dystonic reactions (acute dyskinesias). An acute dystonia is often the earliest extrapyramidal disorder to appear, the great majority occurring within 4½ days of starting therapy, and an appreciable number of cases occur within the first few hours. This is perhaps the most dramatic of the drug-induced disorders of striopallidal function. The syndrome consists of intermittent or sustained muscular spasms and abnormal postures which are both clinically striking and profoundly distressing to the patient. The five commonest manifestations of acute dystonia are torticollis, contraction of the tongue, trismus, occulogyric crisis and opisthotonus.

Occulogyric crisis is characterized by a brief prodromal fixed stare followed by upward and lateral rotation of the eyes. If the eyelids are forced open against blepharospasm, the irides are typically found to be hidden beneath the upper canthus of the eye, leaving only the sclera visible. Associated with these alarming ocular signs, the head is usually tilted backwards and laterally, the mouth is open and the tongue protruded. Erroneous diagnoses for acute dystonia have included tetanus, status epilepticus, meningitis and encephalitis.

Acute dystonic reactions are most likely to occur in young males under the age of 30 years, and are clearly dose related. Care should be exercised over the choice of initial dose, particularly when instituting depot therapy, and account should be taken of the patient's age, sex and weight rather than blind adherence to the manufacturer's recommended test dose. Acute dystonias are spontaneously reversible as plasma drug concentrations fall but the urgency of the clinical situation usually demands positive therapeutic action in the form of an intramuscular injection of an anticholinergic drug such as procyclidine, to which the dystonia will respond rapidly and dramatically.

Akathisia. This is a state of motor restlessness of which the cardinal diagnostic feature is a *subjective* feeling of motor unease or inner tension (*'impatience musculaire'*: van Putten 1975). The unfortunate patient feels unable to keep still but must constantly move in an attempt to relieve his discomfort. The subject constantly shifts his legs and taps his feet and, in severe, cases, may pace up and down. Such florid agitation may be misinterpreted as an exacerbation of psychotic behaviour, leading to an inappropriate increase in drug dosage. Akathisia is probably grossly underdiagnosed. Following the administration of antischizophrenic drugs it appears more slowly than acute dystonia but more rapidly then parkinsonism. Women are almost twice as frequently affected as men. Unlike the other acute extrapyramidal syndromes it tends to respond poorly to anticholinergic medication. Reduction in dosage is the most effective method of management but if this is not possible, benzodiazepines have been found beneficial. It has been proposed that this rather odd but common extrapyramidal syndrome is caused by inhibition of DA transmission not in the nigrostriatal tract but in mesocortical DA pathways projecting from the ventral tegmentum to the frontal cortex (Marsden and Jenner 1980).

Parkinsonism. Antischizophrenic drugs can induce an exact facsimile of classic Parkinson's disease; the cardinal signs of rigidity, tremor, bradykinesia, with a variety of subsidiary clinical features such as changes in gait and posture, excessive salivation, difficulty in speaking and swallowing, characteristic frozen facies and greasy skin.

Bradykinesia is especially common, occurring soon after starting treatment, and frequently the only sign of parkinsonism to occur. The face is blank and expressionless, accessory movements are lost, the arms fail to swing on walking and gesture on talking disappears. Voluntary movement becomes slow in initiation and execution, and reduced in amplitude. The voice becomes soft and handwriting small (micrographia is a sensitive and easily recorded clinical sign). Like akathisia, bradykinesia may pose problems of diagnosis and interpretation. The lack of spontaneity and general slowness may be interpreted as part of the defect state of chronic schizophrenia. 'Akinetic depression' is a term coined by van Putten and May (1978) to capture the negative subjective accompaniment to bradykinesia. It is vital to distinguish a drug-induced parkinsonian syndrome, which may be amenable to anticholinergic drug therapy, from a natural feature of schizophrenic illness. A brief diagnostic trial with an anticholinergic anti-Parkinson drug probably represents the only straightforward means available by which to make such a distinction.

Drug-induced parkinsonism occurs roughly twice as commonly in women as in men of the same age. The majority of cases will appear within 2 weeks of starting treatment but this is quite variable and it is not uncommon for signs to develop after weeks or months with no change in dose level and for no apparent reason. The incidence of drug-induced parkinsonism rises steeply after middle age and there is a suggestion that a family history of Parkinson's disease raises the likelihood of the drug-induced syndrome (Marsden et al. 1981).

The ideal management of drug-induced parkinsonism is reduction in dose of the antischizophrenic agent. Where this may not be possible, for example in the early stages of treatment of the acute psychosis, the prescription of an anti-Parkinson drug may be required for a limited period. Anticholinergic agents are the most widely used drugs for this purpose. Surprisingly, the published evidence for their effectiveness in Parkinson's disease itself is rather sparse, and procyclidine is one of the few of this class which has been compared favourably with placebo (Mindham 1976). While some evidence exists for the effectiveness of orphenadrine and benztropine in the treatment of drug-induced parkinsonism, the evidence in favour of procyclidine again seems the clearest.

Anticholinergic medication is not without dangers and considerable draw-backs. A toxic confusional state may occur, particularly in the elderly, as may all the autonomic effects of atropine-like drugs. Anticholinergic drugs will usually exacerbate an existing tardive dyskinesia and may unmask latent dyskinesia (see below). They may also contribute to the development of hyperthermic episodes, which can be fatal. Hyperpyrexia may result from a combination of peripheral inhibition of sweating by the anticholinergic, and a central effect on thermoregulatory centres by concurrently administered phe-nothiazines (Westlake and Rastegar 1973). A number of reports have claimed that anticholinergics attenuate the therapeutic actions of antischizophrenic drugs. Such an attenuation may be explicable on a pharmacokinetic basis, the anticholinergic causing a reduction in plasma concentrations of the antipsychotic drug by impairing its intestinal absorption (Rivera-Calimlim 1976a) although this effect has been disputed (see Cooper 1978).

There is considerable evidence that chronic anti-Parkinson medication is not required by the vast majority of patients receiving antischizophrenic drugs. Where originally indicated by definite neurological signs, the need for anticholinergic medication usually disappears even if the patient continues to receive the same dose of antipsychotic medication. In about 90% of patients the anticholinergic drug can be withdrawn after 3 months with no return of parkinsonian signs. The following is a summary based on current evidence (Marsden et al. 1981):

(1) Routine prescription of anticholinergic drugs should be *avoided*. This practice results in many patients receiving them who do not need them and it robs the clinician of a valuable clinical sign of substantial DA receptor blockade in the nigrostriatal system.

(2) When drug-induced parkinsonism produces real impairment and distress, consideration should first be given to reducing the dose of the offending drug.

(3) When reduction in dosage of the antischizophrenic drug is not possible, an anticholinergic anti-Parkinson drug should be given only for as long as symptoms are unpleasant or functionally limiting.

(4) Anti-Parkinson drugs should not be given for more than 3 or 4 months without careful reassessment.

(5) If parkinsonism reappears after withdrawal of anticholinergic medication, such medication should be reintroduced for a limited period only.

Chronic Toxicity

While some cases of drug-induced parkinsonism may appear late in the course of treatment and may persist for prolonged periods, the commonest long-term extrapyramidal complication, tardive dyskinesia, is of a very different nature.

Tardive dyskinesia. Within 5 years of the introduction of phenothiazine drugs for the treatment of psychoses Schonecker (1957) drew attention to an involuntary choreoathetoid dyskinesia apparently associated with antipsychotic medication, which is distinguishable from the acute dystonias and from parkinsonism on the basis of both phenomenology and time course. Uhrbrand and Faurbye (1960) coined the term tardive dyskinesia to denote an involuntary hyperkinesia which was characteristically late in appearance during treatment with antischizophrenic drugs.

The disorder occurs most commonly after approximately 2 years of uninterrupted drug treatment but individual variability is wide. The core of the disorder is the bucco-linguo-masticatory (BLM) syndrome consisting of involuntary pursing and smacking of the lips, rolling or thrusting of the tongue, puffing of the cheeks and lateral chewing jaw movements. This cephalic dyskinesia may be associated with choreic movements of the limbs and rhythmic dystonic contraction of axial muscles giving rise to paroxysmal torticollis and pelvic thrusting. In the elderly, the BLM syndrome predominates; in children and adolescents the trunk, arms and hands are commonly affected and here the character of the movements is often more dystonic than choreic. Muscle tone is usually reduced but the BLM syndrome can coexist with features of drug-induced parkinsonism such as cog-wheel rigidity in the limbs. It is the exception rather than the rule for patients to report distress from tardive dyskinesia; more commonly a complaint will come from relatives or nursing staff. Arousal plays a key role in determining the severity of movements; tardive dyskinesia disappears during sleep and is intensified by anxiety, although embarrassment may force the patient to suppress, voluntarily, the movements for limited periods.

Estimates of prevalence vary widely but well-executed studies in both the UK and US have recorded prevalence rates between 40 and 50% of all patients receiving antischizophrenic medication, whether in-patients or out-patients (Marsden et al. 1981). Two differential diagnoses may cause some confusion and misunderstanding. Firstly, there may be a superficial similarity between tardive dyskinesia and the bizarre mannerisms and sterotypies of chronic schizophrenia but most authorities agree that the abnormal movements of schizophrenia are of a different character (Mackay 1981a) and are much less common than tardive dyskinesia. Secondly, a BLM syndrome identical to tardive dyskinesia can occur in old people who have never been exposed to antischizophrenic medication and in them the syndrome is a variant of senile chorea. There is, however, no doubt that the incidence of orofacial dyskinesia in all age groups and for all diagnoses is highly significantly increased by chronic exposure to antischizophrenic drugs.

Of the many variables, in both patients and medication history, which have been investigated for a relationship with risk of tardive dyskinesia, the *age* of the patient stands out clearly as increasing the risk. There is a sharp increase in prevalence after middle age and this is not merely related to the length of time a patient has been exposed to medication—the ageing brain seems particularly susceptible to this disorder. There is no clear evidence incriminating any one sort of antischizophrenic drug; any drug which inhibits central DA transmission for long periods runs the risk of inducing tardive dyskinesia.

A particularly serious aspect of tardive dyskinesia is the fact that the dyskinesia is irreversible in between one-third and one-half of patients. Withdrawal of the offending drug usually causes a paradoxical worsening of the condition and in a considerable proportion of cases the movements will then gradually abate; improvement may continue for as long as 3 years. Factors which appear to militate against reversibility are the duration of drug therapy, age and the duration of obvious dyskinesia. Caution needs to be exercised in the use of periodic drug withdrawals ('drug holidays') as a strategy for avoiding irreversible long-term side effects; Jeste et al. (1979) have found that drug holidays may actually make it more likely that a dyskinesia will become irreversible.

The neurobiological basis of tardive dyskinesia is not yet clear, but the most coherent hypothesis suggests that tardive dyskinesia reflects relative dopaminergic overactivity in the nigrostriatal tract. Chronic occlusion of central DA receptors by an antischizophrenic drug results in compensatory proliferation of the DA receptors. The hypothesis states that in tardive dyskinesia this DA receptor 'supersensitivity' may express itself as neurological disorder if there is a failure of normal homeostatic mechanisms. The result is a functional dopaminergic overactivity relative to cholinergic (and perhaps GABAcidic) transmission in the basal ganglia—the diametric opposite of Parkinson's disease.

Since there is no generally acceptable treatment for tardive dyskinesia, *prevention* must be the most important consideration and the following guidelines are suggested:

(1) Antipsychotic drugs should be prescribed for serious indications only.

(2) The minimum dose for the shortest time should be used.

(3) Regular (monthly) neurological examination should be carried out. Early detection and drug withdrawal will maximize chances of reversibility. The earliest signs are often detected in the tongue, which should be observed retracted in the open mouth.

(4) Particular care should be taken with patients over the age of 50.

Once a tardive dyskinesia has appeared, any concomitant anticholinergic medication should be withdrawn since this will tend to intensify the abnormal movements. The antischizophrenic drug should, if possible, be withdrawn gradually. If complete withdrawal is clinically unjustifiable then dose reduction is the next best strategy. In cases where tardive dyskinesia is irreversible in the face of drug withdrawal or dose reduction (and this may take months or years to assess), a therapeutic trial of a benzodiazepine (such as clonazepam) may evoke some improvement (Sheppard et al. 1981).

In the case of a serious iatrogenic disorder such as tardive dyskinesia it seems prudent to advise all clinicians using long-term antischizophrenic drugs to make a clear statement in the case notes of the clinical indications for such therapy. If, as will often be the case, it is judged clinically inadvisable to withdraw the offending drug in the face of emergent tardive dyskinesia, recognition of the disorder should be made in the case notes along with a statement explaining why, in that particular case, the psychiatric risks of drug withdrawal outweigh the neurological benefits.

Other CNS Effects

EEG effects. The EEG frequency slows, with increased theta and delta waves, a decrease in alpha waves and fast beta activity, and some increase in burst activity and spiking. The seizure threshold is lowered, particularly by the aliphatic phenothiazines such as chlorpromazine. Butyrophenones have variable and unpredictable effects. The likelihood of frank epileptic fits is more in patients with a history of epilepsy or a condition which predisposes to seizures. Therefore the aliphatic phenothiazines are to be avoided in patients prone to epileptic attacks or in withdrawal from general CNS depressants such as alcohol or the barbiturates. High potency agents (such as fluphenazine) can be used relatively safely in epileptic patients if the dose is increased gradually and if concomitant anticonvulsant medication is maintained.

Sedation. This may be particularly noticeable over the first few days of treatment with agents such as chlorpromazine and thioridazine. Tolerance develops fairly rapidly to this effect.

Paradoxical worsening of psychotic symptoms. This may occasionally occur at relatively high doses. It is a phenomenon quite distinct from akathisia or toxic confusion.

Toxic confusional states. These can occur, with typical clouding of consciousness, particularly in the elderly and with the highly atropinic agents such as thioridazine. The confusion usually resolves rapidly after withdrawal or dose reduction.

Autonomic Effects

These are due to the anticholinergic and antinoradrenergic actions of the drugs and are expressed in a wide range of troublesome signs and symptoms, including abnormalities of the ECG.

Atropinic activity can cause dry mouth, inhibition of sweating, blurred vision (mydriasis), constipation (even paralytic ileus), inhibition of ejaculation and urinary retention. Antinoradrenergic effects include cutaneous flushes, blurred vision (miosis) and postural hypotension. The blurring of vision caused by chlorpromazine is due to miosis (anti-NA effects outweight anti-Ach effects) whereas with thioridazine the reverse is true and blurring is due to mydriasis. Postural hypotension is most commonly associated with sudden elevation of plasma drug concentrations resulting from systemic administration. Tolerance to this side effect develops after a few days. The ECG may show broadening and flattening of T waves and increased QR intervals. T-wave changes are commonest with thioridazine and least common with high potency agent. Sudden death, presumed to be of cardiovascular origin, has very occasionally been reported in phenothiazine-treated patients.

Endocrine Effects

Antischizophrenic agents may cause a variety of endocrinological abnormalities due to their interaction with central DA receptors, and probably to a lesser extent with NA and 5-HT receptors. The sites of these actions lie mainly in the hypothalamus and pituitary. The clinically important effects are irregular menstruation, lactation and male impotence.

Drug-induced hyperprolactinaemia seems to underlie most of these problems. Through antagonistic action at DA receptors in the anterior pituitary, antischizophrenic drugs induce substantial rises in circulating prolactin concentrations. The ability of these drugs to do this is related to their potency as DA receptor antagonists, there is a low ceiling to this effect (maximal hyperprolactinaemia can occur at subtherapeutic doses of drug) and no tolerance occurs with chronic treatment (Gruen et al. 1978). High circulating prolactin concentrations may interfere with the actions of gonadotrophins at their end organs, resulting in hypogonadism in males and amenorrhoea in females (Thorner and Besser 1976). Impotence and anovulatory bleeding may also occur. Breast engorgement is not uncommon and lactation can be evoked by gentle pressure on the breast. Male gynaecomastia has also been reported. Phenothiazine-induced male impotence may have two sources; hyperprolactinaemia and inhibition of ejaculation with eventual loss of erectile ability due to autonomic interference (especially with thioridazine). There is no clear evidence that prolonged drug-induced hyperprolactinaemia should be avoided in cases of established breast cancer. It is said that glucose tolerance curves may show some shift into the diabetic range. Weight gain on phenothiazine drugs is not unusual and while the effect probably results from a hypothalamic action, it has not yet been clearly explained.

Skin and Eye Effects

There are three sorts of dermatological complication: allergic (urticarial, maculopapular, petechial or oedematous), contact dermatitis and photosensitivity. Urticaria has been reported to occur in approximately 5% of patients receiving chlorpromazine. Contact dermatitis used to be common in ward staff who handled phenothiazine syrups but this is now rare. A phototoxic sensitivity reaction may occur in patients receiving chlorpromazine. It resembles severe sunburn and direct sunlight should be avoided. A very chronic side effect (occurring after 10 to 15 years) may be blue-grey metallic discolouration of the skin over areas exposed to sunlight. Deposits of melanin-like material may be seen in the dermis after skin biopsy.

Lens and corneal opacities may occur as part of an 'epithelial keratopathy' especially after chronic chlorpromazine treatment. Light-brown, granular deposits occur in the anterior lens and posterior cornea and are visible only at slit-lens examination of the eye. The lesions may progress to opaque brown stellate granules found in the lens. Occasionally, the conjunctivae show brown discolouration. Statistically, lens opacities occur more frequently in patients with skin discolouration. Vision is very rarely impaired. The opacities are dose related and related to chronicity of drug exposure. Sunlight plays a role in both the skin and eye complications of the phenothiazines.

Thioridazine is guilty of a much more serious ophthalmic complication. In doses in excess of about 800 mg/day a retinitis pigmentosa can occur and this is accompanied by substantial visual impairment and even blindness. The retinitis does not remit if the drug is stopped.

Idiosyncratic Reactions

These are relatively rare, are not clearly dose related, and tend to occur early in the course of drug treatment.

Jaundice. This can be associated with the use of phenothiazines and in the 1960s the incidence was reported to be as high as 1%. More recently, for reasons unknown, the incidence has fallen to 0.1% at most. Clinical jaundice is preceded by 'flu-like malaise, abdominal pain, fever, nausea, vomiting and diarrhoea—a picture resembling infectious hepatitis. The biochemical picture is of obstructive jaundice (raised serum bilirubin and alkaline phosphatase) and the pathological picture is one of intrahepatic centralobular cholestasis. There is pericanalicular inflammation with oedema and local infiltration by eosinophils as well as generalized eosinophilia. Most cases have been reported in association with chlorpromazine but it may also occur with thioridazine, promazine, prochlorperazine and, very rarely, fluphenazine.

Blood dyscrasias. Agranulocytosis is probably the most serious of all the side effects, but it is luckily very rare—variously quoted as occurring in between 1 in 10 000 and 1 in 500 000 patients treated with phenothiazines such as chlorpromazine and thioridazine. The mortality rate may be as high as 30%. The polymorphonuclear leucocyte count falls rapidly and this is associated with sore throat, ulcerations and fever. Cross-sensitivity between phenothiazines should be assumed.

Phenothiazines quite often reduce the circulating white cell count by 40–80% but this is a temporary and quite innocuous effect. Transient leucocytosis has also been reported. Thrombocytopenic purpura, eosinophilia, haemolytic anaemias and pancytopenia may rarely occur with the phenothiazines.

Drug Interactions

Interaction with other drugs may affect the circulating plasma levels of antipsychotic drugs and the possible interaction of antischizophrenic and anti-Parkinson agents has already been mentioned. Many *hypnotic* and sedative drugs (such as phenobarbitone) are known to induce drug metabolizing enzymes of the hepatic endoplasmic reticulum and so increase the rate of drug metabolism and reduce the plasma concentrations of a wide variety of psychoactive drugs, including most antischizophrenic agents.

Apparent impairment of absorption of chlorpromazine has been reported to occur with concomitant administration of *antacids* such as aluminium hydroxide gels. This effect may be due to delayed gastric emptying and it is thus not desirable to give antacids and chlorpromazine simultaneously, if possible spacing administration a few hours apart.

The metabolism of *tricyclic antidepressants* may be inhibited by various phenothiazines and by haloperidol, and vice versa. This suggests the possibility of mutual potentiation but the clinical implications of this remain to be evaluated. The mutual metabolic inhibition between phenothiazines and *propranolol* may render the toxicity of propranolol more likely while increasing the circulating plasma levels of the phenothiazine. *Lithium* has been shown to lower the plasma concentrations of chlorpromazine, an effect caused by delayed gastric emptying (Rivera-Calimlim 1976*b*).

Serious doubts about the safety of *haloperidol-lithium* combinations have been raised since the original report by Cohen and Cohen (1974) of four cases of severe extrapyramidal toxicity and irreversible brain damage allegedly due to the combination. However, the results of subsequent systematic investigation and of clinical experience suggest that haloperidol and lithium may be given together at *routine* clinical doses without risk of severe toxicity (Ayd 1978). There may be an enhanced risk of quick-onset extrapyramidal impairment and, at high dose levels of both drugs, an increased risk of lithium CNS toxicity, so it is prudent to monitor more carefully the patient receiving this combination.

References

ATSMON, A., BLUM, I., WIJSENBECK, H., MAOZ, B., STEINER, M. & ZIEGELMAN, G. (1971) The short-term effects of adrenergic blocking agents in a small group of psychiatric patients. *Psychiat. Neurol. Neurochir.*, **74**, 251.

ANGRIST, B., SATHANANTHAN, G., WILK, S. & GERSHON, S. (1974) Amphetamine psychosis: behavioural and biochemical aspects. *J. Psychiat. Res.*, **11**, 13.

AYD, F.J. (1978) Haloperidol: twenty years' clinical experience. *J. clin. Psychiat.*, **39**, 807.

BERGER, P.A. (1981) Clinical studies on the role of endorphins in schizophrenia. In: *Proceedings of the Third World Congress of Biological Psychiatry* (Stockholm, 1981), Amsterdam: Elsevier/North Holland Biomedical Press.

BERGER, P.A., WATSON, S.J., AKIL, H., ELLIOTT, G.R., RUBIN, R.T., PFEFFERBAUM, A., DAVIS, K.L., BARCHAS, J.D. & LI, C.H. (1980) β-endorphin and schizophrenia. *Archs gen. Psychiat.*, **37**, 635.

BORENSTEIN, P. & BLES, G. (1965). Effets cliniques et électroencéphalographiques du métaclopramide en psychiatrie. *Thérapie*, **20**, 975.

BUCHSBAUM, M.S., DAVIS, G., NABER, D., PICKAR, D., BALLANGER, R., WATERS, R., GOODWIN, F.K., VAN KAMMEN, D., POST, R., & BUNNEY, W., Jr. (1981) Pain appreciation, somatosensory evoked potentials and endorphins in normals and patients with schizophrenia and affective disorders. In: *Proceedings of Third World congress of Biological Psychiatry* (Stockholm, 1981), Amsterdam: Elsevier/North Holland Biomedical Press.

CALDWELL, A.E. (1970) History of Psychopharmacology. In: *Principles of Psychopharmacology*, ed. Clark, W.G. & del Guidice, J. New York: Academic Press.

CASEY, J.F., BENNETT, I.F., LINDLEY, C.J., HOLLISTER, L.F., GORDON, M.H., & SPRINGER, N.N. (1960a) Drug therapy in schizophrenia. *AMA Archs gen. Psychiat.*, **2**, 210.

CASEY, J.F., et al. (1960b) Treatment of schizophrenic reactions with phenothiazine derivatives. *Am. J. Psychiat.*, **117**, 97.

CHANG, K.J., HAZUM, E. & CUATRECASAS, P. (1980) Multiple opiate receptors. *Trends in Neuroscience (July)*, 160.

CHEUNG, H.K. (1981) Schizophrenics fully remitted on neuroleptics for 3–5 years—to stop or continue drugs? *Br. J. Psychiat.*, **138**, 490.

CHOUINARD, G. & JONES, B.D. (1980) Neuroleptic-induced supersensitivity psychosis: clinical and pharmacologic characteristics. *Am. J. Psychiat.*, **137**, 16.

CIOMPI, L. (1980) The natural history of schizophrenia in the long term. *Br. J. Psychiat.*, **136**, 413.

COHEN, W.J. & COHEN, N.H. (1974) Lithium carbonate, haloperidol and irreversible brain damage. *JAMA*, **230**, 1283.

CONNELL, P.H. (1958) *Amphetamine Psychosis*. London: Chapman & Hall.

COOPER, T.B. (1978) Plasma level monitoring of anti-psychotic drugs. *Clin. Pharmacokinet.*, **3**, 14.

CREESE, I., BURT, D.R. & SNYDER, S.H. (1976) Dopamine receptor binding predicts clinical and pharmacological potencies of antischizophrenic drugs. *Science*, **192**, 481.

DAVIS, J.M. (1965) Efficacy of tranquilizing and antidepressant drugs. *Archs gen. Psychiat.*, **13**, 552.

DAVIS, J.M. (1975) Overview: maintenance therapy in psychiatry: I. Schizophrenia. *Am. J. Psychiat.*, **132**, 1237.

DAVIS, J.M. & COLE, J.O. (1975) Antipsychotic drugs. In: *Comprehensive Textbook of Psychiatry*, Vol. 2, eds Freedman, A.M., Kaplan, H.I. & Sadock, B.J. 2nd ed. Baltimore: Williams & Wilkins.

DAVIS, J.M. & GARVER, D.L. (1978) Neuroleptics: Clinical use in psychiatry. In: *Handbook of Psychopharmacology*, Vol. 10, ed. Iversen, L.L., Iversen, S.D., & Snyder, S.H. New York: Plenum Press.

DENIKER, P. (1978) Impact of neuroleptic chemotherapies on schizophrenic psychoses. *Am. J. Psychiat.*, **135**, 923.

DIAZ-BUXO, J.A., CAUDLE, J.A., CHANDLER, J.T., FARMER, C.D. & HOLBROOK, W.D. (1980) Dialysis of schizophrenic patients: a double-blind study. *Am. J. Psychiat.*, **127**, 1220.

DONLON, P.T., HOPKIN, J.T., TUPIN, J.P., WICKS, J.J., WAHBA, M. & MEADOW, A., (1980) Haloperidol for acute schizophrenic patients. *Archs gen. Psychiat.*, **37**, 691.

FALLOON, I., WATT, D.C. & SHEPHERD, M. (1978) A comparative controlled trial of pimozide and fluphenazine decanoate in the continuation therapy of schizophrenia. *Psychol. Med.*, **8**, 59.

FJALLAND, B., CHRISTENSEN, A.V. & HYTTEL, J. (1977) Peripheral and central muscarinic receptor affinity of psychotropic drugs. *Naunyn-Schmiedebergs Arch. exp. Path. Pharma.*, **301**, 5.

FORSMAN, A., FOLSCH, G., LARSON, M. & OHMAN, R. (1977) On the metabolism of haloperidol in man. *Curr. Ther. Res.*, **21**, 606.

FREEMAN, H. (1979) Pimozide as a neuroleptic. *Br. J. Psychiat.*, *135*, 82.

FRITH, C.D., STEVENS, M., JOHNSTONE, E.C. & CROW, T.J. (1979) Skin conductance responsivity during acute episodes of schizophrenia as a predictor of symptomatic improvement. *Psychol. Med.*, **9**, 101.

GARVER, D.L., DEKIRMENJIAN, H., DAVIS, J.M., CASPER, R. & ERICKSEN, S. (1977) Neuroleptic drug levels and therapeutic response: preliminary observations with red blood cell bound butaperazine. *Am. J. Psychiat.*, **134**, 304.

GERNER, R.H., CATLIN, D.H., GORELICK, D.A., HUI, K.K. & LI, C.H. (1980) β-Endorphin. *Archs gen. Psychiat.*, **37**, 642.

GOLDBERG, S.C., KLERMAN, G.L. & COLE, J.O. (1965). Changes in schizophrenic psychopathology and ward behaviour as a function of phenothiazine treatment. *Br. J. Psychiat.*, **111**, 120.

GREEN, A.R. & GRAHAME-SMITH, D. (1976) Propranolol inhibits the behavioural responses of rats to increased 5-hydroxytryptamine in the central nervous system. *Nature*, **262**, 594.

GREENBLATT, D.J., SHADER, R.I. & KOCH-WESTER, J. (1976) The psychopharamcology of β-adrenergic blockade: pharmacokinetic and epidemiologic aspects. In: *Advances in Clinical Pharmacology*, Vol. 12, ed. Carlsson, C., Engel, J. & Hansson, L. Berlin: Urban and Schwarzenberg.

GROVES, J.E. & MANDEL, M.R. (1975) The long-acting phenothiazines. *Archs gen. Psychiat.*, **32**, 893.

GRUEN, P.H., SACHAR, E.J., LANGER, G., ALTMAN, N., LEIFER, M., FRANTZ, A. & HALPERN, F.S. (1978) Prolactin responses to neuroleptics in normal and schizophrenic subjects. *Archs gen. Psychiat.*, **35**, 108.

HOGARTY, G.E. & ULRICH, R.F. (1977) Temporal effects of drug and placebo in delaying relapse in schizophrenic outpatients. *Archs gen. Psychiat.*, **34**, 297.

HOLLISTER, L.E. (1977) Antipsychotic medications and the treatment of schizophrenia. In: *Psychopharmacology*, ed. Barchas, J.D., Berger, P.A., Ciaranello, R.D. & Elliott, G.R. New York: Oxford University Press.

IVERSEN, S.D. (1980) Brain chemistry and behaviour. *Psychol. Med.*, **10**, 527.

JANSSEN, P., BRUGMANS, J., DONY, J. & SCHUERMANS, V. (1972) An international double-blind evaluation of Pimozide. *J clin. Pharmacol.*, **12**, 26.

JESTE, D.V., POTKIN, S.G., SINHA, S., FEDER, S. & WYATT, R.J. (1979) Tardive dyskinesia—reversible and persistent. *Archs gen. Psychiat.*, **36**, 585.

JOHNSON, D.A.W. & FREEMAN, H. (1973) Drug defaulting by patients on long-acting phenothiazines. *Psychol. Med.*, **5**, 115.

JOHNSTONE, E.C., CROW, T.J., FRITH, C.D., CARNEY, M.W.P. & PRICE, J.S. (1978) Mechanism of action of the antipsychotic effect in the treatment of acute schizophrenia. *Lancet*, **i**, 848.

KELLY, P.H., SEVIOUR, P.W. & IVERSEN, S.D. (1975) Amphetamine and apomorphine responses in the rat following 6-OHDA lesions of the nucleus accumbens septi and corpus striatum. *Brain Res.*, **94**, 507.

KNIGHTS, A., OKASHA, M.S., SALIH, M.A. & HIRSCH, S.R. (1979) Depressive and extrapyramidal symptoms and clinical effects: a trial of fluphenazine versus flupenthixol in maintenance of schizophrenic outpatients. *Br. J. Psychiat.*, **135**, 515.

LADER, M., (1980) In: *Drug Concentrations in Neuropsychiatry*, Ciba Foundation Symposium 74 (New Series). Oxford: Excerpta Medica.

LASKY, J.J., KLETT, C.J., CAFFEY, E.M., BENNETT, J.L., RORSENBLUM, M.P., & HOLLISTER, L.E. (1962) Drug treatment of schizophrenic patients. *Dis. nerv. Syst.*, **23**, 698.

MANCHANDA, R. & HIRSCH, S.R. (1981) (Des-Tyr')-γ-endorphin in the treatment of schizophrenia. *Psychol. Med.*, **11**, 401.

McCREADIE, R.G., HEYKANTS, J.J.P., CHALMERS, A. & ANDERSON, A.M. (1979) Plasma pimozide profiles in chronic schizophrenics. *Br. J. Clin. Pharmacol.*, **7**, 533.

McCREADIE, R.G. & MacDONALD, I.M. (1977) High dosage haloperidol in chronic schizophrenia. *Br. J. Psychiat.*, **131**, 310.

MACKAY, A.V.P. (1980a) Endorphins: implications for psychiatry. *Advanced Medicine*, Vol. 17, ed. Jewell, D.P. (Royal College of Physicians of London). London: Pitman Books.

MACKAY, A.V.P. (1980b) Neurotransmitters in psychiatry. *Medicine*, **35**, 1799.

MACKAY, A.V.P. (1981a) Controversies in tardive dyskinesia. In: *Neurology*, Vol. 2., *Movement Disorders*, ed. Marsden, C.D. & Fahn, S. London: Butterworths.

MACKAY, A.V.P. (1981b) Assessment of antipsychotic drugs. *Br. J. Clin. Pharmacol.*, **11**, 225.

MACKAY, A.V.P., BIRD, E.D., SPOKES, E.G., ROSSOR, M., IVERSEN, L.L., CREESE, I. & SNYDER, S.H. (1980) Dopamine receptors and schizophrenia: drug effect or illness? *Lancet*, **ii**, 915.

MACKAY, A.V.P. & CROW, T.J. (1980) Positive and negative schizophrenic symptoms and the role of dopamine. *Br. J. Psychiat.*, **137**, 379.

MACKAY, A.V.P., HEALEY, A.F. & BAKER, J. (1974) The relationship of plasma chlorpromazine to its 7-hydroxy and sulphoxide metabolites in a large population of chronic schizophrenics. *Br. J. Clin. Pharmacol.*, **1**, 425.

MANCHANDA, R. & HIRSCH, S.R. (1981) (Des-Tyr')-γ-endorphin in the treatment of schizophrenia. *Psychol. Med.*, **11**, 401.

MARCHAND, W.E. (1955) Occurrence of painless myocardial infarction in psychotic patients. *New Engl. J. Med.*, **253**, 51.

MARSDEN, C.D. & JENNER, P. (1980) The pathophysiology of extrapyramidal side-effects. *Psychol. Med.*, **10**, 55.

MARSDEN, C.D., MINDHAM, R.H.S. & MACKAY, A.V.P. (1981) Extrapyramidal movement disorders produced by antipsychotic drugs. In: *The Pharmacology and Treatment of Schizophrenia*, ed. Bradley, P.B. & Hirsch, S.R. Oxford: Oxford University Press.

MIDDLEMISS, D.N., BLAKEBOROUGH, L. & LEATHER, S.R. (1977) Direct evidence for an interaction of β-adrenergic blockers with the 5-HT receptor. *Nature*, **267**, 289.

MINDHAM, R.H.S. (1976) Assessment of drug-induced extrapyramidal reactions and of drugs given for their control. *Br. J. Clin. Pharmacol.*, **3**, 395.

MOUNTAIN, H.E. (1963) Crash tranquilisation in a milieu therapy setting. *J. Fort Logan Ment. Health Centre*, **1**, 43.

MYERS, D.H., CAMPBELL, P.L., COCKS, N.M., FLOWERDEW, J.A. & MUIR, A. (1981) A trial of propranolol in chronic schizophrenia. *Br. J. Psychiat.*, **139**, 118.

NEBORSKY, R., JANOWSKY, D., MUNSON, E., & DEPRY, D. (1981) Rapid treatment of acute psychotic symptoms with high and low dose haloperidol. *Archs gen. Psychiat.*, **38**, 195.

NIMH-PSC Collaborative Study Group (1964) Phenothiazine treatment in acute schizophrenia. *Archs gen. Psychiat.*, **10**, 246.

OLDHAM, A.J. & BOTT, M. (1971) The management of excitement in a general hospital psychiatric ward by high dosage haloperidol. *Acta psychiat. scand.*, **47**, 369.

PALMOUR, R.M., ERVIN, F.R. & WAGEMAKER, H. (1977) Characterisation of a peptide derived from the serum of psychiatric patients. *Abstr. Soc. Neurosci.*, **7**, 32.

PEET, M., BETHELL, M.S., COATES, A., KHAMNEE, A.K., HALL, P., COOPER, S.J., KING, D.J. & YATES, R.A. (1981a) Propranolol in schizophrenia: I. Comparison of propranolol, chlorpromazine and placebo. *Br. J. Psychiat.*, **139**, 105.

PEET, M., MIDDLEMISS, D.N. & YATES, R.A. (1981b) Propranolol in schizophrenia: II. Clinical and biochemical aspects of combining propranolol with chlorpromazine. *Br. J. Psychiat.*, **139**, 112.

PEROUTKA, S.J. & SNYDER, S.H. (1980) Differential effects of neuroleptic drugs at brain dopamine, serotonin, α-adrenergic and histamine receptors: relationship to clinical potency.

PEROUTKA, S.J., U'PRICHARD, D.C., GREENBERG, D.A. & SNYDER, S.H. (1977) Neuroleptic drug interactions with norepinephrine alpha receptor binding sites in rat brain. *Neuropharmacology*, **16**, 549.

PHILLIPSON, O.T., McKEOWN, J.M., BAKER, J., & HEALEY, A.F. (1977) Correlation between plasma chlorpromazine and its metabolites and clinical ratings in patients with acute relapse of schizophrenic and paranoid psychosis. *Br. J. Psychiat.*, **131**, 172.

PICKAR, D. & BUNNEY, W.E. Jr (1981) Acute Naloxone in schizophrenic patients. A World Health Organisation Collaborative Project. In: *Proceedings of the Third World Congress of Biological Psychiatry* (Stockholm, 1981). Amsterdam: Elsevier/North Holland Biomedical Press.

QUACH, T.T., DUCHENIN, A.M., ROSE, C., & SCHWARTZ, J.C. (1979) In vivo occupation of cerebral histamine H_1-receptors evaluated with ^3H-mepyramine may predict sedative properties of psychotropic drugs. *Eur. J. Pharmacol.*, **60**, 391.

RANDRUP, A. & MUNKVAD, I. (1974) Pharmacology and physiology of stereotyped behaviour. *J. psychiat. Res.*, **11**, 1.

RIVERA-CALIMLIM, L. (1976a) Impaired absorption of chlorpromazine in rats given trihexyphenidyl. *Br. J. Pharmacol.*, **56**, 301.

RIVERA-CALIMLIM, L. (1976b) Effect of lithium on gastric emptying and absorption of oral chlorpromazine. *Psychopharm. Communs*, **2**, 263.

RUTHER, E., GERD., J. & NEDOPIL, N. (1981) Clinical effects of the synthetic analogue of methionine enkephalin Fk-33-824. In: *Proceedings of the Third World Congress of Biological Psychiatry* (Stockholm, 1981). Amsterdam: Elsevier/North Holland Biomedical Press.

SANGIOVANNI, F., TAYLOR, M.A., ABRAMS, R. & GAZTANAGA, P. (1973) Rapid control of psychotic excitement states with intramuscular haloperidol. *Am. J. Psychiat.*, **130**, 1155.

SCHONECKER, M. (1957) Ein Eigenümliches Syndrome in oralen Bereich bei Megaphenapplikation. *Nerventarzt*, **28**, 35.

SHEPHERD, M., LADER, M. & RODNIGHT, R. (1968) *Clinical Psychopharmacology*. London: English Universities Press.

SHEPPARD, G., MACKAY, A.V.P. & KITSON, M. (1981) Clonazepam in the treatment of tardive dyskinesia; a controlled study. In: *Proceedings of the Third World Congress of Biological Psychiatry* (Stockholm, 1981). Amsterdam: Elsevier/North Holland, Biomedical Press.

SNYDER, S.H. (1973) Amphetamine psychosis: a 'model' schizophrenia mediated by catecholamines. *Am. J. Psychiat.*, **130**, 61.

SNYDER, S.H. (1981) Dopamine receptors, neuroleptics and schizophrenia. *Am. J. Psychiat.*, **138**, 460.

SNYDER, S.H., GREENBERG, D. & YAMAMURA, H.I. (1974) Antischizophrenic drugs and brain cholinergic receptors. *Archs gen. Psychiat.*, **31**, 58.

STANLEY, M. & WILKS, S. (1979) Striatal DOPAC elevation predicts antipsychotic efficacy of metoclopramide. *Life Sci.*, **24**, 1907.

STURGEON, D., KIUPERS, L., BERKOWITZ, R., TURPIN, G. & LEFF, J.P. (1981 Psychophysiological responses of schizophrenic patients to high and low expressed emotion relatives. *Br. J. Psychiat.*, **138**, 40.

TARRIER, N., VAUGHN, C., LADER, M.H. & LEFF, J.P. (1979) Bodily reactions to people and events in schizophrenics. *Arch. gen. Psychiat.*, **36**, 311.

THORNER, M.O. & BESSER, G.M. (1976) Bromocriptine. In: *Proceedings of a Symposium at the Royal College of Physicians, London*, ed. Bayliss, R.I.S., Turner, P. & Maclay, W.P. Kent: MCS Consultants.

TYRER, P.J. (1980) Use of β-blocking drugs in psychiatry and neurology. *Drugs*, **20**, 300.

UHRBRAND, L. & FAURBYE, A., (1960) Reversible and irreversible dyskinesia after treatment with perphenazine, chlorpromazine, reserpine and electroconvulsive therapy. *Psychopharmacologia*, **1**, 408.

VAN PUTTEN, T. (1974) Why do schizophrenic patients refuse to take their drugs? *Archs gen. Psychiat.*, **31**, 67.

VAN PUTTEN, T. (1975) The many faces of akathisia. *Compreh. Psychiat.*, **16**, 43.

VAN PUTTEN, T. & MAY, P.R.A. (1978) Akinetic depression in schizophrenia. *Archs gen. Psychiat.*, **35**, 1101.

VAUGHN, C.E. & LEFF, J.P. (1976) The influence of family and social factors on the course of psychiatric illness. *Br. J. Psychiat.*, **129**, 125.

VENABLES, P.H. & WING, J.K. (1962) Level of arousal and the subclassification of schizophrenia. *Archs gen. Psychiat.*, **7**, 114.

WATSON, G.D., CHANDARANA, P.C. & MERSKEY, H. (1981) Relationship between pain and schizophrenia. *Br. J. Psychiat.*, **138**, 33.

WESTLAKE, R.J. & RASTEGAR, A. (1973) Hyperpyrexia from drug combinations. *JAMA*, **225**, 1250.

WIED, D. DE, BOHUS, B., VAN REE, J.M., KOVACS, G.L. & GREVEN, H.M. (1978) Neuroleptic-like activity of [Des-Tyr']-endorphin in rats. *Lancet*, **i**, 1046.

WING, J.K., COOPER, J.E. & SARTORIUS, N. (1972) *The Measurement and Classification of Psychiatric Symptoms*. London: Cambridge University Press.

WISTEDT, B., WILES, D. & KOLAKOWSKA, T. (1981) Slow decline of plasma drug and prolactin levels after discontinuation of chronic treatment with depot neuroleptics. *Lancet*, **i**, 1163.

YORKSTON, N.J., GRUZELIER, J.H., ZAKI, S.A., HOLLANDER, D., PITCHER, D.R. & SERGEANT, H.G.S. (1977) Propranolol as an adjunct to the treatment of schizophrenia. *Lancet*, **ii**, 575.

YORKSTON, N.J., ZAKI, S.A., WELLER, M.P., GRUZELIER, J.H. & HIRSCH, S.R. (1981) DL-propranolol and chlorpromazine following admission for schizophrenia. *Acta psychiat. scand.*, **63**, 13.

3

Antidepressant Drugs

J.H. Dowson

TRICYCLIC ANTIDEPRESSANTS AND RELATED DRUGS

The range of these compounds is shown in Table 3.1. The main pharmacological property shared by the tricyclic antidepressants is their ability to inhibit the reuptake by neurones of the monoamines serotonin (5-HT) and noradrenaline, thereby enhancing monoaminergic neurotransmission.

Side effects and drug interactions, which are shown in Tables 3.2 and 3.3, are relatively severe in the elderly, in whom smaller doses are usually indicated. Although there is no evidence of teratogenic effects, tricyclic antidepressants should be routinely avoided in early pregnancy. If they are given in later pregnancy, the dose should be reduced before delivery, as cardiac and respiratory side effects in the neonate have been reported. Amitriptyline is said not to be excreted in breast milk. Tolerance to many of the initial side effects often develops within several days.

The distinction between the syndromes of endogenous and neurotic depression has been widely used in studies of response to treatment. An endogenous depressive syndrome includes such phenomena as psychomotor retardation, diurnal variation (worse in the morning), early morning wakening, delusions and hallucinations. The neurotic syndrome, on the other hand, may consist of such features as reactivity of mood to pleasant or unpleasant situations, with evening worsening and initial insomnia, often accompanied by various phenomena which are not syndrome specific. However, this distinction is only one aspect of the classification of depressive syndromes (see Chapter 15).

In depressive syndromes with endogenous features there is clear evidence that tricyclics are effective, but in severe cases they may be less effective or ineffective (Glassman et al. 1975; Bielski and Friedel 1976). There is also substantial evidence that tricyclics exert a prophylactic effect in recurrent endogenous depressive syndromes (Davis 1976).

In the neurotic syndrome, and for nonspecific depressive phenomena, the value of tricyclics is less clear. In general, tricyclics are of more limited value, but some patients respond well (Trethowan 1975; Bielski and Friedel 1976).

Table 3.1. Tricyclic antidepressants and related drugs

Iminodibenzyls
   Imipramine—a tertiary amine which is less sedative than amitriptyline
   Desipramine—a secondary amine metabolite of imipramine; one of the most potent inhibitors of noradrenaline uptake with minimal sedative and anticholinergic effects
   Trimipramine—one of the most sedative tricyclics; a tertiary amine
   Clomipramine—inhibits both serotonin and noradrenaline uptake; drowsiness and postural hypotension are often relatively pronounced; a tertiary amine

Dibenzocycloheptenes
   Amitriptyline—a tertiary amine with relatively pronounced sedative and anticholinergic effects
   Nortriptyline—secondary amine metabolite of amitriptyline with relatively little sedative action
   Protriptyline—the least sedative of the tricyclics with stimulant properties; a secondary amine
   Butriptyline—produces minimal inhibition of noradrenaline and serotonin uptake

Other tricyclics
   Doxepin—a tertiary amine with a significant sedative action; it probably has the least cardiotoxic activity of the tricyclics
   Dibenzepin—a tertiary amine
   Dothiepin—may produce fewer side effects than amitriptyline or imipramine; has sedative properties; a tertiary amine
   Iprindole—has minimal inhibitory effects on neuronal noradrenaline and serotonin uptake but may enhance monoaminergic transmission in other ways
   Nomifensine—a potent inhibitor of dopamine and noradrenaline uptake
   Opipramol

Related drugs
   Maprotiline—a tetracyclic selective inhibitor of noradrenaline uptake with little effect on serotonin uptake; it may have relatively less cardiotoxicity. Grand mal seizures are a side effect.
   Mianserin—a tetracyclic with minimal inhibitory effects on neuronal uptake of noradrenaline and serotonin, but may act by increasing noradrenaline release from neurones; also a postsynaptic blocker of serotonin action; it is claimed that it produces relatively little cardiotoxicity or anticholinergic effects. Agranulocytosis and arthropathy have been reported.
   Viloxazine—a bicyclic drug which appears to have imipramine-like and amphetamine-like properties
   Zimeldine—a relatively specific inhibitor of serotonin uptake; claimed to have minimal anticholinergic activity and no antihistaminic action

---

   Tricyclics are of uncertain efficacy for depression occurring in the course of a schizophrenic illness, but some patients with schizo-affective syndromes may benefit (Siris et al. 1978). Clomipramine and imipramine have also been advocated for certain sleep disorders, phobic anxiety, and in obsessive–compulsive disorders. Tricyclic antidepressants have also been used for childhood hyperactivity (Quinn and Rapoport 1975).

   The drug of first choice is often amitriptyline or imipramine depending on the degree of sedation required. It has been suggested that the neurophysiological basis of some endogenous depressive syndromes mainly involves disordered noradrenaline metabolism, while in others serotonin metabolism is principally affected. Thus, there are theoretical grounds for prescribing clomipramine or nomifensine if a course of amitriptyline or imipramine has failed

Table 3.2. Side effects of tricyclic antidepressants

Gastrointestinal
  Common—dry mouth, constipation, nausea
  Less common—paralytic ileus, hiatus hernia (probably due to an anticholinergic action on the oesophageal sphincter), epigastric pain, vomiting, anorexia, odd taste, diarrhoea

Cardiovascular
  Common—postural hypotension, palpitations, sinus tachycardia, ECG changes (e.g. prolongation of PR/QRS/QT, T wave flattening and ST depression) due to delayed conduction
  Less common—hypertension, atrial fibrillation, AV block, bundle-branch block, ventricular tachycardia or fibrillation, aggravation of heart failure, decreased myocardial contractility, cardiomyopathy, sudden death

Neuropsychiatric
  Common—sedation (not with all tricyclics), tremor, blurred vision, paraesthesiae, impaired cognition, EEG changes
  Less common—confusion, restlessness, agitation, insomnia, nightmares, delirium (with hallucinations, due to central anticholinergic activity), aggressive behaviour, epilepsy, parkinsonism, ataxia, dysarthria, choreoathetoid movements, buccofaciolingual movements, nystagmus, myoclonus, peripheral neuropathy, tinnitus, precipitation of hypomania

Genitourinary
  Common—hesitancy, impaired sexual function (delayed orgasm, impaired ejaculation/erection)
  Less common—retention, testicular swelling

Haematological
  Common—eosinophilia
  Less common—agranulocytosis, leucopenia, purpura, thrombocytopenia

Metabolic/endocrine
  Common—weight gain
  Less common—gynaecomastia, amenorrhoea, breast enlargement and galactorrhoea, blood sugar elevation or depression, altered antidiuretic hormone secretion

Other
  Aggravation of glaucoma (especially of the narrow angle type), allergic cholestatic jaundice, allergic skin reactions (e.g. cutaneous vasculitis, urticaria, angioneurotic oedema, pruritus, photosensitivity), headache, oedema, elevation of liver transaminases and alkaline phosphatase, reduction of serum cholesterol, hepatic necrosis, accident-proneness, increases in frequency of mood cycling, a withdrawal syndrome (anxiety, akathisia, nausea, vomiting, sweating, insomnia and headache)

Interactions with the following disease states
  A recent myocardial infarct (an absolute contraindication for tricyclic use), cardiac pathology, prostatic hypertrophy, glaucoma, epilepsy, diabetes, hypertension, liver failure, impaired renal function, the schizophrenias, bipolar affective disorders

---

(Iversen and Mackay 1979; Kessler 1978; Editorial 1981). Clomipramine has relatively greater effect on 5-HT uptake by neurones, while nomifensine has a relatively greater effect on noradrenaline uptake. Nomifensine has been advocated for depressive syndromes in parkinsonian patients, because of its inhibitory effect on dopamine uptake, and clomipramine is claimed to be of use in syndromes involving obsessional or phobic phenomena (Editorial 1978b; Shaw 1977; Paykel 1979). Doxepin is considered to be the drug of choice if the patient has cardiovascular disease.

Table 3.3. Drugs which interact with tricyclic antidepressants

---
Drugs which potentiate tricyclics
 Phenothiazines—compete with tricyclics for hepatic metabolism, and elevate plasma levels
 Methylphenidate—can elevate tricyclic plasma levels

Drugs potentiated by tricyclics
 CNS depressants, including alcohol
 Coumarin derivatives—prothrombin times must be carefully monitored
 Anticholinergic drugs—the anticholinergic effect of a tricyclic may summate with those of a phenothiazine and/or an antiparkinsonian agent
 Adrenaline, noradrenaline—the pressor effects of these drugs (which may be constituents of local anaesthetics) may be potentiated, thus inducing hypertension
 Vasoconstrictors in nasal decongestants—hypertension may result
 Phenothiazines

Drugs antagonized by tricyclics
 Guanethidine, bethanidine, debrisoquine, reserpine, clonidine. Careful monitoring of blood pressure is essential and, when the tricyclic is discontinued, the dose of the antihypertensive drug may need revision

Drugs which antagonize tricyclics
 Barbiturates—cause increased tricyclic metabolism (and reduced plasma levels)

Drugs which interact with tricyclics
 MAO inhibitors—severe hypertension, CNS excitation, hyperpyrexia and coma can occur; if a tricyclic is prescribed following an MAO inhibitor, a drug-free period of at least 14 days must usually be observed
 Phenothiazines—the hypotensive actions may summate; thioridazine with a tricyclic may be liable to induce ventricular arrhythmias
 Lithium—the tremor resulting from lithium and a tricyclic may summate
 Amphetamine and related drugs—this combination may produce hypertension, excitement, hyperpyrexia and cardiac arrhythmias

---

Evidence suggests that there is a range of plasma nortriptyline levels which is associated with therapeutic efficacy and that levels above or below this 'window' are ineffective. It is possible that other secondary amine tricyclics share this property, while the available evidence suggests that for tertiary amines, such as amitriptyline or imipramine, there is a lower, but no upper, threshold plasma level (Editorial 1978*a*; Glassman and Perel 1978).

Different preparations of the same drug can produce variations in target biological activity in the same individual. Changes in a patient's diet can alter plasma levels of tricyclics, and a given dose of drug can produce an enormous variation between individuals with respect to plasma levels of the parent drug and its metabolites, and their ratios.

Routine plasma tricyclic estimation is not yet available, and although the appropriate dose regimen of nortriptyline can be estimated from a single blood sample taken 24 h after an initial dose (Cooper and Simpson 1978*a*), nortriptyline is not usually considered to be a drug of first choice. In the case of amitriptyline or imipramine, the appearance of mild side effects, such as visual accommodation difficulties and postural hypotension, is used to indicate a therapeutic plasma level; dry mouth is not used in this context.

The estimation of plasma levels is useful in determining the bioavailability of both the parent drug and any active metabolites. For example, although clomipramine is relatively effective as a serotonin reuptake inhibitor compared with its action on noradrenaline uptake, it has been reported that the latter action can be enhanced by an accumulation of its metabolites. In a few centres, plasma levels are used routinely for such categories as elderly patients, those with cardiac disease, individuals who develop severe side effects on routine dose regimens, and those who are unresponsive to treatment. In the latter group, noncompliance may be revealed. Another factor which may be of clinical relevance is that hepatic enzymes involved in the metabolism of tricyclics can be induced during a course of treatment, which may lead to the development of reduced plasma levels at a given dose regimen, compared with the initial steady-state values.

A pretreatment ECG should often be performed (Bigger et al. 1978). Amitriptyline should be started on a twice or three times daily regimen and the initial dose may be 75 mg daily (e.g. 25 mg a.m. and 50 mg nocte), less in the elderly. The daily dose is then increased, side effects permitting, by 25 mg every 3 days, so that after 9 days the patient is taking 50 mg a.m. and 100 mg nocte. After a week at this dose, it may again be increased, every 3 days, until mild side effects develop or until a daily dose of 300 mg is reached. In this context it should be stressed that tricyclics are frequently prescribed at an inadequate dose. It is generally considered that a once-daily (nocte) regimen is of comparable efficacy when compared with a divided daily dose, and that patient compliance is increased. Thus, an initial division of the daily dose can be gradually converted to a once-daily regimen. However, administration once daily (nocte) may produce a period of relatively severe side effects during the following morning and should be used with caution in the elderly. In addition, a single bedtime dose may induce more nightmares than a divided dose regimen (Flemenbaum 1976). There is no evidence that slow-release preparations have more efficacy, but they reduce the peaks of tricyclic plasma levels. If anticholinergic side effects are a particular problem, they can sometimes be relieved by concomitant bethanechol chloride administration (Everett 1975).

In those patients who respond, there is a delay of between 1 and 3 weeks before a tricyclic antidepressant begins to exert its therapeutic effects, but if there is no improvement after 4–6 weeks on the maximum tolerated dose within the permitted dose range, the drug should be gradually discontinued. If improvement has occurred, treatment is often continued for about 10 weeks, or longer in some cases. Because of the risk of overdose, not more than a few days supply should be available to the potentially suicidal patient. There is evidence that once recovery from a depressive syndrome has been achieved as a result of chemotherapy or ECT, the continued administration of a tricyclic antidepressant for up to 9 months will significantly reduce the probability of relapse within that time, while clinicians may administer such prophylactic treatment for even longer periods (see Chapter 15).

The patient should be told that there will be a delay before the beneficial effects of the drug can be expected, and that he may feel worse before he feels better. The common side effects should be outlined and the patient should be warned about the possible dangers of driving, drinking alcohol and working with machinery while taking the drug. Where compliance is doubtful, the aid of a relative or friend should be sought.

MONOAMINE OXIDASE INHIBITORS

The hydrazine inhibitors comprise phenelzine, isocarboxazid and iproniazid, which has a high incidence of hepatotoxic effects. Tranylcypromine is a

Table 3.4. Side effects of monoamine oxidase inhibitors

Gastrointestinal
    Common—dry mouth, constipation, nausea

Cardiovascular
    Common—postural hypotension, which is often a particular problem
    Rare—a hypertensive crisis can follow the ingestion of amines (usually tyramine) in foodstuffs, or an interaction with another drug; hypertension is associated with a throbbing headache, increased heart rate, palpitations, throbbing in the neck and a feeling of suffocation; fatal subarachnoid or cerebral haemorrhage can occur

Neuropsychiatric
    Common—blurred vision, drowsiness (e.g. with phenelzine), tremor
    Less common—weakness, paraesthesiae, insomnia (e.g. with tranylcypromine), nightmares, excitement, reduced appetite, hyperreflexia, oculomotor paralysis, muscle spasms, neck rigidity, peripheral neuropathy, epilepsy, ataxia, confusional state with hallucinations, precipitation or aggravation of hypomania, the schizophrenias and migraine

Genitourinary
    Common—hesitancy
    Less common—retention, impaired orgasm/ejaculation, impotence

Haematological
    Leucopenia

Metabolic/endocrine
    Weight gain, hypoglycaemia

Other
    Increased sweating, peripheral oedema of unknown aetiology, increased secretion of antidiuretic hormone, hepatocellular jaundice (which can be fatal and has been associated with the hydrazine MAO inhibitors, especially iproniazid), skin disorders (e.g. maculopapular eruptions), tranylcypromine abuse (due to its euphoriant properties)

Interactions in disease states
    Infective hepatitis, jaundice or cirrhosis contraindicate the use of MAO inhibitors; MAO inhibitors should be used with care in alcoholism, hypertension, parkinsonism, diabetes, congestive cardiac failure, cerebral arteriosclerosis, bipolar affective disorder and the schizophrenias. Some preparations of MAO inhibitors contain gluten and are, therefore, contraindicated in coeliac disease or gluten enteropathy

Food containing amines (especially tyramine) which may interact with MAO inhibitors: these include
    Cheese (except cottage, cream), yeast and meat extracts (often in stews, sausages or soups), alcohol (Chianti is to be particularly avoided but a limited amount of some beverages, other than beer or wine, may be tolerated), nonfresh meat or fish, offal, banana skins, broad bean pods, avocado, caviar, pickled or smoked herring.

Table 3.5. Drugs which interact with monoamine oxidase inhibitors

---

Drugs which can induce a hypertensive crisis
    Decongestants/cold remedies containing pseudoephedrine, ephedrine, phenylethylamine, pheny-
lephrine, phenylpropranolamine or dextromethorphanhydrobromide
    Amphetamine, mephentermine, metaraminol and other antiobesity agents
    Levodopa
    Adrenaline, noradrenaline
    Tricyclics (an appropriate drug-free interval is necessary if the patient has recently received an
MAO inhibitor)

Drugs potentiated by MAO inhibitors
    Pethidine and other narcotic analgesics (e.g. morphine, meperidine)—collapse and death have
occurred; pethidine inhibits serotonin uptake
    Hypoglycaemic agents, including insulin
    Barbiturates, ether, chloral hydrate, alcohol, cocaine, procaine and phenytoin

Other drugs which interact with MAO inhibitors
    Some antihypertensives—potentiation or antagonism has been reported
    Suxamethonium
    Antiparkinsonian drugs—may induce excitement
    Methyldopa or reserpine—may induce excitement

---

non-hydrazine with amphetamine-like actions and is probably the most clinically effective of this class of drugs (Robinson et al. 1978; Tyrer 1979).

Some patients (usually out-patients) with neurotic or nonspecific depressive
syndromes (especially if associated with anxiety) are helped by monoamine
oxidase (MAO) inhibitors, but it is usually difficult to predict which patients
will respond from this heterogeneous group (Robinson et al. 1978). It has also
been claimed that MAO inhibitors are of value for agoraphobia and for some
patients with chronic facial pain, obsessive–compulsive disorders or encapsulated delusions of infestation with parasites. The place of MAO inhibitors for
the syndrome of endogenous depression and other syndromes of probable
endogenous aetiology is uncertain, but some patients who are not helped by
tricyclic antidepressants may respond to MAO inhibitors. The side effects and
drug interactions are summarized in Tables 3.4 and 3.5 (McCabe and Tsuang
1982).

If an MAO inhibitor is to be prescribed, the choice usually lies between
phenelzine and tranylcypromine, a drug which may cause euphoria. It has been
claimed that tranylcypromine is the most clinically effective MAO inhibitor,
although it has been studied less extensively than phenelzine, which is generally
the drug of first choice. Isocarboxazid has been claimed to be the MAO
inhibitor of choice in the elderly.

It has been shown that the activity of liver acetyltransferase varies between
individuals and it has been reported that this enzyme may inactivate hydrazine
MAO inhibitors. The sulphamethazine test assesses 'acetylator status' by
measuring the percentage of a test dose which has been acetylated after a
standard time. However, it is not in routine use, and its value as a predictor of
response to routine doses of MAO inhibitors is controversial (Davidson et al.

1978). Nevertheless, the wide variation in the metabolism of MAO inhibitors between individuals suggests that the clinician must be flexible in his prescribing habits.

Phenelzine can be started at a dose of 15 mg twice daily (once daily in the elderly) and is increased, side effects permitting, to 30 mg A.M. and 15 mg P.M. after 5 days and to 30 mg twice daily after 10 days. The daily dose should then be increased by 15 mg, at weekly intervals, until mild postural hypotension develops or until 90 mg/day is reached. Therapeutic effects would not be expected for about 2 weeks.

Tranylcypromine is usually given in two daily doses, in the morning and mid-afternoon; doses given later in the day may cause insomnia. The starting dose is often 10 mg twice daily rising to 20 mg A.M. and 10 mg P.M. after 7 days. The daily dose should then be increased by 10 mg at weekly intervals, until mild postural hypotension develops or until a dose of 60 mg/day is reached.

The maximal effect of an MAO inhibitor usually occurs before about 6 weeks on the final dose regimen. Very occasionally, higher doses are required. An MAO inhibitor is often continued for at least 6–8 weeks after recovery but this practice is not based on clear evidence. The drug should be discontinued gradually and the patient should be warned that dietary and drug restrictions should be observed for at least 14 days after the final dose.

The likely time course of therapeutic activity and the common side effects should be explained. The patient is given a card stating the dietary restrictions and should be told not to take any other medication, including proprietary preparations and drugs from other doctors or dentists, without consulting his doctor.

LITHIUM CARBONATE

The role of lithium carbonate as a prophylactic agent for some recurrent affective disorders is established, particularly with manic–depressive psychosis in which both manic and depressive episodes occur. In such cases there is evidence that lithium is the best drug for this purpose. Lithium can also have a prophylactic action in recurrent depressive syndromes with endogenous aetiology, although its superiority over a tricyclic antidepressant in this role has not been established (Fieve et al. 1976; Quitkin et al. 1976). In addition, lithium may have a role in the prophylaxis of some schizoaffective syndromes (Reiser and Willett 1976).

Lithium can also be used for treatment of mania or hypomania, periodic catatonia, hyperactivity, and of some schizoaffective syndromes with a manic component (Petursson 1976). There have also been claims that lithium has an antidepressant effect, especially in bipolar affective psychosis, but this is uncertain (House and Martin 1975; Mendels 1976). Lithium has also been used for some of the schizophrenias and for personality disorders who display

Table 3.6. Side effects of lithium carbonate

Neuropsychiatric

Common—fine tremor, made worse by voluntary movement, and resistant to anti-parkinsonian medication. (This mainly affects the hands, although the jaw and lower limbs may be affected.) Also: fasciculation, and mild cognitive or volitional impairment

Less common—dysphoria, clinically significant cognitive impairment, headache, parkinsonian symptoms including 'cog-wheel' rigidity (which does not respond to anti-parkinsonian drug treatment), dizziness, blurred vision, restlessness, irritability, coarse tremor, difficulty in swallowing, tinnitus hyperreflexia, clonus, nystagmus, facial spasms, and transient facial paralysis

Toxicity (serum lithium levels are usually above 1.8 mmol/litre but may be lower.)

Slurred speech, ataxia, incoordination, apraxia, coarse tremor, muscle spasms, vertigo, disorientation, drowsiness, delirium, aphasia, coma, fits, permanent cerebellar defect.

(EEC shows generalized slow waves and reduced alpha activity, with increased theta and delta waves). Serum levels may rise after treatment is stopped (Sellers et al. 1982)

Gastrointestinal

Common—transient nausea, gastric discomfort and loose stools, dry mouth

Less common—vomiting and diarrhoea (usually associated with an excessive dose) constipation, metallic taste, poor appetite

Cardiovascular

Ankle oedema, reversible ECG changes (T wave depression, inversion or amplification), extrasystoles, tachy–bradycardia syndrome. Sinus node dysfunctions.

Genitourinary

Common—reversible polyuria. (However this can persist for months or years after discontinuation)

Less common—proteinuria and impaired erection. Lithium can produce structural renal changes and impaired water reabsorption; there is usually no evidence of associated renal insufficiency, but reversible nephrotic syndrome and a degree of renal insufficiency have been reported.

Haematological

Leucocytosis—mainly neutrophilic

Pregnancy and lactation

A higher than expected incidence of fetal cardiac malformations has been reported associated with maternal lithium treatment during pregnancy. Lithium toxicity in the neonate whose mother received lithium in the period before delivery can include goitre, absent Moro reflex, poor sucking, hypotonia, increased heart rate and increased respiration. Lithium is excreted in breast milk, so breast feeding is contraindicated

Other

Common—increased thirst, weakness and fatigue (which may be transient), increased weight, hypothyroidism (more common in women) and goitre (with or without hypothyroidism)

Less common—pretibial oedema, acneiform eruptions, folliculitis, exacerbation of psoriasis, maculopapular lesions, hypotonus, exacerbation of myasthenia gravis, precipitation of thyrotoxicosis, a reversible exophthalmos, and a withdrawal syndrome involving a degree of cognitive impairment. Rapid relapse after sudden discontinuation. Hyperparathyroidism.

---

impulsive and aggressive behaviour, but there is not sufficient evidence to warrant the routine use of lithium in an attempt to modify such behaviour (Sheard et al. 1976; Gerbino et al. 1978).

The side effects of lithium are shown in Table 3.6 (Coppen and Peet 1979). A fine tremor, increased thirst, polyuria and fatigue are common, and may lessen in severity after several days. EEG changes and a degree of mild cognitive and volitional impairment has also been found in patients and in normal volunteers.

These effects may be of clinical significance even though they may not be apparent to the clinician or the patient (Judd et al. 1977a,b; Heninger 1978; Kropf and Müller-Oerlinghausen 1979). Common longer term side effects include weight gain and thyroid dysfunction, while signs of toxicity, which occur in association with plasma levels which are variable, but are usually above 2 mmol/litre, indicate the need for the drug to be temporarily discontinued and sometimes require in-patient management. Rare examples of severe cognitive deficit, dysarthria, dyskinesia, tremor or dystonia have been reported in association with a combination of lithium and haloperidol, when relatively large doses of the latter have been given, usually in excess of 30 mg/day (Editorial 1977). However, this combination is often required for the management of manic patients, when it would seem prudent not to exceed about 30 mg haloperidol a day. An interaction between lithium and methyldopa has also been described involving increased toxicity and reduced plasma concentrations, while drugs which reduce renal lithium clearance, such as diuretics or tetracyclines, can increase side effects by increasing plasma levels. Chlorpromazine has been claimed to reduce plasma lithium concentrations, while postoperative apnoea has been reported in association with lithium and succinylcholine. In general lithium should be discontinued prior to an elective anaesthetic.

Before lithium treatment is started, the urine should be examined, and serum creatinine, blood urea and electrolytes and thyroid function should be estimated. Dehydration, a low sodium diet, cardiac failure, renal insufficiency, Addison's disease and hypothyroidism are not absolute contraindications to the prescription of lithium, but suggest the need to avoid treatment unless there are strong clinical indications. In such cases, relatively low doses should be used, and additional monitoring should take place. Before commencing treatment, careful explanation and advice must be given to the patient and relatives.

The daily dose of lithium carbonate used as a prophylactic agent usually lies between 800 and 1600 mg, although smaller doses are often appropriate for elderly patients. When lithium is used for the treatment of mania or hypomania, larger doses may be required (Cooper and Simpson 1978b). About two-thirds of a daily dose is usually excreted within 24 h, but as the rest is eliminated over several days, an accumulation of lithium can occur. The starting dose for prophylactic lithium is usually within the range 400–800 mg daily and can be taken as a single daily dose (A.M. or P.M.) or in a twice-daily dose regimen. After about 5 days, a serum lithium level is determined, and if necessary the dose is reviewed. When the appropriate dose of lithium is found which gives consistent serum levels within the range 0.5–1.0 mmol/litre, when estimated 12–16 h after the previous dose, the daily dose can be continued in a twice- or thrice-daily dose regimen. Some preparations of lithium are designed to give a more sustained release, but, in some patients, comparison of these with non-sustained-release brands have not yielded any clear differences as shown by serum levels. However for some patients, sustained release preparations may reduce peak serum levels, and, in combination with a divided daily dose regimen, reduce the gradient of lithium level changes. Peaks and/or gradients have been associated with increased severity of side effects such as tremor and nausea (Persson 1977) and in some patients dividing the daily dose into three or even four parts may produce a further reduction of discomfort. Gradients can be relatively independent of dose. Tablets should be taken after meals as this reduces gastrointestinal side effects and increases absorption (Jeppsson and Sjögren 1975). They should not be chewed or crushed or taken with hot liquids.

After the initial serum lithium level has been determined, after about 5 days, this is repeated weekly until a stable level has been obtained. Thereafter, the interval between measurements can be increased to about 8 weeks (or longer, in some cases) if no complications arise. A blood sample should be taken 12–16 h after the last dose, and the timing of the previous day's lithium intake should be carefully noted to aid the interpretation of changes in a series of values. If 16 h have elapsed since the last dose, levels at the lower end of the therapeutic range would be equivalent to higher levels in blood samples taken after 12 h, and serum levels will also be influenced by the timing of a once-daily regimen, and the distribution of the daily dose in a twice-daily dose schedule. Many patients on a twice-daily regimen take a relatively large dose in the evening, to reduce side effects during the day. Some elderly patients may be adequately controlled on serum levels below the usually quoted therapeutic range. The optimum dose schedule is often determined by clinical experience with the individual patient, but a target serum level of 0.8 mmol/litre, measured 12 h after the last dose of a twice-daily regimen, is often appropriate (Prien and Caffey 1976).

Every patient receiving prophylactic lithium should, if possible, be seen regularly within a psychiatric service (Fieve 1975). Serum lithium and creatinine are examined every 2–4 months and any side effects should be monitored. A persistent tremor is often found in association with serum levels which are within the therapeutic range, and if this is causing problems, it will often be alleviated by propranolol in a dose of 10 mg thrice daily. Treatment-resistant cog-wheel rigidity may also be found (Shopsin and Gershon 1975). The patient should be weighed regularly, as increased weight is a common problem and can be partly due to increased intake of drinks rich in calories, secondary to dry mouth, polyuria and increased thirst. Advice and encouragement to go on a strict calorie-controlled diet may be required. Measurements of thyroid function (serum TSH) should be routinely carried out at 6-monthly intervals, but hypothyroidism often develops relatively suddenly. This is sometimes reversible if lithium is discontinued and in some patients prophylactic treatment should not be restarted unless indicated by further relapse. Even if thyroid function returns to normal, restarting lithium will often produce hypothyroidism once again, which may need treatment with thyroxine. A goitre may develop which may not be associated with hypothyroidism, but which may be treated with thyroxine if necessary. It has been claimed that monitoring serum creatinine phosphokinase can indicate underlying cerebral dysfunction despite normal mood (Kerry 1975), while Vestergaard et al. (1982) have advocated routine serum creatinine estimations as an index of renal function.

In view of the increased incidence of fetal cardiac abnormalities in infants whose mothers took lithium during pregnancy (Weinstein and Goldfield 1975) female patients of childbearing age should be warned of the danger of becoming pregnant while taking lithium, and their contraceptive measures should be reviewed. If, despite this, pregnancy occurs, lithium should be discontinued and the question of termination of the pregnancy should be considered. If the pregnancy continues, lithium should, if possible, not be restarted especially within the first trimester, but in a few cases the clinical requirements for lithium for the treatment of mania are imperative. Lithium clearance increases during pregnancy and decreases after delivery so that in the rare instances when lithium is used during pregnancy the frequent monitoring of serum lithium is essential and the dose should be decreased after delivery. Regimens should involve relatively frequent doses and the target serum lithium level should be reduced. The dose of lithium should, if possible, be reduced in the week or two before delivery, to minimize the effects on the neonate. As lithium is excreted in milk, breast feeding is contraindicated.

Although polyuria of up to 3 litres/day is a common side effect, a few patients develop a more marked polyuria due to a nephrogenic diabetes insipidus which usually responds to lithium withdrawal. At this point additional tests of renal function should be carried out, and if lithium is restarted a lower dose should be prescribed. Although renal biopsy in such patients has been reported to show histological changes, a recent review could not find a single account of death due to renal failure which was caused by lithium administration. However, the possible dangers of renal damage in patients maintained on prophylactic lithium merit further research and clinical caution (Uldall 1981).

Patients taking lithium should be advised that various factors may influence serum levels. Increased sweating associated with a change in the weather, a holiday abroad, a sauna, exercise or fever may significantly reduce lithium clearance and require a reduction of dose. Diets low in sodium may have the same effect. The patient should also be encouraged to avoid dehydration and ensure that any other doctor who is consulted is aware of the lithium regimen before prescribing other medication, particularly diuretics. Digoxin may impair lithium's efficacy.

L-TRYPTOPHAN

There have been claims that L-tryptophan has antidepressant and antimanic properties, but these are not yet proven (Mendels et al. 1975; Herrington et al. 1976; D'Elia et al. 1978). However, there is some evidence that L-tryptophan can potentiate the effects of MAO inhibitors (Walinder et al. 1976). Tricyclic antidepressants (especially if they predominantly block serotonin uptake) may also be potentiated. Supplements of vitamin B_6 (pyridoxine), ascorbic acid and nicotinamide have been given (without clear justification) with L-tryptophan. Pyridoxal phosphate is a coenzyme for serotonin synthesis, while nicotinamide and ascorbic acid inhibit hepatic tryptophan metabolism (Mindham 1979).

L-Tryptophan administration is relatively safe and if an antidepressant is prescribed mainly to provide a placebo in patients who have taken previous overdoses, then L-tryptophan is the drug of choice.

FLUPENTHIXOL

Although flupenthixol is mainly used for the schizophrenias, it has been reported to have antidepressant properties.

HORMONES AND VITAMIN B_6

There is evidence that L-tri-iodothyronine, thyrotropin (TSH), or thyroxine can potentiate tricyclic antidepressants, and it has been suggested that thyrotropin-releasing hormone may have a similar effect (Karlberg et al. 1978). Oestrogen has been used for persistent depression in women, and pyridoxine may be used to treat depressive symptoms associated with oral contraceptives.

STIMULANTS

In general there is no place for dexamphetamine and related drugs in the treatment of depressive syndromes. However, it is possible that some depressed parkinsonian patients and some patients with a chronic 'treatment-resistant' syndrome of neurotic or non-specific depression may benefit. It has recently been reported that age and hypoestrogenism may alter the behavioural response to amphetamine (Halbreich et al. 1981).

ANTIDEPRESSANT COMBINATIONS

It has been said that the dangers of combining an MAO inhibitor with a tricyclic antidepressant have been overstated and the advantages underestimated (Spiker and Pugh 1976). However, this combination can, unless carefully administered, lead to a hypertensive crisis. Tranylcypromine, clomipramine and non-sedative tricyclics should generally be avoided in such combinations and the patient should start with a combination of low doses of phenelzine and amitriptyline. A prior drug-free interval may be appropriate, depending on the previous medication. Other antidepressant combinations have involved two compounds, one of which is a relatively selective inhibitor of the reuptake of noradrenaline, while the other mainly affects the reuptake of serotonin; for example, maproptiline (or nomifensine) and clomipramine (or zimelidine) (see Chapter 15). In theory, the combination of two drugs with different pharmacological profiles may have a greater chance of efficacy against an unknown biological subtype of depression with endogenous aetiology, compared with a single compound. However, this 'broad spectrum' approach should be redundant when the various subtypes can be reliably identified, unless such a combination of drugs has a mutually potentiating effect.

Other possible combinations include:

(1) L-tryptophan (e.g. 2 g three times daily) (or 5-hydroxytryptophan), plus an MAO inhibitor.

(2) Lithium plus a tricyclic, for the prophylaxis of recurrent unipolar endogenous depression; however, it has been claimed that this combination can have a destabilizing effect.

(3) L-tryptophan (or 5-hydroxy tryptophan), plus a tricyclic antidepressant.

(4) L-tryptophan plus lithium.

(5) Thyroxine or tri-iodothyronine plus a tricyclic.

(6) MAO inhibitor plus lithium.

References

BIELSKI, R.J. & FRIEDEL, R.O. (1976) Prediction of tricyclic antidepressant response. A critical review. *Archs gen. Psychiat.*, **33**, 1479.

BIGGER, J.T., KANTAR, S.J., GLASSMAN, A.H. & PEREL, J.M. (1978) Cardiovascular effects of tricyclic antidepressant drugs. In: *Psychopharmacology: A Generation of Progress*, ed. Lipton, M.A., DiMascio, A., Killam, K.F. New York: Raven Press.

COOPER, T.B. & SIMPSON, G.M. (1978a) Prediction of individual dosage of nortriptyline. *Am. J. Psychiat.*, **135:3**, 333.

COOPER, T.B. & SIMPSON, G.M. (1978b) Kinetics of lithium and clinical response. In: *Psychopharmacology: A Generation of Progress*, ed. Lipson, M.A., DiMascio, A. & Killam, K.F. New York: Raven Press.

COPPEN, A. & PEET, M. (1979) The long-term management of patients with affective disorders. In: *Psychopharmacology of Affective Disorders*, ed. Paykel, E.S. & Coppen, A., p. 248. Oxford: Oxford University Press.

DAVIDSON, J., McLEOD, M.N. & BLUM, R. (1978) Acetylation phenotype, platelet monoamine oxidase inhibition, and the effectiveness of phenelzine in depression. *Am. J. Psychiat.*, **135:4**, 467.

DAVIS, J.M. (1976) Overview: maintenance therapy in psychiatry: II Affective disorders. *Am. J. Psychiat.*, **133:1**, 1.

D'ELIA, G., HANSON, L. & RAOTMA, H. (1978) L-tryptophan and 5-hydroxytryptophan in the treatment of depression. A review. *Acta psychiat. scand.*, **57**, 239.

Editorial (1977) Adverse effects of lithium treatment. *Br. med. J.*, **ii**, 346.

Editorial (1978a) Tricyclic antidepressant concentrations and clinical response. *Br. med. J.*, **ii**, 783.

Editorial (1978b) Choosing an antidepressant. *Br. med. J.*, **i**, 128.

Editorial (1981) The new psychiatry. *Br. med. J.*, **ii**, 513.

EVERETT, H.C. (1975) The use of bethanechol chloride with tricyclic antidepressants. *Am. J. Psychiat.*, **132:11**, 1202.

FIEVE, R.R. (1975) The lithium clinic: a new model for the delivery of psychiatric services. *Am. J. Psychiat.*, **132:10**, 1018.

FIEVE, R.R., KUMBARACI, T. & DUNNER, D.L. (1976) Lithium prophylaxis of depression in bipolar I, bipolar II, and unipolar patients. *Am. J. Psychiat.*, **133:8**, 925.

FLEMENBAUM, A. (1976) Pavor nocturnus: A complication of single daily tricyclic or neuroleptic dosage. *Am. J. Psychiat.*, **133:5**, 570.

GERBINO, L., OLESHANSKY, M. & GERSHON, S. (1978) Clinical use and mode of action of lithium. In: *Psychopharmacology: A Generation of Progress*, ed. Lipton, M.A., DiMascio, A. & Killam, K.F. New York: Raven Press.

GLASSMAN, A.N., KANTOR, S.J. & SHOSTAK, M. (1975) Depression, delusions and drug response. *Am. J. Psychiat.*, **132:7**, 716.

GLASSMAN, A.H. & PEREL, J.M. (1978) Tricyclic blood levels and clinical outcome: a review of the art. In: *Psychopharmacology: A Generation of Progress*, ed. Lipton, M.A., DiMascio, A. & Killam, K.F. New York: Raven Press.

HALBREICH, U., ASNIS, G., ROSS, D. & ENDICOTT, J. (1981). Amphetamine-induced dysphoria in postmenopausal women. *Br. J. Psychiat.*, **138**, 470.

HENINGER, G.R. (1978) Lithium carbonate and brain function. *Archs gen. Psychiat.*, **35**, 228.

HERRINGTON, R.N., BRUCE, A., JOHNSTONE, E.C. & LADER, M.N. (1976) Comparative trial of L-tryptophan and amitriptyline in depressive illness. *Psychol. Med.*, **6**, 673.

HOUSE, K.M. & MARTIN, R.L. (1975) MMPI delineation of a subgroup of depressed patients refractory to lithium carbonate therapy. *Am. J. Psychiat.*, **132:6**, 644.

IVERSEN, L.L. & MACKAY, A.V.P. (1979) Pharmacodynamics of antidepressants and antimanic drugs. In: *Psychopharmacology of Affective Disorders*, ed. Paykel, E.S. & Coppen, A. Oxford: Oxford University Press.

JEPPSSON, J. & SJÖGREN, J. (1975) The influence of food on side effects and absorption of lithium. *Acta psychiat. scand.*, **51**, 285.

JUDD, L.L., HUBBARD, B., JANOWSKY, D.S., HUEY, L.Y. & ATTEWELL, P.A. (1977a) The effect of lithium carbonate on affect, mood, and personality of normal subjects. *Archs gen. Psychiat.*, **34**, 346.

JUDD, L.L., HUBBARD, B., JANOWSKY, D.S., HUEY, L.Y. & TAKAHASKY, K.I. (1977b) The effect of lithium carbonate on the cognitive functions of normal subjects. *Archs gen. Psychiat.*, **34**, 355.

KARLBERG, B.E., KJELLMAN, B.F. & KÅGEDAL, B. (1978) Treatment of endogenous depression with oral thyrotropin-releasing hormone and amitriptyline. *Acta psychiat. scand.*, **58**, 389.

KERRY, R.J. (1975) The management of patients receiving lithium treatment. In: *Lithium Research and Therapy*, ed. Johnson, F.N. London: Academic Press.

KESSLER, K.A. (1978) Tricyclic antidepressants: mode of action and clinical use. In: *Psychopharmacology: A Generation of Progress*, ed. Lipton, M.A., DiMascio, A. & Killam, K.F. New York: Raven Press.

KROPF, D. & MÜLLER-OERLINGHAUSEN, B. (1979) Changes in learning, memory, and mood during lithium treatment. *Acta psychiat. scand.*, **59**, 97.

McCABE, B., TSUANG, M.T. (1982) Dietary consideration in MAO inhibitor regimens. *J. clin. Psychiat.* **43**, 178.

MENDELS, J. (1976) Lithium in the treatment of depression. *Am. J. Psychiat.*, **133:4**, 373.

MENDELS, J., STINNETT, J.L., BURNS, D. & FRAZER, A. (1975) Amine precursors and depression. *Archs gen. Psychiat.*, **32**, 22.

MINDHAM, R.H.S. (1979) Tricyclic antidepressants and amine precursors. In: *Psychopharmacology of Affective Disorders*, ed. Paykel, E.S. & Coppen, A., p. 123. Oxford: Oxford University Press.

PAYKEL, E.S. (1979) Management of acute depression. In: *Psychopharmacology of Affective Disorders*, ed. Paykel, E.S. & Coppen, A., p. 235. Oxford: Oxford University Press.

PERSSON, G. (1977) Lithium side-effects in relation to dose and to levels and gradients of lithium in plasma. *Acta psychiat. scand.*, **55**, 208.

PETURSSON, H. (1976) Lithium treatment of a patient with periodic catatonia. *Acta psychiat. scand.*, **54**, 248.

PRIEN, R.F. & CAFFEY, E.M. (1976) Relationship between dosage and response to lithium prophylaxis in recurrent depression. *Am. J. Psychiat.*, **133:5**, 567.

QUINN, P.O. & RAPOPORT, J.L. (1975) One-year follow-up of hyperactive boys treated with imipramine or methylphenidate. *Am. J. Psychiat.*, **132:3**, 241.

QUITKIN, F., RIFKIN, A. & KLEIN, D.F. (1976) Prophylaxis of affective disorders: current status of knowledge. *Archs gen. Psychiat.*, **33**, 337.

REISER, D.E. & WILLETT, A.B. (1976) A favourable response to lithium carbonate in a 'schizo-affective' father and son. *Am. J. Psychiat.*, **133:7**, 824.

ROBINSON, D.S., NIES, A., RAVARIS, L.L., IVES, J.O. & BARTLETT, D. (1978) Clinical psychophar-macology of phenelzine: MAO activity and clinical response. In: *Psychopharmacology: a generation of progress.* ed. Lipton, M.A., DiMascio, A. & Killam, K.F. New York: Raven Press.

SELLERS, J., TYRER, P., WHITELEY, A., BANKS, D.C. & BARER, D.H. (1982) Neurotoxic effects of lithium with delayed rise in serum lithium levels. *Brit. J. Psychiat.* **140**, 623.

SHAW, D.M. (1977) The practical management of affective disorders. *Br. J. Psychiat.*, **130**, 432.

SHEARD, M.H., MARINI, J.L., BRIDGES, C.I. & WAGNER, E. (1976) The effect of lithium on impulsive aggressive behaviour in man. *Am. J. Psychiat.*, **133:12**, 1409.

SHOPSIN, B. & GERSHON, S. (1975) Cogwheel rigidity related to lithium maintenance *Am. J. Psychiat.*, **132:5**, 536.

SIRIS, S.G., VAN KAMMEN, D.P. & DOCHERTY, J.P. (1978) Use of antidepressant drugs in schizophrenia. *Archs gen. Psychiat.*, **35, 1368.**

SPIKER, D.G. & PUGH, D.D. (1976) Combining tricyclic and monoamine oxidase inhibitor antidepressants. *Archs gen. Psychiat.*, **33**, 828.

TRETHOWAN, W.H. (1975) Pills for personal problems. *Br. med. J.*, **iii**, 749.

TYRER, P. (1979) Clinical use of monoamine oxidase inhibitors. In: *Psychopharmacology of Affective Disorders,* ed. Paykel, E.S. & Coppen, A., p. 159. Oxford: Oxford University Press.

ULDALL, P.R. (1981). Renal function in patients receiving long-term lithium therapy. *Can. Med. Assoc. J.* **124**, 1471.

VESTERGAARD, P., SCHOU, M. & THOMSEN, K. (1982) Monitoring of patients in prophylactic lithium treatment. *Br. J. Psychiat.*, **140**, 185.

WALINDER, J., SKOTT, A., CARLSSON, A., MAGY, A. & ROOS, B.E. (1976) Potentiation of the antidepressant action of clomipramine by tryptophan. *Archs Gen. Psychiat.*, **33**, 1384.

WALDSTEIN, M.R. & GOLDFIELD, M.D. (1975) Cardiovascular malformations with lithium use during pregnancy. *Am. J. Psychiat.*, **132:5**, 529.

4

Treatments for Chronic Cognitive Impairment

J.H. Dowson

Impaired cognitive function occurs in disorders which have been described by such terms as acute or chronic brain failure, delirium, confusion, acute or chronic organic brain syndrome, and dementia (Stedeford 1978). This chapter will consider treatments for those mental disorders caused by a recognized biological process which affects brain function, excluding the schizophrenias, manic–depressive disorders and other so-called functional psychoses. As an aetiological diagnosis is the first step in the consideration of treatment, the main causes of chronic cognitive impairment will be reviewed.

CAUSES OF CHRONIC COGNITIVE IMPAIRMENT

Structural Changes in the Brain

These include senile Alzheimer dementia, arteriosclerotic or multi-infarct dementia, presenile dementias, subcortical dementia, cerebral haemorrhage or infarction, chronic alcoholism, cerebral tumour, subdural haematoma, cerebral infections, normal pressure hydrocephalus, the effects of trauma, and cerebral cysts. Over 50% of chronic brain disorder in the elderly results from Alzheimer dementia, while multi-infarct dementia is responsible for about 20%. In a further 20% these two diseases occur together (Prien 1973; Hachinski et al. 1974; Corsellis 1977; Butler 1978).

Toxic Effects on the Brain

Iatrogenic or self-inflicted brain disorder is a common phenomenon and can be the result of unnecessary medication, a withdrawal syndrome, the prescribing of excessive doses, or the simultaneous administration of several drugs which lead to complex and unforeseen interactions. In addition, the presence of tissue necrosis or extracerebral infection can exacerbate brain failure, as can the absorption of blood from a haematoma or a gastrointestinal haemorrhage. A toxic effect on the nervous system can also be produced by some carcinomas even if there are no cerebral metastases.

Metabolic Disorders

These include electrolyte changes (significant potassium depletion is not always associated with abnormal serum values), hypoxia, dehydration, uraemia, adrenocortical disorder, hypercarbia, acidosis, nutritional deficiency (e.g. of vitamin B_{12}, folate or thiamine), myxoedema, thyrotoxicosis, hypercalcaemia, hypocalcaemia, hepatic failure, cardiac failure, hypoglycaemia, hyperglycaemia, hypothermia and hypoxia. Anaemia and pulmonary pathology may contribute to the latter.

Disorders of Cerebral Blood Flow

A reduced cerebral blood flow may be associated with systemic hypotension, carotid stenosis, cardiac arrhythmias, or congestive cardiac failure. The latter may follow a 'silent' myocardial infarction. Short periods of impaired memory can precede a cerebrovascular accident, and cranial arteritis or migraine can present with confusion or episodes of amnesia. The rare syndrome of transient global amnesia may also be due to a cerebrovascular disorder (Whitty 1978; Ponsford and Donnan 1980). This can present with a sudden inability to retain new memories for more than a few minutes, together with anxiety and confusion, and it has been suggested that more subtle changes in the vascular supply to the hippocampus may play a role in the aetiology of some cases of chronic cognitive deficit (Hachinski 1979).

Epileptic Disorders

Epileptic disorders in elderly patients are often due to the effects of cerebral arteriosclerosis. Amnesia and confusion may be associated with a pre-ictal, or post-ictal state, and memory impairment may present as part of a twilight state (which can last for several hours) or petit mal status (Whitty 1978); there may be subsequent amnesia for twilight states. These should be distinguished from post-ictal confusion, which is associated with relatively more confusion.

Other Disorders Associated with Chronic Cognitive Impairment

Reversible brain disorder has been reported in patients undergoing renal dialysis, and may be due to changes in cerebral aluminium (Sullivan et al. 1977; Glen 1980).

Immediately following cerebral trauma, a patient may appear to be aware of his surroundings and respond to questions, but subsequently will not remember events during this period. In addition, retrograde amnesia may occur for varying periods prior to a head injury. In some cases, retrograde amnesia is not present immediately after the injury but develops within several minutes (Whitty 1978).

POSSIBLE MECHANISMS OF DRUG ACTION IN CHRONIC COGNITIVE IMPAIRMENT

Drugs may be prescribed in an attempt to improve various cognitive functions in brain disorder or to modify secondary psychiatric phenomena, such as mood change or behavioural disturbances. Pharmacological agents may act directly on the brain or may produce their cerebral effects as a result of an extracerebral action such as an improvement of cardiac function, which may relieve cerebral anoxia.

Memory and the other cognitive functions might be improved by various pharmacological means, and there are several possible sites of action. The activity of normal or dysfunctioning neuronal systems may be facilitated, or a pathological process may be prevented, slowed down or reversed. Drugs may act on neurones which contribute to the maintenance of memory traces, or on neuronal systems which have a nonspecific role in memory processes such as those involved in activation and arousal. There is evidence that there are several neurophysiological stages in the learning process, and that certain drugs can be either facilitatory or disruptive, depending on several variables such as the timing of administration, or the size of the dose (Lishman 1971; Alpern and Jackson 1978; Rigter and van Riezen 1978).

CEREBRAL VASODILATORS

Certain drugs cause vasodilation by relaxing the smooth muscle in the walls of both cerebral and extracerebral vessels. Several studies have reported that Alzheimer and multi-infarct dementia are associated with a reduction in cerebral blood flow (CBF) (Melamed et al. 1978), but an important determinant of CBF is the rate of cerebral metabolism which, if decreased, may lead to a reduced concentration of carbon dioxide and to vasoconstriction (Yesavage et al. 1979b). It has been reported that loss of brain substance is not an important correlate of the reduction of CBF in Alzheimer dementia (Melamed et al. 1978), so that abnormal metabolism of the remaining neurones may be largely responsible for the reduced CBF in this disease. Thus, vasodilation would not necessarily be expected to improve cerebral function in Alzheimer dementia.

The value of vasodilation for ischaemia in the setting of multi-infarct dementia has also been called into question. It has been argued that local changes in ischaemic areas, such as lactosis and a decrease in pH, produce the maximal degree of vasodilation (Sathananthan and Gershon 1975), which may be limited by arteriosclerotic changes, as these reduce the capacity of vessel walls to dilate. Also, any increase in CBF may not necessarily result in increased neuronal efficiency, and it is possible that selective vasodilation of relatively healthy vessels may divert blood away from ischaemic areas, thus worsening the condition, while peripheral vasodilation may shunt blood away from the brain (Editorial 1979). However, the term 'cerebral vasodilators' is somewhat misleading, as some of these drugs also induce changes in neuronal metabolism, for example, by rendering the brain less vulnerable to anoxia (Yesavage et al. 1979b), so it is possible that a cerebral vasodilator may exert beneficial effects in either multi-infarct dementia or senile Alzheimer dementia by improving neuronal function or by influencing a pathogenic mechanism.

Vasodilator drugs which have been used for the treatment of chronic cognitive impairment will now be considered. Their evaluation has been beset with two major difficulties: the problem of diagnosing and selecting an aetiologically homogeneous group of patients, and the inadequate assessment of outcome. A review by Yesavage et al. (1979b) of the literature on the efficacy of cerebral vasodilators noted that about half the reported studies of cerebral vasodilators lacked controls despite the likelihood of significant placebo effects. Also more than 60 different ways of assessing outcome were identified. Crossover studies were rare, although this design would have increased the statistical power of the many trials which had a relatively small group of patients.

Dihydroergotoxine Mesylate

Dihydroergotoxine is the most extensively studied of all the cerebral vasodilators and has both vasodilator and metabolic effects. It has an α-adrenergic blocking action but no oxytocic activity. It produces a generalized peripheral vasodilation but does not lower the blood pressure in normotensive patients. It consists of a combination of three hydrogenated ergopeptide alkaloids: dihydroergocornine mesylate, dihydroergocristine mesylate and dihydroergokryptine mesylate, in equal proportions.

Many studies in animals and man have shown that dihydoergotoxine can reverse changes in the EEG which are associated with impaired cerebral function (Roubicek et al. 1972; Cerletti et al. 1973; Matejcek et al. 1979). It has also been claimed that this drug increases cerebral oxygen consumption and cerebral blood flow in the cat and man (Geraud et al. 1963; Yesavage et al. 1979b). Dihydroergotoxine may also interfere with the reuptake of norepinephrine, act as a dopamine agonist, increase the cerebral pyruvate/lactate ratio, and inhibit the enzymes involved in the breakdown of adenosine triphosphate (ATP) and cyclic adenosine monophosphate (cAMP) (Meier-Ruge et al. 1975; Ban 1978; Torack 1978; Maclay 1979).

It has been suggested that neuroglia may sometimes play an important role in the development of impaired cerebral circulation if disordered neuronal metabolism leads to swelling of astrocytic processes, which are wrapped around cerebral capillaries. Such swelling could lead to vasoconstriction and a reduction in CBF, while change in neuronal metabolism induced by dihydroergotoxine might be followed by a reduction in astrocytic swelling.

Clinical efficacy. In a recent review of cerebral vasodilators (Yesavage et al. 1979*b*), about half of the studies were not controlled, and the outcome criteria involved a variety of signs and symptoms and several aspects of cognitive function. Greater efforts could often have been made to diagnose underlying pathology, in particular to separate patients with Alzheimer dementia from those with clear evidence of cerebrovascular pathology. It should also be noted that severely impaired patients were often selected for clinical trials, although more favourable results might have been obtained if patients had been studied at an earlier stage of their disorders.

It has been claimed that dihydroergotoxine can produce a variety of beneficial effects involving many signs or symptoms such as confusion, impaired alertness, disorientation, impaired recent memory, mood disorders (anxiety, depression, emotional lability or lack of motivation), disordered social behaviour and somatic complaints such as loss of appetite, dizziness or fatigue. However, a consistent pattern for the beneficial effects of dihydroergotoxine has not been identified.

Yesavage et al. (1979*a*) reviewed 33 studies of dihydroergotoxine of which 22 were considered to be well-designed controlled trials. All these 22 studies reported significant improvement in some behavioural or psychological measure, and in 18 of these the improvement was considered to be of practical benefit. Studies which employed the highest doses, up to 4.5 mg/day, claimed the best results. Overall, it was considered that dihydroergotoxine has the best confirmed efficacy of all the cerebral vasodilators and that this drug should be used in comparison studies involving other drugs for chronic brain disorder. Another recent review of 26 studies (McDonald 1979) concluded that 13 symptoms, involving cognitive dysfunction, depression and behaviour, were significantly improved in at least 50% of the studies. One study by Rao and Norris (1972) involved 57 patients with presumed cerebrovascular insufficiency who received 3 mg dihydroergotoxine daily. These authors reported various significant effects compared with placebo, and reductions of hostility and irritability were considered to be of practical importance, as many patients became more sociable and manageable.

Thibault (1974) reported the effects of dihydroergotoxine on a group of patients with either senile Alzheimer dementia or arteriosclerotic dementia.

The results indicated that the drug had a significant effect, relative to placebo, in 13 out of 18 symptoms, but also illustrated the importance of the placebo effect in elderly patients with chronic brain failure, as 13 out of the 18 symptoms showed a significant improvement on placebo alone. Gaitz et al. (1977) also examined a group of patients with either Alzheimer dementia or arteriosclerotic dementia (or both) who received 3 mg dihydroergotoxine daily for 6 months. The group which had received the drug showed statistically significant improvements over the placebo group in the following areas: confusion, alertness, recent memory, disorientation, depression, emotional lability, hostility, 'bothersomeness', uncooperativeness, dizziness and anxiety.

Dihydroergotoxine is available as tablets, each containing 1.5 mg, and the recommended dose is one tablet three times daily. Dihydroergotoxine can also be given sublingually or by injection. There is evidence that improvement does not appear for about 3–6 weeks and that there may be further gradual improvement for at least 3 months (Venn 1980). It appears to be of value for some patients with either Alzheimer dementia or multi-infarct dementia.

Naftidrofuryl Oxalate

Naftidrofuryl has a sympathetic blocking activity at ganglionic and postganglionic levels and is a vasodilator which has been used to treat peripheral and cerebral vascular disorders (Fontaine et al. 1969). Its other actions include a local anaesthetic effect, a papaverine-like effect, an antiserotonin effect and an antibradykinin effect. When the rat brain is rendered hypothermic, naftidrofuryl administration leads to a rise in temperature in the cerebral cortex (Fontaine et al. 1969), and it has been claimed that the drug can protect the rat brain from the effects of oxygen deprivation, despite other reports of an increase in oxygen consumption. It has also been claimed that this drug can be associated with activation of succino-dehydrogenase, an increase in cerebral ATP, a reduction in cerebral ADP, less inhibition of hexokinase and an increase in the passage of glucose into neurones. It has been suggested that the increase in oxygen consumption and glucose metabolism leads to an increase in tissue levels of carbon dioxide, which then reinforces the direct vasodilator effect of the drug. After radioactive ^{14}C-glucose was given to rats which had received naftidrofuryl, there was a greater degree of incorporation of radioactivity into the brains of the treated animals compared with untreated controls (Meynaud et al. 1973).

In man, the degree of improvement in EEG abnormalities has been claimed to be associated with clinical efficacy and, by using a radioactive trace, the drug has been shown to increase CBF.

Clinical efficacy. Yesavage et al. (1979a) cited eight reports, seven of which fulfilled criteria for well-designed trials and reported practical benefits.

A double-blind trial by Robinson (1972) claimed that there were significant improvements over placebo in a variety of intellectual functions, including memory functions, and it has also been reported that the drug can lead to improvement in anxiety, mood, activity, sphincter control and disordered behaviour (Judge and Urquhart 1972). Measurements of increased cerebral blood flow have been reported to correlate with clinical improvement.

The indications for the use of this drug have usually been the presence of various forms of cerebrovascular disease, and the current prescribing information recommends its use for cerebral or peripheral vascular disorders, without mentioning Alzheimer dementia. However, if the metabolic effects of dihydroergotoxine are beneficial in Alzheimer dementia, the metabolic effects of naftidrofuryl may also be beneficial in this disorder.

In conclusion, naftidrofuryl can be considered to be a promising drug which has not yet been subjected to sufficient clinical investigation. It may have therapeutic effects in various types of chronic brain failure and not just in cerebrovascular disease.

Other Drugs with Mixed Vasodilator and Metabolic Actions

There is evidence that pyritinol can improve impaired cerebral metabolism, increase glucose uptake by the brain, and improve cerebral blood flow (Flood 1979; Goncalves 1979). Pentifylline may also increase glucose uptake. However, although claims of clinical benefit have been made, relatively little information is available for either of these drugs (Yesavage et al. 1979b).

Papaverine Hydrochloride

Papaverine, together with cyclandelate, isoxsuprine and cinnarizine, is considered to have predominantly vasodilator effects (Yesavage et al. 1979b).

Papaverine has been widely prescribed for the treatment of arteriosclerotic dementia but although there is evidence that this drug increases CBF, the reported effects on cerebral oxygen consumption are variable (Ban 1978). Although this drug is considered to have predominantly vasodilator activity, it has been suggested that any therapeutic effects are due to phosphodiesterase inhibition or dopamine receptor blockade. If the latter action is confirmed, this might account for the recurrence of parkinsonian symptoms in patients receiving L-dopa which has been reported to occur when papaverine is added to their medication (Duvoisin 1975).

Papaverine is a derivative of opium and relaxes smooth muscle, although it can decrease cerebrovascular resistance without significantly affecting mean arterial pressure (Prien 1973). It is readily absorbed from the gastrointestinal tract and peak plasma levels have been reported at 1–2 h after administration, falling to low levels after about 6 h.

Clinical efficacy. Yesavage et al. (1979*a*) reviewed 13 studies of which nine were considered to be well-designed. Six of these claimed that the drug produced some improvement over placebo but in only one study was this considered to be of practical benefit. In addition there are five studies which compared papaverine with dihydroergotoxine, and in all these dihydroergotoxine produced greater benefit.

It appears that papaverine does not usually produce clinically significant improvement in chronic brain disorder, although some uncontrolled studies suggest that it may be relatively more effective in less severe forms of dementia (Prien 1973).

Clyclandelate

This drug has similar properties to those of papaverine and is primarily a vasodilator; it relaxes smooth muscle and can increase CBF (Prien 1973). It is readily absorbed from the gastrointestinal tract and its maximal effect occurs within 1½ h.

Clinical efficacy. Yesavage et al. (1979*a*) considered 18 studies but only seven were rated as being well designed. Six of these seven studies reported some positive results in the treatment of brain disorder but only three claimed practical benefit. The effects of this drug on cognitive deficit are therefore uncertain, and while Ban (1978) considered that beneficial effects have been clearly demonstrated, Yesavage et al. (1979*a*) stressed the controversy regarding its use in cerebrovascular disorders.

Isoxsuprine Hydrochloride

This drug is absorbed from the gastrointestinal tract and maximal plasma levels occur from about 1–4 h after administration. It can produce β-adrenergic stimulation (Ban 1978), but its predominant actions as a vasodilator may be due to a direct action on vascular smooth muscle (Dukes 1979). It also reduces blood viscosity.

Clinical efficacy. Five clinical trials have been reported, three of which have been considered to be well designed. (Yesavage et al. 1979*a*). However, only two of the three claimed beneficial effects in brain disorder and these were not considered to be of practical importance. One study has indicated that it can cause a reduction in CBF (Martin 1979).

Cinnarizine

Clinical efficacy. Three investigations into this vasodilator and labyrinthine sedative have been considered to be well designed (Yesavage et al. 1979*b*), and all these three reported beneficial effects in chronic brain disorder. In two of the studies the benefits were considered to be of practical significance.

Other Drugs with Vasodilator Action

Bencyclane has had four trials with mixed results, and betahistine hydrochloride, a treatment for Ménières syndrome, has had one trial for vertebrobasilar artery insufficiency with positive results (Yesavage et al. 1979*b*). Nicotinyl alcohol and nicotinic acid have also been reported to have beneficial effects in cerebral arteriosclerosis (Prien 1973; Ban 1978).

Carbon dioxide (5–7%) is a potent cerebral vasodilator, and carbonic anhydrase inhibitors can produce cerebral vasodilation. It has been confirmed that acetazolamide increases CBF, but habituation to the vasodilator effects of this drug soon develops, while side effects, such as a marked diuresis, are troublesome (Ban 1978). However, another carbonic anhydrase inhibitor with a more selective action on the brain has been shown to increase cerebral blood flow in 'mildly demented patients' over a 6-week period, although no consistent improvement in cognitive functions was detected (Wyper et al. 1976).

It has been pointed out that if well-designed studies involving drugs with mixed vasodilator and metabolic effects are compared with those of drugs with a predominantly vasodilator action, 27 out of 31 trials of drugs with mixed actions reported practical benefits, while such claims were made in only six of the 22 studies of the latter group of drugs (Yesavage et al. 1979*b*).

It can be concluded that the published evidence suggests that dihydroergotoxine and naftidrofuryl oxalate have modest clinical efficacy in some cases of chronic cognitive impairment.

CEREBRAL STIMULANTS

Cerebral stimulants have been used in elderly patients in an attempt to reverse fatigue, motor retardation, apathy, depression and impaired concentration or memory (Ban 1978). There is evidence that ageing is associated with a decline in performance in tasks which assess speed of response, and this may reflect a decrease in the speed of information processing in the CNS (Crook et al. 1977). If this is the case, CNS stimulation is a possible means to improve cerebral functioning in the elderly.

Pentelenetetrazol

It has been reported that this drug improves visual discrimination learning in mice and it is the most extensively studied CNS stimulant for the treatment of chronic brain disorder. It has also been used as a circulatory or respiratory stimulant, a barbiturate antagonist and for the management of Stokes–Adams attacks. It has been claimed that the drug stimulates vasomotor and respiratory centres, as well as the cerebral cortex.

Clinical efficacy. There have been at least 50 studies on the effects of pentelenetetrazol in brain disorder and all but 12 reported positive results. However of the 16 controlled studies, only five claimed beneficial effects (Ban 1978). Although some improvement in cognitive functioning was reported, the effects were mainly related to behaviour or other psychiatric symptomatology (Leckman et al. 1971).

Several studies have investigated the effects of the drug in combination with vitamin supplements, and it has been claimed that pentelenetetrazol combined with nicotinic acid had more beneficial effects than either substance alone.

Pipradrol hydrochloride

Clinical efficacy. This drug has been considered to be more promising than pentelenetetrazol, although it has been less extensively studied (Ban 1978). Of six clinical trials, only one was controlled in which a high dose of pipradrol (5 mg daily) was associated with significant improvement in behaviour, while a low dose (2 mg daily) or placebo produced no significant effect (Turek et al. 1969).

Methylphenidate

This drug is a sympathomimetic agent and cerebral stimulant (Crook et al. 1977). It is readily absorbed from the gastrointestinal tract, and is rapidly metabolized.

Clinical efficacy. Beneficial effects were reported in five out of seven clinical trials, but there is little evidence that methylphenidate produces clinically significant benefits in most cases of chronic brain disorder (Ban 1978). However, this drug, or other stimulants, may be of value in those patients who have a degree of subcortical dementia, in which subcortical impairment may be associated with a relatively intact neocortex. While memory can appear to be grossly impaired, patients with this syndrome may invariably produce the correct answer to a question after a delay which may be as long as several minutes (Albert et al. 1974).

Methylphenidate is available as tablets (10 mg) or ampoules (20 mg) and the prescribing information recommends its use in 'apathetic or withdrawn senile behaviour'. However it has been argued that the increased cardiac work, irritability, decreased appetite and possible exacerbation of psychotic states usually outweigh any beneficial effects (Ban 1978). The recommended dose is 10 mg twice or thrice daily, but in elderly patients the initial dose should not exceed 10 mg daily, and the patient should be carefully monitored for side effects.

Dexamphetamine

The amphetamines are sympathomimetic agents which increase cardiac output, blood pressure and blood flow in skeletal muscle and kidney. They also have a stimulant effect on the central nervous system, elevate mood and induce increased physical and mental activity.

Clinical efficacy. Although the use of stimulants is not generally advocated for chronic brain disorder, it has been claimed that some patients with Alzheimer or arteriosclerotic dementia benefit from 5 mg dexamphetamine in the morning, although this should be discontinued if irritability, anxiety, tremor, dizziness or confusion develop (de Wied et al. 1976; Pradhan 1980).

HORMONES

Fluoxymesterone (α-fluoro-11β-hydroxyl-1,7-methyltestosterone)

This substance has a greater anabolic and androgenic effect compared with methyltestosterone but is less toxic.

Clinical efficacy. Fluoxymesterone (4–5 mg) was administered daily over 6–9 months to elderly patients with mild memory impairment, and this regimen was reported to produce sedation, a feeling of well-being, an increase in purposeful activity, an increased appetite and an improvement in the recall of logical and meaningful material (Rigter and Van Riezen 1978). However no changes were detected in patients with more severe impairment.

Steroids

Clinical efficacy. Chynoweth and Foley (1969) reported three patients whose chronic cognitive impairment developed under the age of 65, who apparently responded to intramuscular hydrocortisone 100 mg three times daily for 2 days, then 50 mg three times daily for 2 weeks, then oral prednisone 5 mg three times daily. In one case the improvement was described as dramatic.

The authors reviewed previous case reports of cerebral sarcoidosis and suggested that their three cases of presenile dementia may have been examples of this condition. The clinical phenomena included fluctuating confusion, behavioural changes, headaches, muscle cramps, focal trembling attacks, transient disturbance of vision, cranial nerve changes, motor and sensory changes in the limbs, hyperreflexia and increased limb tone of a parkinsonian type. ESR was raised to over 20 mm per hour and all three cases showed abnormalities of their serum proteins.

ACTH-like Peptides

There is considerable evidence from animal studies that the hypothalamic peptides which are associated with the control of pituitary function [i.e. vasopressin, adrenocorticotrophic hormone (ACTH) and the related melano-cyte-stimulating hormone (MSH)], also have effects on memory functions (de Wied et al. 1976; Rigter and Van Riezen 1978). Although it is not certain that ACTH and related substances are involved in the specific processes of memory formation and retrieval, they may influence functions such as arousal, motiva-tion, excitability and vigilance. In addition, there is evidence from animal studies that elevated plasma adrenocorticoids are associated with the develop-ment of neuropathological changes such as thickening of hippocampal astro-cytes (Landfield et al. 1978).

Clinical efficacy. There is no convincing evidence that ACTH-like peptides have a role in the treatment of brain disorder but a study of human volunteers reported improved performance on the digit symbol substitution test, digit span and visual reproduction subscales of the Wechsler test, although there were no detectable effects on immediate or short-term verbal memory (Rigter and Van Riezen 1978). Another study of the use of ACTH4-10 in 18 patients with mild cognitive impairments suggested that this compound produced some improve-ment in both mood and cognitive function (Branconnier et al. 1979).

Vasopressin-like Peptides

Vasopressin from pig pituitary contains lysine, while that from most other mammals, including man, contains arginine. Both are active in man, and arginine vasopressin (AVP), lysine vasopressin (LVP), or desglycinamide lysine vasopressin (DGLVP) can improve memory function in rats (Rigter and Van Riezen 1978).

Clinical efficacy. There is some evidence that vasopressin may alleviate memory impairment in aged patients (Legros et al. 1978).

CHOLINERGIC AGENTS

Much evidence indicates that cholinergic neurones have a specific role in the neurophysiological substrate of memory, and that in Alzheimer dementia there is a relatively selective disorder of cholinergic neurones (Bowen et al. 1976; Davies and Maloney 1976; Ghoneim and Mewaldt 1977; Zornetzer 1978; Perry 1980).

The activity of choline acetyltransferase (CAT), which is principally found in nerve terminals, has been reported to be reduced in the cerebral cortex of patients with Alzheimer dementia, while low levels of acetylcholinesterase (ACE) have been associated with reduced CAT. These reductions were most marked in cortical areas which contained the greatest density of senile plaques and neurofibrillary tangles (Perry et al. 1978). Davis and Maloney (1976) reported that the activity of glutamic acid decarboxylase (GAD), which is believed to be in neurones containing γ-aminobutyric acid (GABA), was not reduced in Alzheimer dementia, which suggested that a relatively selective degenerative process had taken place, involving cholinergic neurones. However, GABA-receptor binding is claimed to be reduced in the frontal cortex and caudate nucleus in Alzheimer dementia, indicating that there is some impairment of GABA-ergic neurotransmission in this disorder, while abnormalities of dopamine, serotonin and noradrenaline metabolism have also been reported in this disease (Kristensen et al. 1977; Reisine et al. 1978; Glen 1980; Mann et al. 1980). Another study has reported normal muscarinic cholinergic receptor binding (MCRB) in the cerebral cortex of Alzheimer dementia (Perry et al. 1977), and it has been concluded that neocortical postsynaptic muscarinic receptors are intact in Alzheimer dementia, although this may not be the case in other primary dementias such as Pick's disease (Wisniewski and Terry 1976; Glen 1980). However, there is evidence that MCRB in the hippocampus is reduced in Alzheimer dementia (Reisine et al. 1978).

In addition to the biochemical evidence which has suggested that impaired cholinergic neurotransmission is associated with Alzheimer dementia, anticholinergic drugs (including phenothiazines), can cause confusion in elderly patients with brain disorder and produce cognitive impairment in normal volunteers (Perry et al. 1978).

There are several ways in which drugs could be used to influence cholinergic transmission. The rate of ACh release by neurones might be increased, ACh receptor sites might be activated by other means, or the activity of ACh could be enhanced by the inhibition of acetylcholinesterase.

Physostigmine

It has been claimed that a 1 mg dose of physostigmine salicylate injected subcutaneously is destroyed in 2 h, and, unfortunately, there is no long-acting cholinesterase inhibitor which crosses the blood–brain barrier. Physostigmine has both central and peripheral cholinergic effects but the latter can be alleviated by methylscopolamine, which does not cross the blood–brain barrier (Glen 1980; Marchbanks 1980). Physostigmine prolongs the postsynaptic actions of ACh by inhibiting cholinesterase activity, and has been successfully used in the treatment of toxicity induced by anticholinergic agents. Also, there are reports that physostigmine produced improved memory functions in normal volunteers (Davis et al. 1978), while Drachman (1978), found that physostigmine was able to reverse the effects of scopolamine. This latter drug presumably produced impaired memory functions as a result of its blockade of muscarinic ACh receptors (Ghoneim and Mewaldt 1977). There is a report that physostigmine improved memory functions in a patient with herpes simplex encephalitis (Peters and Levin 1977), and a significant dose-dependent improvement in a recall test has been reported in patients with Alzheimer dementia (Glen 1980). Another report on a single case of Alzheimer dementia described clear improvement in a task involving copying figures, after physostigmine administration (Muramoto et al. 1979), while Peters and Levin (1978) claimed that a combination of physostigmine and lecithin enhanced memory storage and retrieval in Alzheimer dementia. These authors suggested that the effects of a combination of a cholinergic agonist with a choline precursor deserves further investigation. Christie et al. (1981) reported a significant improvement on a picture recognition test with either physostigmine or the muscarinic agonist arecholine, but dose was critical and the benefits were modest.

Choline

Choline, the precursor of ACh, has been reported to improve memory functions in normal volunteers (Sitaram et al. 1978a,b), and choline has been claimed to enhance cholinergic transmission in animal studies (Perry et al. 1978). However, the effects of choline or lecithin in man are uncertain. Although their administration can increase ACh turnover (Glen 1980), dietary lecithin provides choline by the action of hepatic enzymes (Marchbanks 1980), and the plasma and CSF levels of choline have been reported as normal in demented patients. Nevertheless, there is some evidence that choline or lecithin may produce modest beneficial effects (Christie et al. 1981).

Clinical efficacy. Boyd et al. (1977), gave choline chloride, 5 g daily for 2 weeks, followed by 10 g daily, to seven hospitalized patients with severe Alzheimer dementia in an uncontrolled study. No change could be detected by psychological assessment, while a behavioural rating scale indicated no change in four cases, change for the better in two cases and for the worse in one case.

Etienne et al. (1978) reported on three patients with Alzheimer dementia who received choline bitartrate 8 g daily for 1 month and this regimen was associated with a significant increase in plasma choline concentration. One patient became incontinent, withdrawn and suspicious, one patient was unaffected, while the least severely demented patient became able to produce a design in a block designs test. She had not been able to do this prior to treatment and was unable to do so afterwards. This improvement coincided with her peak plasma choline level.

Smith et al. (1978), studied the effects of choline bitartrate, at a dose of 9 g daily for 2 weeks, and placebo for 2 weeks, in ten patients with Alzheimer dementia using a double-blind placebo-controlled crossover design. The test battery included immediate and delayed memory for verbal and visual material. There were no significant differences between drug and placebo but it was noted that three patients seemed less confused after 2 weeks of choline treatment. Pre-existing urinary incontinence was exacerbated in three patients, gastrointestinal side effects were a problem in some patients, and one patient was increasingly depressed. Taminga et al. (1976) described severe depression occurring in two patients who were given choline for tardive dyskinesia. Mohs et al. (1979) also reported that choline chloride did not improve memory impairment in eight elderly patients; however, Fovall et al. (1980) claimed that choline bitartrate, 12 g/day for 2 weeks, produced significant improvement for auditory and visual word recognition in early Alzheimer dementia.

In conclusion, the results of all the strategies for enhancing cholinergic transmission have not produced results of clinical importance, although there is some evidence that there have been modest beneficial effects in certain patients.

1-ACETAMINE-2-PYRROLIDONE (PIRACETAM)

In animals, this drug has been shown to improve memory functions and to give some protection against the effects of hypoxia. It has been claimed that it restores the ATP/ADP ratio, which normally declines with age, and that it does not show toxic or stimulant effects. However, a recent double-blind study did not confirm earlier reports that the drug improved cognitive functions in brain-damaged patients (Glen 1980).

Clinical efficacy. Piracetam has been claimed to alleviate fatigue and improve alertness in a controlled study of 196 patients with an average age of 67 (Stegink 1972), and in another study the drug produced an improvement in mental performance which had been impaired by reducing the firing rate of cardiac pacemakers (Lagergren and Levander 1974).

Mindus et al. (1976) reported on a double-blind placebo-controlled trial of the drug in 18 normal volunteers with a median age of 56 years who had reported that there had been a slight reduction in their memory over several years. Although the self-rating results did not distinguish treatment and placebo groups, the results indicated that the drug had improved performance on both a Digit Symbol Test and a cancellation test ($p<0.001$), so that the authors suggested that the drug may improve the functioning of neurones which are not diseased. Another study by Dimond (1977) on 16 young, healthy volunteers also reported improved recall following a verbal learning task.

Thus piracetam may help to alleviate chronic brain disorder by improving the performance of cells which are functioning normally or which are only mildly impaired. However, Lloyd-Evans et al. (1979) concluded that piracetam was not useful in a study of 109 aged patients with chronic cognitive deficit, although a transitory initial improvement was found.

MECLOFENOXATE (CENTROPHENOXINE)

This substance was synthesized by combining dimethylaminoethanol (DMAE, Deaner, Deanol) with p-chlorophenoxyacetic acid, which is related to the plant growth hormone auxin. The hydrochloride of 2-dimethylaminoethyl 4-chlorophenoxyacetate has been given the approved name meclofenoxate by the World Health Organization. It is also known as centrophenoxine.

There is evidence that at least some of this compound is metabolized to DMAE and p-chlorophenoxyacetic acid, and although it has been suggested that DMAE is mainly responsible for the pharmacological activity of meclofenoxate, p-chlorophenoxyacetic acid and the combined molecule may also have pharmacological activity.

There is histochemical evidence from animal studies that meclofenoxate reduces the activity of succinic and lactic dehydrogenases while causing an increase in the activity of glucose-6-phosphate dehydrogenase. Thus, it has been suggested that meclofenoxate increases the activity of the pentose phosphate pathway (Nandy 1968). Other animal studies have reported that meclofenoxate alleviated the ill-effects of cerebral oxygen deprivation which were produced by a reduced atmospheric pressure or cyanide administration (Marcer and Hopkins 1977). A clinical study has claimed that the drug produced an increase in CBF in grey matter 15 min after an intravenous injection of meclofenoxate, and the drug has been claimed to shorten the postanaesthetic recovery period after thiopentone anaesthesia (Kugler et al. 1973).

Lipofuscin is a complex mixture of intracellular substances which probably represent the accumulated waste products of cellular metabolism, and another effect of meclofenoxate, which has been demonstrated in animal studies, is a reduction in the amount of lipofuscin in the cell bodies of neurones (Glees and Hasan 1976). An increasing accumulation of neuronal lipopigment has been correlated with age and the ceroid-lipofuscinoses, and it has been stated that neuronal lipofuscin is increased in Alzheimer dementia (Malamud 1972). Although there are claims to the contrary (Mann and Sinclair 1978), a recent study has demonstrated an increase in intraneuronal lipofuscin in the inferior olivary nucleus in Alzheimer dementia (Dowson 1982), and if lipofuscin accumulation is one factor which can contribute to neuronal death or impaired function in ageing or some cases of chronic brain disorder, meclofenoxate could have a prophylactic action in some neuropathological processes, in addition to any effects due to its metabolic actions.

Clinical efficacy. Many of the early clinical studies on the effects of the drug on cognitive impairment in the elderly were not properly controlled; however, three double-blind placebo-controlled studies have been published.

Oliver and Restell (1967) used a cross-over design and tested various functions which included digit-span, counting backwards, continuous subtraction in steps of 3, and the ability to retrieve remote memories. No significant effect of meclofenoxate was detected, but this study did not investigate the process of learning new material. However, Gedye et al. (1972) reported that administration of the drug to patients showing clinical evidence of a mild Alzheimer or arteriosclerotic dementia led to a significant improvement in the performance of a task involving new learning.

Marcer and Hopkins (1977) examined the effects of meclofenoxate on memory for new information in 'normal' elderly volunteers who were recruited with the help of their general practitioners. Thirty-one subjects received the drug and 29 received placebo. The trial was double-blind, the dose was 600 mg twice daily for 6 months, and the subjects were tested at 0, 3, 6 and 9 months. As in Oliver and Restell's study, the drug did not improve remote memory functions or immediate memory as measured by digit span; however, in accordance with the results of Gedye et al. (1972), there was a significant improvement in memory for new information as measured by the delayed free recall test. (Subjects listened to a list of ten words which were repeated until seven could be immediately recalled; recall was then retested after an interval of about half an hour.) Also, several patients who were receiving the drug reported a feeling of well-being and increased alertness. This finding of a significantly increased performance on a delayed free recall test was again found in a double-blind multi-centre trial over 12 months (Morton and Goldberg 1979).

The prescribing information suggests that meclofenoxate can be used to improve cognitive impairment in the elderly, to aid recovery of consciousness after head injury and to facilitate recovery after strokes, but it may also be of value in other forms of chronic brain failure. Until recently it has been available in the UK as tablets of 300 mg and the recommended dose for adults was 300 mg three times daily; it is still available in West Germany.

It has been stated that irritability or lassitude may occasionally occur, which usually disappears spontaneously within a few days. There are anecdotal accounts of agitation and insomnia being associated with the drug, and although this association is not clear, it has been suggested that meclofenoxate should not be given in the evening. It has also been stated, but without good evidence, that it should not be given to hyperexcitable patients or to children with extrapyramidal disorders. One study has reported that administration of the drug was associated with a significant increase in the white-cell count but this has not been confirmed.

The possible existence of cardiac side effects, including arrhythmias, has been considered. An unpublished study of patients with cerebrovascular disease has been quoted in which there were 11 deaths among 130 meclofenoxate-treated patients compared with four among 130 controls; at least five of the deaths in the drug-treated group were due to cerebrovascular accidents (Dukes 1978). However, subsequent trials have shown no significant difference in the death rate between placebo and drug-treated groups (Marcer and Hopkins 1977; Exton-Smith 1979). In summary, there is no substantive evidence of cardiac side effects but it would seem advisable not to prescribe meclofenoxate for patients with clinically significant cardiac pathology.

OTHER TREATMENTS FOR CHRONIC COGNITIVE IMPAIRMENT

Many drugs can be indicated for brain disorders which occur secondary to a diagnosable and treatable disease. Infections, anaemia, epilepsy, thyroid or parathyroid dysfunction and diabetes are examples of disorders which can respond to treatment. There is evidence that lack of the vitamins thiamine, B_{12}, or folic acid can contribute to cognitive impairment, and when this is due to alcoholism a course of high-dosage multivitamin preparation containing thiamine is usually given. It is also common practice to seek evidence of B_{12} or folic acid deficiency in every undiagnosed case of chronic brain disorder, although the role of vitamin B_{12} and folic acid deficiency is unclear (Cameron et al. 1963; Reynolds et al. 1973). Amantidine has been given to several patients with Creutzfeldt–Jakob dementia because of its antiviral action, and improvements in both clinical status and EEG have been reported. The apparently dramatic improvement in a few patients has indicated the need for further research with this compound (Sanders and Dunn 1973; Torack 1978).

Other substances which have been used in an attempt to treat chronic brain disorder include anticoagulants, corn oil emulsion, glutamic acid, ribaminol, tricyanoaminopropene, procaine, anticholesterol agents, lipotropic enzymes, ascorbic acid, and ribonucleic acid (RNA) (Beckett 1976; McGaugh and Petrinovich 1965; Prien 1973). Many animal studies have claimed that RNA facilitates learning, and a controlled study in geriatric patients with chronic brain disorder reported that RNA produced beneficial results (Cameron et al. 1963); magnesium pemoline was also said to give rise to beneficial effects and it was suggested that these might have been due to increased RNA production (Kalinowsky and Hippius 1971). However, subsequent studies did not replicate these findings (Prien 1973; Torack 1978). A heavy metal chelating agent, calcium EDTA, has been reported to produce improvement in Pick's disease in an uncontrolled study (Glen 1980), and an abnormality of zinc metabolism in this disorder has been postulated.

L-DOPA has been given to patients with presenile dementia in a placebo-controlled trial, but no effects on a variety of aspects of cognitive functioning could be demonstrated after 6 months (Kristensen et al. 1977), although another trial of L-DOPA in 14 patients with Alzheimer dementia reported small but significant gains in intellectual performance (Lewis et al. 1978). In addition, L-DOPA may have a role in the treatment of subcortical dementia (Albert et al. 1974).

A variety of non-drug treatments have also been advocated for some cases of brain failure. One controlled study reported a significant improvement in cognitive functioning after daily exposure to 3 h of 2.5 atmospheres of pure oxygen, for 15 days, but a subsequent study did not confirm these results (Rashkin et al. 1978). A ventriculoatrial shunt operation can lead to clinical improvement in patients with normal pressure hydrocephalic dementia (Gustafson and Hagberg 1978), and surgical intervention may be indicated for cerebral cysts, neoplasms or subdural haematoma. Finally, in some cases of cerebral arteriosclerosis, various surgical procedures, including extracranial to intracranial bypass surgery, have produced improvement in both neurological and cognitive functions (Greenhalgh et al. 1979; Torack 1978).

CONCLUSIONS

It has been convincingly demonstrated that dihydroergotoxine and naftidrofuryl oxalate can produce modest improvements in groups of patients with chronic cognitive impairment, and there is some evidence that several other drugs including piracetam and meclofenoxate may also be of value in certain patients. Although, in general, the drug treatment of chronic brain disorder has not produced dramatic results, a minority of patients with either Alzheimer dementia or multi-infarct dementia (and perhaps other kinds of dementia) may benefit to a modest but clinically significant extent (Yesavage 1979a). Even in severe cases, improved cognitive function may be reflected by a reduction in the nursing care which is required (Yesavage 1979b).

Proprietary preparations

Dihydroergotoxine mesylate	Hydergine
Naftidrofuryl oxalate	Praxilene
Clyclandelate	Clyclospasmol
Isoxsuprine hydrochloride	Duvadilan, Defencin, C.P.
Cinnarizine	Stugeron
Methylphenidate	Ritalin
Dexamphetamine	Dexedrine, Durophet
Meclofenoxate	Helfergin

References

ALBERT, M.L., FELDMAN, R. & WILLIS, A.L. (1974) The 'subcortical dementia' of progressive supranuclear palsy. *J. Neurol. Neurosurg. Psychiat.*, **37**, 121.

ALPERN, H.P. & JACKSON, S.J. (1978) Stimulants and depressants: Drug effects on memory. In: *Psychopharmacology: A Generation of Progress*, ed. Lipton, M.A., DiMascio, A. & Killam, K.F. New York: Raven Press.

BAN, T.A. (1978) Vasodilators, stimulants, and anabolic agents in the treatment of geropsychiatric patients. In: *Psychopharmacology: A Generation of Progress*, ed. Lipton, M.A., DiMascio, A. & Killam, K.F. New York: Raven Press.

BECKETT, H.D. (1976) Regression of atherosclerosis. *Br. med. J.*, **I**, 1208.

BOWEN, D.M., SMITH, C.B., WHITE, P. & DAVISON, A.N. (1976) Neurotransmitter-related enzymes and indices of hypoxia in senile dementia and other abiotrophies. *Brain*, **99**, 459.

BOYD, W.D., GRAHAM-WHITE, J., BLACKWOOD, G., GLEN, I. & McQUEEN, J. (1977) Clinical effects of choline in Alzheimer senile dementia. *Lancet*, **ii**, 711.

BRANCONNIER, R.J., COLE, J.O. & GARDOS, G. (1979) ACTH4-10 in the amelioration of neuropsychological symptomatology associated with senile organic brain syndrome. *Psychopharmacology*, **61**, 161.

BUTLER, R.N. (1978) In: *Alzheimer's Disease: Senile Dementia and Related Disorders* (Ageing. Vol. 7) ed. Katzman, R., Terry, R.D. & Bick, K.L. New York: Raven Press.

CAMERON, D.E., SVED, S. & SOLYOM, L. (1963) Effects of ribonucleic acid on memory defects in the aged. *Am. J. Psychiat.*, **120**, 320.

CERLETTI, A., EMMENEGGER, H., ENZ, A., IWANGOFF, P. & MEIER-RUGE, W. (1973) In: *Central Nervous System, Studies on Metabolic Regulation and Function*, ed. Genazzani, E., & Herkan, H. Berlin/Heidelberg/New York: Springer Verlag.

CHRISTIE, J.E., SHERING, A., FERGUSON, J. & GLEN, A.I.M. (1981) Physostigmine and arecholine: Effects of intravenous infusions in Alzheimer presenile dementia. *Br. J. Psychiat.*, **138**, 46.

CHYNOWETH, R. & FOLEY, J. (1969) Pre-senile dementia responding to steroid therapy. *Br. J. Psychiat.*, **115**, 703.

CORSELLIS, J.A.N. (1977) Observations on the neuropathology of dementia. *Age Ageing*, **6** (Suppl.), 20.

CROOK, T., FERRIS, S., SATHANANTHAN, G., RASKIN, A. & GERSHON, S., (1977) The effect of methylphenidate on test performance in the cognitively impaired aged. *Psychopharmacology*, **52**, 251.

DAVIES, P. & MALONEY, A.T.F. (1976) Selective loss of central cholinergic neurones in Alzheimer's disease. *Lancet*, **ii**, 1403.

DAVIS, K.L., MOHS, R.C. & TINKLENBERG, J.R. (1978) Physostigmine: Improvement of long-term memory processes in normal humans. *Science*, **201**, 272.

DIMOND, S.J. (1977) Drugs to improve learning in man. In: *The Neuropsychology of Learning Disorders*, ed. Knights, R.M. & Bakke, D.J. Baltimore: University Park Press.

DOWSON, J.H. (1982) Neuronal lipofuscin accumulation in ageing and Alzheimer dementia. *Br. J. Psychiat.* **140**, 142.

DRACHMAN, D.A. (1978) Central cholinergic system and memory. In: *Psychopharmacology: A Generation of Progress*, ed. Lipton, M.A., DiMascio, A. & Killam, K.F. New York: Raven Press.

DUKES, M.N.G. (1978) In: *Side Effects of Drugs. Annual 2* pp. 4, 183. Amsterdam/Oxford: Excerpta Medica.

DUKES, M.N.G. (1979) In: *Side Effects of Drugs. Annual 3* pp. 5, 177. Amsterdam/Oxford: Excerpta Medica.

DUVOISIN, R.C. (1975) Antagonism of levodopa by papaverine. *JAMA*, **231**, 845.

Editorial (1979) Vasodilators in senile dementia. *Br. med. J.*, **2**, 511.

ETIENNE, P., GAUTHIER, S., JOHNSON, G., CLLIER, B., MENDIS, T., DASTOOR, D., COLE, M. & MULLER, H.F. (1978) Clinical effects of choline in Alzheimer's disease. *Lancet*, **i**, 508.

EXTON-SMITH, A.N. (1979) Personal communication.

FLOOD, M.K. (1979) Pyritinol hydrochloride and senile dementia. *Br. med. J.*, **1**, 1148.

FONTAINE, L., GRAND, M., SZARVASI, E. & BASSAT, M. (1969) A study of the vasodilator effect of naftidrofuryl. *Bull. Chim. Ther.*, **1**, 39.

FOVALL, P., DYSKEN, M.W., LAZARUS, L.W., DAVIS, J.M., KAHN, R.L. et al. (1980) Choline bitartrate treatment of Alzheimer-type dementias. *Communs Psychopharmac.*, **4**, 141.

GAITZ, C.M., VARNER, R.V. & OVERALL, J.E. (1977) Pharmacotherapy for Organic Brain Syndrome in Late Life. *Archs gen. Psychiat.*, **34**, 839.

GEDYE, J.C., EXTON-SMITH, A.N. & WEDGEWOOD, J. (1972) A method for measuring mental performance in the elderly and its use in a pilot clinical trial of meclofenoxate. *Age Ageing*, **1**, 74.

GERAUD, J., BESS, A., DELPHA, M., MARC-VERGNES, J.P. & RASCAL, A.L. (1963) Measurement of cerebral blood flow using Krypton 85. *Revue neurol.* **108**, 547.

GHONEIM, M.M. & MEWALDT, S.P. (1977) Studies on human memory: The interactions of Diazepam, Scopolamine and Physostigmine. *Psychopharmacology*, **52**, 1.

GLESS, P. & HASAN, M. (1976) Lipofuscin in neuronal aging and disease. *Norm. Pathol. Anat.* (Stuttg.), **32**, 1.

GLEN, A.I.M. (1980) The Pharmacology of Dementia. *Hosp. Update, Oct.*, 977.

GONCALVES, N. (1979) Pyritinol bei ambulanten geriatrischen Patienten. *Med. Welt*, **30**, 494.

GREENHALGH, R.M., ILLINGWORTH, R.D. MCFIE, J., MILLS, S.P., PERKIN, G.D. & ROSE,F.C. (1979) Extracranial to intracranial micro-vascularisation for the treatment of completed ischaemic stroke. *Br. med. J.*, **2**, 18.

GUSTAFSON, L. & HAGBERG, B. (1978) Recovery in hydrocephalic dementia after shunt operation. *J. Neurol. Neurosurg. Psychiat.*, **41**, 940.

HACHINSKI, V.C. (1979) Relevance of cerebrovascular changes to mental function. *Mech. Ageing Devel.*, **9**, 173.

HACHINSKI, V.C., LASSER, N.A. & MARSHALL, J. (1974) Multi-infarct dementia. *Lancet*, ii, 207.

HUDGE, T.G. & URQUHART, A. (1972) Naftidrofuryl—A double-blind cross-over study in the elderly. *Curr. med. Res. Opin.*, **1**, 166.

KALINOWSKY, L.B. & HIPPIUS, H. (1971) In: *Pharmacological, Convulsive and Other Somatic Treatments in Psychiatry*. New York: Grune and Stratton.

KRISTENSEN, V., OLSEN, M. & THEILGAARD, A. (1977) Levodopa treatment of presenile dementia. *Acta. psychiat. scand.*, **55**, 41.

KUGLER, VON J., DOENICKE, A. & HARKER, E. (1973) Course of thiopental anaesthesia under the influence of centrophenoxine. *Arzneimittel- Forsch.*, **23**, 82.

LAGERGREN, K. & LEVANDER, S.E. (1974) A double-blind study on the effects of Piracetam upon perceptual and psychomotor performance at varied heart rates in patients treated with artificial pacemakers. *Psychopharmacology*, **39**, 97.

LANDFIELD, P.W., WAYMIRE, J.C. & LYNCH, G. (1978) Hippocampal aging and adrenocorticoids: quantitative correlations. *Science*, **202**, 1098.

LECKMAN, J., ANANTH., J.V. & BAN, T.A. (1971) Pentelenetetrazol in the treatment of geriatric patients with disturbed memory function. *J. clin. Pharmacol.*, **11**, 301.

LEGROS, J.J., GILOT, P., SERON, X., CLAESSENS, J., ADAM, A., MOEGLEN, J.M., AUDBERT, A. & BERCHIER, P. (1978) Influence of vasopressin on learning and memory. *Lancet*, i, 41.

LEWIS, C., BALLINGER, B.R. & PRESLY, A.S. (1978) Trial of levodopa in senile dementia. *Br. med. J.*, i, 550.

LISHMAN, W.A. (1971) Amnestic syndromes and their neuropathology. *Br. J. Psychiat. Special publ.*, **No. 6**, 25.

LLOYD-EVANS, S., BROCKLEHURST, J.C. & PALMER, M.K. (1979) Piracetam in chronic brain failure. *Curr. med. Res. Opin.*, **6**, 351.

MACLAY, W.P. (1979) Vasodilators in senile dementia. *Br. med. J.*, **2**, 866.

MALAMUD, N. (1972) Neuropathology of organic brain syndromes associated with aging. *Adv. Behav. Biol.*, **3**, 63.

MANN, D.M.A., LINCOLN, J., YATES, P.O., STAMP, J.E. & TOPER, S. (1980) Changes in the monoamine containing neurones of the human CNS in senile dementia. *Br. J. Psychiat.*, **136**, 533.

MANN, D.M.A. & SINCLAIR, K.G.A. (1978) The quantitative assessment of lipofuscin pigment, cytoplasmic RNA and nucleolar volume in senile dementia. *Neuropath. Appl. Neurobiol.*, **4**, 129.

MARCER, D. & HOPKINS, S.M. (1977) The differential effects of meclofenoxate on memory loss in the elderly. *Age Ageing*, **6**, 123.

MARCHBANKS, R.M. (1980) Choline, acetylcholine and dementia. *Psychol. Med.*, **10**, 1.

MARTIN, A.J. (1979) Vasodilators in senile dementia. *Br. med. J.*, **2**, 866.

MATEJCEK, M., KNOR, K., PIGUIT, P. & WEIL, C. (1979) Electroencephalographic and clinical changes as correlated in geriatric patients treated three months with an ergot alkaloid preparation. *J. Am. Geriat. Soc.*, **27**, 198.

MCDONALD, R.J. (1979) Hydergine: A review of 26 clinical studies. *Pharmakopsychiatr.*, **12**, 407.

MCGAUGH, J.L. & PETRINOVICH, L.F. (1965) In: *International Review of Neurobiology*, Vol. 8, ed. Pfeiffer, C.C. & Smythies, J.R. New York: Academic Press.

MEIER-RUGE, W., ENZ, A., GYGAXP., HUNZIKER, O., IWANOFF, P. & REICHLMEIER, K. (1975) Experimental pathology in basic research of the aging brain. In: *Ageing, 2, Genesis and Treatment of Psychologic Disorders in the Elderly*, ed. Gershon, S. & Raskin, A., pp. 55–126. New York: Raven Press.

MELAMED, E., LAVY, S., SIEW, F., BENTIN, S. & COOPER, G. (1978) Correlation between regional cerebral blood flow and brain atrophy in dementia. *J. Neurol. Neurosurg. Psychiat.*, **41**, 894.

MEYNAUD, A., GRAND, M. & FONTAINE, L. (1973) Effects of naftidrofuryl upon energy metabolism of the brain. *Arzneimittel-Forsch.*, **23**, 1431.

MINDUS, P., CHRONHOLM, B., LEVANDER, S.E. & SCHALLING, D. (1976) Piracetam-induced improvement of mental performance. *Acta psychiat. scand.*, **54**, 150.

MOHS, R.C., DAVIS, KL., TINKLENBERG, J.R., HOLLISTER, L.E., YESAVAGE, J.A. & KOPELL, B.S. (1979) Choline chloride treatment of memory deficits in the elderly. *Am. J. Psychiat.*, **136:10**, 1275.

MORTON, O. & GOLDBERG, A. (1979) Unpublished data from Reckitt and Colman Ltd, Hull, England.

MURAMOTO, O., SUGISHITA, M., SUGITA, H. & TOYOKURA, Y. (1979) Effect of physostigmine on constructional and memory tasks in Alzheimer's Disease. *Archs Neurol., Chicago*, **36**, 501.

NANDY, K. (1968) Further studies on the effects of centrophenoxine on the lipofuscin pigment in the neurones of senile guinea pigs. *J. Geront.*, **23**, 82.

OLIVER, J.E. & RESTELL, M. (1967) Serial testing in assessing the effect of meclofenoxate on patients with memory defects. *Br. J. Psychiat.*, **113**, 219.

PERRY, E.K. (1980) The cholinergic system in old age and Alzheimer's disease. *Age Ageing*, **9**, 1.

PERRY, E.K., PERRY, R.H., BLESSED, G. & TOMLINSON, B.E. (1977) Necropsy evidençe of central cholinergic deficits in senile dementia. *Lancet*, **i**, 189.

PERRY, E.K., TOMLINSON, B.E., BLESSED, G., BERGMAN, K., GIBSON, P.H. & PERRY, R.H. (1978) Correlation of cholinergic abnormalities with senile plaques and mental test scores in senile dementia. *Br. med. J.*, **2**, 1457.

PETERS, B.H. & LEVIN, H.S. (1977) Memory enhancement after physostigmine treatment in the amnestic syndrome. *Archs Neurol., Chicago*, **34**, 215.

PETERS, B.H. & LEVIN, H.S. (1978) Effects of physostigmine and lecithin on memory in Alzheimer disease. *Ann. Neurol.*, **6**, 219.

PONSFORD, J.L. & DONNAN, G.A. (1980) Transient global amnesia—a hippocampal phenomenon? *J. Neurol. Neurosurg. Psychiat.*, **43**, 85.

PRADHAN, S.N. (1980) Central neurotransmitters and ageing. *Life Sci.*, **26**, 1643.

PRIEN, R.F. (1973) Chemotherapy in chronic organic brain syndrome. A review of the literature. *Psychopharm. Bull.*, **9** No. 4, 5.

RAO, D.B. & NORRIS, J.R. (1972) A double-blind investigation of hydergine in the treatment of cerebrovascular insufficiency in elderly patients. *Johns Hopkins med. J.*, **130**, 317.

RASKIN, A., GERSHON, S., CROOK, T.H., SATHANANTHAN, G. & FERRIS, S. (1978) The effects of hyperbaric and normobaric oxygen on cognitive impairment in the elderly. *Archs gen. Psychiat.*, **35**, 50.

REISINE, T.D., BIRD, E.D. & SPOKES, E. (1978) Pre- and post-synaptic neurochemical alterations in Alzheimer's disease. *Trans. Am. Soc. Neurochem.*, **9**, 203.

REYNOLDS, E.H., ROTHFELD, P. & PINCUS, J.H. (1973) Neurological disease associated with folate deficiency. *Br. med. J.*, **2**, 398.

RIGTER, H. & van RIEZEN, H. (1978) Hormones and memory. In: *Psychopharmacology: A Generation of Progress*, ed. Lipton, M.A., DiMascio, A. & Killam, K.F. New York: Raven Press.

ROBINSON, K. (1972) A double blind clinical trial of naftidrofuryl in cerebrovascular disorders. *Med. Dig., Lond.*, **17**, 50.

ROUBICEK, J., GEIGER, C. & ABT, K. (1972); An ergot alkaloid preparation (Hydergine) in geriatric therapy. *J. Am. Geriat. Soc.*, **20**, 222.

SANDERS, W.L. & DUNN, T.L. (1973) Creutzfeldt-Jakob disease treated with Amantidine. *J. Neurol. Neurosurg. Psychiat.*, **86**, 581.

SATHANANTHAN, G.L. & GERSHON, S. (1975) In: *Ageing vol. 2 Genesis and Treatment of Psychologic Disorders in the Elderly*, ed. Gershon, S. & Raskin, A. New York: Raven Press.

SITARAM, N., WEINGARTNER, H. & CAINE, E.D. (1978a) Selective enhancement of serial learning and encoding of low imagery words in man. *Life Sci.*, **22**, 1555.

SITARAM, N., WEINGARTNER, H. & GILLIN, J.C. (1978b) Human serial learning: Enhancement with arecholine and choline and impairment with scopolamine. *Science*, **201**, 274.

SMITH, C.M., SWASH, M., EXTON-SMITH, A.N., PHILLIPS, M.J., OVERSTALL, P.W., PIPER, M.E. & BAILEY, M.R. (1978) Choline therapy in Alzheimer's disease. *Lancet*, **ii**, 318.

STEDEFORD, A. (1978) Understanding confusional states. *Br. J. Hosp. Med.*, 694.

STEGINK, A.J. (1972) The clinical use of Piracetam, a new nootropic drug. *Drug Res.*, **22**, 975.

SULLIVAN, P.A., MURNAGHAN, D.J. & CALLAGHAN, N. (1977) Dialysis dementia: recovery after transplantation. *Br. med. J.*, **ii**, 740.

TAMINGA, C., SMITH, R.C., CHANG, S., HARAZTI, J.S. & DAVIA, J.M. (1976) Depression associated with choline. *Lancet*, **ii**, 905.

THIBAULT, A. (1974) A double-blind evaluation of 'hydergine' and placebo in the treatment of patients with organic brain syndrome and cerebral arteriosclerosis in a nursing home. *Curr. med. Res. Opin.*, **2**, 482.

TORACK, R.M. (1978) Treatment of senile dementia. In: *The Pathologic Physiology of Dementia*. Berlin, Heidelberg, New York: Springer-Verlag.

TUREK, I., KURLAND, A.A. & OTA, K.Y. (1969) Effects of pipradrol hydrochloride on geriatric patients. *J. Am. Geriat. Soc.*, **17**, 408.

VENN, R.D. (1980) In: *Ergot Compounds and Brain Function: Neuroendocrine and Neuropsychiatric Aspects*, ed. Goldstein, M. New York: Raven Press.

WHITTY, C.W.M. (1978) Loss of memory as a clinical problem. *Br. J. Hosp. Med.*, 276.

de WIED, D., VAN WIMERSMA, G., BOHUS, B., URBAN, I. & GISPEN, W.H. (1976) Vasopressin and memory consolidation. *Progr. Brain Res.*, **45**, 181.

WISNIEWSKI, H.M. & TERRY, R.D. (1976) In: *Neurobiology of Ageing*, ed. Terry, R.D. & Gershon, S. pp. 265–280. New York: Raven Press.

WYPER, D.J., McALPINE, C.J., JAWAD, K. & JENNETT, B. (1976) Effects of carbonic anhydrase inhibitor on cerebral blood flow in geriatric patients. *J. Neurol. Neurosurg. Psychiat.*, **39**, 885.

YESAVAGE, J. ET AL. (1979a) Dementia: differential diagnosis and treatment. *Geriatrics. Sept.*, 51.

YESAVAGE, J.A., TINKLENBERG, J.R., HOLLISTER, L.E. & BERGER, P.A. (1979b) Vasodilators in senile dementias. *Archs gen. Psychiat.*, **36**, 220.

ZORNETZER, S.F. (1978) Neurotransmitter modulation and memory. In: *Psychopharmacology: A Generation of Progress*, ed. Lipton, M.A., DiMascio, A. & Killam, K.F., New York: Raven Press.

5

Other Drugs Relevant to Psychiatric Practice

C.Q. Mountjoy

HYPNOTICS

The most favoured hypnotics are benzodiazepines, which have been described in a previous chapter. Other hypnotics which are occasionally of use are chloral, dichloralphenazone, promethazine and chlormethiazole.

Chloral hydrate, which may be useful in treatment of the elderly, is available as capsules of 500 mg or as a mixture containing 500 mg chloral hydrate in 5 ml. The dose ranges between 0.5 and 2 g. Chloral can cause gastritis, and the closely related dichloralphenazone, which is less prone to cause this side effect, may be preferred. The usual dose is two to three tablets each containing 650 mg dichloralphenazone.

Antihistamines such as promethazine in a dose of 20–50 mg may prove useful where other treatments have failed. Chlormethiazole in a dose of 0.5–1 g at night may be useful for the elderly confused patient, but it should be used cautiously in patients who have shown previous signs of being prone to addiction.

BROMOCRIPTINE

Bromocriptine (2-bromo-α-ergocriptine) suppresses prolactin secretion by acting on the pituitary as a functional analogue of endogenous prolactin-inhibiting factor. In addition it is known to be a dopamine agonist. Bromocriptine has been used to suppress lactation and for a variety of conditions including acromegaly, Parkinson's disease, secondary amenorrhoea and infertility. Horrobin et al. (1976) drew attention to the relationship between raised prolactin and a number of types of mental illness and suggested that reduction of prolactin levels by bromocriptine could be useful.

In the treatment of mania, Dorr and Sathananthan (1976) reported improvement in two patients with severe mania in whom phenothiazines and lithium were contraindicated. Saran and Acharya (1977) reported improvement in three out of four patients with mania who were also receiving more conventional antimanic treatment. This study was uncontrolled and the use of other antimanic agents makes interpretation difficult. Smith et al. (1980) reported a placebo-controlled double-blind trial with bromocriptine 2.5 mg three times daily for 3 days, then 5 mg three times daily for 4 days. They were unable to demonstrate any significant effect due to the bromocriptine in the management of the manic patient. On the basis of the studies so far completed it seems unlikely that bromocriptine has any significant part to play in the treatment of mania.

Agnoli et al. (1978) reported an uncontrolled trial of bromocriptine given in a dose of 30 mg for 10 days to ten patients with monopolar endogenous depression. The results were reported as being good in five patients and excellent in two, but comparison with tricyclics in this uncontrolled study favoured the superiority of the tricyclic antidepressants. Colonna et al. (1979), in another uncontrolled study of 12 patients with differing types of depression, were only able to show improvement in three of the patients. These findings, together with personal unpublished experience with bromocriptine in the treatment of depression, suggest that it has no part to play in the treatment of depressive disorders.

Case reports relating to treatment of schizophrenia are confined to very small groups. King (1978) reported the result of treatment in two patients with 'residual' schizophrenia; one of whom got worse while one remained unchanged. Colonna et al. (1978) also described two schizophrenic patients; one improved, while the other, who did not take his tablets as prescribed, deteriorated.

Harrower et al. (1977) treated a group of eight patients with anorexia nervosa with bromocriptine for 2–4 weeks, but only one of the eight, who relapsed following withdrawal of the drug, appeared to improve.

Phuapradit et al. (1978) studied nine patients with early presenile dementia in a single-blind trial for a period of 4 weeks. Bromocriptine failed to improve cognitive disabilities, and side effects, including confusion and nausea, were common, with only six patients able to attain the maximum dose of 20 mg per day.

In summary, there appears to be no evidence for the use of bromocriptine in treatment of depression, mania, anorexia nervosa, schizophrenia or presenile dementia.

Bromocriptine has been reported as being useful in the treatment of some types of hypogonadism, though success is only found in patients who had an associated hyperprolactinaemia (Thorner et al. 1974; Bommer et al. 1979; March 1979). The place of bromocriptine in the treatment of the premenstrual tension syndrome will be mentioned later in this chapter.

Bromocriptine produces a number of side effects, which are dose dependent and include nausea, vomiting and postural hypotension. The side effects can usually be avoided if a small dose is given at the start of the treatment and then increased slowly. Preferably the dose should be taken in the evening with food.

Gastrointestinal complications do not seem to be a major problem, though Wass et al. (1976) have reported increased ulceration and bleeding in acromegalic patients. Although some rats developed endometrial hyperplasia progressing to tumours with long-term treatment with bromocriptine, Besser et al. (1977) found no gynaecological abnormality in women who had been treated with bromocriptine.

Women have an increased risk of pregnancy while on treatment with bromocriptine. There is no increase in the rate of spontaneous abortion, multiple gestations or congenital abnormalities (March 1979).

The usefulness of bromocriptine in psychiatry is confined to patients with hyperprolactinaemia associated with impotence, hypogonadism, or premenstrual tension.

APPETITE DEPRESSANTS

The main treatment of obesity is diet with or without support from 'weight-watching' groups or help from behaviour therapists.

A number of drugs have been used as appetite depressants, the first of which was amphetamine, which was shown in experimental animals to reduce the frequency of eating though not the rate at which food was consumed. It had no effect on stress-induced eating. It exerts a neuropharmacological effect on the adrenergic pathways in the hypothalamus and related structures. Because of the danger of addiction and induction of psychotic episodes, amphetamine and phenmetrazine are controlled by the Misuse of Drugs Act and should not be prescribed for their weight-reducing effects. Diethylpropion, mazindol and phentermine have anorectic properties similar to amphetamine but their stimulant action and associated risk of dependence is less (Garattini et al. 1978). In contrast, fenfluramine shows a sedative action mediated through the serotoninergic system and has peripheral effects such as increased glucose utilization (Kirby and Turner 1976). A side effect of the withdrawal of fenfluramine is a feeling of depression which appears about 4 days after cessation of treatment (Oswald et al. 1971; Steel and Briggs 1972). However, this particular problem is not a major clinical difficulty and can be overcome by gradually reducing the dose of fenfluramine. None of the drugs included in this section should be combined with monoamine oxidase inhibitors because of the danger of a hypertensive crisis.

Fenfluramine and diethylpropion appear to be equally effective in causing reduction of weight in obese patients (Follows 1971). Both drugs are effective in causing weight loss in trials lasting approximately 3 months (Lele et al. 1972; Sainani et al. 1973; Stunkard et al. 1973; Abramson et al. 1980). The usual dosage in these trials was fenfluramine 60 mg daily and diethylpropion 75 mg daily. Innes et al. (1977) have demonstrated a high correlation between weight loss and plasma levels of fenfluramine and so they recommend that the dose of the drug is increased until some weight loss is evident or side effects develop; in some cases as much as 160 mg a day is required to produce results.

Weight loss is greatest in the first few weeks of drug administration; the actual duration of treatment is difficult to decide, as the rate of decrease in weight gradually diminishes, while the potential danger of dependence and addiction increases. Unfortunately, the advantages gained during the use of the anorectic drug are usually eroded over the course of the next few months or years, as the patient tends to return to his former weight (Hudson 1977). Stunkard et al. (1980) followed 120 females and 14 males who were randomly allocated to one of three treatments: behaviour therapy, fenfluramine (with Rogerian group therapy), or behaviour therapy combined with fenfluramine. The dose of fenfluramine was determined by the patient's improvement or by the development of side effects, and the maximum dose permitted was 120 mg per day. After 6 months' treatment the mean weight loss in the fenfluramine-treated group was 14.5 kg, the behaviour therapy and fenfluramine group, 15.3 kg, and the behaviour therapy group, 10.9 kg. However, 1 year after treatment, the fenfluramine-treated group had a mean increase in weight of 8.2 kg, the behaviour therapy and fenfluramine group of 10.7 kg, while the behaviour therapy group had increased by only 1.9 kg.

The results of this study with its admittedly complex design suggest that behaviour therapy is probably a more satisfactory treatment of obesity than anorectic drugs.

In summary, anorectic drugs may have a small part to play in the treatment of difficult and refractory obese patients, but the effects that can be expected from therapy are limited, and usually of short duration. Anorectic drugs should not be prescribed for patients who have shown signs of misuse of drugs or alcohol.

DRUGS FOR THE LONG-TERM TREATMENT OF ALCOHOLISM

Drugs which produce an unpleasant interaction with alcohol have been used in the treatment of alcoholic patients to try and prevent further drinking. Disulfiram, citrated calcium carbimide and metronidazol have been used in such a way, though the latter drug has been found to be ineffective (Gelder and

Edwards 1976). Disulfiram and calcium carbimide reduce the rate of oxidation of acetaldehyde by the enzyme aldehyde dehydrogenase. The result is an increase in circulating acetaldehyde, which leads to hot flushes, intense throbbing in the head and neck, nausea, vomiting, sweating, thirst, hypertension, blurred vision and sometimes confusion. This unpleasant reaction may be deliberately induced whilst the patient is an in-patient, so that he is aware of the consequences of drinking while taking medication.

Calcium carbimide is available in 50-mg tablets and the usual dose is 50 mg twice daily as its duration of action is approximately 12 h. Disulfiram is available in 200 mg tablets and it is usually taken in the maintenance dose of 200 mg daily.

The evaluation of the efficacy of these drugs is made difficult by the alcoholic patient's unreliability in reporting his drinking habits, and the frequent absence of objective evidence of compliance in treatment. Disulfiram has been shown by Robichaud et al. (1979) to cause a significant reduction in days absent from work, compared with the numbers of days lost in a pretreatment phase. Fuller and Roth (1979) studied 128 alcoholic men who were randomly assigned to one of three groups. The first received disulfiram 250 mg daily (which is a pharmacologically active dose), the second received an inactive dose of 1 mg daily, while the third received no disulfiram but a 50 mg riboflavin tablet daily. Each subject from the first two groups was told he was receiving disulfiram and the possible disulfiram–ethanol reaction was vividly described. Patients were followed up for 1 year and independent accounts of drinking behaviour were obtained from a relative. There were no statistically significant differences between the three treatment groups with regard to total abstinence, percentage of drinking days, days worked, family stability as assessed by time spent living with the same relative, or to the percentage of scheduled appointments with a physician which were kept. However, 21% of those who received a regular dose of disulfiram and 25% who received the pharmacologically inactive dose remained abstinent, whereas only 12% of those who received riboflavin did so. Although not statistically significant, the results suggest that fear of the reaction is important in preventing drinking, and if patients are willing to comply they are more likely to be abstinent if given the drug. A deficiency of this study was that patients did not experience a deliberately-induced initial reaction following a test dose of alcohol.

The duration of compliance can be increased by the use of subcutaneous or intramuscular disulfiram implantations, and Malcolm and Madden (1973) and Whyte and O'Brien (1974) found significant improvement in the 6 months following implantation compared with the same preceding period. However, they felt this was unlikely to be due to a pharmacological effect, as significant blood levels of disulfiram are found only in the first week after implantation. This view has been contested by Wilson et al. (1976), who studied 20 alcoholic patients who had been randomly allocated either to a disulfiram implant or sham operation. Despite the fact that a 'challenge' with ethanol 120 h following operation did not elicit any reaction in either group, six patients with sham operations and five with disulfiram implants subsequently began to drink, and only those with implants experienced reactions. Apparently as a result of this pharmacological effect, four of the five implant recidivists remained abstinent. However, Wilson et al.'s study did not show a significant difference between the disulfiram implant and sham operation in terms of postintervention abstinence.

These drugs have been widely used over many years and are regarded by a number of specialists as being a useful part of a more generalized programme of treatment by reducing any immediate temptation to start drinking again (Costello 1975; Ritson 1975; Hore 1977).

In some cases alcoholism has developed secondary to other illness, particularly affective disorders. Merry et al. (1976) have shown that lithium was effective in reducing the drinking and incapacity due to alcohol in a group of alcoholic patients with depressive syndromes, in a prospective placebo-controlled double-blind trial conducted over 1 year. (Lithium had no effect on nondepressed patients.) However, as alcohol abuse is associated with an increased incidence of self-harm incidents, lithium is best avoided because of its high toxicity in overdose, unless it is specifically indicated.

HORMONAL TREATMENT OF AFFECTIVE DISORDERS

Thyroid Hormones

The relationship between thyroid disorder and psychiatric illness has interested clinicians since the time of Graves (1835), who associated the syndrome of globus hystericus with the thyroid gland. In 1888 the Committee of the Clinical Society of London reported on the mental changes observed in over a hundred cases of myxoedema, and noted the general retardation, sluggishness and slowness of apprehension which was associated with insanity in the form of melancholia, chronic mania or dementia. Interest in the therapeutic aspects of thyroid hormones started with the observation by Prange and Lipton (1962) and Prange et al. (1963) that imipramine toxicity was enhanced in hyperthyroidism and reduced in hypothyroidism in animals. The interactions in animals suggested that treatment with tricyclic antidepressants might be enhanced by the use of thyroxine or tri-iodothyronine. In practice, the latter has been used more frequently because of its shorter half-life and its availability in standard oral doses. A number of studies have now reported that there is a therapeutically positive drug–hormone interaction which leads to a more rapid improvement than when a tricyclic is given alone. These studies include those by Prange et al. (1969); Earle (1970); Wilson et al. (1970); Coppen et al. (1972) and Wheatley (1972). A trial with a negative result has been reported by Feighner et al. (1972).

Although the majority of studies do show this positive interaction, the evidence for clinical efficacy is limited, as results reported depend usually on a single statistical significant observation derived from a variety of rating scales on many occasions, and Prange (1972) in a discussion following Feighner's paper, admits that a similar effect to that produced by the introduction of T_3 can be produced by giving larger doses of imipramine. In view of the potential toxicity of tri-iodothyronine given to euthyroid patients over a long period, it would seem sensible to confine the enhancement of the effects of a tricyclic with tri-iodothyronine to the management of some treatment-resistant depressive syndromes.

Thyrotrophin releasing hormone (TRH) is widely distributed within the central nervous system, and Metcalf and Dettmar (1981) have suggested that it is an endogenous ergotropic substance (i.e. that induces anabolism) in the brain. Studies by Plotnikoff et al. (1974) reported that mice showed some reactions which were typical of those induced by antidepressants, after treatment with TRH. In 1972 Prange et al. and Kastin et al. published findings obtained in double-blind trials, in which TRH was administered intravenously to depressed patients and produced a rapid improvement in depressed mood. However, subsequent experience with both intravenous and oral TRH has failed to confirm these original findings (Takahashi et al. 1973; Dimitrikoudi et al. 1974; Mountjoy et al. 1974; Ehrensing et al. 1974; Coppen et al. 1974; Hollister et al. 1974; Benkert et al. 1974; Hall et al. 1975; Evans et al. 1975; van den Burg et al. 1976; Schmidt 1977; Vogel et al. 1977). Loosen et al. (1979) reported that intravenous TRH produced a beneficial effect on mood state during acute alcoholic withdrawal states, but the clinical significance of this report, which is concerned with a self-limiting syndrome, is uncertain. Thus, there is no evidence that TRH has a place in the treatment of depressive syndromes.

Other Hormones

Klaiber et al. (1979) reported that treatment with oestrogen, in doses of up to 25 mg daily for a period of 3 months, was partially effective in relieving the symptoms of chronic endogenous depression in a group of female patients who had failed to respond to other treatments; oestrogen-treated patients improved irrespective of their menopausal status. Because of the danger of endometrial cancer, biopsies were taken and the oestrogens were administered cyclically with a progesterone. The place of oestrogen treatment in the menopause is discussed elsewhere in this chapter.

Gold et al. (1979) reported partial improvement in depressive symptoms in four severely depressed patients treated with the 1-desamino-8-D-arginine vasopressin synthetic analogue of vasopression. However, this hormone has to be administered intranasally, and as the improvement in depressive symptomatology was not great, it is unlikely to be a useful treatment.

Melatonin produces tranquillization with mild euphoria and eventually sleep in normal subjects, but when used in a clinical trial with depressed patients it caused a dramatic worsening in the patients' symptomatology (Carman et al. 1976).

Several studies have failed to show that gonadotrophin-releasing hormone is effective in the treatment of depressed patients (Benkert et al. 1974; Brambilla et al. 1978; Linnoila et al. 1979; Amsterdam et al. 1979), or that it has any effect on the mood of non-depressed sexually impotent men (Davies et al. 1976).

DRUG TREATMENT OF SEXUAL OFFENDERS

Sexual drive can be reduced by increasing the amount of oestrogen or effectively reducing the amount of circulating androgen. Oestrogens have been widely used and may be administered either by mouth, injection or implant (Golla and Hodge 1949; Whitaker 1959; Field and Williams 1970). If the patient can be relied upon to take oral medication, then ethinyloestradiol can be prescribed in a dose of 0.01–0.05 mg a day, which does not usually cause significant nausea. The majority of patients, however, are unreliable, and depot injections of oestradiol undecylenate in a dose of 50–100 mg administered every 3 or 4 weeks may be appropriate (Gunn 1976).

The side effects of oestrogen therapy include testicular atrophy, possible osteoporosis and breast enlargement, with occasional reports of carcinoma of the breast (Symmers 1968).

Cyproterone acts as an antiandrogen by blocking androgen receptors. It also has progestogenic activity which exerts a feedback effect on the hypothalamic receptors, so leading to a reduction in gonadotrophin release and hence to diminished production of testicular androgens. It inhibits spermatogenesis and produces reversible infertility. Gynaecomastia occurs in about 20%, while tiredness and fatigue are common in the first few weeks of treatment. Special precautions have to be taken in case of liver disease, diabetes, and adrenocortical disorder. It is available only as 50-mg tablets and the usual dose is 50 mg twice daily.

Assessment of libido in sexual offenders is particularly difficult, as most studies rely on the patient's own account. However, the use of the penile plethismograph does give some objective indication of the efficacy of treatment. Bancroft et al. (1974) compared ethinyloestradiol 0.01 mg twice daily with cyproterone 50 mg twice daily in 12 patients using a Williams square design. Both drugs were equally effective in reducing the frequency of sexual thoughts and activity, whereas only cyproterone produced a modest reduction of erectile and subjective responses to erotic stimuli. In these doses, for a period of 5 weeks, neither drug caused troublesome side effects. There are many other reports of the efficacy of cyproterone, but in the main they are uncontrolled or lack objective criteria for improvement. A disadvantage of cyproterone is that it is only available as an oral preparation and furthermore, alcohol appears to reduce the effect of the drug, which becomes ineffective in chronic alcoholics.

Other drugs such as the butyrophenone benperidol and other phenothiazine drugs have been used in the treatment of sexual offenders. Tennent et al. (1972) compared benperidol, chlorpromazine and placebo and found benperidol to be superior to placebo in reducing the frequency of sexual thoughts. It is likely that the butyrophenones and phenothiazines merely act as sedatives rather than having any specific effect on libido.

The oestrogens and antiandrogens appear to be effective in reducing libido but, because of their feminizing properties, it is essential that the patient is made aware of the nature of the treatment and its side effects.

TREATMENTS FOR THE PREMENSTRUAL TENSION SYNDROME

This syndrome was first described by Frank (1931). The symptoms are of headache, feelings of tension, irritability, depression, together with a bloated sensation and discomfort in the breasts, abdomen and legs, probably associated with fluid retention. Pruritis, backache, muscle pain and joint pains may also occur (Dalton 1977). In addition, subclinical problems related to personality and neurotic disturbances are often exacerbated in the premenstrual period (Haskett et al. 1980). The symptoms usually develop in the 10 days before the period, and if the diagnosis is to be made it is important that the patient is symptom-free at some stage of the menstrual cycle. Because different authors have used different definitions of the premenstrual syndrome and because many studies have only examined women through a small number of menstrual cycles, it is difficult to obtain a consistent view of frequency of the condition, its aetiology or the response to treatment. The latter is especially difficult to establish because of the high placebo response in studies of just one to two menstrual cycles (Clare 1979).

Depending on the diagnostic criteria and the population studied, between 33% and 95% of women suffer from premenstrual tension. Clare (1977) studied a general practice sample and found that 75% of 521 women complained of at least one premenstrual symptom on the modified version of the menstrual distress questionnaire (Moos 1968). He was also able to show by their response to the General Health Questionnaire (Goldberg 1972) that there were as many psychologically healthy as disturbed women complaining of premenstrual symptoms.

Possible mechanisms causing premenstrual tension have been reviewed by Brush (1977). Among endocrine factors the following have been suggested: (1) progesterone deficiency in the second half of the cycle; (2) raised levels of oestradiol; (3) raised levels of aldosterone; (4) raised levels of prolactin; or (5) lack of balance between two or more hormones within their normal ranges.

Greene and Dalton (1953) suggested that the premenstrual syndrome is associated with low progesterone levels or an abnormal elevation of the oestradiol:progesterone ratio. Munday (1977) found plasma progesterone reduced in the 8 days premenstrually, but that the symptoms of the premenstrual tension started before the reduction in progesterone. O'Brien et al. (1980) claimed that women with premenstrual symptoms had higher progesterone concentrations in the postovulatory phase of the cycle compared with controls. These authors concluded that progesterone deficiency was probably not the cause of premenstrual tension and that treatment with progesterone was illogical unless a deficiency was detected. Dalton has taken issue with this paper because of the lack of clear definition of premenstrual tension and because free progesterone, most important in her opinion, was not measured.

Greene and Dalton (1953) claimed that treatment with progesterone was almost invariably successful. Rees (1953) also claimed in an uncontrolled study that the administration of progesterone such as ethisterone, or an androgen such as methyltestosterone, during the second half of the menstrual cycle was the most effective form of treatment. Taylor (1977) reported a 70% improvement in women treated with a synthetic progesterone, dydrogesterone, in a dose of 10 mg twice daily given from the 12th to the 20th day of the menstrual cycle. However, a controlled trial by Sampson (1979) failed to show any significant difference between placebo and progesterone 200 mg twice daily.

Plasma aldosterone has been found to be elevated in the premenstrual phase of the cycle but there was no significant difference in levels between symptomatic and asymptomatic groups (O'Brien et al. 1979; Munday 1977). In a double-blind clinical trial of spironolactone 25 mg taken four times daily from day 18 to 26, active treatment was shown to be superior to placebo and was effective in reducing weight and relieving psychological symptoms (O'Brien et al. 1979).

Raised levels of prolactin in the premenstrual phase have been shown by Munday (1977), Halbreich et al. (1976), Graham et al. (1978), and Andersen and Larsen (1979). Treatment of the premenstrual syndrome with bromocriptine has proved successful, when the dose is greater than 5 mg a day, in the trials of Benedek-Jaszmann and Hearn-Sturtevant (1976), Andersen et al. (1977) and Graham et al. (1978). Treatment with a dose of less than 5 mg a day (Harrison and Letchworth 1976; Ghose and Coppen 1977) was not effective. The higher dose of bromocriptine reduces psychiatric symptoms as well as reducing premenstrual weight gain and breast enlargement.

Pyridoxine has been tried in the treatment of premenstrual tension after it had been claimed that this substance can relieve depression in patients taking oral contraceptives. Pyridoxine has been claimed, in a controlled but non-blind study (Kerr 1977) to produce a 72% improvement. However, Stokes and Mendels (1972), in a double-blind comparison of pyridoxine and placebo, were unable to show any advantage due to treatment with pyridoxine. Lithium has also been used in an attempt to treat the premenstrual syndrome (Singer et al.

1974; Mattsson and von Schoultz, 1974; Steiner et al. 1980); but was found to be ineffective against the physical symptoms of the syndrome. In addition, most women suffered significant drug-related side effects.

There have been claims that oral contraceptives can be helpful in the treatment of premenstrual tension, but Clare (1977) failed to show any significant difference between the proportion of women suffering premenstrual tension who were taking these preparations and those who were not.

At present there is insufficient evidence to determine the most suitable treatment of premenstrual tension. Where progesterone deficiency is established, then treatment with progesterone would appear to be most appropriate while if prolactin levels are significantly raised, treatment with bromocriptine in a dose greater than 5 mg a day should be considered. If fluid retention is a problem, a diuretic may be helpful. More controlled trials, using clear operational diagnostic criteria and conducted over several cycles, are necessary.

VITAMINS

Pyridoxine may have a role in the treatment of depression associated with the oestrogen–progestogen oral contraceptives which are known to cause abnormalities of tryptophan and pyridoxine metabolism in some patients. Such effects could influence 5-hydroxytryptamine, which has been implicated in the genesis of depression.

Although depression has been regarded as a side effect of oral contraceptives, Goldzieher et al. (1971a,b) and Fleming and Seager (1978) were unable to show any evidence that oral contraceptive takers as a group were more depressed than non-takers. Herzberg et al. (1971) found that depression, headaches and loss of libido were the most common reasons for stopping oral contraceptives; however, the patients who stopped or changed their oral contraceptives had higher mean depression and neuroticism scores before starting treatment, and were more likely to have had a previous psychiatric history of depression.

Adams et al. (1973) studied 22 women without a history of previous psychiatric disorder who had developed depression in association with oral contraceptives. Approximately half had an absolute deficiency of pyridoxine and their depression was shown to improve with pyridoxine 20 mg twice daily in a double-blind cross-over trial. Pyridoxine was ineffective in patients without pyridoxine deficiency.

Treatment with pyridoxine should be considered for patients whose first depressive syndrome started in association with the use of an oral contraceptive, but the disorder may be coincidental and more conventional management may be indicated.

Administration of other vitamins in psychiatric disorder involves the correction of deficiency states. For example, thiamine may be indicated in chronic alcoholics with a poor diet to prevent the complication of Korsakoff's psychosis, while in some patients presenting with a chronic brain syndrome, a deficiency of B_{12} or folate may be found (Reynolds et al. 1973). Appropriate treatment may reverse or at least stop the progress of cognitive deficit, depending on the underlying pathology.

TREATMENTS FOR DEPRESSION AFTER HYSTERECTOMY

Richards (1973, 1974) reported an increased incidence of depression in the 5 years following hysterectomy compared with that of a similar group of women who had had other operations. However, Meikle (1977) was unable to show such a difference and, in a prospective study, Coppen et al. (1981) were unable to demonstrate any alteration in mood or sexual difficulties following hysterectomy. The women in this study were premenopausal and a controlled trial of 3 mg piperazine oestrone sulphate daily compared with placebo showed no advantage in outcome related to treatment with oestrogen.

TREATMENTS FOR MENOPAUSAL STATES

Although a number of current textbooks in gynaecology (cited by Wood 1979) refer to a menopausal syndrome with psychological features such as depression, nervousness, irritability, headache and insomnia, there is doubt whether these symptoms are significantly associated with the time of the menopause (Wood 1979; Bungay et al. 1980), and there is no difference in the pattern of symptomatology between males and females in the relevant age group (Bungay et al. 1980). However, an increased prevalence of minor psychiatric symptoms prior to the menopause has been noted (Ballinger 1975; Bungay et al. 1980) and Ballinger (1975) claimed that these were particularly related to environmental factors, especially to troubles with children. Ballinger (1976) studied patients of menopausal age who were receiving psychiatric treatment and concluded that there was no specific combination of psychiatric symptoms and signs peculiar to the menopause, and that women developing psychiatric symptoms at the time of the menopause appeared to belong to a vulnerable subgroup of the general population, and to have had a history of previous psychiatric illness.

Similar findings by other workers (Fessler 1950; Donovan 1951; Chakravarti et al. 1979) and the absence of evidence of an increase in suicide or hospitalization for affective disorder associated with the menopause (Winokur and Cadoret 1975), suggests that women with psychological problems at the time of the menopause may be selectively attracted to the gynaecological clinic. This explanation is supported by the finding of Worsley et al. (1977) that about 50%

of a sample of women attending out-patient gynaecological clinics suffered from evident psychological abnormality.

Although there is no evidence of any unusual or special psychiatric syndrome associated with the menopause, there seems to be general agreement that the symptoms of hot flushes (McKinlay et al. 1972; Ballinger 1975; Wood 1979) and dyspareunia due to atrophic vaginitis, do occur (Utian 1972; Beard 1975; Hutton et al. 1978; Chakravarti et al. 1979; Bungay et al. 1980).

Chakravarti et al. (1979) have shown that vasomotor symptoms are associated with low plasma oestradiol concentrations in women approaching the menopause. Hutton et al. (1978) compared plasma oestrone and oestradiol concentrations in menopausal women with both superficial dyspareunia and hot flushes, in women with flushes only, and in symptomless women. Women with superficial dyspareunia had significantly lower mean concentrations of plasma oestradiol compared with symptomless women, but intergroup differences in oestrone levels were not found. Flushes were not related to plasma oestrogen.

Clinical evaluation of treatment of the postmenopausal syndrome with natural oestrogen suggests that its primary value is in the treatment of women with hot flushes and superficial dyspareunia and that any alteration in affect is secondary to the suppression of these symptoms (Fessler 1950; Utian 1972; Chakravarti et al. 1979; Wood 1979). Thomson and Oswald (1977) found that piperazine oestrone did reduce the number of episodes of wakefulness in perimenopausal women complaining of insomnia but that it had no significant advantage over placebo for the treatment of flushes or psychological symptoms.

Oestrogens do not seem to be superior to placebo in the treatment of women whose depressive illness coincides with the menopause and who have little in the way of hot flushes or dyspareunia (Chakravarti et al. 1979) and the treatment of any woman with a clear psychiatric syndrome should be no different at the menopause than at any other time. However, if hot flushes and dyspareunia are an additional problem, treatment of these symptoms with oestriol 0.5–1 mg a day or oestradial valerate or oestrone sulphate up to 2 mg daily may be beneficial (Klopper 1976). The British National Formulary (1981) recommends ethinyloestriol as the treatment of choice in a dose of $10/20\,\mu$g daily. An alternative treatment for menopausal flushing is clonidine 2.5 mg twice daily to a maximum of 7.5 mg twice daily (Clayden et al. 1974).

References

ABRAMSON, R., GARG, M., CIOFFARI, A. & ROTMAN, P.A. (1980) An evaluation of behavioural techniques reinforced with an anorectic drug in a double-blind weight loss study. *J. clin. Psychiat.*, **41(7)**, 234.

ADAMS, P.W., ROSE, D.P., FOLKARD, J., WYNN, V., SEED, M. & STRONG, R. (1973) Effect of pyridoxine hydrochloride (vitamin B$_6$) upon depression associated with oral contraception. *Lancet*, i, 7809.

AGNOLI, A., RUGGIERI, S. & SASACCHIA, M. (1978) Restatement and prospectives of ergot alkaloids in clinical neurology and psychiatry. *Pharmacology*, **16**, (Suppl. 1), 174.

AMSTERDAM, J.D., WINOKUR, A., MENDELS, J. & CAROFF, S. (1979) Effect of gonadotropin-releasing hormone on depressed mood, *Lancet*, **ii**, 1138.

ANDERSEN, A.N. & LARSEN, J.F. (1979) Bromocriptine in the treatment of the premenstrual syndrome. *Drugs*, **17**, 383.

ANDERSEN, A.N., LARSEN, J.F., STEENSTRUP, O.R., SVENSTRUP, B. & NIELSEN, J. (1977) Effect of bromocriptine on the premenstrual syndrome. A double-blind clinical trial. *Br. J. Obstet. Gynaecol.*, **84**, 370.

BALLINGER, C.B. (1975) Psychiatric morbidity and the menopause: screening of general population sample. *Br. med. J.*, **3**, 344.

BALLINGER, C.B. (1976) Psychiatric morbidity and the menopause: clinical features. *Br. med. J.*, **1**, 1183.

BANCROFT, J., TENNENT, G., LOUCAS, K. & CASS, J. (1974) The control of deviant sexual behaviour by drugs: 1. Behavioural changes following oestrogens and anti-androgens. *Br. J. Psychiat.*, **125**, 310.

BEARD, R.J. (1975) The menopause. *Br. J. hosp. Med.*, vol. **13**, no. 5, 631.

BENEDEK-JASZMANN, L.J. & HEARN-STURTEVANT, M.D. (1976) Premenstrual tension and functional infertility. Aetiology and treatment, *Lancet*, **ii**, 1095.

BENKERT, O., GORDON, A. & MARTSCHKE, D. (1974) The comparison of thyrotrophin releasing hormone, luteinising hormone-releasing hormone and placebo in depressive patients using a double-blind cross-over technique. *Psychopharmacologia*, **40**, 191.

BESSER, G.M., THORNER, M.O., WASS, J.A.H., DONIACH, I., CANTI, G., CURLING, M., GRUDZINIS-KAS, J.G. & SETCHELL, M.E. (1977) Absence of uterine neoplasia in patients on bromocriptine. *Br. med. J.*, **2**, 868.

BOMMER, J., DEL POZO, E., RITZ, E. & BOMMER, G. (1979) Improved sexual function in male haemodialysis patients on bromocriptine. *Lancet*, **ii**, 496.

BRAMBILLA, F., SMERALDI, E., SACCHETTI, E., et al. (1978) Deranged anterior pituitary responsiveness to hypothalamic hormone in depressed patients. *Archs gen. Psychiat.*, **35**, 1231.

BRITISH NATIONAL FORMULARY, 1981, Number 1. British Medical Association and the Pharmaceutical Society of Great Britain.

BRUSH, M.G., (1977) The possible mechanisms causing the premenstrual tension syndrome. *Curr. Med. Res. Opin.*, **4**, *Suppl. 4*, 9.

BUNGAY, G.T., VESSEY, M.P. & McPHERSON, C.K. (1980) Study of symptoms in middle life with special reference to the menopause. *Br. med. J.*, **1**, 181.

BURG, W. VAN DEN, PRAAG, H.M. VAN, BOS, E.R.H., PIERS, D.A., ZANTEN, A.K. VAN, & DOORENBOS, H. (1976) TRH by slow, continuous infusion: an antidepressant? *Psychol. Med.*, **6**, (3) 393.

CARMAN, J.S., POST, R.M., BUSWELL, R. & GOODWIN, F.K. (1976) Negative effects of melatonin on depression. *Am. J. Psychiat.*, **133**(10), 1181.

CHAKRAVARTI, S., COLLINS, W.P., THOM, M.H. & STUDD, J.W.W. (1979) Relation between plasma hormone profiles, symptoms, and response to oestrogen treatment in women approaching the menopause. *Br. med. J.*, **1**, 983.

CLARE, A.W. (1977) Psychological profiles of women complaining of premenstrual symptoms. *Curr. Med. Res. Opin.*, **4**, *Suppl. 4*, 23.

CLARE, A.W. (1979) The treatment of premenstrual symptoms. *Br. J. Psychiat.*, **135**, 576.

CLAYDEN, J.R., BELL, J.W. & POLLARD, P. (1974) Menopausal flushing: double-blind trial of a non-hormonal medication. *Br. med. J.*, **1**, 409.

COLONNA, L., PETIT, M. & LKEPINE, J.P. (1978) Intérêt de la bromocriptine dans les schizophrénies dysthymiques. *Encéphale*, **4**, 115.

COLONNA, L., PETIT, M. & LEPINE, J.P. (1979) Bromocriptine in affective disorders. A pilot study. *J. Affect. Dis.*, **1**, 173.

COMMITTEE OF THE CLINICAL SOCIETY OF LONDON (1888) Report on myxoedema. *Trans. Clin. Soc. London*, Vol. **21** (Suppl.), 30.

COPPEN, A., BISHOP, M., BEARD, R.J., BARNARD, G.J.R. & COLLINS, W.P. (1981) Hysterectomy, hormones and behaviour. A prospective study. *Lancet*, **i**, 126.

COPPEN, A., MONTGOMERY, S., PEET, M., BAILEY, J., MARKS, V. & WOODS, P. (1974) Thyrotrophin-releasing hormone in the treatment of depression. *Lancet*, **ii**, 433.

COPPEN, A., WHYBROW, P.C., NOGUERA, R., MAGGS, R. & PRANGE, A.J. Jr. (1972) The comparative antidepressant value of -tryptophan and imipramine with and without attempted potentiation by liothyronine. *Arch. Gen. Psychiat.*, **26**, 234.

COSTELLO, R.M. (1975) Acoholism treatment and evaluation: in search of methods. *Int. J. Addict.*, **10**, 251.

DALTON, K. (1977) *The Premenstrual Syndrome and Progesterone Therapy*. London: Heinemann Books.

DAVIES, T.F., MOUNTJOY, C.Q., GOMEZ-PAN, A., WATSON, M.J., HANKER, J.P., BESSER, G.M. & HALL, R. (1976) A double-blind cross over trial of gonadotrophin releasing hormine (LHRH) in sexually impotent men. *Clin. Endoc.*, **5**, 601.

DIMITRIKOUDI, M., HANSON-NORTY, E. & JENNER, F.A. (1974) TRH in psychoses. *Lancet*, **i**, 456.

DONOVAN, J.C. (1951) Menopausal syndrome: a study of case histories. *Am. J. Obstet. Gynec.*, **62**, 1281.

DORR, C. & SATHANANTHAN, K. (1976) Treatment of mania with bromocriptine (letter to the editor). *Br. med. J.*, **i**, 1342.

EARLE, B.V. (1970) Thyroid hormone and tricyclic antidepressants in resistant depressions. *Am. J. Psychiat.*, **126**, 1667.

EHRENSING, R.H., KASTIN, A.J., SCHALCH, D.S., FRIESEN, H.G., BARGAS, J.R. & SCHALLY, A.V. (1974) Affective state and thyrotrophin and prolactin responses after repeated injections of thyrotrophin-releasing hormone in depressed patients. *Am. J. Psychiat.*, **131**, 714.

EVANS, L.E.J., HUNTER, P.R., HALL, R., JOHNSTON, M. & ROY, V.M. (1975) A double-blind trial of intravenous thyrotrophin-releasing hormone in the treatment of reactive depression. *Br. J. Psychiat.*, **127**, 227.

FEIGHNER, J.P., KING, L.J., SCHUCKIT, M.A., CROUGHAN, J. & BRISCOE, W. (1972) Hormonal potentiation of imipramine and ECT in primary depression. *Am. J. Psychiat.*, **128**, 1230.

FESSLER, L. (1950) The psychopathology of climacteric depression. *Psychoanal. Q.*, **19**, 28.

FIELD, L.H. & WILLIAMS, M. (1970) The hormonal treatment of sexual offenders. *Medicine, Sci. Law*, **13**, 195.

FLEMING, O. & SEAGER, C.P. (1978) Incidence of depressive symptoms in users of the oral contraceptive. *Br. J. Psychiat.*, **132**, 431.

FOLLOWS, O.J. (1971) A comparative trial of fenfluramine and diethylpropion in obese, hypertensive patients. *Br. J. clin. Pract.*, **25**(5), 236.

FRANK, R.T. (1931) The hormonal causes of premenstrual tension. *Arch. Neurol. Psychiat.*, **26**, 37.

FULLER, R.K. & ROTH, H.P. (1979) Disulfiram for the treatment of alcoholism. An evaluation in 128 men. *Ann. intern. Med.*, **90**, 901.

GARATTINI, S., BORRONI, E., MENNINI, T. & SAMANIN, R. (1978) Differences and similarities between anorectic agencts. In: *Central Mechanisms of Anorectic Drugs*, ed. S. Garattini & R. Samanin. New York: Raven Press.

GELDER, M.G. & EDWARDS, G. (1976) Metronidazole in the treatment of alcohol addiction: a controlled trial. In: *Alcohol Dependence and Smoking Behaviour*, ed. Edwards, G., Russell, M.A.H., Hawks, D. & MacCafferty, M., pp. 95–97. Farnborough: Saxon House.

GHOSE, K. & COPPEN, A. (1977) Bromocriptine and premenstrual syndrome: controlled study. *Br. med. J.*, **i**, 147.

GOLD, P.W., BALLENGER, J.C., WEINGARTNER, H., GOODWIN, F.K. & POST, R.M. (1979) Effects of 1-desamino-8-D-arginine vasopressin on behaviour and cognition in primary affective disorder. *Lancet*, **ii**, 992.

GOLDBERG, D. (1972) 'The Detection of Psychiatric Illness by Questionnaire'. Maudsley Monograph No. 21. London: Oxford University Press.

GOLDZIEHER, J.W., MOSES, L.E., AVERKIN, E., SCHEEL, C. & TABER, B.Z. (1971a) A placebo-controlled double-blind crossover investigation of the side effects attributed to oral contraceptives. *Fertility Sterility*, **22**, 609.

GOLDZIEHER, J.W., MOSES, L.E., AVERKIN, E., SCHEEL, C. & TABER, B.Z. (1971b) Nervousness and depression attributed to oral contraceptives: a double-blind placebo-controlled study. *Am. J. Obstet. Gynec.*, **111**, 1013.

GOLLA, F.L. & HODGE, S.R. (1949) Hormone treatment of sex offenders. *Lancet*, **i**, 1006.

GRAHAM, J.J., HARDING, P.E., WISE, P.H. & BERRIMAN, H. (1978) Prolactin suppression in the treatment of premenstrual syndrome. *Med. J. Aust. Special Suppl.*, 18.

GRAVES, R.J., (1835) Newly observed affection of the thyroid gland in females. *Lond. Med. Surg. J.*, **7**, 516.

GREENE, R. & DALTON, K. (1953) The premenstrual syndrome. *Br. med. J.*, **i**, 1007.

GUNN, J. (1976) Sexual offenders. *Br. J. hosp. Med.*, **15**(1), 57.

HALBREICH, J., ASSAEL, M., BEN-DAVID, M. & BORNSTEIN, R. (1976) Serum prolactin in women with premenstrual syndrome. *Lancet*, **ii**, 654.

HALL, R., HUNTER, P.R., PRICE, J.S. & MOUNTJOY, C.Q., (1975) Thyrotrophin-releasing hormone in depression. *Lancet*, **i**, 162.

HARRISON, P. & LETCHWORTH, A.T. (1976) Bromocriptine in the treatment of the premenstrual syndrome. Proceedings from a Symposium held at the Royal College of Physicians, London, p. 103.

HARROWER, A.D.B., YAP, P.L., NAIRN, I.M., WALTON, H.J., STRONG, J.A. & CRAIG, A. (1977) Growth hormone, insulin, and prolactin secretion in anorexia nervosa and obesity during bromocriptine treatment. *Br. med. J.*, **ii**, 156.

HASKETT, R.F., STEINER, M., OSMUN, J.N. & CARROLL, B.J. (1980) Severe premenstrual tension—Delineation of the syndrome. *Biol. Psychiat.*, **15**(1), 121.

HERZBERG, B.N., DRAPER, K.C., JOHNSON, A.L. & NICOL, G.C. (1971) Oral contraceptives, depression and libido. *Br. med. J.*, **3**, 485.

HOLLISTER, L.E., BERGER, P., OGLE, F.L., ARNOLD, R.C. & JOHNSON, A. (1974) Protirelin (T.R.H.) in depression. *Archs gen. Psychiat.*, **31**, 468.

HORE, B.D. (1977) Clinical features and treatment of alcoholism. *Br. J. Hosp. Med.*, **18**, 106.

HORROBIN, D.F., KARMALI, R.A., MTABAJI, J.P., MANKU, M.S. & NASSAR, B.A. (1976) Prolactin and mental illness, *Postgrad. med. J.*, **52** (Suppl. 3), 79.

HUDSON, K.D. (1977) The anorectic and hypotensive effect of fenfluramine in obesity. *J. Roy. Coll. G.P..*, **27**, 497.

HUTTON, J.D., JACOBS, H.S., MURRAY, M.A.F. & JAMES, V.H.T. (1978) Relation between plasma oestrone and oestradiol and climacteric symptoms. *Lancet*, **i**, 678.

INNES, J.A., WATSON, M.L., FORD, M.J., MUNRO, J.F., STODDART, M.E. & CAMPBELL, D.B. (1977) Plasma fenfluramine levels, weight loss and side effects. *Br. med. J.*, **2**, 1322.

KASTIN, A.J., EHRENSING, R.H., SCHALCH, D.S. & ANDERSEN, M.S. (1972) Improvement in mental depressed with decreased thyrotrophin response after administration of thyrotrophin-releasing hormone, *Lancet*, **ii**, 740.

KERR, G.D. (1977) The management of the premenstrual syndrome. *Curr. Med. Res. Opin.*, **4**, Suppl. 4, 29.

KING, D.J. (1978) Dopamine agonists for negative symptoms in schizophrenia. *Br. J. clin. Pharmacol.*, **6**, 541.

KIRBY, M.J. & TURNER, P. (1976) Do 'anorectic' drugs produce weight loss by appetite suppression? *Lancet*, **i**, 566.

KLAIBER, E.L., BROVERMAN, D.M., VOGEL, W. &KOBAYASHI, Y. (1979) Estrogen therapy for severe persistent depressions in women. *Archs gen. Psychiat.*, **36**, 550.

KLOPPER, A. (1976) Endocrine and metabolic diseases. Treatment of infertility and menopausal symptoms. *Br. med. J.*, **2**, 414.

LELE, R.D., JOSHI, V.R. & NATHWANI, A.N., (1972) A double-blind clinical trial of fenfluramine. *Br. J. Clin. Pract.*, **26**, 79.

LINNOILA, M., LAMBERG, B.A., ROSBERG, G. et al. (1979) Thyroid hormones and TSH, Prolactin, and LH responses to repeated TRH and LRH injections in depressed patients. *Acta psychiat. scand.*, **59**, 536.

LOOSEN, P.T., PRANGE, A.J. Jr. & WILSON, I.C. (1979) TRH (Protirelin) in depressed alcoholic men: Behavioural changes and endocrine responses. *Archs gen. Psychiat.*, **36**, 540.

MALCOLM, M.T. & MADDEN, J.S. (1973) The use of disulfiram implantation in alcoholism. *Br. J. Psychiat.*, **123**, 41.

MARCH, C.M. (1979) Bromocriptine in the treatment of hypogonadism and male impotence. *Drugs*, **17**, 349.

MATTSSON, B. & SCHOULTZ, B. VON (1974) A comparison between lithium, placebo and a diuretic in premenstrual tension. *Acta psychiat. scand.*, (*Suppl.*) **225**, 75.

MCKINLAY, S., JEFFERYS, M. & THOMPSON, B. (1972) An investigation of the age at menopause. *J. Biosoc. Sci.*, **4**, 161.

MEIKLE, S., BRODY, H. & PYSH, F. (1977) An investigation into the psychological effects of hysterectomy. *J. nerv. ment. Dis.*, **164**(1), 36.

MERRY, J., REYNOLDS, C.M., BAILEY, J. & COPPEN, A. (1976) Prophylactic treatment of alcoholism by lithium carbonate. *Lancet*, **ii**, 481.

METCALF, G. & DETTMAR, P.W. (1981) Is thyrotrophin releasing hormone an endogenous ergotropic substance in the brain? *Lancet*, **i**, 586.

MOOS, R.H. (1968) The development of a menstrual distress questionnaire. *Psychosom. Med.*, **30**, 853.

MOUNTJOY, C.Q., PRICE, J.S., WELLER, M., HUNTER, P, HALL, R. & DEWAR, J.H. (1974) A double-blind crossover sequential trial of oral thyrotrophin-releasing hormone in depression. *Lancet*, **i**, 958.

MUNDAY, M. (1977) Hormone levels in severe premenstrual tension. *Curr. Med. Res. Opin.*, **4**, *Suppl. 4*, 16.

O'BRIEN, P.M.S., CRAVEN, D., SELBY, C. & SYMONDS, E.M. (1979) Treatment of premenstrual syndrome by spironolactone. *Br. J. Obstet. Gynaecol.*, **86**, 142.

O'BRIEN, P.M.S., SELBY, C. & SYMONDS, E.M. (1980) Progesterone, fluid and electrolytes in premenstrual syndrome. *Br. med. J.*, **280**, 1161.

OSWALD, I., LEWIS, S.A., DUNLEAVY, D.L.F., BREZINOVA, V. & BRIGGS, M. (1971) Drugs of dependence though not of abuse: fenfluramine and imipramine. *Br. med. J.*, **3**, 70.

PHUAPRADIT, P., PHILLIPS, M., LESS, A.J. & STERN, G.M. (1978) Bromocriptine in presenile dementia (letter). *Br. med. J.*, **1**, 1052.

PLOTNIKOFF, N.P., PRANGE, A.J., BREESE, G.R., ANDERSON, M.S. & WILSON, I.C. (1974) The effects of thyrotrophin-releasing hormone on dopa response in normal, hypophysectomised and thyroidectomised animals. In: *The Thyroid Axis, Drugs and Behaviour*, ed. Prange, A.J. Jr. New York: Raven Press.

PRANGE, A.J. Jr. & LIPTON, M.A. (1962) Enhancement of imipramine mortality in hypothyroid mice. *Nature (Lond.)*, **196**, 588.

PRANGE, A.J. Jr., LIPTON, M.A. & LOVE, G.N. (1963) Diminution of imipramine mortality in hypothyroid mice. *Nature (Lond.)*, **197**, 1212.

PRANGE, A.J. Jr., WILSON, I.C., LARA, P.P., ALLTOP, L.B. & BREESE, G.R. (1972) Effects of thyrotrophin-releasing hormone in depression. *Lancet*, **ii**, 999.

PRANGE, A.J. Jr., WILSON, I.C., RABON, A.M. & LIPTON, M.A. (1969) Enhancement of imipramine antidepressant activity by thyroid hormone. *Am. J. Psychiat.*, **126**, 457.

REES, L. (1953) The premenstrual tension syndrome and its treatment. *Br. med. J.*, **1**, 1014.

REYNOLDS, E.H., ROTHFIELD, P. & PUICUS, J.H. (1973) Neurological disease associated with folate deficiency. *Br. med. J.*, **2**, 398.

RICHARDS, D.H. (1973) Depression after hysterectomy. *Lancet*, **ii**, 430.

RICHARDS, D.H. (1974) A post-hysterectomy syndrome. *Lancet*, **ii**, 983.

RITSON, E.B., (1975) Psychological medicine. Treatment of alcoholism. *Br. med. J.*, **2**, 124.

ROBICHAUD, C., STRICKLER, D., BIGELOW, G. & LIEBSON, I. (1979) Disulfiram maintenance employee alcoholism treatment: A three-phase evaluation. *Behav. Res. Ther.*, **17**, 618.

SAINANI, G.S., FULAMBARKAR, A.M. & KHURANA, B.K. (1973) A double-blind clinical trial of fenfluramine in the treatment of obesity. *Br. J. Clin. Pract.*, **27**(4), 136.

SAMPSON, G.A. (1979) Premenstrual syndrome: A double-blind controlled trial of progesterone and placebo. *Br. J. Psychiat.*, **135**, 209.

SARAN, B.M. & ACHARYA, S. (1977) Bromocriptine in treating mania. *Am. J. Psychiat.*, **134**(6), 702.

SCHMIDT, J. (1977) Treatment of endogenous depressions with thyrotrophin-releasing hormone. *Acta. psychiat. scand.*, **55**, 142.

SINGER, K., CHENG, R. & SCHOU, M. (1974) A controlled evaluation of lithium in the premenstrual tension syndrome. *Br. J. Psychiat.*, **124**, 50.

SMITH, A.W., CHAMBERS, C. & NAYLOR, G.J. (1980) Bromocriptine in mania—a placebo-controlled double-blind trial. *Br. med. J.*, **280**, 86.

STEEL, J.M. & BRIGGS, M. (1972) Withdrawal depression in obese patients after fenfluramine treatment. *Br. med. J.*, **3**, 26.

STEINER, M., HASKETT, R.F., OSMUN, J.N. & CARROLL, B.J. (1980) Treatment of premenstrual tension with lithium carbonate. *Acta. psychiat. Scand.*, **61**, 96.

STOKES, J. & MENDELS, J. (1972) Pyridoxine and premenstrual tension. *Lancet*, **i**, 1177.

STUNKARD, A.J., CRAIGHEAD, L.W. & O'BRIEN, R. (1980) Controlled trial of behaviour therapy, pharmacotherapy, and their combination in the treatment of obesity. *Lancet*, **ii**, 1045.

STUNKARD, A., RICKELS, K. & HESBACHER, P. (1973) Fenfluramine in the treatment of obesity. *Lancet*, **i**, 503.

SYMMERS, W. ST. C. (1968) Carcinoma of breast in transsexual individuals after surgical and hormonal interference with primary and secondary sex characteristics. *Br. med. J.*, **2**, 83.

TAKAHASHI, S., KONDO, H., YOSHIMURA, M. & OCHI, Y. (1973) Antidepressant effect of thyrotrophin-releasing hormone (T.R.H.) and the plasma thyrotrophine levels in depression. *Folia psychiat. neurol. Jap.*, **27**, 305.

TAYLOR, R.W. (1977) The treatment of premenstrual tension with dydrogesterone ('Duphaston'). *Curr. Med. Res. Opin.*, **4**, *Suppl. 4*, 35.

TENNENT, G., BANCROFT, J. & CASS, J. (1972) The Control of Deviant Sexual Behaviour by Drugs: A Double-Blind Controlled Study of Benperidol, Chlorpromazine and Placebo. Special Hospitals Research Report No. 5. London: Special Hospitals Research Unit.

THOMSON, J. & OSWALD, I. (1977) Effect of oestrogen on the sleep, mood and anxiety of menopausal women. *Br. med. J.*, **2**, 1317.

THORNER, M.O., MCNEILLY, A.S., HAGAN, C. & BESSER, G.M. (1974) Long-term treatment of galactorrhoea and hypogonadism with bromocriptine. *Br. med. J.*, **2**, 419.

UTIAN, W.H. (1972) The true clinical features of postmenopause and oöphorectomy and their response to oestrogen therapy. *S afr. med. J.*, **46**, 732.

VOGEL, H.P., BENKERT, O., ILLIG, R., MÜLLER-OERLINGHAUSEN, B. & POPPENBERG, A. (1977) Psychoendocrinological and therapeutic effects of TRH in depression. *Acta. psychiat. scand.*, **56**, 223.

WASS, J.A.H., THORNER, M.O., BESSER, G.M., MORRIS, D., STUART MASON, A., LIUIZZI, A. & CHIODINI, P.G. (1976) Gastrointestinal bleeding in patients on bromocriptine. *Lancet*, **ii**, 851.

WHEATLEY, D. (1972) Potentiation of amitriptyline by thyroid hormone. *Archs gen. Psychiat.*, **26**, 229.

WHITAKER, L.H. (1959) Oestrogen and psychosexual disorders. *Med. J. Aust.*, **2**, 547.

WHYTE, C.R. & O'BRIEN, P.M.J. (1974) Disulfiram implant: a controlled trial. *Br. J. Psychiat.*, **124**, 42.

WILSON, A., DAVIDSON, W.J. & WHITE, J. (1976) Disulfiram implantation: placebo, psychological deterrent, and pharmacological deterrent effects. *Br. J. Psychiat.*, **129**, 277.

WILSON, I.C., PRANGE, A.J. Jr., MCCLANE, T.K., RABON, A.M. & LIPTON, M.A. (1970) Thyroid-hormone enhancement of imipramine in now retarded depressions. *New Eng. J. Med.*, **282**, 1063.

WINOKUR, G. & CADORET, R. (1975) The irrelevance of the menopause to depressive illness. In: *Topics in Psychoendocrinology*, ed. Sachar, E.J. Seminars in Psychiatry. London: Grune & Stratton.

WOOD, C. (1979) Menopausal myths. *Med. J. Aust.*, **1**, 496.

WORSLEY, A. & WALTERS, W.A.W., WOOD, E.C. (1977) Screening for psychological disturbance amongst gynaecology patients. *Aust. N.Z. J. Obstet. Gynaecol.*, **17**, 214.

6

The Convulsive Therapies

G.E. Berrios

INTRODUCTION

Artificially induced seizures in humans alter cognition, level of arousal, quality of consciousness and mood. The former three effects are short lived and considered as clinically undesirable. Mood change, on the other hand, is longer lasting and may result from modifications in the sensitivity of certain populations of brain receptors. In spite of claims that electro-convulsive therapy (ECT) produces brain damage, no substantial evidence is available.

Electricity is the most commonly used convulsive agent. Camphor in oil, picrotoxine or metrazol are no longer used, as control of the timing and number of seizures is difficult. Flurothyl, an ether derivative, is as effective as electricity, and produces less memory impairment but more headache and nausea.

The original technique of ECT has been modified by the introduction of drugs and oxygenation. However, the belief that these ameliorate side effects is not yet fully substantiated. It may even be that the modifications themselves produce (or worsen) side effects.

The quality of research into the effectiveness of ECT has of late improved, and a number of double-blind controlled trials (i.e. real vs. simulated ECT) have been carried out. Experimental work into its mode of action is also taking place.

ECT started as a treatment for schizophrenia, but it soon became apparent that it had a better and more sustained effect on some forms of affective disorder. However, catatonic schizophrenia is still treated by ECT, as are some severe and neuroleptic-resistant forms of schizophrenic, schizoaffective, and cycloid psychoses. Persisting organic delirious states may also, on occasions, require ECT.

INDICATIONS

Depression

The primary indication for ECT is those depressive states which are characterized by such features as delusions, guilt, remorse, nihilistic ideas, hallucinations, psychomotor retardation, biological shift (i.e. disturbance of appetite, bowel habit, sleep, weight, sexual drive), suicidal risk, and stuporous behaviour. It is accepted that severe depression of endogenous aetiology is often not responsive to, or may be made worse by, tricyclic antidepressants. If the patient does not respond to these drugs this is also considered as an indication for ECT.

Although methodological deficiencies have bedevilled the literature (Riddell 1963; Barton 1977; Scovern and Kilmann 1980) the available evidence supports the firm belief of most clinicians that ECT is more effective than other antidepressant treatments for certain forms of depression (Turek and Hanlon 1977; Scovern and Kilmann 1980). Freeman et al. (1978) gave two simulated ECTs in the course of ECT treatment and found that patients so treated took longer to recover compared with a group who received genuine ECT throughout. Lambourn and Gill (1978) gave unilateral simulated ECT to 16 depressives and found no difference with controls, but the diagnosis was unclear, as was the severity of the disorder; also, there was no EEG monitoring to ascertain if bilateral seizures had taken place. Johnstone et al. (1980) gave real or simulated ECT to 'endogenous' depressives but variations in the severity of illness may have affected the results. Both groups 'improved considerably during the course of treatment but the improvement was greater in the real ECT group'. However, the advantage of real over simulated ECT was not retained, and at the 1-month and 6-month follow-ups the Hamilton scores of the two groups were almost the same. West (1981) gave simulated ECT to a sample of 22 'primary' depressives, while a matched group received real ECT. The latter group improved markedly on three different measures, in contrast to the control group, and the patients who had received simulated ECT improved when switched to real ECT. Although, in general, this evidence supports the value of ECT in certain depressive disorders, it would seem that in most of these studies the patients involved did not consistently present the type of depressive disorder which would be generally considered as 'almost certain to respond' to this form of treatment. It has also been reported that ECT normalizes the Dexamethasone Suppression Test in unipolar depressives (Albala et al. 1981).

Attempts have been made to identify depressive phenomena that might predict successful outcome, and clinical, personality, neurophysiological and pharmacological aspects have been studied. The results have been disappointing. For example, predictive scales based on clinical features do not seem superior to clinical assessment. The predictive value of subjective and physiological responses to methedrine, methacholine, and amylobarbitone have also been investigated, but the response scatter, false positives and false negatives, prevent their use in clinical practice. Neurophysiological predictors, such as an early appearance of EEG slow wave activity following ECT (Roth et al. 1957) or following an injection of amylobarbitone (Shagass and Jones 1958) have been claimed to predict positive outcome; this has since been challenged (Volavka 1974).

It is unclear whether ECT reduces the likelihood of a future relapse (Kalinowsky 1980), and whether there is a crucial time during the depressive episode in which the condition is more susceptible to ECT. Some believe that ECT is less successful when given too early or too late in relation to onset. Others claim that the earlier the application of ECT, the fewer the treatments that are required to achieve improvement (Snaith 1981). The belief that extra applications of ECT (after clinical improvement) 'stabilize outcome' (Kalinowsky and Hippius 1969) has not been substantiated (Barton et al. 1973).

If required, ECT may be given in the presence of severe physical conditions such as heart disease (Regestein and Lind 1980; Bidder 1981). In the case of Parkinson's disease, it has been claimed that it may even improve the physical condition (Asnis 1977; Yudofsky 1979; Balldin et al. 1981).

Schizophrenia

The question of the efficacy of ECT in schizophrenia remains unanswered. While reviewers agree on the dearth of hard evidence in favour of a sustained effect (Greenblatt 1977; Turek and Hanlon 1977; Freeman 1979; Fink 1979*a*; Salzman 1980; Taylor 1981), clinicians continue using it in selected cases. It is considered as a 'mood modifier' (Müller 1960), an 'adjuvant' (Angst 1975), a controller of 'hyperactivity' (Baruk 1960), a 'life saving' treatment in catatonic stupor, and as the 'last resort' in severe schizophrenia refractory to neuroleptics (Ey et al. 1974).

ECT reduces hallucinations, anxiety, hyperactivity, aggression, suicidal behaviour, mood disorder and stupor but has less effect on thought disorder, delusions, apathy and incongruency (Fink 1979*a*). For these latter phenomena, a combination of ECT and neuroleptics may be more effective (Salzman 1980). Early comparisons of real and simulated ECT in schizophrenia did not show the former to be superior (Brill 1959), but a recent double-blind study on ten 'paranoid schizophrenics' indicated that the group which received ECT improved significantly in comparison with a group which received simulated treatment (Taylor and Fleminger 1980). Chronicity and 'negative' symptoms (e.g. lack of initiative or drive) carry a bad response to ECT (Fink 1979*a*). Flurothyl-induced convulsions have been reported as superior to ECT in the treatment of both schizophrenia (Freund and Warren 1965) and schizoaffective disorders (Ries et al. 1981). Protracted delirium may also be treated by ECT (Kramp and Bolwig 1981).

Mania

Few controlled studies exist on the efficacy of ECT in mania (Fink 1979*b*), but it is widely accepted that manic patients (especially those with acute onset and good premorbid adjustment), respond favourably, particularly in relation to symptoms such as acute excitement, aggression and exhaustion (Schiele and Schneider 1949). ECT compares well with neuroleptics (Langsley et al 1959; McCabe and Norris 1977) and is better than no treatment on outcome variables such as mental state, duration of hospitalization and social recovery (McCabe 1976). ECT is used in the USA for the treatment of mania (Asnis et al. 1978) and is recommended in the UK in selected cases (Ashcroft et al. 1978; Kendell 1981).

CONTRAINDICATIONS

Near-absolute contraindications to ECT are myocardial infarction and cerebrovascular accident during the previous 6 weeks, although when it is considered as life saving, ECT may occasionally be given to such patients or to those with high 'anaesthetic risk' (Gerring and Shields 1982). For example, ECT may be the only method to save the life of a patient with stuporous depression who is refusing food or drink even though he may have had a myocardial infarction 3 weeks previously (Regestein and Lind 1980). In most cases monitoring equipment and a consultant anaesthetist must be at hand.

Cerebral oedema (for example following carbon monoxide poisoning) and raised intracranial pressure are contraindications to ECT, and, in general, ECT should not be given to a patient with a brain tumour, although it may be prescribed as a last resort in cases of severe depression when no surgical solution is available (Dressler and Folk 1975). The mortality resulting from neurological complications associated with ECT in a series of patients with brain tumours was 28% within 1 month of the treatment (Maltbie et al. 1980). However, no correlation was found between tumour type, size or location, and increased risk of mortality.

Pregnancy is not a contraindication to ECT (Smith 1956; Sobel 1960). It has been reported that there were no adverse effects on a group of children whose mothers were given ECT during pregnancy (Forssman 1955).

Age is not considered as a crucial excluding factor. There is a natural reluctance to give ECT to infants or children although this has occasionally been done in cases of severe depression unresponsive to pharmacotherapy (Frommer 1968), or in rare cases of schizophrenia (Hift et al. 1960). Combinations of ECT and lithium may sometimes reduce the therapeutic effect of the former (Small et al. 1980).

The elderly or the mildly demented should be given unilateral ECT to the non-dominant hemisphere, which mitigates memory impairment and post-ECT confusion (Fraser and Glass 1978; Gaspar and Samarasinghe 1982). Patients fitted with heart pacemakers can also receive ECT (Abuiso 1978). Patients with severe arterial hypertension are at risk of cerebrovascular accident, as critical increases in blood pressure take place during ECT particularly in atropinized hypertensives (Bodley and Fenwick 1966); but in life-threatening situations ECT can be given provided that the hypertension is treated by a nitroprusside microdrip and the atropine omitted (Regestein and Lind 1980). Patients suffering from severe cardiac arrhythmias must be carefully monitored, as ECT increases heart rate, and may be associated with an increased QT interval and decreased P–R interval (Troup et al. 1978). The occasional cardiovascular complications of ECT should not be allowed to obscure the fact that this treatment is safer than many tricyclic antidepressant drugs, which may induce a persistent conduction disorder (Burrows et al. 1976). A temporary increase in blood–brain barrier permeability takes place immediately after ECT (Bolwig et al. 1977; Bradbury 1979), and this may constitute a potential contraindication in patients taking neurotoxic drugs. The therapeutic use of this phenomenon has not yet been explored.

TECHNIQUE

Before the convulsive stimulus the patient is given a short-acting anaesthetic, an antimuscarinic agent, a muscle relaxant and oxygen. These 'modifications' are believed to minimize anxiety, excessive salivation, vagal overstimulation, fractures, hypoxaemia, confusion and headaches. ECT in the UK is given in special treatment units (Pippard and Ellam 1981) and in most centres an anaesthetist, psychiatrist and nurse are in attendance.

Preparation of the patient is important and should involve a full assessment of anaesthetic risk. Potential interactions between current (and recent) medications and the drugs used in the ECT procedure must be considered, and it should also be remembered that some drugs modify the convulsive threshold. Fasting for at least 6 h before treatment is mandatory, and dentures and prostheses must be removed. Physical handicaps (e.g. hemiplegic limbs) must be recorded as these may not show the motor activity which indicates that a seizure has been successfully induced. Since age, sex, mental state, diagnosis and medications directly influence seizure threshold, these factors must be taken into consideration to adjust the 'dose' of electricity. A rubber mouth 'gag' should be used to protect gums, teeth and tongue.

Informed consent must be obtained if this is possible, and the Royal College of Psychiatrists (1977) has provided the following guidance: 'Consent is a matter between patient and doctor and it is a medical responsibility to ensure that the patient has been given an explanation of the procedure, benefits and dangers'. In case of refusal to provide consent (or inability to do so, for example, if the patient is in a depressive stupor), a decision has to be made whether there are grounds to attempt to overrule this objection by compulsorily administering treatment. If the psychiatrist feels that compulsory treatment is justified, it is the College's recommendation that Section 26 of the Mental Health Act 1959 be applied and that ECT should not be given under Section 25. A further recommendation was that a second consultant opinion should be sought, and the matter discussed with staff and relatives, unless immediate treatment seems imperative. Consent warrants only one series of treatments; if an interval (the length of which has not yet been stipulated) elapses, then another consent must be obtained.

The Anaesthetic

Intravenous thiopentone sodium in a 2.5% solution (150–250 mg) is commonly used, although it occasionally causes arrhythmias (Pitts et al. 1965; Woodruff 1969). Intravenous methohexitone in a 1% solution (60–100 mg) allows a quicker recovery, and this drug has fewer cardiac side effects (Allen and Pitts 1979). Spontaneous breathing occurs earlier with methohexitone (mean interval = 59.4 s) than with thiopentone (mean interval = 80.0 s) (Tresise and Stenhouse 1968). Methohexitone, however, shortens EEG seizure duration by 42% when compared with ketamine (Lunn et al. 1981). Barbiturate anaesthetics raise seizure threshold and may therefore reduce the efficacy of unilateral ECT (d'Elia and Rastma 1975). The use of anaesthesia does not affect the efficacy of ECT nor prolong length of stay in hospital (Seager 1959).

Ventilation

Pretreatment ventilation with O_2 prevents hypoxaemia (McAndrew and Hauser 1967), lessens confusion and memory impairment (Ottosson 1974; Blachly and Gowing 1966), but prolongs seizure intensity and duration (Holmberg et al. 1956; Posner et al. 1969). By preventing hypoxaemia it may also attenuate breakdown of the blood–brain barrier (Clemedson et al. 1958; Bradbury 1979). Although hypoxaemia does not seem relevant to the clinical efficacy of ECT, it may be related to the intensity of post-ECT memory impairment, in view of hippocampal susceptibility to reduced O_2 tension (Berlyne and Strachan 1968). This could explain the mild Korsakoff-like state observed after ECT (Ottosson 1974).

Muscle Relaxant

Occasional bone fractures involving the low dorsal spine, humerus, and femur, led to the use of curare (Bennett 1940), and later to succinylcholine (suxamethonium chloride, Scoline) (Holmberg and Thesleff 1952), which is a neuromuscular blocking agent. Some centres in the UK use suxethonium

(Pippard and Ellam 1981). Within 40–50 s of the i.v. administration of succinylcholine (20–60 mg) (which is given in a separate syringe to prevent hydrolysation by the alkaline barbiturate solution), chest and neck fasciculations appear. The ensuing paralysis and apnoea last for about 2 min. Subsequent muscle ache is a frequent side effect.

Prolongation of the neuromuscular blockade may result from the additive effect of other neuromuscular blocking agents given concurrently, or from a decreased ability to hydrolyse succinylcholine resulting from a pseudocholinesterase deficiency syndrome (Liddell 1968). This is carried as a recessive trait, and in its homozygous form occurs in about 1 in 2800 of the population; heterozygotes, which form about 3.8% of the population, show a variety of responses to the drug, and such individuals may require intermittent positive respiration. The effect of a 3-mg test dose on tendon reflex responsiveness has been suggested as a screening device (Porter 1964; Impastato 1965), but the rarity of the condition may not warrant this precaution (Detre & Jarecki 1971).

The concentration of plasma and hepatic pseudocholinesterase may be increased in renal disorder (Hurwitz 1974), and reduced in liver disease, (McArdle 1940), severe anaemia, malnutrition (Hodges and Harkness 1954), and carcinoma. Concomitant exposure to succinylcholine and a cholinesterase inhibitor (e.g. physostigmine) may precipitate a syndrome characterized by prolonged apnoea, bronchial secretion, bradycardia, bronchospasm, histamine release and hyperkalaemia (Packman et al. 1978; Marco and Randels 1979). Sulfates of neomycin, streptomycin, kanamycin, polymyxin B and colistin (Pittinger et al. 1970), and eye drops containing ecothiophate iodide (Cavallaro et al. 1968), may also prolong post-ECT apnoea if succinylcholine has been administered. Quinidine may decrease motor end-plate sensitivity to acetylcholine (Schmidt et al. 1963). Succinylcholine increases the probability of cardiac arrhythmia in digitalized patients (Dowdy and Fabian 1963), and may prolong apnoea in patients receiving phenelzine (Bodley et al. 1969), lithium carbonate (Hill et al. 1976) and promazine (Regan and Aldrete 1967).

If muscle relaxation is complete, visual monitoring of the clonic movements is not possible. If EEG monitoring is not available, the cuff from a sphygmomanometer may be used to block the circulation into the ipsilateral arm (in the case of unilateral ECT) before the muscle relaxant is given; motor evidence of a seizure can then be observed (Addersley and Hamilton 1953). It should be noted that evidence of seizure on the ipsilateral side demonstrates that a unilateral electrode placement has induced a seizure which has spread to the other hemisphere. EMG seizure duration, however, is shorter (43–89%) than EEG seizure duration (Sørensen et al. 1981).

Anticholinergic Agents

ECT produces sialorrhoea, bronchorrhoea, vagal overstimulation (which may lead to bradycardia and arrhythmias), and sympathetic stimulation associated with tachycardia. Cardiac rate changes during the seizure from an initial slowing to a sudden increase before a terminal fall. Thus, anticholinergic agents have been used to block parasympathetic stimulation, although the evidence for the 'cardioprotective' action of these agents is not clear. Bankhead et al. (1950) injected 1.2 mg atropine subcutaneously 20 min before ECT to patients who were used as their own controls, and found that there were fewer arrhythmias in the treated group. Also, Nowill et al. (1954) found a 1.5-mg dose of atropine to be correlated with a smaller number of arrhythmias than 0.4 mg, while Parry Jones (1964) compared oral and intravenous atropine and found that the latter afforded more protection. However, Rich et al. (1969) found no difference between 1 mg and 2.5 mg atropine, using patients as their own controls, and more recently Troup et al. (1978) carried out recordings showing that tachycardia occurred after atropinization (106±3.2 to 142±6 beats/min). The cardioprotective use of atropine has, therefore, been called into question (Wyant and MacDonald 1980). There is even some evidence that it may precipitate a paradoxical bradycardia as a result of early vagal stimulation (Vickers et al. 1978), and that it magnifies the hypertensive response during ECT (Bodley and Fenwick 1966). The latter side effect is partly due to a comcomitant severe sympathetic stimulation (Anton et al. 1977). Arrhythmias of sympathetic origin are not modified by anticholinergic medication.

Tricyclic antidepressants seem to produce a marked anticholinergic effect; for example, Snyder and Yamamura (1977) have shown that the antimuscarinic action of an average dose of a tertiary tricyclic such as amitriptyline or imipramine is probably more potent, even during chronic treatment, than the dose of atropine given as protection before ECT. Assuming that antimuscarinic action does have a cardioprotective effect, then there is no need to administer anticholinergics in patients already on tricyclic antidepressants.

The presumed antisalivation effect of atropine during ECT is also poorly established; for example, although Bhattacharya and Wested (1963) found that i.v. or oral atropine were 'equally effective' in preventing salivation, no controls were used. Wyant and MacDonald (1980) have not confirmed this finding.

There is some evidence that atropine may worsen ECT-induced memory impairment (Zornetzer 1978), alter EEG pattern (Ulett and Johnson 1957), and prolong confusion (Frankel 1978). More evidence is therefore needed if atropine is to continue in routine use. If its value eventually becomes established, then there is a case for considering the use of an antimuscarinic agent that does not cross the blood–brain barrier (e.g. methylscopolamine).

Convulsive Agents

Flurothyl. This compound can be administered by inhalation or injection, and is excreted unmetabolized by the lungs (Adler 1975). It is a safe alternative when electricity cannot provoke a fit (Small and Small 1972), or when it is contraindicated (e.g. in certain patients with cardiac pacemakers) (Small

1974). The flurothyl-induced seizure is longer (mean 100 s), is therapeutically equivalent to ECT (Small 1974), and offers a marginal 'psychological' advantage as it may be described as 'drug treatment' (Kafi and Dennis 1966).

Flurothyl produces less memory impairment and confusion, but more salivation, headache, nausea, vomiting and EEG changes than ECT (Small and Small 1975). It is also more susceptible to the antagonistic effects of barbiturates, and hence produces more 'missed' seizures; also, spontaneous seizures and the occasional status epilepticus are more frequent with flurothyl (Fink 1979a). It is contraindicated in pregnancy, although its teratogenic effects are not well established. The industrial production of flurothyl ceased some time ago and this is to be regretted, as it has a place in convulsive therapy (Kalinowsky 1980).

Patients are premedicated in the same way as for ECT. It is administered in a 1-litre breathing bag connected to an oxygen supply and vaporizer. One millilitre flurothyl is placed into the vaporizer, which leads to a mask tightly fitted onto the patient's face. A mixture of oxygen and flurothyl is squeezed at a rate of once every 3 s, and this is continued until a few tonic contractions appear (usually after six to eight inhalations). After a latency period, of about 40 s from the beginning of the procedure, a grand mal seizure appears, heralded by a few myoclonic contractions. Failures to achieve seizures are more common with flurothyl, and are usually related to variations in circulation time and rate of absorption (Small and Small 1975).

Electricity. This is the convulsive agent most commonly used. In general, the type of electricity and amount of energy are not related to efficacy so long as a threshold is reached which induces a bilateral seizure. This is necessary for the full therapeutic effect. However, the wave type and amount of energy of the applied electricity are relevant to the intensity of post-ECT confusion, memory impairment, muscle ache, headache and malaise (Maxwell 1968; Valentine et al. 1968; Weaver et al. 1974; Robin and de Tissera 1982). The 'glissando' technique, in which the amount of electrical energy is gradually increased, was once required to avoid sudden muscle contraction, but has been made redundant by the use of muscle relaxants. There is some evidence that this procedure delivers more energy than is required (Weaver 1977; Robin 1981).

ECT machines may use a transformer or a capacitor as the source of electricity. Capacitors are safer and deliver a more constant energy value (Gordon 1981). A commonly used British machine (Duopulse MK4) delivers modified bidirectional or unidirectional sinewave currents; it takes an input of 100–150 volts and has an output of between 1 and 36 J. A time switch can be built into the machine upon request; a suitable duration of unidirectional current is often between 0.5 and 4 s. Machines should conform with British Standard 5724, Part I, and should be serviced quarterly.

Suboptimal doses of electricity result in 'missed' or 'aborted' seizures. These are useless and can produce side effects; no more than two shocks per treatment should be given, even if no seizure is obtained.

The 'optimal' stimulus can be defined as the minimal amount of electricity required to produce a bilateral seizure, but this is not helpful in practice, as an individual's convulsive threshold varies from day to day under the influence of bodily and environmental variables. For example, factors such as young age, male sex, water retention, vasopression, withdrawal states, hypoglycaemia, and wet, cold days are associated with a relatively low convulsive threshold, which requires less electric energy. On the other hand, old age, female sex, excitement, dehydration, benzodiazepines, antiepileptic medication, and cold, dry days are associated with a relatively high convulsive threshold (Hurwitz 1974).

One crucial variable is the current that actually reaches the brain after the resistance of the head tissues has been overcome. For example, during bilateral ECT, up to 70% of the current may spread along scalp shunts due to the high resistance of the skull, which is of the order of up to 5000 ohms per millimetre of thickness (Hayes 1950; Weaver 1976). This shunting effect is even more marked in unilateral ECT, and may explain the frequent number of missed ECTs in this form of treatment. It has therefore been suggested that skull X-rays be used to determine vault thickness (Gordon 1981).

Unidirectional wave forms (Friedman and Wilcox 1942) and pulse currents are therapeutically equivalent and produce less memory impairment, confusion and malaise than the standard sinewave current (Gordon 1982; Valentine et al. 1968).

The Seizure

A bilateral seizure (whether or not accompanied by a motor fit) is necessary for therapeutic effect (Cronholm and Ottosson 1960). The routine method to determine whether such a seizure has been induced is by visual inspection of attenuated bilateral clonic movements of the hands and feet. However, such movements can be deceiving, as succinylcholine fasciculations or the tonic contraction of the mandible resulting from the direct stimulation of the masticatory muscles, may be mistakenly regarded as a positive response. Hence, electromyographic monitoring of ipsilateral muscles (in unilateral ECT) by means of visual or auditory signals has been advocated (Ives et al. 1976; Williams et al. 1978). EEG monitoring has the advantage of providing information about brain seizure duration (Berrios and Katona 1983). Recent evidence suggests that total seizure time (obtained by summating the duration of all the seizures in one series of treatments) may be correlated with clinical efficacy. Totals of less than 210 s seem to predict bad response (Maletzky 1978). This retrospective study needs replication, as patients received multiple seizures (mean 3.5) per session, and were drawn from a heterogeneous population taking varied medication. The reason why ECT was stopped early in the cases that did not reach the 210-s total is not clear.

After the current has been delivered, the usual response pattern consists of a latent phase (2–5 s), followed by a tonic phase (10–20 s), and then a clonic phase (30–50 s). There is marked inter- and intrapatient variability (Tresise and Stenhouse 1968). Correlation between electric and motor seizure is not good and the former tends to last an average of 40 s longer than the latter (Maletzky 1978; Sørensen et al. 1981). After the clonic phase, a refractory period of 1–3 min ensues, which may be accompanied by an isoelectric EEG during its early stage (Blachly and Gowing 1966). It has been claimed that successive seizures tend to be shorter and require more energy to be produced (Kurland et al. 1976; Small et al. 1978); however, Maletzky (1978) found a tendency for EEG seizure duration to increase from a mean of 81.5 s for the first seizure to a mean of 92.4 s for the tenth seizure. There is no evidence, however, that ECT produces kindling (Small et al. 1981).

Placing of Electrodes

These are attached to cotton wool and lint soaked in saline. Placing is not crucial to clinical efficacy, provided that an optimal stimulus reaches the brain. Bilateral placing is still popular, although unilateral placing is generally considered to have an equivalent therapeutic effect (Lancaster et al. 1958). Memory impairment, confusion and EEG changes are least marked with unilateral placing over the nondominant hemisphere (Heshe et al. 1978). However, clinicians who continue using bilateral placing claim that more unilateral treatments are required. This may be because optimal results with unilateral placing depend upon factors such as adequate determination of dominance, generalization of seizural activity to both hemispheres, and a sufficient separation of electrodes (±9 cm) to avoid excessive shunting of the electrical stimulation. Since EEG monitoring is not routinely performed, a higher number of false positives may result from unilateral ECT, because motor evidence of a unilateral seizure may be mistaken for a bilateral seizure. This may reduce total treatment efficacy and thus lead to more treatments being given. In spite of these disadvantages, unilateral nondominant placing is indicated in the elderly (Fraser and Glass 1978), in patients suffering from dysphasia, or in those who rely on a high standard of memory performance.

The temporal position is a site 4 cm above and perpendicular to the mid-point of a line connecting the outer angle of the eye to the external auditory meatus. The parietal position is 9 cm posterosuperior to the temporal position, at an angle of 70° with this line. Bilateral ECT usually employs the temporal position, on each side, while unilateral ECT generally involves the temporal and parietal sites. Frontoparietal placing has been reported to produce less memory impairment compared with the temporoparietal positions (Inglis 1969); however, this claim has been challenged (d'Elia and Widepalm 1974). Electrode placement should avoid any skull defects (Gardon 1982).

The dominant hemisphere can be determined by asking which hand is used for writing, and by observing which leg is moved first when the patient is told to start walking, which hand is used for a penknife to cut a piece of card in half, and which hand is used to throw a ball of paper. If there is doubt, bilateral ECT should be given, as unilateral ECT to the dominant hemisphere produces relatively severe side effects.

The brain does not behave as a homogeneous conductor as its various structures have different levels of resistance; the electricity usually travels along blood vessels and axonal bundles (Lorimer et al. 1949). It is unclear what brain structures should be reached for optimal clinical results, but the centrencephalic nuclei have been mentioned in this context (Fink 1979a). The fact that plasma levels of hypothalamic hormones increase after ECT lends some support to this view (Skrabanek et al. 1981). However, more recent work on the mode of action of ECT has implicated receptor sensitivity (Grahame-Smith et al. 1978; Lerer and Belmaker 1982).

SIDE EFFECTS

Fractures, dislocations, and excessive fear have been brought under control by the pharmacological modifications of ECT. However, memory impairment, confusion, headache and muscle ache have been less well controlled, and the effects of electricity, atropine, succinylcholine, and the anaesthetic on these are unclear. Anecdotal reports from countries where unmodified ECT is still being used seem to indicate that the pharmacological modifications themselves (e.g. atropine and barbiturate) may be making these symptoms worse. Although it was once claimed that patients feared ECT, (Barnett 1973; Kalinowsky 1980), recent research shows that this is generally not the case (Freeman et al. 1980; Hughes et al. 1981).

Short-Term Side Effects of ECT

Seizures may be followed by subjective and behavioural changes which may last from minutes to months. These include confusion, dyspraxia, impairment of perceptual motor skills, patchy forgetfulness, defects in learning, and impaired sequencing of retrieved memories. Headache and muscle ache, paraesthesiae, nausea and vomiting may also occur.

Other physiological changes may include arrhythmias and transient increases in heart rate (Troup et al. 1978), in blood pressure (Hamilton et al. 1979), in haemoconcentration, and in cerebral blood flow. The function of the blood–brain barrier is impaired (Bradbury 1979), and there is an increase in cerebral arterial vasoconstriction (Matakas et al. 1977). These changes result from a combined effect of autonomic activation, hypoxaemia and muscular spasm. The hypertension can be attenuated by β-receptor blockade (Jones and Knight 1981).

Evidence regarding cardiac arrhythmias with unmodified ECT is scanty, but the incidence of premature beats after modified ECT has been variously reported as 39% (Green and Woods 1955), 43% (Woodruff et al. 1968), and 78% (Lewis et al. 1955). The latter study reported 21 patients all suffering from organic heart disease; however, in the first study, ten cases with known heart disease produced no abnormalities. The incidence of post-ECT arrhythmias peaks immediately after the seizure, prior to the onset of spontaneous breathing. The most common phenomenon is premature ventricular contraction. Tele-monitoring shows that an increase in premature beats may once again take place in the late afternoon on the day of ECT (Small et al. 1978).

Factors such as sympathetic overstimulation, hypoxia, thiopentone anaesthesia, hypercapnia, respiratory acidosis and organic heart disease may increase the likelihood of arrhythmias (McKenna et al. 1970). These are in most cases self-terminating, and cause no recognized morbidity or mortality after ECT.

Hyperglycaemia, increased plasma levels of cortisol (Sachar et al. 1973), and raised plasma ACTH (Allen et al. 1974) have also been reported after ECT. Hypercortisolaemia, however, may be related to an underlying depressive illness (Carroll 1981). Prolactin plasma levels peak about 25 min after ECT (Öhman et al. 1976), and correlate with an increased risk of experiencing another epileptic fit (Trimble 1978). It has also been reported that the metabolites of serotonin (Valzelli and Garattini 1974), dopamine (Ilaria and Prange 1975), and noradrenaline (Modigh 1976) are increased after ECT. It has been suggested that ECT stimulates the pituitary adrenocortical axis and that ECT could be a method of treatment for some cases of hypothalamic hypopituitarism (Pitts and Patterson 1979). However, the neuroendocrinological effects of ECT are still uncertain, as no consistent changes can be recognized (Fink 1981). Other clinical effects have also been attributed to ECT; for example, that it improves tardive dyskinesia (Price and Levin 1978), or can alleviate diabetes mellitus (Fakhri et al. 1980), but evidence is limited. Amongst the biochemical changes which have been described in relation to ECT are a marked increase in CSF proteins (Alexopoulos et al. 1978), an increase in CSF pyruvate concentration (Molnar et al. 1979), and an increase in CSF total creatine phosphokinase, which peaks 6 h after ECT (Braash and Demaso 1980).

Medium-Term Side Effects of ECT

Memory impairment. A similar degree of memory impairment follows both unmodified and modified ECT, but it does not seem to be necessary for its therapeutic effect (d'Elia 1974). Both impaired retrieval of pre-ECT information (retrograde amnesia) and impaired retention of new material after the treatment (anterograde amnesia) are involved (Harper and Wiens 1975). Memory for information acquired just before the treatment is particularly vulnerable. Recovery follows 'Ribot's law', in that older information is recollected first; other variables, such as the 'meaning' or the 'emotional charge' of memories do not seem relevant, and ECT-induced memory impairment is not influenced by the psychological importance of the information (Williams 1966). Squire and Slater (1975) constructed a test based on recollection of American television programmes shown only once between 1957 and 1972, and found that ECT caused a temporal gradient of impairment in long-term memory; namely that programmes broadcast 1–3 years before ECT were more likely to be forgotten than those shown 4–17 years before. The same team also found that, after ECT, time sequencing of events was more impaired than other aspects of memory (Squire 1977).

The duration of memory impairment is variable. Summers et al. (1979) found that about 48% of 31 patients developed detectable impairment after the fifth ECT and that this lasted, on average, 20.1 days. In another study Weeks et al. (1980) found that little memory impairment could be detected at 4 months and none at 6 months. These authors summarized a number of studies and found that the mean recovery time (to pre-ECT cognitive functioning or better) was of 72 days, with a range of 7–270 days.

In clinical practice, the patient's report of memory disorder may not always coincide with objective assessment. Thus, a patient may complain of being forgetful, despite an ability to perform well on testing, or may feel quite happy about his memory when objective impairment can be found. Malloy et al. (1982) have shown an improvement in cognitive function after ECT.

Certain factors are related to the intensity of the memory impairment. For example, unilateral electrode placing to the non-dominant hemisphere, and a relatively low frequency of treatments, produce relatively less memory defect (Squire and Slater 1978). Also, the total amount of electricity administered is associated with the severity of the memory defect (Abrams 1974; d'Elia and Raotma 1977).

The advantages of unilateral non-dominant ECT with regard to memory impairment are offset, to some extent, by its effect on visuospatial and constructional tasks. Also, unilateral non-dominant ECT may be followed by transitory reflex asymmetry, hemiparesis, tactile and visual inattention and homonymous hemianopia (Cohen et al. 1968; Ashton and Hess 1976; Heshe et al. 1978; Kriss et al. 1978).

Piracetam (Mindus et al. 1975), pemoline (Small et al. 1968) and amphetamine (Mah and Albert 1975) have been reported to attenuate the amnesic effect of ECT, while tryptophan does the converse (d'Elia et al. 1978).

The type of electricity which is utilized is of relevance, as the production of a seizure by pulse currents requiring relatively less energy, produces less cognitive impairment than the 60-Hz main currents (Weaver et al. 1977).

Tardive seizures. These are rare, and occur some time after ECT (Stensrud 1958). Up to 1955, 63 cases had been reported in the literature (Blumenthal 1955), and were mainly related to treatment involving convulsive drugs or unmodified ECT (Karliner 1956). 'Kindling', i.e. the gradual lowering of seizure threshold after repeated convulsions, has been suggested as an explanation, but this hypothesis does not explain the finding that consecutive treatments reduced mean seizure duration from 44 to 40 s (Small et al. 1978), and required increasing current for their induction (Green 1960).

EEG changes. ECT can affect the EEG between treatments while, during the sessions, the EEG exhibits a pattern which is indistinguishable from that found in a grand mal seizure with tonic and clonic stages. The seizure may be followed by an isoelectric period, although on occasions there is no abrupt cessation of the paroxysmal high voltage slow waves (bilateral and diffuse) that characterize the clonic stage. It has been suggested that ECT-induced seizural activity is synchronized from subcortical structures; an alternative hypothesis involves cortical spread (Berrios and Katona 1983).

After a course of ECT the patient is left with a generalized EEG slowing which frequently returns to baseline after 1 month and almost always in 3 months (Chusid and Pacella 1952; Weiner 1980). However, 21 days after the last bilateral or unilateral nondominant ECT, about 75% of patients still show slow activity (Sutherland et al. 1969). After unilateral placing of electrodes, delta activity tends to be more prominent on the treated side (Small et al. 1969). Some clinical groups such as older depressives exhibit a greater degree of slowing than younger schizophrenics (Fink 1979a), while the severity and persistence of the EEG slowing seem proportional to the number of ECTs received (Stein et al. 1968).

Time of onset and duration of post-ictal EEG changes have been related to therapeutic outcome; for example, the larger the percentage of delta activity (as elicited by thiopentone), the lower the probability of relapse within 6 months (Roth et al. 1957; Fink and Kahn 1957). Kurland et al. (1976) reported that treatment failures showed a relatively longer EEG isoelectric period.

Flurothyl produces longer seizures than ECT (mean 120 s), but myoclonic jerking and incomplete seizures are also more common (Fink 1979a). Laurell and Perris (1970) found the EEG changes are more marked, appear earlier and last longer with flurothyl; this has been challenged by Small (1974).

Long-Term Side Effects of ECT

The claim that ECT produces severe brain damage is based on a number of uncontrolled postmortem reports and some experimental animal evidence (Frankel 1977; Freidberg 1977). The changes described in these reports include glial, neuronal and blood vessel changes (Alpers and Hughes 1942), petechial haemorrhages and palatal myoclonus secondary to pons bleeding (Baruk 1960).

Computed tomography shows no specific changes in the brain of elderly patients after various courses of ECT (Calloway et al. 1981).

Animal studies have identified similar changes. However, the dubious stimulus equivalence used in these studies (Bini 1938; Hartelius 1952), precludes meaningful extrapolation to humans, the more so as most of these changes appear to be reversible (Frankel 1977; Garcia and Cervos Navarro 1980).

Mortality is rare with ECT, and the reported figure is between 1 and 3 per 30 000 treatments (Barker and Baker 1959; Heshe and Roeder 1976). These figures must be compared with the probable mortality amongst depressed patients who would be expected to benefit, but who are not offered ECT; for example, Avery and Winokur (1976) found that ECT-treated patients had a lower mortality than those treated with tricyclic antidepressants or who remained untreated, and that this effect was more marked in the elderly. However, methodological difficulties, in particular the problems in relation to the selection of groups of patients with the types of depressive syndrome which are usually responsive to ECT, make it impossible to draw firm conclusions from such comparisons.

References

ABRAMS, R. (1974) Multiple E.C.T.: What have we learned? In: *Psychobiology of Convulsive Therapy*, ed. Fink, M. et al. New York: J. Wiley and Son.

ABUISO, P. et al. (1978) E.C.T. in patients with pacemakers. *J. Am. med. Ass.*, **240**, 2459.

ADDERSLEY, D.J. & HAMILTON, M. (1953) Use of succinylcholine in E.C.T. *Br. med. J.*, **i**, 195.

ADLER, M.W. (1975) Pharmacology of Flurothyl: Laboratory and Clinical Applications. In: *Current Developments in Psycho-Pharmacology*, Vol. 2, ed. Essman and Valzelli. New York: Spectrum.

ALBALA, A.A., GREDEN, J.F., TARIKA, J. & CARROLL, B.J. (1981) Changes in serial dexamethasone suppression tests among unipolar depressives receiving ECT. *Biological Psychiatry*, **16**, 551.

ALEXOPOULOS, G.S. et al. (1978) Increase in C.S.F. protein in association with ECT. *J. Neurol. Neurosurg. Psychiat.*, **41**, 1145.

ALLEN, J.P. et al. (1974) Corticotropine release during E.C.T. in man. *Am. J. Psychiat.*, **131**, 1225.

ALLEN, R.E. & PITTS, N. (1979) Drug modification of E.C.T.: Methohexital and Diazepam. *Biol. Psychiat.*, **14**, 69.

ALPERS, B.J. & HUGHES, J. (1942) The brain changes in electrically induced convulsions in cats. *J. Neuropath. exp. Neurol.*, **1**, 173.

ANGST, quoted in HIPPIUS, H. (1975) Rôle de la sismothérapie à l'ère de la psychopharmacologie. *l'Encéphale*, **i**, 195.

ANTON, A.H. et al. (1977) Autonomic blockade and the cardiovascular and catecholamine response to electroshock. *Anaesth. Analg.*, **56**, 46–54.

ASHCROFT, G.W. et al. (1978) Affective disorders. In: *Companion to Psychiatric Studies*, ed. Forrest, A.D. et al. 2nd ed. Edinburgh: Churchill Livingstone.

ASHTON, R. & HESS, N. (1976) Amnesia for random shapes following unilateral and bilateral electroconvulsive shock therapy. *Percept. Mot. Skills.*, **42**, 669.

ASNIS, G (1977) Parkinson's disease, depression and E.C.T.: a review and case study. *Am. J. Psychiat.*, **134**, 191.

ASNIS, G. et al. (1978) E.C.T. in Metropolitan New York hospitals: A survey of practice 1975–76. *Am. J. Psychiat.*, **135**, 479.

AVERY, D. & WINOKUR, G. (1976) Mortality in depressed patients treated with E.C.T. and antidepressants. *Archs gen. Psychiat.*, **33**, 1029.

BALLDIN, J. (1982) Factors influencing prolactin release by ECT. *Acta psychiat. scand.*, **65**, 365.

BALLDIN, J. et al. (1981) Predictors for improvement after ECT in parkinsonian patients with on-off symptoms. *J. neurol. Transmission*, **52**, 199.

BANKHEAD, A.J. et al. (1950) The anticipation and prevention of cardiac complications in electroconvulsive therapy. *Am. J. Psychiat.*, **106**, 911.

BARKER, J.C. & BAKER, A.A. (1959) Deaths associated with electroplexy. *J. ment. Sci.*, **105**, 339.

BARTON, J.L. (1977) E.C.T. in depression: the evidence of controlled studies. *Biol. Psychiat.*, **12**, 687.

BARTON, J.L. et al. (1973) The prophylactic value of extra E.C.T. in depressive illness. *Acta psychiat. neurol. scand.*, **49**, 386.

BARUK, H. (1960) *Les thérapeutiques psychiatriques*. Presses Universitaires de France.

BENNETT, A.E. (1940) Preventing traumatic complications in convulsive shock therapy by curare. *J. Amer. med. Ass.*, **114**, 322.

BERLYNE, N. & STRACHAN, M. (1968) Neuropsychiatric sequelae of attempted hanging. *Br. J. Psychiat.*, **114**, 411.

BERRIOS, G.E. & KATONA, C. (1983) EEG and ECT, the current position. *J. Neurol. y Psiquiat. (Lima).* (In press).

BHATTACHARYA, A. & WEST, E.D. (1963) Comparison of salivary suppression by intravenous and subcutaneous atropine before ECT. *Br. J. Psychiat.*, **109**, 631.

BIDDER, T.G. (1981) ECT in the medically ill patient. *Psychiat. Clin. North Am.*, **4**, 391.

BINI, L. (1938) Experimental researches on epileptic attacks induced by an electric current. *Am. J. Psychiat.*, **94**, 172.

BLACHLY, P. & GOWING, D. (1966) Multiple monitored electroconvulsive treatment. *Compreh. Psychiat.*, **7**, 100.

BLUMENTHAL, I.J. (1955) Spontaneous seizures and related E.E.G. findings following shock therapy. *J. nerv. ment. Dis.*, **122**, 581.

BODLEY, P.O. & FENWCK, P.B.C. (1966) The effect of E.C.T. on patients with essential hypertension. *Br. J. Psychiat.*, **112**, 1241.

BODLEY, P.O. et al. (1969) Low serum pseudocholinesterase levels complicating treatment with phenelzine. *Br. med. J.*, **ii**, 510.

BOLWIG, T.G. et al. (1977) The permeability of the blood brain barrier during electrically induced seizures in man. *Europ. J. clin. Invest.*, **7**, 87.

BRAASH, E.R. & DEMASO, D.R. (1980) Effects of E.C.T. on serum isoenzymes. *Am. J. Psychiat.*, **137**, 625.

BRADBURY, M. (1979) *The concept of a blood brain barrier*. New York: John Wiley.

BRILL, N.O. et al. (1959) Relative effectiveness of various components of E.C.T. *Arch. Neurol. Psychiat., Chicago.*, **81**, 627.

BURROWS, G.C. et al. (1976) Cardiac effects of different tricyclic antidepressant drugs. *Br. J. Psychiat.*, **129**, 335.

CALLOWAY, S.P. et al. (1981) ECT and cerebral atrophy. *Acta psychiat. scand.*, **64**, 442.

CARROLL, B.J. et al. (1981) A specific laboratory test for the diagnosis of melancholia. *Archs gen. Psychiat.*, **38**, 15.

CAVALLARO, R.J. et al. (1968) Effect of Ecothiophate therapy on the metabolism of succinylcholine in man. *Anesth. Analg.*, **47**, 570.

CHUDIS, J.G. & PACELLA, B.L. (1952) The E.E.G. in E.C.T. *J. nerv. ment. Dis.*, **116**, 95.

CLEMEDSON, C.J. et al. (1958) The influence of CO_2 inhalation on the cerebral vascular permeability to trypan blue (the blood barrier). *Acta path. microbiol. scand.*, **42**, 137.

COHEN, B. et al. (1968) Functional asymmetry of the human brain. *Science*, **162**, 475.

CRONHOLM, B. & OTTOSSON, J.O. (1960) Experimental studies of the therapeutic action of electroconvulsive therapy in endogenous depression. *Acta psychiat. neurol. scand. (Suppl.)*, **35**, 69.

D'ELIA, G. (1974) Unilateral E.C.T. In: *Psychobiology of Convulsive Therapy*, ed. Fink, M. et al. New York: Wiley.

D'ELIA, G. & RAOTMA, H. (1975) Is unilateral E.C.T. less effective than bilateral E.C.T.? *Br. J. Psychiat.*, **126**, 83.

D'ELIA, G. & WIDEPALM, K. (1974) Comparison of frontoparietal and temporoparietal unilateral electroconvulsive therapy. *Acta psychiat. scand.*, **50**, 225.

D'ELIA, G. et al. (1978) Influence of tryptophan on memory functions in depressive patients treated with unilateral E.C.T. *Acta psychiat. scand.*, **57**, 259.

DETRE, T.P. & JARECKI, H.G. (1971) *Modern Psychiatric Treatment*. Philadelphia: Lippincott.

DOWDY, E.G. & FABIAN, L.W. (1963) Ventricular arrhythmias induced by succinylcholine in digitalized patients. *Anesth. Analg.*, **42**, 501.

DRESSLER, D.M. & FOLK, J. (1975) The treatment of depression with E.C.T. in the presence of brain tumour. *Am. J. Psychiat.*, **132**, 1320.

EY, H. et al. (1974) *Manuel de Psychiatrie, 4th ed.* Paris: Masson et Cie.

FAKHRI, O. et al. (1980) Effect of E.C.T. on diabetes mellitus. *Lancet*, **ii**, 775.

FINK, M. (1979a) *Convulsive Therapy: Theory and Practice*. New York: Raven Press.

FINK, M. (1979b) Mania and electroseizure therapy. In: *Manic Illness*, ed. Shopsin, B. New York: Raven Press.

FINK, M. (1981) Neuroendocrinology and E.C.T.: A review of recent developments. *Compreh. Psychiat.*, **21**, 450.

FINK, M. & KAHN, R.L. (1957) Relation of E.E.G. delta activity to behavioural response in electroshock. Quantitative serial studies. *Arch. Neurol. Psychiat., Chicago.*, **78**, 516.

FORSSMAN, H. (1955) Follow up study of sixteen children whose mothers were given E.C.T. during gestation. *Acta Psychiat. Scand.*, **30**, 437.

FRANKEL, R.H. (1977) Current perspective of E.C.T.: A discussion. *Am. J. Psychiat.*, **134**, 1014.

FRANKEL, F.H. (ed.) (1978) *Report No. 14 of the American Psychiatric Association Task Force on Convulsive Therapy*. Washington D.C.: A.P.A.

FRASER, R.M. & GLASS, I.B. (1978) Recovery from E.C.T. in elderly patients. *Br. J. Psychiat.*, **133**, 524.

FREEMAN, C.P.L. (1979) Electroconvulsive therapy: its current clinical use. *Br. J. hosp. Med.*, **21**, 281.

FREEMAN, C.P.L. et al. (1978) Double blind controlled trial of E.C.T. and simulated E.C.T. in depressive illness. *Lancet*, **i**, 738.

FREEMAN, C.P.L. et al. (1980) E.C.T. II: Patients who complain. *Br. J. Psychiat.*, **137**, 17.

FREUD, J.D. & WARREN, F.Z. (1965) A clinical impression of hexfluorodiathyl ether (Indoklon) following more than 800 treatments. *Dis. nerv. Syst.*, **25**, 56.

FRIEDBERG, J. (1977) Shock treatment, brain damage and memory loss: A neurological perspective. *Am. J. Psychiat.*, **134**, 1010.

FRIEDMAN, E. & WILCOX, P.H. (1942) Electrostimulated convulsive doses in intact humans by means of unidirectional currents. *J. nerv. ment. Dis.*, **96**, 56.

FROMMER, E.A. (1968) Depressive illness in childhood. In: *Recent Developments in Affective Disorders*, ed. Coppen, A. & Walk, A. Kent: Headley Brothers.

GARCIA, J.H. & CERVOS-NAVARRO, J. (1978) Electroconvulsive therapy (E.C.T.). Its effects on the brain and other tissues (a review). *Conference on E.C.T., Efficacy and Impact*. New Orleans, Feb. 23rd 1978.

GASPAR, D. & SAMARASINGHE, L.A. (1982) ECT in psychogeriatric practice. *Compreh. Psychiat.*, **23**, 170.

GERRING, J.P. & SHIELDS, H.M. (1982) The identification and management of patients with a high risk for cardiac arrhythmias during modified ECT. *J. clin. Psychiat.*, **43**, 140.

GORDON, D. (1981) The electrical and radiological aspects of E.C.T. In: *Electroconvulsive Therapy: An Appraisal*, ed. Palmer, R.L. Oxford: Oxford University Press.

GORDON, D. (1982) Electro-convulsive therapy with minimum hazard. *Brit. J. Psychiat.*, **141**, 12.

GRAHAME-SMITH, D.G. et al. (1978) Mechanism of the antidepressant action of E.C.T. *Lancet*, **i**, 254.

GREEN, M.A. (1960) Relation between threshold and duration of seizures and electrographic change during convulsive therapy. *J. nerv. ment. Dis.*, **131**, 117.

GREEN, R. & WOODS, A. (1955) Effects of modified E.C.T. on the electrocardiogram. *Br. med. J.*, **i**, 1503.

GREENBLATT, M. (1977) Efficacy of E.C.T. in affective and schizophrenic illness. *Am. J. Psychiat.* **134**, 1001.

HAMILTON, M. et al. (1979) E.C.T. cognitive defect and elevation of blood pressure. *Br. J. Psychiat.*, **135**, 77.

HARPER, R.G. & WIENS, A.N. (1975) E.C.T. and memory. *J. nerv. mental Dis.*, **161**, 245.

HARTELIUS, H. (1952) Cerebral changes following electrically induced convulsions. *Acta psychiat. neurol. scand.* (Suppl.), 77.

HAYES, K.J. (1950) The current path in electric convulsive shock. *Arch. Neurol. Psychiat.*, **63**, 102.

HESHE, J. & ROEDER, E. (1976) Electroconvulsive therapy in Denmark. *Br. J. Psychiat.*, **128**, 241.

HESHE, J. et al. (1978) Unilateral and Bilateral E.C.T. *Acta psychiat. scand.* (Suppl. 275).

HIFT, E. et al. (1960) Results of shock therapy on schizophrenics in childhood. *Schweiz. Arch. Neurol. Psychiat.*, **86**, 256.

HOILL, G.E. et al. (1976) Potentiation of succinylcholine neuromuscular blockade by lithium carbonate. *Anesthesiology*, **44**, 439.

HODGES, R.J.H. & HARKNESS, J. (1954) Suxamethonium sensitivity in health and disease: A clinical evaluation of pseudocholinesterase levels. *Br. med. J.*, **ii**, 18.

HOLMBERG, G. & THESLEFF, S. (1952) Succinyl-choline-iodide as a muscular relaxant in electroshock therapy. *Am. J. Psychiat.*, **108**, 842.

HOLMBERG, G. et al. (1956) Experiments in the prolongation of convulsions induced by electric shock treatment. *Acta psychiat. neurol. scand.*, **31**, 61.

HUGHES, J. et al. (1981) Are patients shocked by E.C.T.? *J. Roy. Soc. Med.*, **74**, 283.

HURWITZ, T.D. (1974) Electroconvulsive therapy: a review. *Compreh. Psychiat.*, **15**, 303.

ILARIA, R. & PRANGE, A.J. (1975) Convulsive therapy and other biological treatments. In: *The Nature and Treatment of Depression*, ed. Flack, F.F. and Droghi, S.S. New York: Wiley & Son.

IMPASTATO, D.J. (1965) The safest possible clinical use of succinylcholine in electroshock therapy. *Acta psychiat. scand.*, **41**, 294.

INGLIS, J. (1969) Electrode placement and the effect of E.C.T. on mood and memory in depression. *Can. psychiat. Ass. J.*, **14**, 463.

IVES, J.O. et al. (1976) Portable electromyograph monitoring of unilateral E.C.T. *Am. J. Psychiat.*, **133**, 1340.

JOHNSTONE, E.C. et al. (1980). The Northwick Park Electroconvulsive therapy trial. *Lancet*, **ii**, 1317.

JONES, R.M. & KNIGHT, P.R. (1981) Cardiovascular and hormonal responses to ECT. *Anaesthesia*, **36**, 795.

KAFI, A. & DENNIS, M. (1966) Advantages of Indoklon convulsive therapy. *Hosp. Comm. Psychiat.*, **17**, 297.

KALINOWSKY, L.B. (1980) Convulsive therapies. In: *Comprehensive Textbook of Psychiatry*, ed. Kaplan, T. et al., 3rd ed. New York: William and Wilkins.

KALINOWSKY, L.B. & HIPPIUS, H. (1969) *Pharmacological, Convulsive and other Treatments in Psychiatry.* New York: Grune and Stratton.

KARLINER, W. (1956) Epileptic states following electroshock therapy. *J. Hillside Hosp.*, **5**, 1.

KARLINER, W. & PADULA, L. (1959) Indoklon combined with Penthothal and Anectine. *Am. J Psychiat.*, **115**, 1041.

KENDELL, R.E. (1981) The contribution of E.C.T. to the treatment of affective disorders. In: *Electroconvulsive Therapy: An Appraisal*, ed. Palmer, R.L. Oxford: Oxford University Press.

KRAMP, P. & BOLWIG, T.G. (1981) ECT in acute delirious states. *Compreh. Psychiat.*, **22**, 368.

KRISS, A. et al. (1978) Neurological asymmetries immediately after unilateral E.C.T. *J. Neurol. Neurosurg. Psychiat.*, **41**, 1135.

KURLAND, A.A. et al. (1976) Electroconvulsive therapy and E.E.G. correlates in depressive disorders. *Compreh. Psychiat.*, **17**, 581.

LAMBOURN, J. & GILL, D. (1978) A controlled comparison of simulated and real E.C.T. *Br. J. Psychiat.*, **133**, 514.

LANCASTER, N.P. et al. (1958) Unilateral electroconvulsive therapy. *J. ment. Sci.*, **104**, 221.

LANGSLEY, D.G. et al. (1959) Comparison of CPZ and ECT in treatment of acute schizophrenic and manic reactions. *Arch. Neurol. Psychiat.*, **81**, 384.

LAURELL, B. & PERRIS, C. (1970) Seizure and post seizure electroencephalographic pattern. *Acta psychiat. scand.* (Suppl.), **213**, 8.

LERER, B. & BELMAKER, R.H. (1982) Receptors and the mechanism of action of ECT. *Biol. Psychiat.*, **17**, 497.

LEWIS, W.H. Jr. et al. (1955) Cardiovascular disturbances and their management in modified electrotherapy for psychiatric illness. *New Engl. J. Med.*, **252**, 1016.

LIDDELL, J. (1968) Cholinesterase variants and suxamethonium apnoea. *Proc. R. Soc. Med.*, **61**, 168.

LORIMER, R. et al. (1949) Path of current distribution in brain during electroconvulsive therapy. *Electroenceph. clin. Neurophysiol.*, **1**, 343.

LUNN, R.J. et al. (1981) Anesthetics and ECT seizure duration. *Biol. Psychiat.*, **16**, 1163.

MAH, C.J. & ALBERT, D.J. (1975) Reversal of ECS-induced amnesia by post-ECS injections of amphetamine. *Pharmacol. Biochem. Behav.*, **3**, 1.

MALETZKY, B.M. (1978) Seizure duration and clinical effect in electroconvulsive therapy. *Compreh. Psychiat.*, **19**, 541.

MALLOY, F.W. et al. (1982) Changes in neuropsychological test performance after ECT. *Biol. Psychiat.*, **17**, 61.

MALTBIE, A.A. et al. (1980) Electroconvulsive therapy in the presence of brain tumour. *J. nerv. ment. Dis.*, **168**, 400.

MARCO, L.A. & RANDELS, P.M. (1979) Succinylcholine drug interactions during E.C.T. *Biol. Psychiat.*, **14**, 433.

MATAKAS, F. et al. (1977) Spastic constriction of cerebral vessels after E.C.T. *Arch. Psychiat. Nervenkr.*, **224**, 1.

MAXWELL, R. (1968) Electrical factors in E.C.T. *Acta psychiat. scand.*, **44**, 436.

MCANDREW, J. & HAUSER, G. (1967) Preventilation of oxygen in E.C.T.: suggested modification of technique. *Am. J. Psychiat.*, **124**, 251.

MCARDLE, B. (1940) The serum choline esterase in jaundice and diseases of the liver. *Q. J. Med.*, **9**, 107.

MCCABE, M.S. (1976) E.C.T. in the treatment of mania: a controlled study. *Am. J. Psychiat.*, **133**, 688.

MCCABE, M.S. & NORRIS, B. (1977) E.C.T. versus CPZ in mania. *Biol. Psychiat.*, **12**, 245.

MCKENNA, G. et al. (1970) Cardiac arrhythmias during electro-shock therapy: significance, prevention, treatment. *Am. J. Psychiat.*, **127**, 530.

MINDUS, P. et al. (1975) Does piracetam counteract the E.C.T.-induced memory dysfunctions in depressed patients? *Acta psychiat. scand.*, **51**, 319.

MODIGH, K. (1976) Long term effects of E.C.T. on synthesis turnover and uptake of brain monoamines. *Psychopharmacology*, **49**, 179.

MOLNER, L. et al. (1979) Die Wirkung der bilateralen and unilateralen Elektroschocktherapie auf die Zusammensetzung des Liquor cerebrospinalis. *Arch. Psychiat. Nervenkr.*, **227**, 159.

MÜLLER, M. (1960) Die Therapie der Schizophrenien. In: *Psychiatrie der Gegenwart*, Vol. II, Klinische Psychiatrie, ed. Gruhle, H.W. et al. Berlin, Heidelberg, New York: Springer-Verlag.

NOWILL, W.K. et al. (1954) Succinylcholine in electroshock therapy II. Cardiovascular reactions. *Arch. Neurol. Psychiat.*, **71**, 189.

ÖHMAN, R. et al. (1976) Prolactin response to E.C.T. *Lancet*, **i**, 936.

OTTOSSON, J.O. (1974) Systemic biochemical effects of E.C.T. In: *Psychobiology of Convulsive Therapy*, ed. Fink, M. et al. New York: J. Wiley.

PACKMAN, P.M. et al. (1978) Hazards of succinylcholine administration during electrotherapy. *Archs gen. Psychiat.*, **35**, 1137.

PARRY-JONES, W.U. (1964) Oral atropine in premedication for electroconvulsive therapy. *Lancet*, **i**, 1067.

PIPPARD, J. & ELLAM, L. (1981) *ECT in Great Britain, 1980. A Report to the Royal College of Psychiatrists*. London: Gaskell.

PITTINGER, C.B. et al. (1970) Antibiotic-induced paralysis. *Anesth. Analg.* **49**, 487.

PITTS, F.N. et al. (1965) Induction of anaesthesia with methohexital and thiopental in electroconvulsive therapy. *New Engl. J. Med.*, **273**, 353.

PITTS, F.N. & PATTERSON, C.W. (1979) E.C.T. for iatrogenic hypothalamic-hypopituiterism (CRF-ACTH Type). *Am. J. Psychiat.*, **136**, 1074.

PORTER, I.H. (1964) Genetic basis of drug metabolism in man. *Toxic Appl. Pharmacol.*, **6**, 499.

POSNER, J.B. et al. (1969) Cerebral metabolism during electrically induced seizures in man. *Arch. Neurol. Chicago*, **20**, 388.

PRICE, T.R.P. & LEVIN, R. (1978) The effects of E.C.T. on T.D. *Am. J. Psychiat.*, **135**, 991.

REGAN, A.G. & ALDRETE, J.A. (1967) Prolonged apnoea after administration of promazine hydrochloride following succinylcholine infusion. *Anesth. Analg.*, **46**, 315.

REGESTEIN, Q.R. & LIND, L.J. (1980) Management of electroconvulsive treatment in an elderly woman with severe hypertension and cardiac arrhythmias. *Compreh. Psychiat.*, **21**, 288.

RICH, C.L. et al. (1969) Electrotherapy: The effects of atropine on E.K.G. *Dis. nerv. Syst.*, **30**, 622.

RIDDELL, S.A. (1963) The therapeutic efficacy of E.C.T. *Archs gen. Psychiat.*, **8**, 546.

RIES, R.K. et al. (1981) E.C.T. in medication resistant schizoaffective disorder. *Compreh. Psychiat.*, **22**, 167.

ROBIN, A.A. (1981) E.C.T. current status. In: *Electroconvulsive Therapy: An Appraisal*, ed. Palmer, R.L. Oxford: Oxford University Press.

ROBIN, A. & DE TISSERA, S. (1982) A double blind controlled comparison of the therapeutic effect of Low and High Energy ECT. *Brit. J. Psychiat.*, **141**, 357.

RODIN, E. et al. (1971) Neurophysiological mechanisms involved in grand mal seizures induced by Metrazol and Megimide. *Electroenceph. Clin Neurophysiol.*, **30**, 62.

ROTH, M. et al. (1957) Prognosis and pentothal-induced electroencephalographic changes in electro-convulsive treatment. *Electroenceph. clin. Neurophysiol.*, **9**, 225.

ROYAL COLLEGE OF PSYCHIATRISTS (1977) Memorandum on the use of electro-convulsive therapy. *Br. J. Psychiat.*, **131**, 261.

SACHAR, E.J. et al. (1973) Disrupted 24 hour patterns of cortisol excretion in psychotic depression. *Archs gen. Psychiat.*, **28**, 19.

SALZMAN, C. (1980) The use of E.C.T. in the treatment of schizophrenia. *Am. J. Psychiat.*, **137**, 1032.

SCHIELE, B.C. & SCHNEIDER, R.A. (1949) The selective use of E.C.T. in organic patients. *Dis. nerv. Syst.*, **10**, 291.

SCHMIDT, J.L. et al. (1963) The effect of quinidine on the action of muscle relaxants. *J. Amer. med. Ass.*, **183**, 143.

SCOVERN, A.W. & KILMANN, P.R. (1980) Status of electroconvulsive therapy. *Psychol. Bull.*, **87**, 260.

SEAGER, C.P. (1959) Controlled trial of straight and modified electroplexy. *J. ment. Sci.*, **105**, 1022.

SHAGASS, C. & JONES, A.L. (1958) A neurophysiological test for psychiatric diagnosis: results in 750 patients. *Am. J. Psychiat.*, **114**, 1002.

SKRABANEK, P. et al. (1981) ECT increases plasma growth hormone, prolactin, luteinising hormone and follicle-stimulating hormone but not thyrotropin or substance P. *Psychoneuroendocrinology*, **6**, 261.

SMALL, I.F. et al. (1968) Influence of Cylert upon memory changes in E.C.T. *Am. J. Psychiat.*, **125**, 837.

SMALL, I.F. (1974) Inhalant convulsive therapy. In: *Psychobiology of Convulsive Therapy*, ed. Fink, M. et al. New York: Wiley and Sons.

SMALL, J.G. & SMALL, I.F. (1972) Clinical results: Indoklon versus E.C.T. *Seminars in Psychiatry*, **4**, 13.

SMALL, I.F. & SMALL, J.G. (1975) The clinical use of Flurothyl. In: *Current Developments in Psychopharmacology, Vol. 2*, ed. Essman and Valzelli. New York: Spectrum.

SMALL, J.G. et al. (1978) Electrophysiology of E.C.T. In *Psychopharmacology: A Generation of Progress*, ed. Lipton M.A. et al. New York: Raven Press.

SMALL, J.G. et al. (1980) Complication with electroconvulsive treatment combined with Lithium. *Biol. Psychiat.*, **15**, 103.

SMALL, J.G. et al. (1981) Does ECT produce kindling? *Biol. Psychiat.*, **16**, 773.

SMITH, S. (1956) Use of electroplexy (E.C.T.) in psychiatric syndromes complicating pregnancy. *J. ment. Sci.*, **102**, 796.

SNAITH, R.P. (1981) How much E.C.T. does the depressed patient need? In: *Electroconvulsive Therapy: An Appraisal*, ed. Palmer, R.L. Oxford: Oxford University Press.

SNYDER, S.H. & YAMAMURA, H.I. (1977) Antidepressants and the muscarinic acetylcholine receptor. *Archs gen. psychiat.*, **34**, 236.

SOBEL, D.E. (1960). Fetal damage due to ECT, insuline coma, chlorpromazine or reserpine. *Arch. gen. Psychiat.*, **2**, 606.

SØRENSEN, P.S. et al. (1981) ECT: A comparison of seizure duration as monitored with EEG and EMG. *Acta psychiat. scand.*, **64**, 193.

SQUIRE, L.R. (1977) E.C.T. and memory loss. *Am. J. Psychiat.*, **134**, 997.

SQUIRE, L.R. & SLATER, P.C. (1975) Forgetting in very long term memory as assessed by an improved questionnaire technique. *J. exp. Psychol.*, **104**, 50.

SQUIRE, L.R. & SLATER, P.C. (1978) Bilateral and unilateral E.C.T.: Effects on verbal and nonverbal memory. *Am. J. Psychiat.*, **135**, 1316.

STEIN, J. et al. (1968) Die bioelektrisch kontrollierte Krampfbehandlung der endogene Psychosen in Narkose and Relaxation. *Arch. sychiat. Nervenkr.*, **211**, 448.

STENSRUD, P.A. (1958) Cerebral complications following 24 562 convulsion treatments in 893 patients. *Acta psychiat. neurol. scand.*, **33**, 115.

SUMMERS, W.K. et al. (1979) The natural history of acute organic mental syndrome after bilateral E.C.T. *Biol. Psychiat.*, **14**, 905.

SUTHERLAND, E.M. et al. (1969) EEG, memory and confusion in dominant, non-dominant and bi-temporal ECT. *Br. J. Psychiat.*, **115**, 1059.

TAYLOR, P.J. (1981) E.C.T. in schizophrenia: a review. In: *Electroconvulsive Therapy: An Appraisal*, ed. Palmer, R.L. Oxford: Oxford University Press.

TAYLOR, P. & FLEMINGER, J.J. (1980) E.C.T. for schizophrenia. *Lancet*, **i**, 1380.

TRESISE, P.C. & STENHOUSE, N.S. (1968) E.C.T. Phases with and without anaesthesia. *Br. J. Psychiat.*, **114**, 1383.

TRIMBLE, M.R. (1978) Serum prolactin in epilepsy and hysteria. *Br. med. J.*, **ii**, 1682.

TROUP, P.J. et al. (1978) Effect of Electroconvulsive therapy on cardiac rhythm, conduction and repolarization. *Pace*, **1**, 172.

TUREK, I.S. & HANLON, T.E. (1977) The effectiveness and safety of E.C.T. *J. nerv. ment. Dis.*, **164**, 419.

ULETT, G.A. & JOHNSON, D.W. (1957) Effect of atropine and scopolamine upon electroencephalographic changes induced by E.C.T. *Electroenceph. clin. Neurophysiol.*, **9**, 217.

VALENTINE, M. et al. (1968) A comparison of techniques in electroconvulsive therapy. *Br. J. Psychiat.*, **114**, 989.

VALZELLI, L. & GARATTINI, S. (1974) Effect of electroshock on indoleamine metabolism and aggressive behaviour. In: *Psychobiology of Convulsive Therapy*, ed. Fink, M. et al. New York: Wiley and Sons.

VAN PRAAG, H.M. (1976) Amine hypotheses of affective disorders. In: *Handbook of Psychopharmacology, Vol. 10*, ed. Iversen, L. et al. New York: Raven Press.

VICKERS, M.D. et al. (1978) *Drugs in Anaesthetic Practice, 5th ed.* London: Butterworths.

VOLAVKA, J. (1974) Is EEG slowing related to the therapeutic effect of convulsive therapy? In: *Psychobiology of Convulsive Therapy*, ed. Fink, M. et al. New York: Wiley and Son.

WEAVER, L. (1976) Current density in bilateral and unilateral E.C.T. *Biol. Psychiat.*, **11**, 303.

WEAVER, L.A. et al. (1977) A comparison of standard alternating current and low-energy brief pulse electrotherapy. *Biol. Psychiat.*, **12**, 525.

WEAVER, L. et al. (1974) Stimulus parameters in E.C.T. *J. Psychiat. Res.*, **10**, 271.

WEEKS, D. et al. (1980) E.C.T.: III: Enduring cognitive deficits? *Br. J. Psychiat.*, **137**, 26.

WEINER, R.D. (1980) The persistence of E.C.T. induced changes in the E.E.G. *J. nerv. ment. Dis.*, **168**, 224.

WEINER, R.D. et al. (1980) Prolonged confusional state and E.E.G. seizure activity following concurrent E.C.T. and Lithium use. *Am. J. Psychiat.*, **137**, 1452.

WEST, E. (1981) Electric convulsion therapy in depression: a double blind controlled trial. *Br. med. J.*, **i**, 355.

WILLIAMS, M. (1966) Memory disorders associated with E.C.T. In: *Amnesia*, ed. Whitty, C.M. & Zangwill, O.L. London: Butterworth.

WILLIAMS, R. et al. (1978) Application of a muscle-potential monitor to E.C.T. (To be published.)

WOODRUFF, R.A. (1969) Electrotherapy: the effects of barbiturate anaesthesia, succinylcholine and pre-oxygenation on E.K.G. *Dis. nerv. Syst.*, **30**, 180.

WOODRUFF, R.A. Jr. et al. (1968) The drug modification of E.C.T. *Archs gen. Psychiat.*, **18**, 605.

WYANT, G.M. & MACDONALD, W.B. (1980) The role of atropine in ECT. *Anaesth. Intens. Care*, **8**, 445.

YUDOFSKY, S.C. (1979) Parkinson's disease, depressions and electroconvulsive therapy. A clinical and neurobiological synthesis. *Compreh. Psychiat.*, **20**, 579.

ZORNETZER, S.F. (1978) Neurotransmitter modulation and memory: a new neuropharmacological phrenology? In: *Psychopharmacology: A generation of progress*, ed. Lipton, M.A. et al. New York: Raven Press.

7

Psychosurgery

Hilary M. Evans

During the three years from 1974 to 1976, 431 neurosurgical operations were performed for psychiatric disorder in the British Isles (Barraclough and Mitchell-Heggs 1978); this number is steadily decreasing. Fifty-eight per cent of operations were carried out in three psychosurgical units, in which 82% of cases suffered from obsessive–compulsive or affective disorders, 8% from conditions associated with repeated violence (one unit only), and a mere 6% from schizophrenia or schizoaffective psychosis. No operations were performed for psychogenic pain or sexual psychopathology. The high success rate of modern psychosurgery results by and large from skilful selection of patients.

The other important factor has been the introduction of stereotactic methods to replace free-hand techniques. Using a stereotactic atlas of the brain, lesion sites can be located by calculating their coordinates in relation to vertical, horizontal and parasaggital planes to a three-dimensional accuracy of 1 mm. With a stereotactic frame in position, anatomical landmarks can be established and the coordinates translated to the patient's brain. Electrical stimulation can sometimes be used to confirm the accuracy of the siting before a lesion is made. Thus, there is minimal destruction of surrounding tissue and consequently fewer unwanted side effects than in 'open' procedures such as orbital undercutting and bimedial leucotomy.

Contemporary psychosurgical procedures and their contribution to the treatment of a variety of psychiatric disorders will now be reviewed.

NEUROSURGERY FOR OBSESSIVE–COMPULSIVE AND AFFECTIVE DISORDERS

The vast majority of current psychosurgical procedures are intended for treatment of chronic and severe depression or anxiety states. Since the early prefrontal leucotomies became popular (Moniz 1936), it has seemed that disorders of affect can respond more favourably than the psychoses. Nevertheless, the enthusiasm generated by success with depression rapidly led to prescription of similar procedures for schizophrenia, such that this diagnosis accounted for two-thirds of over 10 000 patients operated on in Great Britain between 1942 and 1954 (Tooth and Newton 1961). Although some patients (18%) appeared to be considerably improved by surgery, failures and severe side effects were so common that neurosurgery for the schizophrenias receded with the introduction of phenothiazines in the 1950s. However, new operative procedures continued to be developed and refined for treatment of a wide range of affective disorders, obsessional states and exceptional cases of schizophrenia; these techniques have been reviewed by Valenstein (1973). With more standardization and restriction of operative procedures, the effect of surgical intervention shifted from immediate blunting of affect to a more gradual relief of certain symptoms, especially chronic tension.

Operative Procedures

Stereotactic limbic leucotomy. This procedure was developed at St George's Hospital in London and during 1974–78 accounted for an estimated 13% of patients undergoing psychosurgery in the UK (Barraclough and Mitchell-Heggs 1978). This procedure involves stereotactic placement of lesions, by means of a cryogenic probe or radiofrequency coagulation, into anterior limbic sites shown to produce characteristic autonomic responses to electrical stimulation (Kelly *et al.* 1973). Under light general anaesthesia and following full head-shave, a Leksell stereotactic frame (Leksell 1966) is fitted to the skull and a lumbar air encephalogram is performed to locate ventricular outline and bony landmarks from which lesion coordinates are calculated. The majority of patients receive three or four 7–8 mm lesions in the ventromedial quadrant of each frontal lobe. An additional four lesions are placed in the cingulum bundle bilaterally (Fig. 7.1) in cases of obsessive–compulsive disorder or chronic anxiety state (Richardson 1973). The operation takes about 4 h to complete and the patient returns to the psychiatric ward about 1 week later, after recovering from any side effects of surgery, such as headache, incontinence or mild disorientation. There is often an immediate reduction of tension and depression following limbic leucotomy.

Stereotactic subcaudate tractotomy. This also involves ablation of the basofrontal area but is unique in its lesioning method, developed by Knight at the Brook General Hospital in London from the now outdated orbital undercutting technique of Scoville (1949). Ceramic rods containing radioactive ^{90}Yttrium seeds are inserted in two lines of three into the anterior subcaudate tracts (Fig. 7.1). The seeds, which have a half-life of about 62 h, gradually produce a lesion about 25 mm long. Stereotactic tractotomy is performed with the patient under general anaesthesia and takes about 90 min to complete. An estimated 30% of psychosurgical patients underwent this operation between 1974 and 1976 in the UK (Barraclough and Mitchell-Heggs 1978).

There are several other procedures related to those already described (Fig. 7.1). *Stereotactic anterior cingulotomy* (cingulumotomy, cingulotractomy) has been found very effective in treating disorders of affect, and obsessive–compulsive neurosis. Originally adopting the free-hand, 'open' technique (anterior

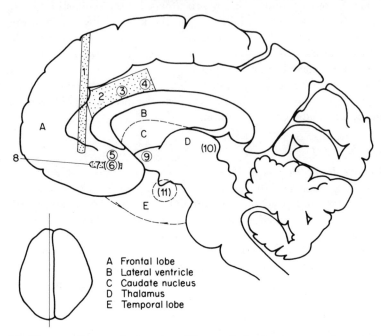

A   Frontal lobe
B   Lateral ventricle
C   Caudate nucleus
D   Thalamus
E   Temporal lobe

Figure 7.1. Diagram of parasagittal section of human brain showing approximate lesion sites unilaterally for various psychosurgical procedures. Dotted lines and figures in brackets indicate regions more lateral to the midline. 1: Bimedial leucotomy (shaded area); 2: anterior cingulectomy (shaded area); 3 & 4: stereotactic limbic leucotomy, cingulate sites; 5 & 6: stereotactic limbic leucotomy, ventromedial frontal lobe sites; 7: stereotactic subcaudate tractotomy (shaded area); 8: orbital undercutting incision; 9: hypothalamotomy; 10: pulvinotomy; 11: amygdalotomy.

cingulectomy), involving bilateral removal of about 3–4 cm of tissue in Brodmann's Area 24 (Whitty et al. 1952), the procedure gradually incorporated stereotactic methods (see below) and lesions have also been produced by radio-yttrium implantation (Knight 1973).

Multifocal leucocoagulation. This procedure employs rather different methods. Developed by Crow (1973) at the Burden Neurological Institute in Bristol, it involves stereotactic implantation into the frontal lobes of sheaves of three to seven gold wire electrodes which are activated selectively and repetitively over about 6 months to produce lesions of gradually increasing size, according to clinical response.

Bimedial leucotomy. This is an open procedure developed by Greenblatt and Solomon (1952) as a substitute for the more radical frontal lobotomies, and has been performed on a large number of patients at the Maudsley Hospital in London, and elsewhere. The operation is carried out under direct vision. Using a metal sucker introduced from above through 4-cm trephine holes on each side of the midline, an incision is made bilaterally in a vertical line just rostral to the lateral ventricles, restricted to a medial 2 cm of tissue and extending into the ventromedial segment of each frontal lobe (Fig. 7.1). Stereotactic methods and radiofrequency coagulation have recently been adopted for this procedure, with lesion sites determined by symptomatic criteria (Post and Schurr 1977).

Clinical Efficacy

Despite the methodological problems of assessment and the absence of control groups, there is evidence that both stereotactic limbic leucotomy and subcaudate tractotomy can be extremely effective in treatment of certain patients with chronic and severe obsessive–compulsive neurosis, anxiety and depressive disorders. The results of the two procedures can be compared by examining the performance of two groups of obsessive–compulsive patients on the Leyton Obsessional Inventory (LOI) (Cooper 1970), a supervised card-sorting inventory yielding scores for obsessive–compulsive symptoms, obsessional personality traits, 'Resistance' and 'Interference' (i.e. disablement produced by symptoms). The limbic leucotomy group (Kelly 1980) comprised 26 patients suffering from obsessive–compulsive neurosis tested before surgery and at least 1 year (but on average nearer 2 years) postoperatively. The subcaudate tractotomy group (Bridges et al. 1973) consisted of 24 obsessive–compulsive patients tested at least 3 years postoperatively. Long-term outcome as measured by the LOI was strikingly similar for both surgical groups (Fig. 7.2), and there were highly significant differences between pre- and postleucotomy scores. To put the scores into perspective, both leucotomy and tractotomy groups' scores decreased markedly towards those of a non-psychiatric sample of 25 'house-proud' housewives (Cooper and McNeil 1968).

In addition to the LOI, both operative groups, including a further 18 obsessive–compulsive patients in the leucotomy group, completed the Taylor Scale of Manifest Anxiety (Taylor 1953). A mean preleucotomy score of 30.3 dropped significantly to 19.7 during the follow-up period ($p < 0.001$), reflecting a marked reduction in anxiety. This score was slightly lower than the post-tractotomy group's mean score of 22.8.

Results of psychological assessment of depressive symptomatology have been reported both following limbic leucotomy and following subcaudate tractotomy. In a prospective study involving 148 leucotomy patients, 36 of whom suffered from primary depressive disorder, Kelly (1980) reported a highly significant ($p < 0.001$), decrease in all mean scores for depression from just before surgery to follow-up a mean of 20 months later. Scales used included the Beck Depression

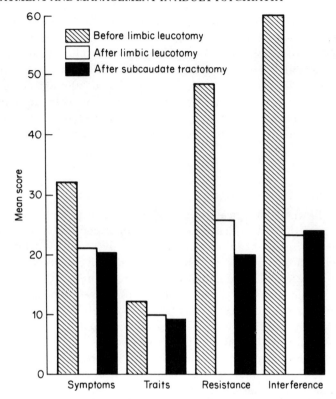

Figure 7.2. Mean scores on the Leyton Obsessional Inventory for 26 obsessive–compulsive patients tested before and at least 1 year (mean 20 months) after stereotactic limbic leucotomy (Kelly 1980). Also shown are mean scores for 24 obsessive–compulsive patients tested at least 3 years after stereotactic subcaudate tractotomy (Bridges et al. 1973).

Scale (Beck et al. 1961), the Hamilton Depression Scale (Hamilton 1967) and the Depression Score of the Middlesex Hospital Questionnaire (MHQ) (Crown and Crisp 1966). Göktepe et al. (1975) employed the Wakefield Inventory (Snaith et al. 1971) to quantify depression after subcaudate tractotomy in 127 patients at least 2½ years postoperatively, but as this was a retrospective study, no preoperative scores had been collected for comparison.

Following limbic leucotomy, anxiety scores for the whole group were also markedly reduced (Kelly 1980). In a diagnostic subgroup comprising 25 cases of chronic anxiety state, follow-up scores dropped significantly on the Taylor Scale ($p < 0.01$), the Hamilton Anxiety Rating Scale (Hamilton 1959) and the Phobic, Somatic and Free-Floating Anxiety subscales of the MHQ ($p < 0.001$). An excellent review of surgical intervention for anxiety has been published by Smith and Kiloh (1980).

Global rating of clinical improvement is the most widely employed method for determining the efficacy of individual surgical procedures, although there have been many methodological difficulties including considerable variation in the rating criteria. Many workers have opted for a five-point rating scale based on that of Pippard (1955), such that patients rated as:

I are symptom free and fully recovered
II are greatly improved with minimal residual symptoms
III are improved, but significant symptoms remain
IV are essentially unchanged
V are worse (though not necessarily as a result of surgery)

Clinical ratings from a number of studies are shown in Table 7.1; some have been adapted for comparison and the reader is advised to consult the source papers for the original methods of rating and presentation.

A 67% overall improvement rate is claimed for limbic leucotomy (Kelly 1980), with 42% of the whole sample rated as 'greatly improved' or 'symptom-free' (categories I and II). For a separate sample of patients, with different raters and rating criteria and a longer follow-up period, Göktepe et al. (1975) claim marked improvement among 58% of subcaudate tractotomy patients. Comparing category I and II ratings among diagnostic subgroups, obsessive −compulsive patients showed greatest clinical improvement (61%) in the limbic leucotomy group, and depressed patients (particularly those with recurrent rather than chronic depression) showed the greatest improvement (68%) in the subcaudate tractotomy group. Limbic leucotomy was associated with a great improvement in 30% of patients with chronic or phobic anxiety and 39% with 'other' diagnoses including schizophrenia; the figures for subcaudate tractotomy were 62% and 7% respectively.

It cannot be overstated that only approximate comparisons can be drawn between these studies, which are beset with methodological problems. For example, the limbic leucotomy study included ten patients who died within the follow-up period (all were rated as 'worse') whereas the 25 patients who died after stereotactic tractotomy were excluded.

Neither procedure has been shown to produce serious undesirable side effects on intellect or personality. Evidence of disinhibition following limbic leucotomy appeared to be limited to a slight increase in Extraversion scores on the Maudsley Personality Inventory (Eysenck 1959) and a few cases of increased outspokenness reported by relatives but considered by all involved with the patient to have been a change for the better (Kelly 1980). After stereotactic tractotomy, slight disinhibition was reported by relatives of 6.7% of patients (Göktepe et al. 1975).

Mean intelligence quotients derived from the Wechsler Adult Intelligence Scale (Wechsler 1955) showed no decline 6 weeks after limbic leucotomy when compared with preoperative scores. On the contrary, mean Full Scale IQ for

Table 7.1 Clinical outcome of various psychosurgical procedures

Diagnosis		n	Minimum follow-up period	No. patients in each clinical category*					% greatly improved
				I	II	III	IV	V	(I and II)
Stereotactic limbic leucotomy (Kelly 1980)	Total sample	148	1 yr.	18	44	37	36	13	42
	Obsessional	49		7	23	11	5	3	61
	Anxiety	27		3	5	9	8	2	30
	Depression	36		7	7	8	11	3	39
	Other	36		1	9	9	12	5	36
Stereotactic subcaudate tractotomy (Göktepe et al. 1975)	Total sample	134	2½ yr.	45	33	33	23	0	58
	Obsessional	18		7	2	6	3	0	50
	Anxiety	24		11	4	5	4	0	62
	Depression	78		27	26	16	9	0	68
	Other	14		0	1	6	7	0	7
Bimedial leucotomy (Post et al. 1968)	Mixed	52	3 yr.	7	7	14	15	9	27
Stereotactic anterior cingulotomy (Ballantine et al. 1967)	Mixed	17	1 yr.	3	6	2	3	3	53
Multifocal leucocoagulation (Crow 1973)	Total sample	90	2 yr.	29	26	18	17	0	61
	Obsessional	49		14	13	11	11	0	55
	Anxiety (fear)	41		15	13	7	6	0	68

* I Symptom-free
II Greatly improved
III Improved
IV Unchanged
V Worse

Kelly's (1980) group of 122 patients rose significantly from 102.5 preoperatively to 105.7 postoperatively ($p < 0.001$). Both Verbal and Performance quotients showed similar highly significant increases, probably due to practice effects and improved concentration. There was no significant decline in scores on any of the 11 subtests.

Anterior cingulotomy (Table 7.1) greatly improved 9 out of 17 (53%) patients rated at least 1 year postoperatively (Ballantine et al. 1967). A decade later the same author reported on long-term clinical outcome of 154 psychiatric patients who underwent this procedure between 1962 and 1975 in the USA. A 'significantly improved' rating, assigned to patients who were symptom free or much improved, including those still under frequent psychiatric care, accounted for 70–80% of cases. The reported absence of permanent side effects has been confirmed elsewhere (Teuber et al. 1977).

Results of multifocal leucocoagulation (with concurrent psychotherapy) were published for a series of 90 patients comprising 49 with obsessive–compulsive disorder and 41 with a particular form of chronic anxiety (Crow 1973). 'Substantial improvement' or better (categories I–III of Table 7.1) was claimed for 81% of patients after the 2- to 12-year follow-up period, with anxious patients doing better than the obsessive–compulsive group. Despite its comparable effectiveness with other operations, this procedure is relatively prolonged, denies patients normal social contact for several months and may increase the risk of infection.

There is evidence that bimedial leucotomy may be effective in relieving much affective symptomatology, but this procedure carries considerable risk of psychiatric complications. Table 7.1 shows global clinical ratings (originally A to E) for 52 patients who underwent surgery between 1953 and 1958 and were followed up approximately 3 years later. Twelve patients are excluded from the figures shown, including all six cases of schizophrenia and two who died. An estimated 56% of patients were improved (27% greatly improved) following bimedial leucotomy and these figures rose to about 62% (37%) after an extended follow-up period. However, long-term side effects were present in almost two-thirds of cases and 29% suffered troublesome or disabling complications such as disinhibition, fits, anergia and incontinence.

A review of contemporary psychosurgery would not be complete without reference to its use for anorexia nervosa. Of five anorectic patients who underwent limbic leucotomy, one became symptom free, three were unchanged and one committed suicide during the 20-month mean follow-up period (Kelly 1980). A detailed report of four of these patients has been published by Crisp and Kalucy (1973). Free-hand bimedial leucotomy was reported to produce 'excellent' results in six out of seven anorectics (the seventh patient committed suicide), 1 month to 4 years (mean 17 months) postoperatively (Post and Schurr 1977). Ballantine et al. (1977) reported that symptoms of anorexia were present in 47% of 84 patients selected for anterior cingulotomy; at follow-up such symptoms had disappeared in all but about 9% of cases. However, as anorexia nervosa often improves without treatment, no firm conclusions can be drawn, and it should also be noted that those patients selected for psychosurgery are likely to be atypical examples (i.e. often the most severe cases) of this syndrome.

Finally, some patients with schizophrenic syndromes have apparently responded well to contemporary surgical intervention in carefully selected cases with associated tension, anxiety, depressions or obsessions. Of 19 patients who underwent limbic leucotomy, Kelly (1980) reported a 63% overall improvement, with markedly reduced affective symptomatology and decreased frequency and severity of psychotic episodes. However, it is doubtful that the underlying schizophrenic process is modified.

NEUROSURGERY FOR PATHOLOGICAL AGGRESSION

Neurosurgery is occasionally employed as a last resort in treating pathological aggression or self-mutilation, often associated with epilepsy, mental subnormality, personality disorder or chronic schizophrenia, although considerable ethical problems exist. Target sites for lesions lie in the temporal lobes, particularly the amygdala (amygdalotomy), or in the hypothalamus (hypothalamotomy).

Operative Procedures

Amygdalotomy or *amygdaloidotomy* evolved from the more radical temporal lobotomies instituted for epilepsy. Stimulation of the amygdala in conscious patients produces rage, restlessness, 'flight' reaction or physically destructive behaviour (Hitchcock and Cairns 1973). Amygdalotomy is performed bilaterally or unilaterally by means of stereotactic bipolar electrocoagulation, with the patient under general anaesthesia. The approach is through frontal burr holes at the coronal suture, 3 cm or 4 cm from the midline (Kiloh et al. 1974). Amygdalotomy has been combined with subcaudate tractotomy (Vaernet and Madsen 1970).

Schvarcz et al. (1972) in Argentina described a technique for performing posteromedial *hypothalamotomy* based on the work of Sano et al. (1966) in Japan. With the aid of sterotactic apparatus, pneumoencephalography and polygraphy of autonomic activity during electrical stimulation, target sites were located bilaterally in the medial section of the posterior hypothalamic area. Electrical stimulation of this site under local anaesthesia produced 'a strong emotional reaction of a fearful quality' (Schvarcz 1977) as well as marked cardiovascular sympathetic responses. Lesions were made through prefrontal burr holes by electrocoagulation, usually under general anaesthesia.

Stereotactic hypothalamotomy has also been recommended for certain individuals with a history of sexual violence. Dieckmann and Hassler (1977) in Germany selected target sites in the 'sexual behaviour centre' and in part of the 'hormonal sexual centre' of the hypothalamus, and lesioned the ventromedial nucleus, preoptic area and tuberomamillary complex unilaterally in four male sexual offenders.

Finally in Czechoslovakia, Nádvorník et al. (1977) lesioned the anterior hypothalamus bilaterally in ten patients with 'hedonia', and claimed consequent reduction of alcoholism and sexual deviance.

Clinical Efficacy

Amygdalotomy is rarely performed in the UK, but a study of 18 patients treated over a 5-year period has been reported by Hitchcock and Cairns (1973) working in Edinburgh. The patient group comprised five females and 13 males aged 8–46 years, of whom all but two had a history of epilepsy. All were referred for abnormally aggressive behaviour, associated in five cases with severe subnormality, in four cases with alcoholism and in four further cases with personality disorder. Shortly after amygdalotomy, three patients suffered fewer and less severe epileptic fits; five patients were less violent and destructive than preoperatively; six showed less psychological disturbance and one showed reduced self-abusive behaviour. However, with regard to discharge into the community, the authors state: '...we cannot claim, as other authors have done, that post-operatively a majority of patients become capable of effective functioning in a social context' (Hitchcock and Cairns 1973, p. 901).

A year after amygdalotomy, Kiloh et al. (1974) in Australia found 50% overall improvement (22% 'markedly improved') in a mixed group of 18 patients showing pathological aggression, but over a 2–6 year follow-up only 39% of the patients were rated as even slightly improved. This result may have been due to the large number of mentally retarded patients in the sample, in whom injurious behaviour is rarely reduced by this method alone, and such behaviour may respond more favourably when amygdalotomy is combined with stereotactic tractotomy (Vaernet and Madsen 1970; Post and Schurr 1977). Also, epileptic patients, who as a group did best overall, numbered only five in the sample of 18.

Side effects of amygdalotomy included convulsions, infection and even permanent hemiparesis. There was no gross impairment of intellect or cognitive function after the immediate postoperative period.

With regard to posteromedial hypothalamotomy, Sano et al. (1972) in Japan claimed 95% overall improvement in a sample of 43 patients, of whom 13 showed marked improvement. They also reported a decrease in frequency and intensity of seizures in over 30% of patients with associated epilepsy.

Schvarcz (1977) reported 80% overall improvement after posterior hypotha-lamotomy among 33 successive patients during a follow-up period of 1–8 years. Of these, 19 (58%) showed marked improvement (without aggressive crises and with reasonable social readjustment); eight were classed as improved (with occasional irritability, but tractable and with reasonable social adjustment); and in six cases the condition neither improved nor worsened. In general, this procedure appeared to be associated with a decrease in violent behaviour, hostility and restlessness, and an increase in calmness and cooperation. Side effects during the first postoperative week included hyperinsomnia, hyperther-mia and lack of spontaneity; however, none of these effects was permanent and performance on intelligence tests was not impaired.

Ventromedial hypothalamotomy was performed for sexual violence in four patients between 1972 and 1974 (Dieckmann and Hassler 1977). All showed a marked reduction in sexual drive postoperatively, with consequent release from prison. The main side effect was augmented appetite resulting in weight gain.

NEUROSURGERY FOR INTRACTABLE PAIN

When chronic and debilitating pain is thought to have a strong psychogenic component, or when it is known to be organic in origin but causes intolerable emotional suffering, psychosurgery may be indicated. Target sites for relief of pain lie in the anterior cingulate area or in the thalamus, which projects to the cingulum. In past years, prefrontal lobotomy has been found effective in treating pain (Watts and Freeman 1948) but the deterioration of personality often accompanying this procedure led to its gradual decline.

Operative Procedures

Stereotactic anterior cingulotomy or *cingulumotomy* has been described in detail by Foltz and White (1962) from the USA. The patient's head is shaved anteriorly and ventricles outlined by means of pneumoencephalography. Under local anaesthesia, burr holes are produced 1.5 cm each side of the midline, 9 cm posterior to the nasion. Electrodes are inserted to a depth of 3.5 cm below the cortex into the anterior cingulate area, and after checking their position on X-ray film, two or three electrocoagulative lesions are made in each cingulum. A marked improvement in affect was usually found to accompany lesion production, and stimulation of target sites in two patients produced feelings of agitation and apprehension which the patients found difficult to describe (Foltz and White 1962).

Thalamotomy is another procedure intended to relieve pain. Stereotactic methods are employed for lesioning various groups of thalamic nuclei, the most common target sites being the pulvinar (pulvinotomy) or the centromedian, dorsomedial or ventrolateral nuclei. Thalamotomy is performed with the patient fully conscious, in order to minimize risks of damaging the motor system.

Stereotactic anterior pulvinotomy has been described by Laitinen (1977). The lateral ventricle contralateral to the side of pain (or both ventricles if pain is bilateral) is outlined by air introduced through a frontal burr hole. Using the posterior commissure, the midline and the intercommissural line as landmarks, the pulvinar is located and destroyed anteriorly by one or two thermocoagulative lesions, often producing immediate pain relief.

Hypophysectomy may be effective in relieving pain caused by carcinoma of the breast or prostate, but this procedure is considered inappropriate for treating 'psychogenic' pain. The operation involves stereotactic placement of a cryogenic probe into the pituitary fossa via the nasal cavities. Alternatively, lesions may be produced by radioactive yttrium, or by free-hand methods following craniotomy (Bond 1979).

Clinical Efficacy

Foltz and White (1962) reported the apparent effects of frontal cingulumotomy on 16 patients and assigned each to one of three groups. Group I comprised five patients with 'psychogenic pain', assessed 5 months to 7 years postoperatively. Of these, one was classed as 'excellent', three as 'good' (but one died), and one as 'fair'. Group II patients (five cases) had 'organic disease with paroxysmal pain related to emotion' and were followed up 1 month to 6 years after operation. Two obtained rating as 'excellent', one was 'fair' and two were rated as 'poor', of whom one was reclassed as 'good' following reoperation. Of six group III patients, with 'neoplastic disease, organic pain and strong emotional factors', two were classed as 'excellent', three as 'good' and one as 'fair'. All group III patients predictably died of their illness within 9 months of operation.

Overall, those patients with severe depression included in their diagnosis showed the most improvement after surgery, whereas there was little change in those with 'inadequate personality'.

The authors commented: 'The perception of pain as such does not appear to be modified, but the patient's total reaction to pain and the threat to existence that it represents is modified markedly'. They concluded that the effectiveness of the operation 'depends primarily on the basic substrate of personality and emotional reactivity of the patient' (Foltz and White 1962).

The therapeutic effects of thalamotomy are strikingly inconsistent, but anterior pulvinotomy may be preferable to centromedian thalamotomy in terms of permanence of pain relief (Laitinen 1977), and to ventrolateral thalamotomy in terms of undesirable effects on cognition (Vilkki and Laitinen 1976). In a series of 41 cases of intractable pain treated by anterior pulvinotomy between

1970 and 1974, 46% of patients were completely free of pain immediately after surgery, 29% complained of residual, dull pain, and 10% obtained no benefit from the operation. However, at follow-up a mean of 29 months later, these figures changed to 29%, 27% and 44%, respectively. Four patients suffered permanent disabling side effects, including numbness and aphasia (Laitinen 1977). These results, in line with long-term results of ablation of other thalamic nuclei, are not very encouraging.

MANAGEMENT OF THE PSYCHOSURGICAL PATIENT

Patients referred for psychosurgery have generally been under the care of a psychiatrist for several years but infrequently there are direct referrals from general practitioners.

To conclude from the studies reviewed, a patient with severe persistent treatment-resistant depression, anxiety or obsessive–compulsive neurosis can be considered for stereotactic limbic leucotomy or stereotactic tractotomy; some patients with uncontrollable pathological aggressiveness associated with a psychiatric or neurological abnormality may occasionally be referred for amygdalotomy or hypothalamotomy; and, rarely, cases of intractable debilitating pain may be referred for cingulotomy or thalamotomy. Such patients should be able to give informed consent, have failed to respond to all other treatments for several years, and not be compulsorily detained.

Unfavourable prognostic signs include psychopathy, antisocial premorbid personality, drug dependency and alcoholism.

Weighed against the operative risks already described, and also the 0.6% risk of chronic epilepsy (Smith 1977), must be the dangers associated with continuing psychiatric morbidity, notably suicide and self-injury.

Preoperatively the psychosurgical team satisfies itself that the patient has undergone energetic attempts with the whole spectrum of routine therapies with no lasting success. The patient and close relatives are made aware of the potential risks and benefits of surgery and informed consent is obtained. It is important that the family understands that the patient's postoperative improvement is often very gradual, taking perhaps 2 years to achieve full benefit.

The patient is usually admitted 1 week prior to operation for clinical and psychological tests and withdrawal of medication. Postoperative headache and nausea may be treated with a codeine compound and generally recover during the first week. Anticonvulsants may be given routinely, but other medication is avoided as far as possible. Behaviour therapy tends to be more effective after surgery and is reintroduced where appropriate, for example with obsessive –compulsive disorders.

Both the patient and his family must be reassured constantly that progress during the first year or so is gradual and that temporary worsening of symptoms does not mean that the operation has failed. If this is not stressed and if support is withdrawn, there may be a considerable risk of suicide.

In the hands of experts, psychosurgery may offer considerable benefits to a highly selected group of patients and its place should not be ignored among the variety of treatments available today. Although previous evaluation of psychosurgery is far from satisfactory from a methodological viewpoint, the psychiatrist must guard against prejudice and inappropriate emotional reactions. The evidence, flawed though it is, suggests that many patients with intractable and distressing conditions have received considerable benefit. The ethical controversy continues.

References

BALLANTINE, H.T., CASSIDY, W.C., FLANAGAN, N.B. & MARINO, R. (1967) Stereotactic anterior cingulotomy for neuropsychiatric illness and intractable pain. *J. Neurosurg.*, **26**, 488.

BALLANTINE, H.T., LEVY, B.S., DAGI, T.F. & GIRIUNAS, I.B. (1977) Cingulotomy for psychiatric illness: report of 13 years' experience. In: *Neurosurgical Treatment in Psychiatry, Pain and Epilepsy*, ed. Sweet, W.H., Obrador, S. & Martín-Rodríguez, J.G. Baltimore: University Park Press.

BARRACLOUGH, B.M. & MITCHELL-HEGGS, N.A. (1978) Use of neurosurgery for psychological disorder in British Isles during 1974–6. *Br. med. J.*, **2**, 1591.

BECK, A., WARD, C., MENDOLSON, M., MARK, J. & ERBAUGH, J. (1961) An inventory for measuring depression. *Archs gen. Psychiat.*, **4**, 561.

BOND, M.R. (1979) Local analgesia, nerve blocks and surgical methods of pain relief. In: *Functional Neurosurgery*, ed. Rasmussen, T. & Marino, R. New York: Raven Press.

BRIDGES, P.K., GÖKTEPE, E.O. & MARATOS, J. (1973) A comparative review of patients with obsessional neurosis and depression treated by psychosurgery. *Br. J. Psychiat.*, **123**, 663.

COOPER, J. (1970) The Leyton Obsessional Inventory. *Psychol. Med.*, **1**, 48.

COOPER, J. & McNEIL, J. (1968) A study of house-proud housewives and their interaction with their children. *J. Child. Psychol. Psychiat.*, **9**, 173.

CRISP, A.H. & KALUCY, R.S. (1973) The effect of leucotomy in intractable adolescent weight phobia (primary anorexia nervosa). *Postgrad. med. J.*, **49**, 883.

CROW, H.J. (1973) Intracerebral polarisation and multifocal leucocoagulation in some psychiatric illnesses. *Folie psychiat. neurol. neurochir. neerl.*, **76**, 365.

CROWN, S. & CRISP, A.H. (1966) A short clinical diagnostic self-rating scale for psychoneurotic patients. *Br. J. Psychiat.*, **112**, 917.

DIECKMANN, G. & HASSLER, R. (1977). Treatment of sexual violence by stereotactic hypothalamotomy. In: *Neurosurgical Treatment in Psychiatry, Pain and Epilepsy*, ed. Sweet, W.H., Obrador, S. & Martín-Rodríguez, J.G. Baltimore: University Park Press.

EYSENCK, H. (1959) *Manual of the Maudsley Personality Inventory*.London.

FOLTZ, E.L. & WHITE, L.E. (1962) Pain 'relief' by frontal cingulumotomy. *J. Neurosurg.*, **19**, 89.

GÖKTEPE, E.O., YOUNG, L.B. & BRIDGES, P.K. (1975) A further review of the results of stereotactic subcaudate tractotomy. *Br. J. Psychiat.*, **126**, 270.

GREENBLATT, M. & SOLOMON, H.C. (1952) Survey of nine years of lobotomy investigations. *Am. J. Psychiat.*, **109**, 262.

HAMILTON, M. (1959) The assessment of anxiety states by rating. *Br. J. med. Psychol.*, **32**, 50.

HAMILTON, M. (1967) Development of a rating scale for primary depressive illness. *Br. J. Soc. clin. Psychol.*, **6**, 278.

HITCHCOCK, E. & CAIRNS, V. (1973) Amygdalotomy. *Postgrad. med. J.*, **49**, 894.

KELLY, D. (1980) *Anxiety and Emotions: Physiological Basis and Treatment.* Springfield, Ill.: Charles C. Thomas.

KELLY, D., RICHARDSON, A. & MITCHELL-HEGGS, N. (1973) Stereotactic limbic leucotomy: neurophysiological aspects and operative technique. *Br. J. Psychiat.*, **123**, 133.

KILOH, L.G., GYE, R.S., RUSHWORTH, R.G., BELL, D.S. & WHITE, R.T. (1974) Stereotactic amygdaloidotomy for aggressive behaviour. *J. Neurol. Neurosurg. Psychiat.*, **37**, 437.

KNIGHT, G. (1973) Further observations from an experience of 660 cases of stereotactic tractotomy. *Postgrad. med. J.*, **49**, 845.

LAITINEN, L.V. (1977) Anterior pulvinotomy in the treatment of intractable pain. In: *Neurosurgical Treatment in Psychiatry, Pain, and Epilepsy*, ed. Sweet, W.H., Obrador, S. & Martín-Rodríguez, J.G. Baltimore: University Park Press.

LEKSELL, L. (1966) Some principles and technical aspects of stereotaxic surgery. In: *Pain*, ed. Knighton, R.S. & Dumke, P.R., Boston: Little, Brown.

MONIZ, E. (1936) *Tentatives opératoires dans le traitement de certaines psychoses*. Paris: Masson et Cie.

NÁDVORNÍK, P., SRAMKA, M. & PATOPRSTÁ, G. (1977) Transventricular anterior hypothalamotomy in stereotactic treatment of hedonia. In: *Neurosurgical Treatment in Psychiatry, Pain and Epilepsy*, ed. Sweet, W.H., Obrador, S. & Martín-Rodríguez, J.G. Baltimore: University Park Press.

PIPPARD, J. (1955) Rostral leucotomy: a report on 240 cases personally followed up after 1½ to 5 years. *J. ment. Sci.*, **101**, 756.

POST, F., REES, L. & SCHURR, P.H. (1968) An evaluation of bimedial leucotomy. *Br. J. Psychiat.*, **114**, 1223.

POST, F. & SCHURR, P.H. (1977) Changes in the pattern of diagnosis of patients subjected to psychosurgical procedures, with comments on their use in the treatment of self-mutilation and anorexia nervosa. In: *Neurosurgical Treatment in Psychiatry, Pain and Epilepsy*, ed. Sweet, W.H., Obrador, S. & Martín-Rodríguez, J.G. Baltimore: University Park Press.

RICHARDSON, A. (1973) Stereotactic limbic leucotomy: surgical technique. *Postgrad. med. J.*, **49**, 860.

SANO, K., SEKINO, H. & MAYANAGI, Y. (1972) Results of stimulation and destruction of the posterior hypothalamus in cases with violent, aggressive or restless behaviors. In: *Psychosurgery*, ed. Hitchcock, E., Laitinen, L. & Vaernet, K. Springfield, Illinois: Charles C. Thomas.

SANO, K. YOSHIOKA, M., OGASHIWA, M., ISHIJIMA, B. & OHYE, C. (1966) Postero-medial hypothalamotomy in the treatment of aggressive behaviors. *Confinia neurol.* **27**, 164.

SCHVARCZ, J.R. (1977) Results of stimulation and destruction of the posterior hypothalamus: A long-term evaluation. In: *Neurological Treatment in Psychiatry, Pain and Epilepsy*, ed. Sweet, W.H., Obrador, S. & Martín-Rodríguez, J.G. Baltimore: University Park Press.

SCHVARCZ, J.R., DRIOLLET, R., RIOS, E. & BETTI, O. (1972) Stereotactic hypothalamotomy for behaviour disorders. *J. Neurol. Neurosurg. Psychiat.*, **35**, 356.

SCOVILLE, W.B. (1949) Selective cortical undercutting as a means of modifying and studying frontal lobe function in man. *J. Neurosurg.* **6**, 65.

SMITH, J.S. (1977) The treatment of anxiety, depression and obsessionality. In: *Psychosurgery and Society*, ed. Smith, J.S. & Kiloh, L.G., Oxford: Pergamon Press.

SMITH, J.S. & KILOH, L.G. (1980) The psychosurgical treatment of anxiety. In: *Handbook of Studies on Anxiety*, ed. Burrows, G. & Davis, B. Amsterdam: Elsevier/North Holland Biomedical Press.

SNAITH, R.P., AHMED, S.N., MEHTA, S. & HAMILTON, M. (1971) Assessment of the severity of primary depressive illness. *Psychol. Med.*, **1**, 143.

TAYLOR, J. (1953) A personality scale of manifest anxiety. *J. abnorm. soc. Psychol.*, **48**, 285.

TEUBER, H.-L., CORKIN, S.H. & TWITCHELL, T.E. (1977) Study of cingulotomy in man: a summary. In: *Neurosurgical Treatment in Psychiatry, Pain and Epilepsy*, ed. Sweet, W.H., Obrador, S. & Martín-Rodríguez, J.G. Baltimore: University Park Press.

TOOTH, G.C. & NEWTON, M.P. (1961) *Leucotomy in England and Wales 1942–54. Reports on Public Health and Medical Subjects No. 104*. London: Ministry of Health, HMSO.

VAERNET, K. & MADSEN, A. (1970) Stereotactic amygdalotomy and basofrontal tractotomy in psychotics with aggressive behaviour. *J. Neurol. Neurosurg. Psychiat.*, **33**, 858.

VALENSTEIN, E.S. (1973) *Brain Control*, p. 264. London: John Wiley.

VILKKI, J. & LAITINEN, L.V. (1976) Effects of pulvinotomy and ventrolateral thalamotomy on some cognitive functions. *Neuropsychologia*, **14**, 67.

WATTS, J.W. & FREEMAN, W. (1948) Frontal lobotomy in the treatment of unbearable pain. *Res. Publ. Ass. nerv. ment. Dis.*, **27**, 715.

WECHSLER, D. (1955) *Manual for the Wechsler Adult Intelligence Scale*. New York: The Psychological Corporation.

WHITTY, C.W.M., DUFFIELD, J.E., TOW, P.M. & CAIRNS, H. (1952) Anterior cingulectomy in the treatment of mental disease. *Lancet*, **i**, 475.

8

Individual Psychotherapy

G.E. Berrios

INTRODUCTION

Psychotherapy can be defined as the modification of abnormal behaviour by psychological means. 'Behaviour' refers to both public demeanour and subjective experience, 'abnormal' to both subjectively unpleasant and statistically deviant dysfunction, and 'psychological means' to forms of communication conveyed by language, or to the provision of certain experiences. Thus behaviour therapy, relaxation techniques and hypnosis can also be considered as forms of psychotherapy. However this chapter will only be concerned with that form of psychotherapy which is dependent upon the nature of the relationship between the patient and the therapist; such a relationship involves an informational and emotional exchange which may modify the behaviour of both participants.

Definitions of psychotherapy are not essential to its practice but are necessary for purposes such as therapeutic outcome studies and organization of training. Some definitions are descriptive: i.e. 'the art of alleviating personal difficulties through the agency of words and a personal professional relationship' (Storr 1979), while others highlight change: i.e. an 'interpersonal process designed to bring about modifications of feelings, cognitions, attitudes and behaviour which have proven troublesome to the person seeking help' (Strupp 1978). Yet others are critical, and psychotherapy has been called an 'undefined technique applied to unspecific problems with unpredictable outcome' (Hinsie and Campbell 1970). As the format of psychotherapeutic practice changes according to theoretical, ethical and professional variables, so there is no homogeneous body of theory and practice which is available for controlled research.

The process of 'individual' psychotherapy consists of the exchange of verbal and non-verbal messages in the context of a relationship between two individuals, and it has been claimed that one possible outcome of this process is a non-random modification of the patient's (or client's) personality resulting from manoeuvres and strategies under the cognitive control of the therapist. The latter is guided by a theoretical model, but although a great deal of debate has taken place on the relative efficacy of the various 'schools' of psychotherapy, there is evidence that, at least for groups of patients, technical procedures and theoretical models are less relevant to outcome than the personal attributes of the therapist, including his capacity for empathy, warmth, flexibility and genuineness (Frank 1974).

Some forms of psychotherapy have the relatively modest aims of supporting the individual in 'the here and now', while other procedures strive for more ambitious goals which can include the provision of insight and the subsequent modification of established patterns of behaviour. Some psychotherapists have even excluded symptomatic change from their primary objectives on the basis that this will lead to 'symptom substitution'. However, this fear may be unwarranted.

Few aspects of psychotherapy are free from controversy. Some find it difficult to accept that 'talking' may constitute, by itself, a means of significant change, while others, although accepting that change may take place, consider psychotherapy as a 'hit and miss' activity, on the basis that little is known about its crucial variables. It has also been pointed out that for any sample of patients treated by psychotherapy, the rate of spontaneous remission is unknown and adequate controls cannot be provided (Rachman and Wilson 1980). In answering these criticisms it has been claimed that it is the ongoing relationship (and not the mere 'talking') that constitutes the main agent of change; that sufficient is known about the psychotherapeutic process to control outcome; and, that the detailed study of individual cases ought to be accepted as a source of evidence as statistical procedures may not be relevant to the study of psychotherapy.

Much controversy also surrounds the assessment of outcome, and it has been suggested that a 'positive' outcome can be judged to have occurred when the patient comes 'to see' his problems in the same way as the therapist. Thus, a judgement of positive outcome may sometimes depend more upon the therapist's powers of persuasion than upon the appropriateness of his interventions.

Most psychiatrists in the UK practise in the context of the National Health Service, which imposes practical constraints upon their psychotherapeutic activity, and although many professionally trained people who are not psychiatrists are engaged in various forms of psychotherapeutic activity, there are no generally accepted standards for their training. The British Psychological Society has advised against registration of psychotherapists on the basis that it would 'not be feasible to establish any generally accepted consensus as to precisely which of these various psychotherapy trainings should be regarded as acceptable for the purposes of registration' (B.P.S. 1980; Shepherd 1980).

If psychotherapy is an effective form of treatment, it follows that undesirable effects may also occur, although some have believed that psychotherapy is, at its best, very effective and, at its worst, innocuous. However, clinical experience suggests that negative effects can occur, and that psychotherapy should be offered only 'on prescription', that is, in response to clear indications, in the same way as all other methods of treatment; it is not the basic panacea upon which the 'symptomatic' treatments are grafted. In the UK, adequate monitoring by experienced psychiatrists of the 'psychotherapy' offered by a psychiatric service is difficult to achieve, and non-medical professionals are taking on an ever larger number of patients for psychotherapy.

This chapter will emphasize the practical aspects of individual psychotherapy in routine psychiatric practice. It will not consider relatively long-term psychotherapy which is based on methods derived from psychoanalytic theories. Psychotherapy will be considered as a form of treatment which is not incompatible with other procedures such as ECT or psychopharmacology (Rosenzweig and Griscom 1978).

GENERAL PRINCIPLES

Urban and Ford (1971) have suggested that 'one of the ways to encompass the heterogeneity that the field of psychotherapy represents is within the framework of the problem solving approach', which involves recognition of the difficulty, definition of its boundaries, search for solutions, selection of a solution, and implementation. The psychotherapeutic process can be analysed from the point of view of the therapist, the patient or the relationship itself. Successful outcome has been shown to correlate positively with high scores in therapist variables such as warmth, empathy, altruism and flexibility (Truax and Carkhuff 1967; Razin 1977; Parloff et al. 1978). It is not clear whether these characteristics may be enhanced by specialized psychotherapeutic training, as they depend to a considerable extent on the therapist's personality.

Various patient variables are important with regard to outcome. In order to enter into a relatively intensive form of psychotherapy, the patient should usually be willing to cooperate, be relatively articulate, accept that the origin of his dysphoria might be 'psychological', and be prepared to consider interpretations designed to illuminate unconscious mental activity. Conversely, indications of poor outcome are chronic alcoholism, drug addiction, long-term hospitalization, serious suicidal behaviour, chronic phobic or obsessive–compulsive disorders, antisocial or self-destructive behaviour, severe endogenous depression, or acute schizophrenic psychosis (Malan 1979). These do not constitute absolute contraindications to intensive psychotherapy and occasional successes have been reported, but for most techniques which include the aim of exploring mental processes of which the patient is unaware, they constitute exclusion criteria. In practice, the type of patient chosen for relatively intensive psychotherapy is different from the chronic attender at psychiatric out-patient clinics.

TYPES OF INDIVIDUAL PSYCHOTHERAPY

Individual psychotherapies may be classified according to objectives, theory, length and setting (Alexander and French 1946; Castelnuovo-Tedesco 1975; Karasu 1977), but for the purposes of this chapter individual psychotherapy will be divided into 'supportive' and 'interpretive' types (Burke et al. 1979; Marmor 1979). Supportive psychotherapy consists of relatively 'common sense' measures such as the provision of advice, encouragement, an opportunity to express emotion, and attention to any modifiable aspect of the environment, while interpretive psychotherapy places an emphasis on producing an increasing awareness of unconscious mental activity (see Chapter 9). However, in practice, there is considerable overlap between these two classes of intervention (Bloch 1977, 1979; Johnson et al. 1980).

Supportive Psychotherapy

This is the most commonly practised form of psychotherapy and is the generic name for a variety of procedures, whose characteristics depend a great deal, as in all psychotherapy, upon the therapist's personal style. Thus attempts to offer a standardized description must be somewhat idealized (Bloch 1979).

Patients with chronic psychiatric problems often lead a precarious social existence due to factors such as residual psychotic symptoms, chronic neurotic disorder, maladaptive personality characteristics and the prevailing attitudes of society. Such individuals, together with those living through short-term crises, constitute the two main groups who receive supportive psychotherapy.

Crisis intervention is a form of supportive psychotherapy which has attracted much theorizing, although it is not clear whether it should be considered as a separate technique. In fact, it has 'as many meanings as there are people writing about it' (Barcroft 1979).

The term 'crisis' originated in Greek medicine as a method for the prediction of change in the course of illness. Among the French psychiatrists of the early nineteenth century it simply meant 'spell' or 'attack'. In our own day its meaning is defined in interactional terms as the loss of a state of dynamic equilibrium (homeostasis) between hypothetical 'coping' mechanisms and external pressures. The term 'crisis' is used to refer both to the change itself and to its psychological consequences; thus it is both an explanatory and a descriptive concept which conveys a sense of transience. It also implies that the patient has a good chance of recovering, that he will suffer psychological distress and that recovery may occur without any outside influence.

The views of Lindeman, Erikson and Caplan have been influential in the development of a theoretical justification for psychotherapeutic interventions in a crisis (Darbonne 1968; Brandon 1970). For example it has been claimed that skilful psychotherapeutic intervention during a crisis can increase the likelihood of a positive outcome, and that it is possible that equilibrium can be regained at a higher level of functioning as a result of learning during the crisis period. The plausibility of these concepts has led to the development of aetiological theories, specialized psychiatric services and new techniques of social therapy (Caplan 1964; Viney 1976; Donovan et al. 1979).

One form of crisis intervention is a period of intensive short-term psychotherapy of between a few days and 6 weeks. This can take place in a variety of settings including special units, a psychiatric unit or a day hospital. The therapist focuses on the crisis itself, its precipitants and future repercussions, and may also use nonpsychotherapeutic treatments such as pharmacotherapy in cases of overwhelming anxiety or disturbed sleep. Treatment is said to facilitate psychological reorganization and the mobilization of internal resources.

Controlled outcome studies on the value of crisis intervention are not available, so that it is still unclear what proportion of the recovery is due to natural spontaneous improvement, to the discontinuation of the source of stress, or to the techniques themselves. A recent study showed that psychiatric 'flying squads' which visit the patient's home seem to make no difference to psychiatric admission rates in neighbouring hospitals (West et al. 1980), and current practices of crisis intervention seem to be based largely on theoretical grounds. However, Stein (1981) has recently claimed that a 24-hour 'walk-in' clinic in an urban setting can reduce hospital readmission rates in those patients with chronic psychoses. Since walk-in clinics, crisis intervention units or psychiatric flying squads are all expensive, further cost–benefit analyses are indicated. Research in this area is difficult as it may be deemed unethical to withhold psychotherapeutic support in times of crisis. Despite the lack of evidence, it seems likely that supportive psychotherapy for short-term crises is worth pursuing (Cooper 1979).

Patients with chronic psychiatric disorders require supportive psychotherapy of a different kind, and some of the most accessible include those attending clinics for regular medication. During these contacts the social and psychological repercussions of the primary condition can be explored, and the patient is offered directive counselling. Two other groups in need of support consist of patients with chronic neurotic symptoms or maladaptive personality traits, which are often combined. For such individuals, regular out-patient attendance may be used to foster a limited dependence which can reduce the degree of decompensation in a crisis, thereby lessening the risk of hospital admission; supportive psychotherapy in this context can involve somewhat ritualized sessions, whose value stems less from their content than from the attendance itself. Another group who attend for supportive psychotherapy do so for what can be called iatrogenic reasons; some doctors find it difficult to discharge patients, and study of chronic attenders often reveals that some no longer require follow-up.

Supportive psychotherapy is inherent to all doctor–patient interactions (Cawley 1977). However, if one of the main variables in relation to outcome is the therapist's capacity for empathy and warmth, then alternative and more economical sources of support, involving other professional disciplines and the voluntary services must be sought (Hornblow and Sloane 1980). Supportive psychotherapy is a heterogeneous activity which encompasses techniques such as advice, encouragement, persuasion, explanation, diversion, reassurance, and an opportunity to display emotion. However, the appropriate advice may be complex and should be based on a detailed appraisal of the patient's personality and relationships. As such interventions take place against a background of community support it can be difficult to assess the extent of the doctor's contribution (Henderson et al. 1980).

In summary, supportive psychotherapy consists of the provision of an appropriate relationship with the therapist, together with interventions designed to modify the patient or his environment. Counselling and the opportunity to express emotions are directed to the patient himself, while attempts to modify the environment may include help with housing, money matters, and relationships within the family. The objectives may include helping the patient to come to terms with his psychological or social handicaps, and no attempt is made to modify fundamental personality traits. The goals of supportive psychotherapy are 'directed towards providing symptomatic improvement and re-establishing the patient's usually adaptive behaviour...This is not to imply that supportive psychotherapy is just a stop-gap measure...For many persons, the use of supportive techniques may constitute the most appropriate treatment approach' (Johnson et al. 1980).

When appropriate, clear advice should be given in the form of recommendations or suggestions. However, an even more directive approach may be appropriate for the severely handicapped patients, in whom decision making is often impaired. During a crisis, patients should be advised not to take any important decisions until some improvement has taken place.

Ventilation, which is the expression of pent-up emotion in a controlled and supportive interaction, may benefit patients who develop a mood disorder as a result of a build-up of distressing or anger-provoking ideas in everyday situations and, if the encouragement of this is appropriate, it should usually precede other interventions. Reassurance should, if possible, be specific, as general or vague reassurance is rarely helpful. Diversion, which involves the deliberate redirection of a patient's attention towards areas which allow him to utilize his assets, or are less likely to produce emotional arousal, may also be useful, for example, in patients whose social functioning is being affected by delusional beliefs. In spite of the occasional claim that patients with a severe schizophrenic illness benefit from relatively intensive psychotherapy designed to produce 'insight' (Benedetti 1980), it is unlikely that this is the case. During a severe psychosis, it is far more constructive to divert the patient's attention towards those areas of his personality and functioning which are relatively intact, thus helping him to regain a hold on reality. During the state of remission, a further goal of supportive psychotherapy may be to help the patient to understand what has happened and to come to terms with any residual symptoms. Strauss and Carpenter (1981) have written: 'the psychotherapy of schizophrenia need not be based on aetiological theory. The therapist who assumes that all aspects of schizophrenia are caused by personally meaningful connections will mislead and ultimately frustrate the patient and himself'.

Supportive psychotherapeutic measures may also be used in the management of neurotic reactions to severe physical illness; this approach may reduce the need for analgesia and facilitate the patient's general management (Johnson et al. 1980).

Interpretive Psychotherapy ('Brief' Psychotherapy)

The concept of brief interpretive psychotherapy is often unclear with regard to its length, theoretical background, techniques and efficacy. If 'brief' is taken to refer to duration of the total therapy, then a definition is not satisfactory unless the number and length of individual sessions are specified, but, in general, brief therapy refers to treatment administered in months rather than years involving 10–40 sessions of about 55 min, although successful outcomes have been reported with the so-called 20 minutes hour (Castelnuovo-Tedesco 1965). The accumulative length of brief interpretive psychotherapy is therefore determined both by the theoretical model that inspires it and by practical factors such as the time available, the psychotherapist's views, and the patient's response and resistance during treatment.

In practice, brief interpretive psychotherapy refers to techniques applied within a time scale as outlined above, which involve the aim of producing an increased awareness of unconscious mental activity. The search for the 'meaning' of behaviour in terms of early life events is not an overriding consideration, although such explanation can sometimes aid the development of insight. Suitable candidates for this approach usually present with neurotic symptoms (with the exception of obsessive–compulsive disorders), or repeated patterns of maladaptive behaviour (often associated with a personality disorder), which involve a degree of unconscious motivation, fear or conflict. (However, this is not to say that unconscious processes are always relevant in the development of these disorders.) With regard to unconscious (or partly conscious) processes, an interpretive approach is not usually undertaken unless their presence and nature are suspected by the therapist as, with the limited time available, it is usually imperative to formulate the focus of treatment at an early stage. In the case of undesirable patterns of behaviour in the setting of personality disorder, although unconscious motivation, fear or conflict may not be relevant, the subject can often be helped to understand the consequences of his behaviour, if these have been obscured by psychological defence mechanisms (see Glossary, Chapter 9). In any context, such defence mechanisms may have prevented the individual from facing up to the insoluble nature of a situation, or from attempting its modification if solutions exist. If the psychotherapist considers that defence mechanisms are maladaptive, he should try to assist the patient to discard them by using various strategies which are outlined in Chapter 9. However, it may be appropriate for certain mental processes to remain unconscious if their disguise represents the best possible adjustment.

The first two or three sessions of interpretive psychotherapy are usually dedicated to exploring the patient's problems, life history and personality, while subsequent sessions help the patient to become increasingly aware of unconscious mental activity. Any intervention on the part of the therapist directed to this end is called an 'interpretation'. During treatment, the patient may undergo what Alexander and French (1946) have called a 'corrective emotional experience'. The most popular brief interpretative psychotherapy techniques are those of Malan (1976), Castelnuovo-Tedesco (1965), Sifneos (1979), Small (1971), Mann (1973) and Rosen (1979).

The importance of Malan's contribution (1976, 1979) is threefold. It provides cogent arguments as to the rationality of his approach and provides the reader with adequate examples; it recognizes that psychotherapy may coexist with other forms of psychiatric treatment, thus departing from the isolationist approach of earlier specialists; and, most importantly, it acknowledges that some kind of outcome assessment is required.

Malan's central tenet is that the gradual learning process of relatively long-term psychotherapy (involving many months or years) can be achieved in a shorter period if technical modifications are introduced. These changes consist of offering to selected patients appropriate interpretations that focus on specific problems or conflicts. His selection criteria are the presence of high motivation, learning ability, and adequate psychological resilience, together with the possession of certain interpersonal and social skills. These, as can be seen, are rather restrictive. His exclusion criteria are a history of serious suicidal attempts, chronic alcoholism or drug addiction, long-term hospitalization, more than one course of ECT, a confirmed homosexual asking to be heterosexual, chronically incapacitating phobic and obsessional symptoms, and gross destructive or self-destructive 'acting out' (Malan 1979). The application of these criteria is qualified by the claim that 'it does not necessarily mean that no patient showing any of these characteristics ever responds to a psychotherapeutic approach but what it does mean is that, statistically speaking, such patients tend to be unsuitable' (Rounsaville et al. 1981; Weissman 1979).

Malan subscribes to the view that psychotherapy should be provided 'on prescription'; the psychotherapist must, therefore, formulate a clear psychiatric diagnosis, assess the relevant psychological and social factors, and formulate realistic goals for psychotherapy. Interpretations are used during the early stages of treatment to test psychopathological hypotheses and also to assess the patient's ability to cope with this form of intervention, but before interpretations are embarked upon, the therapist must make sure that the patient accepts that his problems are amenable to psychological help, is willing to talk about his feelings, can cope with discussion of emotionally charged topics, and is adequately motivated. It should be remembered that brief interpretive psychotherapy can worsen the patient's symptoms during the early stages so that marked psychological fragility may be a contraindication to treatment. At the beginning of treatment it is useful to determine a date for termination of the therapy, rather than to specify the actual number of sessions. In general, Malan has proposed 40 sessions as the upper limit; this is somewhat higher than other 'brief' psychotherapists who have proposed numbers between 10 and 20.

Malan has also tried to obtain validation for his methods by the detailed study of case histories. However, his conclusions have been criticized by Rachman and Wilson (1980), who, after acknowledging Malan's 'exceptional readiness to ask hard and even painful questions', call into question his method of assessing therapeutic outcome. They point out that he did not carry out any controlled comparisons, and that his retrospective assessment of outcome was not 'blind'. Nevertheless, Malan's awareness of the limited resources for the provision of psychotherapy in most psychiatric services cannot be questioned; Skynner and Brown (1981) have recently proposed, on economic grounds, that where possible family and group psychotherapy should be encouraged in preference to individual treatment.

NEGATIVE EFFECTS

From the proposition that psychotherapy is effective in modifying behaviour, it does not follow that the change will always be in the desired direction. Although opinions vary in this respect, it is likely that, as with any treatment, psychotherapy can produce short- and long-term side effects including depressive symptoms, a reversion to immature patterns of behaviour, destructive acts, increased anxiety, hostility, paranoid ideas, complaints of somatic disorders, worsening or generalization of existing phobias, guilt, lowered self-esteem, loss of impulse control and suicide (Hadley and Strupp 1976; Gomez-Schwartz 1982).

Theoretically it might be possible to identify potential sources of failure as originating in the therapist, the patient or the technique. For example, certain personality traits in the therapist have been associated with a poor therapeutic outcome, including emotional 'coldness', marked obsessionality, an excessive desire to make people change, seductiveness, and lack of interest, warmth or genuineness. Likewise, certain aspects of a patient's psychopathology have been claimed to correlate with poor outcome; these include masochistic character traits, lack of motivation for change and an unwillingness to accept treatment. Finally, aspects of technique such as inadequate assessment, or formulation of inappropriate or unrealistic treatment goals can also be relevant to failure.

In order to prevent these effects, the trainee psychiatrist should have the necessary attributes of personality and must receive regular supervision. He must ensure that his early work is with patients whose problems are not beyond his skills by seeking help with the selection of patients and with the type of approach for each case. During the treatment itself every psychiatrist must watch for the exacerbation of ongoing symptoms, the appearance of new ones, and the development by the patient of excessive dependence. The reasons for persistent lack of progress must be actively explored. If the psychiatrist is in training, he should see at least two or three 'long-term' patients (i.e. for about 2 years) and five or six relatively 'short-term' patients.

Not all suitable patients can be offered psychotherapy and, if resources are scarce, it is important that this costly commodity is offered sparingly. The conventional diagnostic categories are not very useful as selection criteria but brain damage, severe schizophrenic, manic or depressive states, psychopathic personality, and drug or alcohol abuse syndromes constitute recognizable groupings which suggest that, while supportive psychotherapy may help to contain and manage the problems, procedures which involve more ambitious treatment goals are not indicated.

The exclusion of these categories still leaves a large group of patients such as those with non-sociopathic personality disorders or with certain of the neuroses, who may be suitable for an interpretive approach. A number of criteria must then be used to select, from amongst this heterogeneous group, those most likely to respond. Such criteria may involve motivation, desire to change, ability to see problems in psychological terms, therapeutic optimism, lack of severe paranoid traits, ability to exercise a degree of self-control and a satisfactory (or potentially satisfactory) social situation.

If an emphasis is put on the external manifestations of behaviour, a common fear is that 'symptom substitution' may occur, that is to say, a symptom which disappears may be replaced by a new one. For example 'behaviour therapy' has been accused of just treating the symptom rather than its causes, and therefore of inviting symptom substitution. However, such evidence as there is does not indicate that this phenomenon is often of clinical significance (Cahoon 1968; Reider 1976), so that behaviour therapy may produce more extensive changes than it is generally believed (Weitzman 1967). This view is also taken by Skynner and Brown (1981) who have considered that patients with 'simple deficiencies in experience' or in whom 'training has been inappropriate' may especially benefit from a direct behavioural approach. Also, Fisher and Greenberg (1977) have pointed out that Freud felt that 'removal of symptoms without insight attainment would not necessarily lead to a new incapacitating dysfunction'.

THE MANIPULATIVE PATIENT

Some patients demand inappropriate medication or interviews (and may get angry or threaten suicide if this is refused), request frequent reassurance and promises of help, telephone the therapist at unreasonable hours, set impossible conditions and objectives for the therapy, and complain bitterly of lack of progress. Other less overtly manipulative patients behave in an obsequious and self-deprecating manner, putting the responsibility for treatment entirely in the therapist's hands, thus encouraging a collusion with the patient's apparent helplessness. Such patients do not usually make significant gains from psychotherapy, and are often rejected by their therapists or at least provoke much negative feeling.

Manipulative behaviour may accompany psychiatric syndromes such as hysterical neurosis (Martin 1971), personality disorder (Zetzel 1971; Bursten 1973), depression (Coyne 1976) and mania (Janowsky et al. 1970) and controversy exists in the literature about its nature, meaning and management.

One model of the nature of manipulative behaviour predicts that if the therapist gives in to the manipulative bid, this reinforces the underlying psychopathology. Thus, limit-setting appears to be the correct therapeutic strategy. The patient's bid must be challenged or uncovered, and his bluff should be called so that he has to endure the reaction to an ungratified manipulation. It is hoped that this may help him to discover that his distress is bearable, and that no major catastrophe takes place as a result of an unfulfilled desire. Even when the patient's 'threats' may lead to undesirable or dangerous actions such as an episode of self-injury, the therapist should not necessarily acquiesce, but this policy must be tempered by common sense, and if the patient shows significant distress or emotional arousal, then a short hospital admission may be appropriate even if this is what the patient is demanding. However, in such cases early discharge must be the aim (Murphy and Guze 1960.

Another model considers manipulation to be an interactional behaviour for which the therapist is equally responsible, and it has been claimed that manipulatory behaviour is, in fact, a 'role violation' perpetrated by the patient (Mackenzie et al. 1978). According to this concept, manipulative patients refuse to accept that the therapist is in charge and do not respect the tacit but clear boundaries of their relationship. This may result from the doctor's inability to make them clear. The challenge to the psychiatrist stems from the fact that the game is no longer being played by his rules, and he responds with outrage and anger, which, it is claimed, may conceal his fear lest he is blamed for the treatment failure. In terms of this model the therapist must develop extra tolerance and learn to live with the fact that he has set inappropriately strict rules of conduct for some patients.

In practice, both views are partially correct. Manipulative behaviours cannot be considered as a homogeneous group; some examples reflect severe psychopathology in the patient, while others may result from inappropriate management by the therapist. It is also true that some psychiatrists are too free in describing the patients as 'manipulative', so that the term loses its descriptive value and becomes a pejorative category. However, some individuals suffering from particular forms of personality disorder may resort to persistent manipulation, when limit setting should constitute the main therapeutic strategy.

LIMIT SETTING

A degree of limit setting takes place in all psychotherapeutic situations, which involve the therapist shaping the behaviour of the patient by verbal and non-verbal means. For example, if a psychotherapeutic process fosters dependence on the therapist, it is not uncommon for certain patients to delay imparting important information until the final stage of the session thus implicitly asking for the session to be extended. Such manoeuvres must be resisted by, for example, acknowledgement of the point in question and telling the patient that this will be considered at the beginning of the next session (Murphy and Guze 1960).

Adequate termination of therapy is often difficult to provide in the context of many psychiatric services. One reason for this is that trainee psychiatrists may change their attachments every 6–12 months, thus leaving large numbers of patients who are automatically transferred to their replacements. Another cause of inadequate termination is that some therapists are inappropriately unwilling to discharge their patients; sometimes this is due to an inability to tolerate the idea that nothing further can be done to help an unresolved problem.

Inadequate termination may be a common cause of chronicity amongst persistent attenders at out-patient clinics, and it is the responsibility of the senior psychiatrist to make sure that trainees deal appropriately with the concluding stages of therapy. Part of the last three sessions must be used to allow the patient to express his feelings about the impending separation. In general it is wise during this period to shift the emphasis from the patient's problems and deficits to his strengths and assets (Pumpian-Mindlin 1958). It is also important for trainee psychiatrists to plan their out-patient clinics so that no patient starts brief interpretive psychotherapy unless there is sufficient time for adequate termination before his planned departure.

SELF-DISCLOSURE

The question of how much the therapist should reveal of his reactions, attitudes and personal situation applies to all situations outside psychoanalysis, in which it is said that minimal disclosure should occur (Cozby 1973). Strassberg et al. (1977) have suggested that psychotherapists who are interested in eliciting adequate levels of self-disclosure by patients should not be excessively reserved, and have pointed out that patients are more likely to self-disclose towards the latter part of the session. However, although self-disclosure by the conductor of a psychotherapeutic group has been found to enhance group participation (Kangas 1971), it is unlikely that a marked degree of self-disclosure by the therapist is important or necessary to positive outcome. The therapist should aim to provide the patient with sufficient information to demonstrate his concern and motivation, but should bear in mind that he is engaged in a professional relationship which is always qualitatively different from purely social interactions (Jourard 1968). Limited physical contact such as touching the patient's hand in a situation where he is expressing genuine distress may sometimes constitute an appropriate part of the process of making the therapist appear 'human'.

OUTCOME STUDIES

Some psychotherapists consider that their work is not accessible to conventional validation procedures and subscribe to Freud's view (1922) that since all cases are unique, statistical methods that deal with group responses cannot be used as measures of outcome. Hence it has been claimed that a comparison of experimental and control groups on the basis of average outcome scores, which is the conventional paradigm, is unhelpful, as the mean score in the experimental sample may cancel out score dispersion in opposite directions (Bergin 1970). In addition it is argued that psychodynamic models of man constitute a new form of rationality and are, therefore, beyond conventional science (Farrell 1981).

Nevertheless, a number of psychotherapists are prepared to undertake outcome studies, although an agreement on the evaluation criteria has proved difficult as categories such as 'cure' or 'improvement' seem too crude and inadequate for the assessment of behavioural change (Rachman and Wilson 1980). Other outcome criteria such as consumer satisfaction and cost–benefit analysis have been proposed (Thomander 1976; Kazdin and Wilson 1978).

It has been suggested that the analysis of relatively simple forms of psychotherapy, such as counselling, should precede the evaluation of more complex forms of treatment (Shapiro 1975; Ryle 1980), and that simple research designs, which are directed towards answerable questions and concentrate on particular disorders, should be selected (Gelder 1976). A promising strategy involves the use of several criteria including patient-related variables, the proportion of patients who improve, the magnitude and durability of various measures of improvement, and a cost–benefit analysis (Kazdin and Wilson 1978).

Recent studies and reviews seem to agree that psychotherapy at its best produces desirable change (Smith and Glass 1977) and at its worst leads to either no change or, occasionally, change for the worse. Evidence that success rates are significantly higher than the rates of spontaneous remissions is not impressive, but evaluation of the latter involves many methodological difficulties (Luborsky et al. 1975; Sloane et al. 1975; Hadley and Strupp 1976; Malan 1976; Strupp 1978; Strupp and Hadley 1979; Rachman and Wilson 1980).

Outcome studies are not necessarily designed to identify the therapeutic ingredients in the range of psychotherapies, and it is not clear whether a psychotherapist's technical skills and theoretical standpoint are usually relevant to outcome. Luborsky et al. (1975) considered that the therapist's theoretical model or his treatment method were not significantly related to therapeutic success. However, it has been repeatedly shown that the therapist's 'warmth, empathy and genuineness' are likely to be correlated with positive change (Razin 1977). Another study which followed up patients a year after the termination of treatment concluded that experienced psychotherapists did not achieve significantly better results than non-qualified college professors (Strupp and Hadley 1979). Therefore, there is doubt as to the relevance of theoretical frameworks and long training to successful outcome in psychotherapy for many patients. However, clinical experience indicates that a knowledge of the phenomena to be found in human relationships, combined with experience, are at times essential attributes for the psychiatrist. This implies that, despite the difficulties in demonstrating specific therapeutic ingredients, the essential non-specific personal qualities of the therapist are not, by themselves, always sufficient (Chodoff 1982).

References

ALEXANDER, F., FRENCH, T.M. (1946) *Psychoanalytic Therapy, Principles and Application* (Ch. 4). New York: Ronald Press.

BARCROFT, J. (1979) 'Crisis Intervention'. In: *An Introduction to the Psychotherapies*, ed. Bloch, S. Oxford: Oxford University Press.

BENEDETTI, G. (1980) Individual psychotherapy in schizophrenia. *Schiz. Bull.*, **6**, 633.

BERGIN, A.E. (1970) The deterioration effect. *J. abnorm. Psychol.*, **75**, 300.

BLOCH, S. (1977) Supportive Psychotherapy. *Br. J. hosp. Med.*, **18**, 63.

BLOCH, S. (1979) 'Supportive Psychotherapy'. In: *An Introduction to the Psychotherapies*, ed. Bloch, S. Oxford: Oxford University Press.

BRANDON, S. (1970) Crisis theory and possibilities of therapeutic intervention. *Br. J. Psychiat.*, **117**, 627.

BRITISH PSYCHOLOGICAL SOCIETY (1980) Statement on statutory registration of psychotherapists. *Bull. Br. psychol. Soc.*, **33**, 353

BURKE, J.D., WHITE, H.S. & HAVENS, L.L. (1979) Which short term therapy? *Archs gen. Psychiat.*, **36**, 177.

BURSTEN, B. (1973) *The Manipulator: A Psychoanalytic Point of View*. Connecticut: Yale University Press.

CAHOON, D.D. (1968) Symptom substitution and the behaviour therapies: a reappraisal. *Psychol. Bull.*, **69**, 149.

CAPLAN, G. (1964) *An Approach to Community Mental Health*. London: Tavistock.

CASTELNUOVO-TEDESCO, P. (1965) *The Twenty Minute Hour*. London: Churchill.
CASTELNUOVO-TEDESCO, P. (1975) Brief Psychotherapy. In: *American Handbook of Psychiatry*, ed. Arieti, S. New York: Basic Books.
CAWLEY, R.H. (1977) The teaching of psychotherapy. *Assoc. Univ. Teach. Psych.*, Newsletter, Jan. 19th, 1977.
CHODOFF, P. (1982) Assessment of psychotherapy. *Arch. gen. Psychiat.*, **39**, 1097.
COOPER, J.E. (1979) *Crisis Admission Units and Emergency Psychiatric Services*. World Health Organization Publication.
COYNE, J.C. (1976) Toward an interactional description of depression. *Psychiatry*, **39**, 28.
COZBY, P.C. (1973) Self-disclosure. *Psychol. Bull.*, **79**, 73.
DARBONNE, A. (1968) Crisis: a review of theory, practice and research. *Int. J. Psychiat.*, **6**, 371.
DONOVAN, J.M. et al. (1979) The crisis, an outcome study. *Am. J. Psychiat.*, **136**, 906.
FARRELL, B.A. (1981) *The Standing of Psychoanalysis*. Oxford: Oxford University Press.
FISHER, S. & GREENBERG, R.P. (1977) *The Scientific Credibility of Freud's Theories and Therapies*. New York: Basic Books.
FRANK, J.D. (1974) Therapeutic components of psychotherapy. *J. Nerv. mentl Dis.*, **159**, 325.
FREUD, S. (1922 ed.) *Introductory Lectures on Psychoanalysis*. London: Allen and Unwin.
GELDER, M.G. (1976) Research methodology in psychotherapy—why bother? *Proc. R. Soc. Med.*, **69**, 505.
GOMEZ-SCHWARTZ, B. (1982) Negative changes induced by psychotherapy. *Brit. J. Hosp. Med.*, **28**, 248.
HADLEY, S.W. & STRUPP, H.M. (1976) Contemporary views of negative effects in psychotherapy. *Archs gen. Psychiat.*, **33**, 1291.
HENDERSON, S. et al. (1980) Social relationship, adversity and neurosis: a study of associations in a general population sample. *Br. J. Psychiat.*, **136**, 574.
HINSIE, L.E. & CAMPBELL, R.J. (1970) *Psychiatric Dictionary*. London: Oxford University Press.
HORNBLOW, A.R. & SLOANE, H.R. (1980) Evaluating the effectiveness of a telephone counselling service. *Br. J. Psychiat.*, **137**, 1377.
JANOWSKY, D.S. et al. (1970) Playing the manic game. *Archs gen. Psychiat.*, **22**, 252.
JOHNSON, C.W. et al. (1980) *Basic Psychotherapeutics*, Chapter 3. London: MTP.
JOURARD, S.M. (1968) *Disclosing Man to Himself*. Princeton, N.J.: Van Nostrand.
KANGAS, J.A. (1971) Group members self-disclosure. *Com. Group Stud.*, **2**, 65.
KARASU, T.B. (1977) Psychotherapies: An Overview. *Am. J. Psychiat.*, **134**, 851.
KAZDIN, A.E. & WILSON, T. (1978) Criteria for evaluating psychotherapy. *Archs gen. Psychiat.*, **35**, 407.
LABORSKY, L. et al. (1975) Comparative studies of psychotherapies. *Archs gen. Psychiat.*, **32**, 995.
MACKENZIE, R.B. et al. (1978) The manipulative patient: an interactional approach. *Psychiatry*, **41**, 264.
MALAN, D.H. (1976) *The Frontier of Brief Psychotherapy*. New York: Plenum Press.
MALAN, D.H. (1979) *Individual Psychotherapy and the Science of Psychodynamics*, pp. 225–6. London: Butterworth.
MANN, J. (1973) *Time Limited Psychotherapy*. Cambridge, Mass.: Harvard University Press.
MARMOR, J. (1979) Short-term dynamic psychotherapy. *Am. J. Psychiat.*, **136**, 149.
MARTIN, P.A. (1971) Dynamic considerations of the hysterical psychosis. *Am. J. Psychiat.*, **128**, 745.
MURPHY, G.E. & GUZE, S.B. (1960) Setting limits: the management of the manipulative patient. *Am. J. Psychotherapy*, **14**, 30.
PARLOFF, M.B. et al. (1978) Research on therapist variable in relation to process and outcome. In: *Handbook of Psychotherapy and Behavioural Change*, ed. Bergin, A.E. & Garfield, S.L., 2nd ed. New York: John Wiley.
PUMPIAN-MINDLIN, E. (1958) Comments on Techniques of Termination and Transfer in Clinical Settings. *Am. J. Psychother.*, **12**, 455.
RACHMAN, S.J. & WILSON, G.T. (1980) *The Effects of Psychological Therapy*, Chapters 2–6. Oxford: Pergamon Press.
RAZIN, A.M. (1977) The A.B. variable: still promising after 20 years. In: *Effective Psychotherapy, A Handbook of Research*, ed. Gurman, A.S. & Razin, A.M. Oxford: Pergamon Press.
REIDER, N. (1976) Symptom substitution. *Bull. Menninger Clin.*, **40**, 629.
ROSEN, B. (1979) A method of structured brief psychotherapy. *Br. J. Med. Psychol.*, **52**, 157.

ROSENZWEIG, N. & GRISCOM, H. (Eds.) (1978) *Psychopharmacology and Psychotherapy Synthesis or Antithesis?* New York: Human Science Press.
ROUNSAVILLE, B.J. et al. (1981) Psychotherapy with depressed patients. *Br. J. Psychiat.*, **138**, 67.
RYLE, A. (1980) Some measure of goal attainment in focussed integrated active psychotherapy: a study of 15 cases. *Br. J. Psychiat.*, **137**, 475.
SHAPIRO, D.A. (1975) Some implications of psychotherapy research for clinical psychology. *Br. J. med. Psychol.*, **48**, 199.
SHEPHERD, M. (1980) Statutory registration of psychotherapists? *Bull. Roy. Coll. Psychiat.* November, pp. 166–8.
SIFNEOS, P.E. (1979) *Short-term Dynamic Psychotherapy, Evaluation and Technique.* New York: Plenum Publishing.
SKYNNER, A.C.R. & BROWN, D.G. (1981) Referral of Patients for Psychotherapy. *Br. med. J.*, **282**, 1952.
SLOANE, R.B., STAPLES, F.R., CRISTOL, A.H. et al. (1975) *Psychotherapy vs. Behaviour Therapy.* Boston: Harvard University Press.
SMALL, L. (1971) *The Briefer Psychotherapies.* London: Butterworths.
SMITH, M.L. & GLASS, G.V. (1977) Analysis of psychotherapy: outcome studies. *Am. Psychol., Sept.*, 752.
STEIN, L. (1981) Community treatment of schizophrenia: an economic cost–benefit analysis. Paper delivered to World Psychiatric Assn. Meeting, New York.
STORR, A. (1979) *The Art of Psychotherapy*, (p. vii). London: Heinemann.
STRASSBERG, D. et al. (1977) Self disclosure. *Compreh. Psychiat.*, **18**, 31.
STRAUSS, J.S. & CARPENTER, W.T. (1981) *Schizophrenia*, p. 178. New York: Plenum Medical.
STRUPP, H.H. (1978) 'Psychotherapy Research and Practice, an overview.' In: *Handbook of Psychotherapy and Behavioural Change: An Empirical Analysis*, eds. Garfield, S.L. & Bergin, A.E. New York: John Wiley.
STRUPP, H.H. & HADLEY, S.W. (1979) Specific vs. nonspecific factors in psychotherapy. *Archs gen. Psychiat.*, **36**, 1125.
THOMANDER, D. (1976) Researching psychotherapy effectiveness in mental health service agencies. *J. Community Psychol.*, **4**, 215.
TRUAX, C.B. & CARKHUFF, R.R. (1967) *Towards Effective Counselling and Psychotherapy* (see Section II). Chicago: Aldine Publishing Co.
URBAN, H.B. & FORD, D.H. (1971) 'Some Historical and Conceptual Perspectives on Psychotherapy and Behavioural Change.' In: *Handbook of Psychotherapy and Behavioural Change*, ed. Bergin, A.E. & Garfield, S.L. New York: John Wiley.
VINEY, L.L. (1976) The concept of crisis. *Bull. Brit. psychol. Soc.*, **29**, 387.
WEISSMAN, M.M. (1979) The psychological treatment of depression. *Archs gen. Psychiat.*, **36**, 1261.
WEITZMAN, B. (1967) Behaviour Therapy and Psychotherapy. *Psychol. Rev.*, **74**, 300.
WEST, D.A. et al. (1980) Emergency psychiatric home visiting: report of four years experience. *J. clin. Psychiat.*, **41**, 113.
ZETZEL, E.R. (1971) A developmental approach to the borderline patient. *Am. J. Psychiat.*, **127**, 867.

9

Group Psychotherapies

J.H. Dowson

GROUP PSYCHOTHERAPY: DEFINITION AND THERAPEUTIC INGREDIENTS

Definition

Group psychotherapy encompasses a variety of forms and goals which include relief of psychological symptoms, modification of social or family relationships, and a permanent change in attitudes or other aspects of the relatively stable organization of an individual's mental activity and behaviour, which comprise personality (de Maré 1972; Yalom 1975).

A group of individuals, who are appropriate called patients within the setting of a psychiatric service, meet regularly with one or more trained professionals to interact by verbal interchange and other communicative behaviour (Jones et al. 1971a; Cawley 1974; Frank 1979).

Therapeutic Ingredients

All the phenomena which are found in individual psychotherapy may also be present in group psychotherapy although some, such as the importance of the relationship between patient and therapist, are attenuated, while others, such as the provision of new interpersonal situations from which the patient may learn, receive an extra dimension in groups.

Individual psychotherapy involves two main approaches which often overlap. The 'supportive' approach implies that the therapist accepts a degree of dependency from the patient and provides an active input to their relationship. The therapeutic ingredients include advice, explanation, instruction, suggestion, a caring attitude with active listening, reassurance, encouragement, persuasion, permission for the display of emotion, and environmental manipulation if this is possible and desirable. The focus is usually on the present and future, rather than on the past. In contrast, the approach derived from psychoanalytic theory is directed towards an awareness and understanding of

181

unconscious mental activity and uses the techniques of free association, overcoming resistance, dismantling psychological defence mechanisms, and analysis of dreams, transference and countertransference (see glossary). Unconscious attitudes, motives and conflicts are discovered and, if necessary, modified. Thus, the focus is on the past.

Several studies have claimed that certain characteristics of a psychotherapist are associated with treatment efficacy, such as an ability to empathize with the patient and to be personally concerned about his welfare, together with emotional warmth and genuineness (Malan et al. 1976). The presence of a 'treatment alliance' (Sandler et al. 1970c), which refers to the common aims of therapist and patient, can also be beneficial as can the provision of new learning situations.

Cognitive and emotional components of a learning process can usefully be distinguished although, in practice, these are never completely separated. Cognitive learning involves conscious mental activity, which may include the registration of new experiences and, by the process of insight, the development of an awareness of attitudes, feelings or conflicts which had not been fully available to consciousness. Insight can be induced or assisted by suggestions (interpretations) from the therapist, which are directed towards the defence mechanisms responsible for the patient's transference or resistance (see glossary); however, even though a patient may develop some insight, perhaps by becoming aware of the maladaptive nature of a behaviour pattern or attitude, this may have little impact if the learning process did not involve an emotional dimension, which was concerned with motivation and mood. If emotional arousal occurs during a series of learning experiences, the effects are more likely to include an emotional as well as a cognitive change, so that emotional arousal has been termed the motive power of psychotherapy. Although cognitive events accompanied by a minimum of emotion can produce beneficial effects, psychological events which are associated with the expression of emotion are usually necessary for significant personality adjustment.

Not all psychological defence mechanisms are maladaptive, and psychotherapy is often directed towards a strengthening of these unconscious manoeuvres to distort reality, if they provide the best method of coping with an insoluble situation or an unmodifiable personality structure.

A patient can often be helped to recognize what he can achieve by his own efforts, and identification with the therapist, involving the patient modelling himself on the therapist's attitudes and behaviour, may also be of benefit. Another therapeutic ingredient in individual psychotherapy is the instillation of hope, but this must not involve making wild promises and predictions which, if unrealized, will produce despair and loss of confidence. A patient's hope is often a reflection of a positive approach by the therapist and, even when severe and intractable problems exist, it may be possible to comment on the patient's fortitude or transient symptomatic relief. Also, the therapist's continued concern and interest encourages a positive attitude in the patient. Another important therapeutic ingredient in individual psychotherapy can be catharsis, involving the expression of anger, depression, anxiety or, more rarely, positive feelings. Catharsis can be therapeutic in itself as was shown by a young man who was admitted to a psychiatric hospital with severe neurotic depression and anxiety following the death of his alcoholic father. Although he clearly recognized his feelings of intense anger towards his father for ruining the life of his family, these conflicted with positive feelings, and it was not until he had repeatedly expressed his anger in a psychotherapeutic setting that his symptoms were relieved. Self-disclosure, particularly if this involves confession, may also provide relief of some neurotic symptoms, even if this does not generate specific advice or other interventions.

Group psychotherapy can provide new learning situations which are derived from a much wider range of interpersonal interactions than is possible in individual psychotherapy. Insight may be obtained by observing unconscious motivation in other group members, while increased self-awareness is produced by the patient finding out, by 'feedback', how he is perceived by others. Each patient is usually encouraged to display his own psychopathology by ensuring that he feels 'safe' enough to do so, and he may have the opportunity to develop and test new patterns of social interaction. Insight can be variable in relation to a beneficial instance of new learning, and may be minimal or non-existent. Thus, a patient with limited capacity for abstract thought may increase his self-confidence by being able to advise or comfort other patients, without being aware that a poor opinion of his value to others was one of his main problems.

Group psychotherapy can also provide therapeutic events which are specific to this form of treatment. An atmosphere of trust, openness, concern, tolerance, and support, with controlled negative feedback, has been termed 'group cohesiveness', and may be therapeutic in itself. It is also well known that any group of individuals can exert powerful pressure to conform to the attitudes of the majority, and this force may be harnessed to the correction of maladaptive behaviour. The experience of universality, in which the patient realizes that other people have problems, sometimes similar to his own, has often been cited by patients to be therapeutic, and the process of sharing problems encourages group members to become less self-absorbed. The opportunity to be altruistic may also reduce self-absorption and increase self-esteem. In some groups, reenactment of family relationships may take place if other group members resemble various members of the patient's family, and this process may assist the development of insight. For some patients, such as those with social phobias, groups provide the feared situation and a setting in which coping strategies can be developed, while a collective approach to problem solving can sometimes lead to the optimum solution for certain problems.

Group psychotherapy usually provides various additional indirect benefits, the importance of which should not be underestimated. If the group meetings take place in a psychiatric unit, the interest and morale of the staff may be increased, and the assessment and monitoring of the patient is improved. For in-patients, the relief of boredom associated with this or any other activity may also be of considerable, if non-specific, value.

GROUP-SPECIFIC PHENOMENA

Psychotherapy in groups incorporates a variety of communication patterns involving both verbal and non-verbal behaviour.

The possible benefits of so-called group pressures have already been considered; groups have the capacity to define, by consensus, acceptable attitudes or behaviour and then to exert pressure to conform to these standards. Behaviour which is generally acceptable may be rewarded by positive regard, while deviance can be punished by criticism, hostility or by being ignored. At times, the overt consensus attitude may be more extreme than the most widely held viewpoint. Another property of groups is their ability to define what appears to be reality to the majority; for example, the staff may be considered to be uncaring, or it may be assumed that all patients have similar problems. Such assumptions may be far from accurate. Resistance may involve the collaboration of group members to prevent the consideration of reality perhaps by means of silence or changing the subject by directing attention to another group member. Although at such times the patients may not be fully aware of what is happening, the author once had the experience of every member of a group making a deliberate decision before the meeting that no-one would utter a word! A common example of an unconscious collaborative defence is that of scapegoating, where one individual receives hostile feelings which have been displaced by several group members from their appropriate target; this often occurs when a new member enters a group.

When emotion is expressed in a group there is a tendency for it to precipitate the experience of a similar feeling in several other group members. Thus, a sharing of expressed emotion often occurs; one angry complaint about the staff may initiate a chorus, while a weeping patient may elicit several complaints of depressed mood.

Another group process has been called the 'chain phenomenon' when several members contribute to a group theme, while an examination of the pattern of interaction in a series of meetings invariably demonstrates a tendency for the form and content of the meetings to undergo constant change. Irregular cycles are often seen in which, for example, a meeting (or series of meetings) characterized by the patients being constructive, caring and active will be followed by withdrawal, hostility and hopelessness, before the original form eventually returns.

Finally, a consideration of group-specific phenomena would not be complete without mention of interactions which may take place at times other than the group meetings, but which would not have occurred if the patients had not been members of the same group.

HISTORICAL DEVELOPMENT

Since Moreno introduced the term 'group psychotherapy' in 1931, many theoretical frameworks and techniques have emerged for use in a wide variety of settings. These include the short-stay psychiatric unit, the out-patient clinic, the medium- and long-stay units of psychiatric hospitals, and specialist psychiatric units for alcoholism and forensic problems (de Maré and Kreeger 1974; Ryle 1976). Regular group meetings may also involve non-patients, such as trainees in those professions where increased self-awareness and an ability to communicate are particularly important.

Unfortunately, the value of research in this field has been limited and, in general, theoretical considerations have determined clinical practice (Malan 1973). Three main theoretical approaches have been derived from psychoanalytic theory; the first examines the relationship of each individual patient to the group or therapist, the second is concerned with the relationship of the group as a whole to the therapist, while the third approach emphasizes treatment by the group itself, focussing on general aspects of the group such as themes, communication patterns, values and cohesiveness. In this last approach, the therapist ignores, as far as possible, his own relationship with individual group members or with the group as a whole. The first two strategies have been termed psychoanalysis 'in' groups and 'of' groups, (Ezriel 1950; Bion 1961; Wolf and Schwartz 1962) while the latter, the so-called group-analytic method (Foulkes and Anthony 1965), encourages the therapeutic ingredients to be provided 'by' the group (de Maré and Kreeger 1974).

Despite the differences between these various schools derived from psychoanalysis, they share the underlying assumption that therapy largely consists of exploring unconscious mental processes by means of interpretations directed towards resistance and transferences. However, although these approaches may be useful with carefully selected groups of out-patients, the group equivalent of 'supportive' individual psychotherapy is important in most types of group psychotherapy which are routinely practised within a psychiatric service.

GROUP PSYCHOTHERAPY IN A PSYCHIATRIC ADMISSION UNIT

The present chapter will focus on a particular type of activity which is practised in the in-patient admission units of many psychiatric services: the twice or thrice-weekly 'open' group (with a turnover of patients) which recruits

its members from a range of diagnoses, problems, ages, intellectual abilities, and social backgrounds. This type of group psychotherapy requires considerable flexibility on the part of group conductor who must use a variety of techniques derived from several theoretical approaches. However a consideration of this type of group psychotherapy will also illustrate the principles of conducting other types of group, including those which result from the application of rigorous criteria to select a more homogeneous membership.

Organization

A psychiatric admission unit caters for in-patients whose average stay in hospital is less than 2 months. Day-patients may also attend, some of whom will have recently received in-patient treatment. The goals of group psychotherapy for individual patients in this setting vary considerably, and although the majority of patients who pass through a psychiatric admission unit may be included in a group at some stage, some are not suitable for this form of treatment and certain principles of selection should be observed. Severely psychotic patients and those with marked paranoid or schizoid personality traits should generally be excluded; the paranoid patient often evokes hostility, which reinforces his pathological ideas, while the severely withdrawn schizoid person will usually find a group too threatening. Also, excessively narcissistic individuals with a minimal capacity to take note of others should not usually be selected. Sociopathic individuals, addicts of both drugs and alcohol and those whose problems centre on sexual deviation must be included only after careful consideration and, in general, there should not be more than one patient with any of these problems in each group (Kadis et al. 1974; Bloch 1979a).

Certain characteristics of a patient imply suitability for group psychotherapy irrespective of the presenting psychiatric syndrome, and a selected patient should be judged to have sufficient psychological reserves to tolerate the anxiety-provoking situations which invariably arise in groups. The patient who is likely to derive significant benefit will usually have had at least one 'meaningful' relationship, have the capacity to participate in discussion and to use abstract concepts, be committed to active cooperation, be able to experience and express emotion, and have a clearly defined area of conflict (Marmor 1979); however, these qualities are not essential for a patient to be included in the type of group under consideration. The group conductor should avoid selecting a patient who would be conspicuously different from the other group members on such dimensions as age, social class, intelligence or verbal ability, and the inclusion of too many patients who are likely to say very little must be avoided. Patients whose major difficulty is that they become emotionally dependent on others to an excessive extent often do better in groups than in individual psychotherapy, as a pathological and disabling dependency upon one individual is usually avoided in a group setting. The group conductor should interview each prospective member and consider the current state of the group, the nature of the patients' problems and personality, and the conductor's attitudes towards the patient; if the conductor feels considerable hostility towards an individual, this may preclude selection. The patient can be asked to provide a written account of his history and presenting problems, which can indicate motivation as well as providing information (Bloch 1979a). If a patient is selected, the conductor must then consider the best time for entry, as joining a group when patients are particularly hostile or apathetic may not be appropriate.

After a patient has been selected, he should be seen individually by the conductor or other staff member for a preparatory session (Yalom 1967). Certain rules are usually made: patients should not meet socially outside the hospital, any significant change in life situation must be reported to the group, notice must be given if attendance is not possible, and confidentiality must be maintained. If necessary it should be made clear that repeated disruptive behaviour other than verbal interchange may lead to exclusion. The patient is told that the meetings have no set agenda and that his tasks will be to talk about his problems, feelings and thoughts, and to interact with other group members. It may be appropriate to ask that the patient commits himself to attendance at a minimum number of meetings.

The optimum number of patients is generally agreed to be about eight, with a range of three to twelve (de Maré and Kreeger 1974). Each meeting lasts for 1 hour and takes place two or three times weekly. Sessions should be as evenly spaced as possible and there is some evidence that time between meetings can be an important variable (Jones et al. 1971b). Group members sit in a circle so that non-verbal communication is apparent.

The group conductor should have some experience and must be assisted by at least one other staff member. During each meeting one individual must be clearly designated as the conductor, but two, or even three co-conductors may alternate this responsibility. Not more than three staff members should accompany a group of about eight patients. One, and preferably two, staff should be regular group members while the third may be a student or trainee who can attend for a limited number of meetings. Although two or three staff members may be sufficiently experienced to share the task of conducting the group, one therapist may wish to retain continual responsibility as the conductor; in this situation other staff members can act as 'participant observers' who are relatively inactive. The staff should meet for about 15 minutes after each session when the conductor can compare his impressions with those of his colleagues. A written summary or report may then be prepared, which can be given to the patients at the next meeting (Yalom et al. 1975). For many group members, group psychotherapy is part of a varied treatment programme and the conductor must ensure that good communications exist between staff in the group and other staff members in the various professional disciplines.

Goals of Group Psychotherapy

Although the patient and therapist may not be able to agree the aims of the treatment, the conductor should formulate realistic goals for each group member during the selection process, bearing in mind the likely capacity for change and the time which will be needed to achieve the desired effects. It is a common mistake to underestimate the time required to produce clinically important changes in a patient's fundamental personality structure. A minimum of 6–12 months is usually necessary to induce even modest changes in the personality traits which comprise the major syndromes of personality disorder, and these are rarely achieved in the the type of group under consideration.

Sometimes the treatment goal does not involve change but an attempt to prop up the patient who cannot manage his life without some help (Bloch 1979*b*). Support may be provided for a limited time during a resolving crisis, but group attendance may also play its part in the management of more chronic problems. In a crisis, attention must be paid to the precipitating events, which may have involved loss, change, interpersonal difficulties or a conflict between alternatives (Caplan 1961; Bancroft 1979).

Group treatment may be concerned with the cause or effects of psychological disorder; thus, attention may be directed towards a lack of trust in others which has led to anxiety and unhappiness, while a patient who has suffered repeated episodes of psychosis may be helped to adjust to his residual deficits and vulnerability to stress.

Treatment goals can involve the relief of symptoms which include what Frank (1974) has called 'demoralization'. This involves a feeling of isolation, shame, and a loss of long-term goals. Group psychotherapy may be used to enhance a patient's capacity to relate to others, so that he may be more able to achieve close personal relationships, perhaps by being less assertive or histrionic, less uncomfortable in company, less mistrustful of others or more independent (Bloch 1979*a*). Another goal may be to modify various aspects of personality (other than those responsible for the major syndromes of personality disorder), such as low self-esteem, lack of purpose and self-confidence, an inability to express emotion, or a tendency to behave impulsively with poor control of emotional expression.

At times, psychological defence mechanisms should be strengthened, perhaps by encouraging avoidance of certain problems but, if defences are maladaptive, a goal may be to assist the patient to discard these or to substitute less harmful manoeuvres. The dismantling of defences usually involves the development of insight; for example a patient may accept that a particular problem is insoluble, or be able to face a decision which has been avoided.

Another important aim of group psychotherapy of the type under consideration is the regular monitoring and assessment of the psychological state and life situation of each group member. Group psychotherapy provides an opportunity for this to be achieved in a way which is particularly valuable if the availability of staff for individual interviews is limited. Group psychotherapy can also encourage staff interaction with patients, improve staff morale and foster cooperation across professional boundaries.

The Patient's Contribution

Each patient is told that his task in the group involves self-disclosure, listening, and interacting with others. The emphasis is on verbal communication by which each patient reveals various aspects of his psychological functioning, such as his attitudes, patterns of social interaction and psychological defences. Transferences to several group members may develop, involving unrealistic feelings and attitudes, which indicate unconscious mental activity.

However, non-verbal behaviour must not be forgotten. When a patient is speaking, the other group members will be engaged in various forms of silent participation: emotions may be shared, self-examination may be taking place and the silent patient may be learning from events which involve others. Overt non-verbal activity such as facial expressions, fidgeting, moving restlessly in the chair, tapping the foot, or playing with an ashtray or cigarette, should be noted and may be most informative. More rarely, unacceptable and dramatic behaviour may occur: objects are thrown, physical violence or attempts at self-harm take place, or the patient rushes out of the meeting.

The Conductor's Role

Tasks. The conductor bears ultimate responsibility for the group and undertakes the various administrative tasks which have been described. The conductor must also open and close each meeting, monitor the proceedings, and intervene appropriately. The relationship of each individual patient to the group must be borne in mind and group processes should be identified. Both verbal and non-verbal behaviour is noted and patterns are sought. The conductor should also be aware of his own emotional reactions.

To achieve the treatment goals for the individual members, and to foster the therapeutic activity of the group, the conductor has a wide range of interventions at his disposal. The first priority must always be to do no harm, and a vulnerable patient who cannot cope with certain stressful situations has to be actively protected and, if necessary, withdrawn from the group. The conductor must set a standard of behaviour involving tolerance, concern, perseverance and, above all, calm in difficult situations. He should encourage an atmosphere of openness, trust and hope which is 'safe' for self-disclosure and will, by a variety of methods, further the specific treatment goals which have been formulated.

Interventions. The conductor's contributions are also both verbal and non-verbal. Various comments and questions facilitate a climate of communication, concern, mutual support and the sharing of experience or emotion. Interventions may be relatively non-directive, or be aimed specifically at one group member or a particular topic. At times the conductor should encourage the sharing and expression of emotion, perhaps by drawing attention to depression or anger in the meeting, and by inviting others to share their own feelings or experiences. However, it is not a good policy constantly to encourage the expression of anger or depression (Bancroft 1979). The opinions of the conductor and other staff are often an important class of intervention, as these may help to counteract pathological opinions and behaviour patterns which are shared by most of the group members. Other types of intervention include clarification, the promotion of problem solving behaviour, confrontation, directives, and interpretations. Clarification of a situation may be the first step in solving a problem; Goldfried and Goldfried (1975) have described subsequent stages in this process: the identification of methods for the solution with an examination of their consequences, the choice of one of these possible methods, and the planning of the various steps for its performance. Confrontation refers to the technique of repeatedly bringing the group face to face with a situation, while directives, although usually kept to a minimum, can be essential. Interpretations are the final major category of verbal input and refer to comments designed to produce insight.

Non-verbal activity includes silent participation involving attentive listening. Gestures, facial expression and movements will convey varying degrees of information about the conductor's underlying thoughts, while another type of non-verbal intervention is that of physical activity. Although the need for this should be rare, the conductor and other staff may occasionally have to stop a fight, or prevent an attempt at self injury.

General principles. A flexible approach to the conductor's role is essential as changes of strategy are often required. Although the conductor may have no alternative but to encourage a leader-centred communication pattern, in which he interacts with several group members in turn, there should be periods when most interactions are between group members. Group communication is encouraged by such techniques as asking a question of the group rather than of an individual, inviting the expression of views from previously silent members and focussing on themes which are of general relevance. In a series of meetings, there should be a balance regarding the content of topics discussed; although events in the remote past and a quest for explanations may be important, the 'here and now', both inside and outside the group, together with an anticipation of the future, should predominate.

At any moment, the conductor has a choice from a range of overall strategy for the conduct of the group (Kadis et al. 1974). At one extreme the conductor is authoritative, active, and freely gives his opinions and reactions. His main aim is to provide a setting in which patients feel minimal anxiety, where conflicts are diffused or avoided, and where sharing of problems, mutual support and group cohesion are encouraged. The focus is on the problems and symptoms of the here and now. At the other end of the spectrum, the conductor is minimally active, non-directive and keeps his views to himself. No attempt is made to avoid any anxiety and hostility, which adversely affects group cohesion. Emotional expression is encouraged, and the focus is on relationships, the awareness of the effects of behaviour on others, defences, and group or individual transferences.

Most group meetings of the type under consideration involve an amalgam of strategies and during each meeting the conductor's tactics may undergo several changes in response to events in the group. However, in general, strategy is weighted towards the former end of the spectrum, so that group psychotherapy in an admission unit should provide a situation in which patients can usually feel safe and do not often experience a high level of anxiety. The members should generally feel able to join in, and have trust in the staff. Unfortunately, some staff members are not suited to be group conductors in this setting by virtue of their personality or theoretical bias; Yalom (1975) has described the aggressive, confronting, excessively self-revealing, controlling and charismatic group conductor, and it is likely that this type of conducting can be harmful. Also, if a group conductor exclusively applies principles derived from psychoanalytic theory, so that he invariably uses the latter strategy outlined above, this generally produces a non-therapeutic group in an admission unit setting. The conductor must strive to ensure that group meetings are usually characterized by attentive concern, so that the members feel relaxed and able to contribute. Of course, emotions are expressed and tensions appear, but these can be tolerated if the background atmosphere is one of calm and trust. The conductor must act naturally and should be prepared to voice his own opinions or to demonstrate his personal concern when this is appropriate. A conductor who displays nothing of his views or reactions encourages the development of marked hostility which may not be adequately resolved in an open group consisting of individuals with a variety of psychiatric disorders. However, the conductor must limit the degree to which his own personality becomes apparent and some formality is required, in keeping with the professional nature of the conductor's role. The conductor must constantly review the degree of his activity, whatever the overall strategy. This must be considered every few minutes, and the staff should not be so active throughout a meeting that the patient members of the group are seldom given a chance to interact. Often it is appropriate for the conductor to say very little during the first part of the meeting, but if interactions do not develop, or break down, a more active and directive approach is usually necessary; in these circumstances a subsequent attempt should be made to provide a period when the staff is minimally active.

Resistance

Resistance has been defined as all the obstacles to the aims and procedures of treatment which arise from within the patient, and may include both conscious and unconscious mental activity (Sandler et al. 1970*a*).

The latter may involve the various defence mechanisms and the 'negative therapeutic reaction' in which improvement, or the expression by the therapist of an opinion that the patient has improved, is followed by a worsening of the patient's condition (Sandler et al. 1970*b*).

Resistance can involve a varying proportion of group members; examples include persistently coming late, refusing to discuss a particular topic, ignoring staff comments, meeting socially outside the psychiatric unit, the formation of subgroups whose interactions persistently exclude other group members, scapegoating, showing hostility to new members, taking turns to speak, and preselecting topics for discussion. Although psychological defence mechanisms may fulfil a useful function, and should not always be considered as resistance, they lead to the avoidance or distortion of reality and may impede the treatment process. Another phenomenon that can result from the use of defences is that of splitting, where the ambivalence of feelings to a person or situation is not recognized and the opposing emotions or attitudes are separated; one or more parts may be masked or distorted by defence mechanisms. Transference and counter-transference also involve unconscious mental activity which, if unresolved, can interfere with treatment; for example, one or several group members may develop unrealistic expectations of treatment, or excessive emotional dependence on the conductor (Sandler et al. 1970).

Several techniques are available for overcoming resistance. The conductor may ignore it, encourage a safe, supportive group atmosphere, mobilize the group members to share their experiences in relation to the topic under discussion, and wait. But if aspects of a particular situation are persistently avoided or distorted, the resistance can be side-stepped by asking a direct question about the topic which is being avoided, if this is known. If this procedure is not effective, the conductor may draw the attention of the group to the resistance itself; for example, if a long silence is considered to be a resistance, the group may be encouraged to consider their feelings about the silence and the possible reasons why this situation has occurred. A fourth technique for overcoming resistance is to provide an interpretation, if unconscious mechanisms are involved. For example, a suggestion was made to a husband who had been deserted by his wife, and who was depressed, tense and excessively protective to his children, that he may have mixed feelings towards his children, as many people in his situation resent such responsibility. This helped the patient to recognize that he felt intensely resentful towards his children as well as towards his wife. Sometimes, all the conductor's efforts to overcome resistance will be in vain, and if the resistance is in the form of a long silence, this will continue. At this stage the conductor has no option but to accept that, for the moment, he has done all he can. The conductor does not bear all the responsibility for the efficacy of the group, as this is shared to some extent between all its members. Thus, in the case of a prolonged silence, the ball can be repeatedly put back into the group's court by the conductor pointing out that he can only do so much and that he hopes some group member will be able to help towards the resolution of the impasse. Sometimes the anxiety provoked by an extended silence is a useful catalyst to increased effort and self-reliance by the group members, but, in general, the conductor should try and help the group to avoid this situation.

Emotionality

Although mental events have both a cognitive and emotional component, it is useful to isolate the emotional content of each group meeting for consideration. Anger, depression and anxiety are of particular relevance, but disgust, positive attraction, happiness and elation should also be noted. If personality change is a goal of treatment for some group members, a degree of emotional arousal may be facilitative and, at times, essential, while varying degrees of emotionality are an inevitable part of all types of group psychotherapy.

Anger may occur in many disguises, such as a show of boredom, sarcasm, or the excessive politeness resulting from the use of the defence mechanism of reaction formation, in which the opposite of an underlying feeling appears in consciousness. The conductor should not necessarily draw the group's attention to signs of anger, which can often be ignored, but if these are persistent, exploration may be indicated. Underlying attitudes can be considered, and group members may be helped to handle the experience or expression of anger more appropriately. When anger is overt, the conductor or other group members may face considerable hostility. If the conductor is on the receiving end he must remain outwardly calm, and wait for the feelings to have been expressed before making any comments. Even after a delay he must not be in too much of a hurry to defend himself; the views of other group members should be invited, and he may decide not to give a specific reply. However, if the anger is directed to another group member, the conductor may need to be actively protective. If the staff are being accused of having various shortcomings, it is usually better not to argue, while an angry response on the part of the conductor is invariably inappropriate, especially if it involves a lack of the self-control which is an essential attribute of his role. It is often helpful to try and identify a pattern of inappropriate emotional arousal or expression, as the group experience may be representative of behaviour which repeatedly occurs in other situations.

A patient who is depressed and tearful is often ashamed at exhibiting emotion and if there are clear signs that a group member is upset it is often reassuring if the conductor indicates that he has noticed. This implies that it is 'all right' to be upset and the conductor may then try and encourage sharing of similar feeling, either past or present, and mobilize the group's support. However, the tearful patient may find it very uncomfortable to remain at the centre of the group's attention, and the conductor should consider shifting the focus without necessarily changing the subject; for example, a patient who had been upset the previous week could be asked how he has been feeling. Talk of suicidal ideas may reduce the likelihood of subsequently putting these thoughts into action, but it may be necessary to arrange to see the patient individually after the meeting, if, at the end, he appears to be actively suicidal. However, the motivation behind some patients' talk of possible self-injury is the expression of anger or an attempt to manipulate the attitudes and behaviour of the group. In such cases it may be necessary to state clearly that the group or staff cannot always accept responsibility for a person's actions. At the same time it is important to maintain a sympathetic approach which can be difficult, as the behaviour of some patients in such situations often arouses hostility.

Emotions can be 'acted-out' by disruptive non-verbal behaviour which, if it is not modified or contained by group pressures, may require a patient's exclusion from the group by the conductor. Physical intervention by the staff may very occasionally be necessary to stop aggression or self-injury, and, if a patient leaves the meeting, it may be appropriate for a member of the group to try and persuade him to return.

The conductor's own emotions must not be forgotten, and a capacity for self-control with regard to their expression is an essential skill which may require experience for its development. If the conductor expresses strong emotions, this should only occur after he has decided that this feedback would be helpful to the group. If, occasionally, this ideal is not realized, and the conductor's involuntary expression of strong feeling is apparent, it is probably best for him to acknowledge to the group that he is feeling angry, depressed or anxious. This tactic may defuse tension or embarassment.

Positive emotions should not be discouraged, but laughter or jokes are often defensive and inappropriate. They should be accepted at their face value only with caution.

The Beginning and End

The conductor should open each group meeting formally, and introduce any new member. He should then state the reasons for any absences and, if these are unknown, should encourage the group to consider if any action is appropriate; in a hospital setting a patient may volunteer to look for a missing individual. At this point the conductor can wait for a patient to start the proceedings, as part of the overall policy for the staff to be minimally active for at least part of the meeting. This allows the group to assume some responsibility for selecting the topics to be considered. However, if an initial silence continues for a minute or more, interactions should be encouraged by non-directive interventions which prompt the group as a whole.

During the final 15 minutes, the conductor should be aware that the end of the meeting is near. He may then decide to prompt previously silent members by directly asking them for their comments and, in the final few minutes, the patients can be invited in turn to give their reactions to the meeting or to each other (Wolf 1949). The conductor should try and ensure that the scheduled time for ending the meeting does not arrive during an unresolved period of emotionality but, if this occurs, the meeting may have to be extended. This should be avoided if possible, and an alternative technique for dealing with a patient who is very distressed or angry at the end of the meeting is to say that, although it is time to finish, a staff member will remain with the patient. This should also be a rare event, and patients should not be encouraged to expect individual attention immediately after a meeting.

The inexperienced conductor often finds it difficult to decide on his concluding remarks. At times, it may be appropriate to summarize the events of the meeting or end on a hopeful and encouraging note. But the conductor must not feel that it is his duty to do either, and when the mood is one of hopelessness or resentment, or when the meeting ends in the middle of the consideration of a problem, a statement can be made which merely clarifies the situation; for example 'one of the main problems seems to be that everyone has given up hope of any improvement', or 'although we have to finish now, we must come back to this problem next time'. On other occasions the conductor need not say anything other than to formally close the meeting by a comment such as: 'I am sorry to interrupt you but we have come to the end of our time'. This may be quite difficult, as he may come under pressure to say something 'clever' or reassuring, or to prolong the meeting. If group members ignore a concluding remark, the conductor may need to repeat his closing statement. If necessary he should interrupt the group, rising to his feet with other staff members.

Patterns of Group Interaction

Various developmental stages have been described in 'closed' groups (which rarely admit new members), and these can also be seen, albeit less predictably, in 'open' groups (Schutz 1958). In a closed group, an initial 'forming' stage has been identified in which members are often anxious, defensive and ambivalent. The group is dependent on the therapist for guidance and takes few risks. Members are on their best socially acceptable behaviour as they attempt to find out what is permitted and the nature of their task (Ryle 1976; Bloch 1979a). The middle stage has been termed the 'working' group and involves several patterns of group activity: 'storming', in which conflicts are expressed (often accompanied by criticism of the conductor for not being sufficiently directive), 'norming', in which cohesion develops, and 'performing', in which self-disclosure occurs and solutions to problems may emerge. In addition there may be periods when defence mechanisms are predominant (Bion 1961; Tuckman 1965). The final stage of a closed group is that of 'termination', which is analogous to the discharge of individual members from an open group.

Termination should occur if no further significant benefits are possible, while leaving the group may be, in itself, a therapeutic process, during which further steps are taken towards an appropriate degree of emotional independence.

Although the above stages are not delineated so clearly in an open group, phases of group interaction, e.g. involving dependency, cohesion or emotionality, are often experienced. Thus, if a group is constructively discussing problems in a relaxed and supportive atmosphere, this does not usually last for more than, at most, a few meetings; conversely, the conductor can tell himself that meetings characterized by despondency, hostility and apathy are likely to become more positive.

Although patterns of communication which involve several group members should be encouraged, lengthy dialogues may also be appropriate, if these do not lead to undue exclusion of other group members. Overt or covert structuring of communications, such as turn taking or assuming that certain questions must never be asked, should be generally avoided but, as previously described, patients may be asked in turn for their comments near the end of the meeting. The conductor should remember that the communication pattern of a group has a life of its own, which is not entirely dependent on the staff activity, and that members interact to a considerable extent outside groups in a hospital setting.

The degree of staff activity is a common topic for discussion in staff meetings. As part of the flexible approach which is required, the conductor must be prepared to vary his pattern of activity; constant intervention by the conductor stifles the group processes, but a directive and active approach by the staff may be needed when the group members lack the capacity to provide a positive input.

Certain themes are commonly encountered, such as previous treatment, symptoms, problems of being a patient, and the relevance, function and difficulties of the group itself. Dependency, trust, self-confidence, loss of hope, future plans, coping with emotions, loneliness, difficulties with authority, childhood experiences, recent life events and marital problems are also often discussed. Responsibility for one's actions is another recurrent theme and group members may share unrealistic expectations of some kind of magical treatment which will involve little effort on their part. Although many psychiatric syndromes respond well to physical treatments, the kind of problems that are considered in groups invariably require some effort and motivation from the patients.

Leaving the Group

If membership has been beneficial, leaving the group can be a significant event, even in patients who hav not participated actively. The setting of a target discharge date is particularly important for those patients who have developed a significant degree of dependency on the group, and the discussion of reactions to discharge may be an important part of treatment. The conductor should mention when it is a patient's last meeting and, if appropriate, emphasize that follow-up arrangements have been made. Psychological defences are often intensified before discharge, so that emotionality and exploration of unconscious processes should be minimized during a patient's final meetings. Timing of discharge is vital, as if it is too late a damaging over-dependence may have resulted. The optimum time for each patient will be determined, to a large extent, on the goals which have been formulated.

The Conductor's Problems

Personality, knowledge and experience determine the efficacy of a group conductor, and it must be recognized that certain traits, such as excessive emotional coldness or obsessionality, disqualify an individual for this task. Conducting a group can be a stressful experience, and the relatively inexperienced conductor must always have the assistance of at least one other staff member, together with regular supervision. Various maladaptive behaviour patterns have been described in trainee psychiatrists (Shershow and Savodnik 1976) who, together with other professionals, often find that working in groups is the most demanding of all their duties. The conductor is himself involved in the group processes and may be caught up in contagious emotion. He may be the focus of hostility and be subjected to unreasonable demands, which require a firm stand against pressures to conform. Faced with stressful situations, the conductor's defence mechanisms may distort his judgement and he may take refuge behind a professional mask, by showing his 'wares' in the form of long summaries, involved interpretations or the use of jargon (Yalom 1966).

One of the main attributes of an effective group psychotherapist is a degree of self-awareness and self-control, together with a confidence which enables him to doubt and question his own actions. The potentially harmful effects of counter-transference or the conductor's defences can be minimized by supervision, feedback from other staff members in the group, and the conductor's increasing recognition of certain characteristics of his own personality. Self-control involves an ability to endure difficult interpersonal situations by 'sitting it out' and keeping calm. This does not imply that the conductor is not experiencing strong emotions, but their expression is being controlled. Reacting with anger and getting caught up with a prevailing feeling of despair are two of the most common pitfalls for the group conductor.

Common Situations in Group Psychotherapy

Group members may sit expectantly, awaiting direction from the conductor in the hope that someone else can sort out their problems without any effort on their part. This attitude may need to be discussed and the conductor should repeatedly clarify what can and cannot be done without the members' active participation. This may reduce the hostility which usually accompanies unrealistic and unfulfilled demands.

There are many kinds of silence which reflect apathy, active consideration, a brooding hopelessness, perplexity, anger, tension, stubbornness, or, especially with new members, uncertainty as to what they should be discussing. In general, long silences are not beneficial, but their resolution will depend on the underlying cause. Of course, it should be remembered that although the predominant mood or attitude of the group in a silence (or any other situation) can often be identified, it is unusual for it to be shared by all the members. Some of those who do not share the prevailing attitude or emotion understandably find repeated references to the opinions of 'the group' rather irritating, and the conductor should always bear in mind that a group is composed of individuals.

If the conductor does not know what to do in any situation, the answer is often 'nothing', apart from putting up with the situation while continuing to try and help the group to function. He may have to remind himself that the burden of responsibility for the proceedings of the group is shared by all its members and that, apart from not giving up, he is not necessarily obliged to 'do something'.

At times the conductor is aware of a major event, such as a recent attempted suicide of one of the members, which he feels is being avoided at the expense of 'safer' topics. In this situation he should usually raise the issue at some time during the meeting.

Another common event is the repeated questioning of the conductor by one or more group members; this poses a problem, because although it is often appropriate to give direct answers, an excess of this type of interaction fosters dependency and impairs group communication. Thus, it may be necessary for the conductor to say that a question will be answered later in another setting, or that he considers an excess of questions and answers to be unhelpful in group meetings. However it is rarely appropriate to completely ignore a question.

Group members may try and strike up a special relationship with the conductor, perhaps by imparting 'confidential' information between meetings, but the conductor should usually make it clear that he is not able to accept information on this basis and that if it is confided, he will reserve the right to bring it to the attention of the group. There are many ways in which members attempt to manipulate the conductor to carry out inappropriate actions and he must be able to refuse certain demands.

The overtalkative group member who monopolizes meetings is another common problem. Often group pressures and firm interventions by the conductor are effective, but in the case of hypomanic patients, who may have relapsed since joining the group, temporary exclusion may be necessary.

The Milieu of the Psychiatric Admission Unit

Small-group psychotherapy of the type under consideration takes place against the background of the so-called admission unit. The importance of the social environment (or milieu) in psychiatric hospitals has long been recognized (Jones et al. 1971d), and Main (1946) introduced the term 'therapeutic community', which has come to imply frequent group meetings, an emphasis on problems involving social relationships, good interpersonal communication, flattening of the pyramid of institutional authority, free emotional expression and examination of institutional roles (Clark and Myers 1970). However this type of organization produces its own problems (Zeitlyn 1967).

Considerable and relatively exclusive emphasis on these principles results in the therapeutic community 'proper', and has been advocated for some long-stay wards of psychiatric hospitals and for specialist units catering for sociopathic personalities and for those who abuse drugs and alcohol. But a typical psychiatric admission unit must cater for a wide range of psychiatric disorders, including the manic–depressive psychoses and the schizophrenias, for which an emphasis on medical treatment is often appropriate. In this setting, a dilution of the senior psychiatrist's ultimate responsibility for the prescription of medical treatment, sometimes against the patient's will, should not occur. In addition, organizing an admission unit as a proper therapeutic community implies that groups provide the focus of treatment for all patients; but this is not the case, and, for some patients in an admission unit, inclusion in groups can produce harmful effects. However, principles derived from the therapeutic community proper are of considerable value in the admission unit setting: a variety of group activities should be available, the patients are encouraged to assume as much responsibility for themselves and their fellow patients as is possible, while staff of all disciplines should be willing to consider constructive and informed criticism, taking decisions in consultation with their colleagues. However, in the case of disagreement, it should be recognized that it is the responsibility of the senior psychiatrist to make the final decision regarding the medical aspects of treatment or management. All staff and patients of an admission unit may be encouraged to meet regularly for an unstructured community meeting, which may involve about 30–50 people for 45 minutes, but the patients should realize that they are free to choose not to attend. Although daily community meetings of this type have been advocated, it is the author's opinion that these should only be held at the beginning and end of the week, with various structured communal activities scheduled for other days.

The large group has been defined as a meeting which comprises more than 30 people (de Maré and Kreeger 1974b; Kreeger 1975), and Schiff and Glassman (1969) have described the consequences of increasing group size: a higher proportion of patients are silent, subgrouping increases, the participation of the less active members is reduced, and the contribution of the conductor and staff is increased. There is some overlap between the activities of community meetings and group psychotherapy, but the former should focus on day-to-day problems in the ward and administrative matters. Community meetings also enable the staff to identify quickly the main management problems of the ward and assess a large number of patients in a short time. All the staff who attend should be urged to participate, although not necessarily in every meeting, and one of their members is designated as the conductor.

Various forms of structured group activity should contribute to the admission unit's programme; a weekly review meeting chaired by a member of the medical staff can discuss non-confidential aspects of treatment, considering each patient in turn, but if patients prefer not to participate, this wish should be respected. Administrative arrangements, including those for weekend leave, can also be clarified. Other forms of structured group activity may involve art, music, psychodrama, and various forms of recreation.

Staff members require their own group activities, although there is a danger that an excess of time is spent in this way. Inexperienced staff who are involved in group psychotherapy must be supervised in weekly meetings and all staff in a group should spend about 15 minutes discussing each session. The overall staff effectiveness depends to a significant extent on adequate communication, and all staff in an admission unit should meet regularly for an administrative meeting. This should be structured, with a chairman and an agenda.

Negative Effects

A negative effect has been defined as a lasting deterioration in a patient, directly attributable to therapy; however transient effects may also be important (Hadley and Strupp 1976).

Existing problems may be magnified: the inability of the passive dependent patient to refuse unreasonable demands may be exploited by group members, the paranoid patient may consistently evoke hostility which strengthens his beliefs, and social phobias may be intensified in a group which lacks cohesion, concern and support. Psychotic patients or those with limited intelligence may not be able to join in, thus compounding a feeling of inadequacy, while exposure to an emotionally charged situation may exacerbate a psychosis. Maladaptive defence mechanisms and behaviour patterns may be reinforced: the withdrawn individual may become more socially isolated, or the group may provide an opportunity to develop a tendency to display undue aggression.

New problems may also arise. A system of defence mechanisms can represent the best possible way of coping and, if these are explored, decompensation may result in further impairment of the patient's adjustment, perhaps involving depression, anxiety or excessive dependence on the group (Neki 1976). In addition, new defences may develop which are even more maladaptive than the originals. Symptom substitution may occur: for example a preoccupation with somatic complaints may be replaced by the overt development of a previously covert paranoid psychosis. The setting of unrealistic goals will lead to frustration, disappointment and loss of hope for both the patient and therapist, while for some patients the pursuit of 'therapy' can become an unproductive end in itself which serves to protect the individual from the need to face up to immediate problems. Breaches of confidentiality may occasionally have serious consequences, for example if they involve extramarital relationships or criminal activity, while for some patients a relapse in the severity of their disorder, perhaps involving suicidal intent, may not be recognized in a group setting.

Emotional arousal may have several harmful effects: heightened emotions can give rise to destructive or antisocial 'acting out' behaviour, such as taking an overdose, and can precipitate an episode of manic–depressive or schizophrenic psychosis in patients who are predisposed to these disorders.

The conductor must monitor the group sessions for harmful effects and take active steps to stop their development. If necessary a patient should be excluded, either temporarily or permanently, for his own good or to prevent harm to others. If meetings are consistently characterized by anger, distrust and lack of concern, the disadvantages will probably outweigh any advantages, and disbanding the group should be considered. However this should not be necessary with an experienced conductor and careful selection of patients.

Finally, the development of a sexual relationship between two group members may occur, usually with adverse consequences, especially if the male patient has pronounced sociopathic personality traits. This potential problem should be anticipated when selecting the members of a group.

Training and Supervision for Group Conductors

A group conductor should have certain attributes of personality, a degree of self-awareness, and some theoretical knowledge and experience.

Self-awareness and theoretical knowledge can be acquired in various ways which often include a meeting of trainee conductors with their supervisor in a group setting (Jones et al. 1971c). In this group, the same phenomena that are found in psychotherapeutic groups may occur; for example, the trainees may show resistance by avoiding discussion of certain aspects of their work, by an inability to monitor group processes, or by avoiding the discussion of covert events. Counter-transferences of trainees to the patients may be apparent to other members of the supervision group; thus, a trainee conductor may inappropriately feel that the problems of a group member have a bad prognosis. A transference on the part of the trainee to the supervisor may show itself in an excessive need for approval, an unresolved hostility to authority, or intense rivalry with fellow trainees.

EFFICACY OF GROUP PSYCHOTHERAPY

Published studies do not provide sufficient evidence to demonstrate the efficacy of various psychotherapeutic techniques, with the exception of behaviour therapy (Shepherd 1979), and a major difficulty which is encountered by investigators of group psychotherapy is that, like individual psychotherapy, the procedure is undifferentiated. In addition, the treatment goals and criteria for the definition of improvement are varied. Beneficial effects may be judged on the basis of changes observed in the group, disappearance of symptoms, improved subjective well-being, the views of the conductor, the opinions of friends or relations of the patient, increased self-knowledge, increased competence at work, or changes in social behaviour (Frank 1968; Jones et al. 1971e; Malan 1973; Weissman 1975; Malan et al. 1976; Yalom et al. 1977; Kazdin and Wilson 1978; Kilman et al. 1979). However, there is often a low correlation between various outcome measures (Luborsky et al. 1975). Apart from the methodological problems in measuring outcome, the results are often affected by spontaneous recovery and many non-treatment variables. Also, if a particular psychotherapeutic method is being investigated, many non-technique variables are relevant, such as the 'helping relationship' with the therapist, although this may be of less importance in groups compared with individual psychotherapy (Gurman and Gustafson 1976). As each group is unique, control data must be interpreted with caution.

Luborsky et al. (1975) in their review of the literature concluded that many therapeutic ingredients are common to various forms of psychotherapy, and that it has not been demonstrated that differences in outcome are associated with different types of psychotherapy. This conclusion was also supported by Sloane et al. (1975). However, although the evidence suggests that most patients in the studies reviewed did benefit, and that psychotherapy in all its forms can be effective, it cannot be concluded that the nature of the technical procedures in groups is irrelevant. In the absence of research data, clinical judgement based on experience is essential.

VARIETIES OF GROUP PSYCHOTHERAPY

Other types of group psychotherapy can be organized within a psychiatric service in addition to the particular type of group which has been considered. Some groups may cater for out-patients alone, or the conductor may select a relatively homogeneous group with regard to treatment goals. Although some group activities for out-patients may involve little more than social contact and a cup of tea, others may have members whose goals include significant personality change (Swenson and Martin 1976). Such groups are usually closed but new members may occasionally be recruited. Each session lasts

90 minutes and may occur weekly for about 12–18 months or more intensively over a shorter period. Sometimes groups may be selected with regard to the homogeneity of presenting problems such as social phobia, agoraphobia, alcoholism, drug addiction or sociopathy (Bloch 1979a). Groups for sociopathic individuals should be in the context of a specialist institution or service. Other groups may comprise couples with marital difficulties, the relatives of patients, or several members of one family.

Additional varieties of group occur outside the setting of a psychiatric service (Kadis et al. 1974a; Bloch 1979a; Frank 1979). 'Marathon' groups have been described, lasting for between 6 and 48 hours, and peer self-help groups such as Alcoholics Anonymous and Depressives Anonymous may not include a professional conductor. The use of so-called alternate (or coordinated) sessions involve the patient/client members of an out-patient group meeting on their own, alternately with the conventional sessions (Kadis 1959; Hurwitz 1970; Dumont 1974; Kadis et al. 1974).

CONCLUSIONS

This chapter has been written in the belief that various forms of group psychotherapy, while so far eluding effective research scrutiny, are a useful part of the range of treatments provided by a modern psychiatric service. Although not all psychiatric patients benefit, groups may form the major part of treatment for some patients, while for many others it is a useful adjunct to other methods. It has the advantage of being cost effective, which is important in view of the increasing demand for psychotherapy.

However, problems can occur if group activities involving individuals with a wide range of psychiatric and social problems are approached with a rigid theoretical viewpoint. Statements such as 'symptoms, after all, are a form of camouflage; why therefore base selection (for inclusion in a group) on disguise?' (de Maré and Kreeger 1974c) are typical of an approach derived from psychoanalysis, which, while valid for some patients, does not take into account other factors such as abnormalities of brain function which are almost certainly necessary for the development of the major psychoses. Although it has been claimed that 'psychoanalysis has shown that neuroses are based on conflict' (Foulkes and Anthony 1965), the relevance of this claim to many patients with the syndrome of obsessive–compulsive neurosis or with certain phobias, is questionable.

Conducting a group is demanding work requiring natural ability, experience, knowledge and technique. It should not be undertaken without sufficient staff who can attend regularly, and supervision for the inexperienced conductor. If groups cannot be conducted properly, it is better that an attempt to provide this form of treatment should not be made.

GLOSSARY OF TERMS

Unconscious Mental Activity

Mental activity which has the potential of entering conscious awareness; an example is an instruction given in a 'hypnotic state' which is subsequently carried out without the individual being consciously aware of the reasons for his actions.

Insight

The awareness of previously unconscious mental events; there are degrees of awareness, so that insight is not an 'all-or-nothing' phenomenon. This term can also be used in a less specific sense to include any discovery which an individual makes about himself.

Free Association

The individual is encouraged to talk about whatever thoughts come into conscious awareness. In a group setting an equivalent phenomenon is a 'chain reaction' of contributions from various members, each contribution being inspired by its predecessor.

Psychological Defence Mechanisms

Forms of unconscious psychological activity which may distort the awareness and expression of mental events, such as emotions or attitudes.
Examples include:

a) Denial (i.e. repression). A special type of denial is known as 'isolation', when different components of an individual's reaction are separated; for example when an emotional reaction to bereavement is not consciously experienced, or delayed.

b) Avoidance

c) Projection; when unconscious mental events (i.e. ideas, attitudes, emotions, drives), are attributed to others.

d) Sublimation; when unconscious mental events produce conscious experiences which are similar but more acceptable to the individual or society.

e) Substitution; when unconscious mental events are expressed indirectly.

f) Intellectualization; when mental events remain unconscious because of distortion or disguise by complex argument and discussion.

g) Rationalization; when mental events are distorted or disguised by apparent explanations which are false.

h) Reaction formation; when the opposite of unconscious mental events appears in conscious awareness.

i) Undoing; which comprises overt behaviour arising from reaction formation. An example would be oversolicitous behaviour towards another individual associated with unconscious dislike.

j) Displacement; when mental events remain unconscious because of the predominance of other mental events which are in conscious awareness.

k) Regression; when an individual may return to a child-like pattern of mental functioning and behaviour, for example, becoming excessively dependent with frequent temper tantrums. Regression may help to keep certain mental events unconscious, by removing motivation for self-scrutiny or resolving problems.

Resistance

Obstacles to the aims and procedures of psychotherapy which arise from within the patient. Resistance generally involves psychological defence mechanisms, although conscious mental events may also contribute.

Transference

Aspects of the patients' emotions, attitudes, motivations, and behaviour which are directed to the therapist (and, in groups, to other group members), which seem inappropriate, and are derived in part from past experience. Transference phenomena may be present at the beginning of a relationship or develop subsequently.

Counter-transference

Inappropriate emotions, attitudes, motivations and behaviour on the part of the therapist which are directed to an individual patient or group of patients.

References

BANCROFT, J. (1979) Crisis intervention. In: *An Introduction to the Psychotherapies*. ed. Bloch, S. Oxford: Oxford University Press.

BION, W.R. (1961) In: *Experiences in Groups and Other Papers*. London: Tavistock Publications.

BLOCH, S. (1979a) Group psychotherapy. In: *An Introduction to the Psychotherapies*, ed. Bloch, S. Oxford: Oxford University Press.

BLOCH, S. (1979b) Supportive psychotherapy. In: *An Introduction to the Psychotherapies*, ed. Bloch, S. Oxford: Oxford University Press.

CAPLAN, G. (1961) *An Approach to Community Mental Health*. London: Tavistock Publications.

CAWLEY, R. (1974) Psychotherapy and obsessional disorders. In: *Obsessional States*, ed. Beech, H.R. London: Methuen.

CLARK, D.H. & MYERS, K. (1970) Themes in a therapeutic community. *Br. J. Psychiat.*, **117**, 389.

EZRIEL, H. (1950) A psychoanalytic approach to group treatment. *Br. J. med. Psychol.*, **23**, 59.

FOULKES, S.H. & ANTHONY, E.J. (1965) *Group Psychotherapy*, 2nd ed. Harmondsworth, England: Penguin Books.

FRANK, J.D. (1968) Methods of assessing the results of psychotherapy. In: *The Role of Learning in Psychotherapy*, ed. Porter, R. London: Churchill.

FRANK, J.D. (1974) The restoration of morale. *Am. J. Psychiat.*, **131**, 271.

FRANK, J.D. (1979) What is psychotherapy? In: *An Introduction to the Psychotherapies*, ed. Bloch, S. Oxford: Oxford University Press.

GOLDFRIED, M.R. & GOLDFRIED, A.P. (1975) Cognitive change methods. In: *Helping People Change*, ed. Kanfer, F.H., Goldstein, A.P. New York: Pergamon Press.

GURMAN, A.S. & GUSTAFSON, J.P. (1976) Patients' perceptions of the therapeutic relationship and group therapy outcome. *Am. J. Psychiat.*, **133, 11**, 1290.

HADLEY, & STRUPP, H.H. (1976) Contemporary views of negative effects in psychotherapy. *Archs gen. Psychiat.*, **33**, 1291.

HURWITZ, N. (1970) Peer self-help psychotherapy groups and their implications for psychotherapy. *Psychother. Theory Res. Pract.*, **7**, 41.

JONES, M., MCPHERSON, F., WHITAKER, D.S., SUTHERLAND, J.D., WALTON, H. & WOOLF, H. (1971a–e) *Small Group Psychotherapy*, ed. Walton, H., pp. 18a, 35b, 66c, 101d, 108e. Harmondsworth, England: Penguin Books.

KADIS, A.L. (1959) The role of co-ordinated group meetings in group psychotherapy. *Acta psychother. psychosom. Orthop. 7: Suppl. 174.*

KADIS, A.L., KRASNER, J.D., WEINER, M.F., WINICK, C. & FOULKES, S.H. (1974) *Practicum of Group Psychotherapy*, 2nd ed., pp. 87a, 123b. New York: Harper and Row.

KAZDIN, A.E. & WILSON, G.T. (1978) Criteria for evaluating psychotherapy. *Archs gen. Psychiat.*, **35**, 407.

KILMAN, P.R., SCOVERN, A.W. & MOREAULT, D. (1979) Factors in the patient–therapist interaction and outcome: a review of the literature. *Compreh. Psychiat.*, **20:2**, 132.

KREEGER, L. (1975) In: *The Large Group*, ed. Kreeger, L. London: Constable.

LUBORSKY, L., SOINGER, B. & LUBORSKY, L. (1975) Comparative Studies of Psychotherapies. *Arch. Gen. Psychiat.*, **32**, 995.

MAIN, T.F. (1946) The hospital as a therapeutic institution. *Bull. Men. Clin.*, **10**, 66.

MALAN, D.H. (1973) The outcome problem in psychotherapy research. *Archs gen. Psychiat.*, **29**, 719.

MALAN, D.H., BALFOUR, F.H.G., HOOD, V.G. & SHOOTER, M.N. (1976) Group psychotherapy. *Archs gen. Psychiat.*, **33**, 1303.

DE MARÉ, P.B. (1972) In: *Perspectives in Group Psychotherapy*. London: Allen and Unwin.

DE MARÉ, P.B. & KREEGER, L.C. (1974) *Introduction to Group Treatments in Psychiatry*, pp. 7a, 14b, 16c, 32d. London: Butterworths.

MARMOR, J. (1979) Short term dynamic psychotherapy. *Am. J. Psychiat.*, **136**, 149.

NEKI, J.S. (1976) An examination of the cultural relativism of dependence as a dynamic of social and therapeutic relationships. *Br. J. med. Psychol.*, **49**, 11.

RYLE, A. (1976) Group psychotherapy. *Br. J. hosp. Med.*, March, 239.

SANDLER, J., DARE, C. & HOLDER, A. (1970) Basic psychoanalytic concepts: transference. *Br. J. Psychiat.*, **116**, 667.

SANDLER, J., HOLDER, A. & DARE, C. (1970a) Basic psychoanalytic concepts: resistance. *Br. J. Psychiat.*, **117**, 215.

SANDLER, J., HOLDER, A. & DARE, C. (1970b) Basic psychoanalytic concepts: the negative therapeutic reaction. *Br. J. Psychiat.*, **117**, 431.

SANDLER, J., HOLDER, A. & DARE, C. (1970c) Basic psychoanalytic concepts: the treatment alliance. *Br. J. Psychiat.*, **116**, 555.

SCHIFF, S.B. & GLASSMAN, S.M. (1969) Large and small group therapy in a state mental health centre. *Int. J. Group Psychother.*, **19:2**.

SCHUTZ, W.C. (1958) In: *Firo: a three-dimensional theory of interpersonal behavior*. New York: Rinehart.

SHEPHERD, M. (1979) Psychoanalysis, psychotherapy, and health services. *Br. med. J.*, **2**, 1557.

SHERSHOW, J.C. & SAVODNIK, I. (1976) Regression in the service of residency education. *Archs gen. Psychiat.*, **33**, 1266.

SLOANE, R.B., STAPLES, F.R., CRISTOL, A.H., YORKSTON, N.J. & WHIPPLE, K. (1975) Short-term analytically orientated psychotherapy vs. behavior therapy. *Am. J. Psychiat.*, **132**, 373.

SWENSON, W.M. & MARTIN, H.R. (1976) A description and evaluation of an outpatient intensive psychotherapy center. *Am. J. Psychiat.*, **133:9**, 1043.

TUCKMAN, B.W. (1965) Developmental sequence in small groups. *Psychol. Bull.*, **63**, 384.

WEISSMAN, M.M. (1975) The assessment of social adjustment. *Archs gen. Psychiat.*, **32**, 357.

WOLF, A. (1949) The psychoanalysis of groups. *Am. J. Psychother.*, **3**, 213.

WOLF, A. & SCHWARTZ, E.K. (1962) *Psychoanalysis in Groups*. New York: Grune and Stratton.

YALOM, I.D. (1966) Problems of neophyte group therapists. *Internat. J. soc. Psychiat.*, **12**, 52.

YALOM, I.D. (1975) *The Theory and Practice of Group Psychotherapy*. New York: Basic Books.

YALOM, I.D., BOND, G., BLOCK, S., ZIMMERMAN, E. & FRIEDMAN, L. (1977) The impact of a weekend group experience on individual therapy. *Archs gen. Psychiat.*, **34**, 399.

YALOM, I.D., BROWN, S. & BLOCH, S. (1975) The written summary as a group psychotherapy technique. *Archs gen. Psychiat.*, **32**,605.

YALOM, I.D., HOUTS, P.S., NEWELL, G. & RAND, K.H. (1967) Preparation of patients for group therapy. A controlled study. *Archs gen. Psychiat.*, **17**, 416.

ZEITLYN, B.B. (1967) The therapeutic community—fact or fantasy? *Br. J. Psychiat.*, **113**, 1083.

10

The Behaviour Therapies

S. Morley

THE CHARACTERISTICS OF BEHAVIOUR THERAPIES

There is no exact definition of behaviour therapy but behavioural approaches to treatment share a number of prominent features (Erwin 1978; Kazdin 1979). The therapies are directed at the modification of symptoms and their current determinants; symptoms are regarded as the problem rather than as a manifestation of some underlying personality dysfunction. Behaviour therapies involve setting specific treatment goals and emphasize the experimental investigation of single cases and the controlled evaluation of general methods of treatment (Gottman and Markman 1978; Shapiro 1966; Kazdin 1978). References to treatments not discussed in this chapter are included in the *Supplementary bibliography*.

THE USE OF 'ANALOGUE STUDIES' OF BEHAVIOUR THERAPIES

A number of studies of the techniques of behaviour therapy have been conducted on 'analogue' populations. These are non-clinical groups with mild symptoms who are often drawn from student populations and are recruited for a particular study. They may be offered an incentive such as financial reward. These subjects may differ from clinical groups on other variables, such as the degree of social support, which can affect the prognosis (Henderson et al. 1978; Huxley et al. 1979). Although analogue studies have been criticized on the grounds that they are less likely to have relevance to clinical problems (Luborsky et al. 1975), they have a role in the development of therapeutic techniques. The initial testing of a therapeutic procedure can be best conducted under controlled conditions which are more easily obtained by using an analogue population, and studies aimed at identifying the effective components of treatment may also be facilitated by using homogeneous groups of subjects under strict experimental control.

There are, however, a limited number of analogue populations available, and while certain disorders such as monosymptomatic fears are well represented in the general population, it seems unlikely that analogues of any other disorders, such as the agoraphobic syndrome or obsessions and compulsions, are identifiable. Although recent research has described the widespread prevalence of intrusive unwanted thoughts (Rachman and De Silva 1978), and treatment procedures have been investigated on this group (Parkinson and Rachman 1980), there are some notable differences between the 'obsessions' of normal and clinical samples (Rachman and De Silva 1978). Another limitation of analogue research is that the relative importance it might attach to any particular treatment component is of uncertain predictive value. For example, Mathews (1978) noted that 'non-specific' factors, which are often a potent source of change in analogue studies and clinical groups with monosymptomatic phobias, are less important determinants of outcome for agoraphobic patients. Mathews (1978) also suggested that the knowledge of improvement and social reinforcement obtained during treatment may be more important in the treatment of severe clinical problems than has been indicated by analogue studies. Ultimately the usefulness of analogue studies can only be empirically determined (Kazdin and Rogers 1978).

METHODS FOR CHANGING FEAR AND AVOIDANCE

Introduction

Much of the behaviour therapy literature is concerned with methods for treating phobic and obsessional states. Systematic desensitization, implosion and flooding are based on the assumption that the abnormal behaviour is motivated by fear and anxiety. In the case of obsessive–compulsive disorders the emotional state may be best described as discomfort (Rachman and Hodgson 1980). Thus treatments should reduce fear so that avoidance is minimized and approach behaviour encouraged. However, there is evidence from experimental and clinical studies that this analysis is not entirely correct as fear and avoidance may not be closely correlated (Rachman 1976a; Bandura 1977; Mineka 1979). For example fear need not be present for avoidance behaviour to be maintained. Two other treatments, modelling and response prevention, pay attention to the elimination of avoidance and the development of approach behaviour.

Systematic Desensitization

Systematic desensitization as introduced by Wolpe (1958) contains three components: firstly, a hierarchy of feared situations is constructed, ranging from those which provoke a mild degree of anxiety to those which elicit maximum fear; secondly, the patient is trained in muscle relaxation; and thirdly, the items are presented by asking the patient to imagine them in order of increasing severity. Items are desensitized when the subject no longer reports feeling frightened while imagining them. In practice, therapy sessions are often accompanied by 'homework assignments' when the patient is instructed to expose himself, in reality, to a previously desensitized item.

Wolpe's explanation of the mechanism of systematic desensitization was based on the principle of reciprocal inhibition, in which sympathetic arousal and fear are repeatedly paired with stimuli associated with relaxation, with the aim of weakening the association between the feared stimuli and the usual pattern of responses. Wolpe's explanation has been challenged, for there is evidence that neither relaxation nor the hierarchy are necessary for the reduction of fear (Rachman 1968; Gillan and Rachman 1974; Marks 1975). Evans (1973) has argued that the procedures involved in systematic desensitization are analogous to those used in extinction, i.e. the presentation of a stimulus without reinforcement, while Watts (1979) has discussed the reasons for considering systematic desensitization as an habituation process. A further type of explanation stresses the relevance of cognitive processes, involving the subject's expectancy of symptomatic improvement, rather than the hypothesized non-conscious, mechanisms which are postulated by the other explanations (Lick and Bootzin 1975; Kazdin and Wilcoxon 1976; Rosen 1976).

Flooding and Implosion

The terms flooding and implosion are often used interchangeably yet they refer to procedures derived from different assumptions. Implosion was developed by Stampfl (Stampfl and Levis 1967, 1968; Levis and Hare 1977) who proposed that phobias and obsessions are products of classical conditioning in which fear has developed as a result of being associated with aversive events. The fear-eliciting stimuli are called 'conditioned stimuli' (CS) and the fear responses the 'conditioned responses' (CR). Extinction of the CR occurs when the CS is repeatedly presented in the absence of reinforcement. Stampfl has argued that there are two classes of CS, namely 'symptom contingent cues' and 'sequential cues'. Symptom contingent cues are those which invariably occur in association with the subject's fear symptoms and usually define the category of a phobia (such as a crowded shop in an agoraphobic syndrome), while sequential cues are those events which only occurred during the original conditioning; for example, a woman who showed avoidance of travelling in cars was found to have initially experienced anxiety 15 years previously when she had to travel a considerable distance to see her acutely ill son. While she presented with a travel phobia, there was also an underlying fear of losing her son; in this case cars were considered as the symptom contingent cue, while her son's illness probably provided the sequential cue.

'Implosion' treatment can begin once the full set of cues has been established by clinical interview, trial and error. The subject is instructed to imagine the cues (including sequential cues) as vividly as possible, and the prolonged exposure to the cues is designed to evoke and maintain a high level of anxiety until a spontaneous reduction (implosion) occurs. This procedure is repeated with variation in the content of the imagined scenes, until no anxiety is elicited. Uncontrolled case studies indicate that implosion is effective for a variety of phobias and obsessional disorders. However, Levis and Hare (1977) noted that there were few controlled studies in which the effects of attempts to modify sequential cues had been adequately evaluated, while there was clear evidence that the presentation of symptom contingent cues, as in flooding (see below), can produce a marked reduction in symptoms (Levis and Hare 1977; Marshall et al. 1979).

'Flooding' is similar to implosion. It is assumed that fear can be reduced by prolonged exposure, either in imagination or reality, to the evoking stimuli. The major differences between flooding and implosion are that flooding does not involve exposure to the hypothesized sequential cues or a requirement that maximum levels of fear should be experienced during exposure.

The practice of flooding has varied considerably (Marshall et al. 1979); for example the term 'prolonged exposure' implies treatment sessions ranging from 2 min (Rachman 1966) to 2 h (Stern and Marks 1973). There are also differences in the mode of presentation of the evoking stimulus (in vivo, imaginal, audio or video tape), the degree of response prevention, the number of subjects treated together (group or individual treatments), and the concurrent administration of pharmacological agents.

Marshall et al. (1979) proposed that fear reactions are self-limiting and that after an initial period of raised fear, there will be a return to prestimulus baseline levels even though the subject is still exposed to the stimulus. Thus, if exposure is prolonged until this later phase, the subject will associate the reduced anxiety level with the fear stimulus, and the procedure should produce 'more adaptive expectations regarding contact with the fearful situation'. Marshall et al. (1979) endorsed Eysenck's proposal that short-duration exposures to intensely fearful stimuli may increase subsequent levels of fear, and the main therapeutic implication of this analysis is that exposure time should be tailored to the individual by prolonging a treatment session until fear is reduced.

Modelling

Learned aspects of behaviour which can be acquired by watching others (modelling) range from simple motor acts to complex cognitive activities

(Rosenthal and Bandura 1978; Rosenthal and Zimmerman 1978). Bandura (1969) identified three main effects of modelling: the transmission of new behaviour, the inhibition of unnecessary and unwanted responses, and the facilitation of established responses. A fourth effect, the setting of cognitive standards of self-regulation, has also been identified (Rosenthal and Bandura 1978). The psychological mechanisms involved in modelling are attention, memory, the production of overt behaviour, and motivation. The presentation of models in behaviour therapy varies with regard to the nature of the model and to the degree of participation by the subject. Models may be 'live' or 'symbolic' as in the case of video tape or film. 'Covert' models, which are imagined by the subject after verbal description, may be equally effective (Kazdin 1974*a,b,c;* 1980). With regard to patient participation, this may range from passivity to active engagement; the latter seems to have greater therapeutic effect (Roper et al. 1975; Bandura et al. 1977). Participant modelling also involves encouragement, social approval, guidance and correction, with the therapist gradually reducing his level of activity (Bandura et al. 1977). Other variations in modelling procedures involve the number of repeated presentations, the presence or absence of a graded hierarchy, and the psychological characteristics of the therapist. It has been concluded that models who are similar to the observer with respect to coping styles are relatively more effective (Meichenbaum 1971; Kazdin 1974*a*; Rosenthal and Bandura 1978).

In summary, modelling can be a therapeutic procedure for reducing fear and avoidance, and increasing appropriate adaptive behaviour in patients with phobic and obsessive–compulsive neuroses (Bandura 1969; Rachman 1976*b*; Rosenthal and Bandura 1978).

Response Prevention

This is defined as the prevention of the maladaptive behaviour initiated by the patient to escape from the fear-evoking stimulus. For example, an agoraphobic patient can be encouraged to remain in a crowded store, or a patient with compulsions is dissuaded from performing his rituals. Repeated and prolonged exposure appears to be necessary (Mills et al 1973; Foa et al. 1980). Current behavioural regimens for treating obsessive–compulsive neuroses vary in the degree to which response prevention is enforced. Patients may merely be asked to refrain from carrying out their rituals (Marks et al. 1975; Rachman et al. 1979), or prevented from performing them by means of a 24-h supervision (Meyer et al. 1974). The superior results achieved by the latter might be attributable to this difference (Beech and Vaughan 1978; Foa and Steketee 1979; Rachman and Hodgson 1980).

Discussion

There are three potential therapeutic ingredients in the behavioural treatment of fear and avoidance; exposure to the fear-evoking stimulus, prevention of escape and avoidance, and induction of appropriate coping behaviour. These methods have been applied to the following phobias: animal, social, object, blood and injury, flying and travel, and agoraphobia (Gelder et al. 1973; Solyman et al. 1973; Marks 1975, 1978; Connolly et al. 1976; Mathews 1978; Emmelkamp 1979; Jannoun et al. 1980). Real life exposure to the phobic stimulus seems preferable to imaginal exposure, relatively prolonged exposure (flooding) may produce a more rapid reduction of fear, and suitable models facilitate the acquisition of coping responses (Bandura 1977; Emmelkamp 1979; Marks 1975, 1978).

The selection of an appropriate technique is determined by practical considerations. For example, exposure in imagination is indicated when the phobic stimulus is imaginary, as in nightmares (Hersen 1972), or unobtainable or uncontrollable, as in a fear of thunder and lightning (Liddell and Lyons 1978). The choice between flooding and graded exposure (desensitization) is largely determined by the wishes of the subject. Many phobic patients display considerable courage in facing intense fear, and there is no evidence that flooding procedures produce untoward side effects (Shipley and Boudewyns 1980). Practice in approaching the phobic stimulus outside formal treatment ensures maintenance of therapeutic gains. Hence recent approaches to treating agoraphobia have made home-based practice their central feature (Mathews et al. 1977; Jannoun et al. 1980).

The treatment of compulsions is most effective when patients are given real life exposure to the provoking stimuli and the compulsive responses are prevented. This treatment is most readily instituted using participant modelling. Checking, cleaning or washing, and repetitive rituals have all been successfully treated with this combination of techniques (Foa and Steketee 1979; Rachman and Hodgson 1980).

Systematic desensitization has not been so effective in treating obsessive –compulsive neurosis, and the efficacy of imaginal-based treatment in these disorders requires further investigation. Foa et al. (1980) have reported that the addition of flooding in imagination enhances the effects of in vivo exposure and response prevention in the treatment of compulsive checking, which is the most refractory of the compulsions to behavioural treatment (Rachman and Hodgson 1980).

The treatment of obsessions which are unaccompanied by compulsive behaviour is relatively unexplored and while there are case reports of successful treatment using procedures such as thought stopping (Stern et al. 1975; Foa and Steketee 1979), it is not clear which patients show the best response to treatment.

METHODS FOR CHANGING SOCIAL BEHAVIOUR

Social Skills Training

Psychiatric syndromes are often associated with difficulties in forming and sustaining interpersonal relationships, or with other impairments of social functioning (Zigler and Philips 1960, 1961; Argyle 1969; Henderson et al. 1978), and an approach known as social skills training is directed at modifying the person's social performance (Argyle 1969). This procedure is concerned with the goals of behaviour, the interpretation of feedback, and the presence of appropriate motor components such as eye contact, voice control and posture. An alternative analysis of deficient social performance has been proposed by Wolpe (1969), who suggested that excessive anxiety can inhibit appropriate social behaviour. Although some people do experience anxiety in social situations, Wolpe's assumption that the appropriate behavioural skills are present should be questioned (Twentyman and Zimering 1979).

Contemporary social skills training includes modelling of the target behaviour by another, rehearsal and role play under controlled conditions, feedback which gives the subject the view of others about the adequacy of his social performance, coaching, guidance, and encouragement from the therapist (Hersen and Bellack 1976; Twentyman and Zimering 1979). The main assessment instruments for social skills training, namely self-report questionnaires and role-play tests, present methodological problems. Furthermore the relationship of these measures to real-life behaviour is unclear (Mischel 1968; Shapiro 1975; Bellack et al. 1978; Twentyman and Zimering 1979). Nevertheless, assessment of gains should be made in relation to the everyday social environment of the subject (Shepherd 1978, 1981).

Studies involving volunteer non-psychiatric subjects (e.g. 'unassertive' and 'heterosexually unskilled' college students) have attempted to identify the therapeutic ingredients of social skills training. It has been concluded that modelling and instructions seem to be the most effective components (Hersen and Bellack 1976). Shepherd (1981) has reviewed 52 studies of social skills training with psychiatric patients published between 1970 and 1980, which included comparisons between groups (Argyle et al. 1974; Marzillier et al. 1976) and single case studies (Marzillier and Winter 1978). However it is not easy to delineate and define the range of social skill problems, and Shepherd found that his evaluation was hampered by lack of sufficient information regarding the psychiatric state and social competence of the patients referred for treatment. It was concluded that, while modelling had been of importance, there had also been an additive effect, so that an increase in the number of treatment components was correlated with the degree of improvement on various measures. Despite these findings, studies which compared social skills training with other treatment have not revealed significant difference in efficacy (Argyle et al. 1974; Hersen and Bellack 1976; Marzillier et al. 1976; Twentyman and Zimering 1979).

In addition to measuring the effects of social skills training on target responses, such as duration of eye contact or speech production, researchers have been concerned with whether these generalize to other situations, or are accompanied by improvement in the person's psychiatric state. Shepherd

(1981) found that eight out of eleven studies provided evidence for such a generalization effect (Bellack et al. 1976), while other studies have detected improvement in the psychiatric state of the individual (Argyle et al. 1974; Percell et al. 1974; Marzillier et al. 1976).

METHODS FOR REDUCING UNWANTED BEHAVIOUR

Aversion Therapy

Aversion therapy is a term applied to procedures in which a noxious stimulus, such as electric shock or drug induced nausea, is used to reduce or eliminate unwanted behaviour, and there are three main methods which have been discussed by Rachman and Teasdale (1969a,b). The first involves classical conditioning, when the stimulus which elicits the unwanted behaviour is repeatedly paired with a noxious stimulus; for example, a fetishist may receive repeated presentations of the fetish paired with shock (Raymond and O'Keefe 1965; Marks and Gelder 1967), with the aim of conditioning unpleasant feelings to the previously attractive stimulus. In the second procedure a noxious stimulus (i.e. punishment), is presented when the person emits the unwanted behaviour (Harris and Ersner-Hershfield 1978); for example, Risley (1968) reported that an autistic girl's dangerous behaviour of climbing to high places could be eliminated by response-contingent shock. The third procedure is known as avoidance conditioning, and involves the presentation of the 'deviant' stimulus which gives rise to the deviant behaviour; this is followed, some seconds later, by a noxious event, which may be avoided if the subject makes a response to remove the deviant stimulus. Feldman and MacCulloch (1971) have used this procedure in an attempt to modify homosexual behaviour, when their subject was presented with a slide of a desirable male which could be removed from the screen by pressing a button to avoid electric shock. An additional feature was that the original slide was replaced by a slide of an attractive female.

The main applications of aversion therapy in adult psychiatric patients have been to various sexual disorders including homosexuality (Feldman and MacCulloch 1971; Adams and Sturgis 1977), fetishism (Raymond and O'Keefe 1965), paedophilia (Josiassen et al. 1980), exhibitionism (Rooth and Marks 1974), transvestism (Blakemore et al. 1963), and to the addictions, in particular smoking (Russell et al. 1976) and alcoholism (Vogler et al. 1970). There is evidence from controlled studies that aversion therapy was superior to psychotherapy in reducing homosexual feelings and behaviour (McConaghy 1977), but many studies involving other sexual disorders have been uncontrolled, so that the efficacy of some aversive techniques is difficult to assess. Although there is some evidence that aversive procedures help some patients who smoke or drink alcohol excessively, it appears that these methods are no better than alternative treatment regimens (Miller et al. 1973; Emrick 1975; Russell et al. 1976; Raw 1978) and despite the success of aversive procedures in some cases, there is no evidence that its efficacy is due to the conditioning processes (Hallam and Rachman 1972, 1976; McConaghy 1977). With respect to alcohol abuse, there is evidence that treatment gains are related to the patient's occupational and family resources (Bromet and Moos 1977) and his attitude to, and participation in, a treatment programme, regardless of the programme's content (Miller et al. 1973; Bromet et al. 1977).

Covert Sensitization

During covert sensitization (Cautela 1967), the subject is instructed to imagine the performance of his deviant act and, at the point when the act is almost completed, the therapist instructs him to switch the image to an unpleasant one. For example, a paedophiliac would imagine undressing and touching his victim until, at the point of sexual gratification, he would be asked to switch his image to one where the child is covered with disgusting, putrefying abscesses. Cautela (1967, 1973) has proposed that the procedures used in covert sensitization are analogous to the classical conditioning and punishment procedures outlined previously, but this has been questioned (Little and Curran 1978; Kazdin and Smith 1979).

Covert sensitization has been used to treat obesity (Janda and Rimm 1972), alcoholism (Ashem and Donner 1968), smoking (Sipich et al. 1974) and a variety of sexual disorders such as homosexuality (Maletsky and George 1973), exhibitionism (Maletsky 1980), and paedophilia (Barlow et al. 1969). Little and Curran (1978) have reviewed the evidence for the efficacy of covert sensitization and concluded that in treating obesity, smoking and alcoholism this method is no more effective than a variety of control procedures. Little and Curran (1978) concluded that some sexual disorders can be modified by covert sensitization, and suggested that this may be partly due to an attenuation of sexual fantasies. This hypothesis remains to be tested.

METHODS BASED ON OPERANT CONDITIONING

Introduction

The central construct of operant theory is that behaviour is a function of its consequences. *Positive reinforcers* are those consequences which increase the probability of a repetition of the behaviour in question, (i.e. the 'target response'), while an increase in the frequency of a target response can also be brought about by *negative reinforcement*, in which the removal of an aversive event is contingent on the correct response being performed. If the onset of the aversive event is contingent on the production of the target response, the probability of the resonse reoccurring is reduced and the procedure is known as *punishment*. Punishment also occurs when a target response is followed by the removal of a positive event. A target response may also be reduced by *extinction*, which is the withdrawal of reinforcement, while behaviour may also be controlled by antecedent stimuli known as *discriminant stimuli*, which provide the individual with information about the future availability of reinforcement. An example of a discriminant stimulus is a red traffic light which indicates that punishing consequences are likely for those who transgress. In developing new behaviour patterns by varying reinforcement, *shaping, prompting* and *fading* techniques can be used. Shaping is carried out by reinforcing small steps organized as successive stages towards the target response. For example, mute schizophrenics might be initially reinforced for making any noise, after which the criteria for reinforcement can be made more stringent until words and then sentences are rewarded (Fraser et al. 1981). Prompts are events which help initiate the desired response, and they may include verbal instruction, physical guidance and modelling. The gradual withdrawal of a prompt is referred to as fading.

These relatively few and simple procedures have been applied to a wide range of human behaviour with considerable success. Ayllon and his colleagues (Ayllon and Michael 1959; Ayllon and Haughton 1964) have demonstrated how disruptive behaviour and bizarre language in institutional settings can be reduced by the application of extinction procedures, and operant conditioning has also been used in the treatment of more acute psychiatric disorders. Blinder et al. (1970) reported that anorexic patients can be induced to gain weight by using the 'Premack Principle' to determine a suitable reinforcer. [The Premack Principles states that a behaviour with a relatively high probability of occurrence will reinforce behaviour with a low probability (Danaher 1974)]. Blinder et al. (1970) gave their patients with anorexia nervosa opportunity to engage in physical exercise if they gained weight which, together with other positive reinforcement programmes, have been successful in producing short-term weight gain in this disorder (Brady and Reiger 1975; Swann Van Buskirk 1977).

Operant conditioning procedures have also been used to modify complaints of pain in 'chronic pain' patients (Fordyce 1976), reduce self-mutilation in children (Carr 1977), reverse inappropriate gender identity behaviour (Rekers et al. 1976), modify classroom behaviour (Ayllon et al. 1975), reduce chronic hyperventilation (Singh et al. 1980), control epileptic seizures (Mostofsky and Balaschak 1977), and modify many other problem behaviours (Rimm and Masters 1979).

Token Economies

Token economies are programmes of behaviour modification which make use of the principle of conditioned reinforcement. Conditioned reinforcers are events which have no intrinsic value but which, by association with reinforcers acquire reinforcing properties. In token economies, tokens (conditioned reinforcers) are dispensed for the performance of appropriate behaviour, and the tokens can then be exchanged for real goods, known as 'backup reinforcers'. Token economies specify exactly what behaviours will earn tokens and how much each behaviour is worth. For example, keeping one's bed area tidy might be worth three tokens, but cleaning the ward lavatories might earn 15 tokens. Undesirable behaviour may be eliminated by instituting a 'response cost' programme, in which a fine is imposed for undesirable behaviours and the patient loses tokens. Token economies have been extensively employed to improve self-care and to increase appropriate social behaviour in chronic schizophrenics and other institutionalized patients (Ayllon and Azrin 1968; Kazdin 1977). Token economies have also been applied to the management of institutions for delinquent youths (Braukman and Fixen 1975).

Controlled studies of token economies are rare, but Hall et al. (1977) compared a token economy regimen with a control condition which included all the elements of the token economy except that the tokens were delivered on a non-contingent basis. Their data clearly showed that the token economy had an immediate beneficial effect on social functioning, personal appearance (dress) and routine behaviour (e.g. shaving), but by the end of a 12-month experimental period the control group had made similar gains. The role of tokens as conditioned reinforcers must therefore be questioned, and the experiment of Hall et al. (1977) suggests that other features of the token economy, such as increased structure in the ward and the feedback and social approval contingent on the production of target behaviour, are also important determinants of change. However, despite these qualifications, a token economy programme can be a powerful procedure for producing and maintaining changes in individuals with chronic psychiatric disorders.

Self-Control and Self-Management

Skinner (1953) argued that self-control could be conceptualized in operant theory as the deliberate arrangement of the environment by a person to change or maintain his behaviour. The major techniques in self-control are *stimulus control, self-reinforcement, self-punishment,* and *self-observation.*

Behavioural excesses and deficits may be thought of as involving inappropriate stimulus control. For example, overweight people may eat in many inappropriate places and as part of their treatment they are asked to change, systematically, the conditions under which they eat. The number of places where they are allowed to eat is reduced (stimulus narrowing), and stimuli which inhibit eating may be displayed in appropriate places. Thus an overweight man might be asked to display a picture of himself inside the biscuit tin. At the same time competing responses, which reduce the desire or the availability of food, are introduced; examples of these might be drinking a large glass of water and going for a walk. In self-reinforcement and self-punishment, the individual is instructed to administer the consequences after he has completed a target, so a student with study problems would be advised to give himself a break filled with a desirable activity after he has completed a piece of work. In the initial stages of a programme, small units of behaviour are reinforced in accord with the principle of shaping. Self-punishment can be employed in a similar way, and failure to achieve a set target might be punished by the person contracting to donate to his least favourite political party or charity. Self-observation is a feature of all self-control programmes, and it often produces desirable changes (Kazdin 1974*d*; Ciminero et al. 1977; Nelson 1977). For example, people who were asked to record the number of cigarettes smoked, reduced their frequency of smoking (McFall and Hammen 1970), and such procedures have been used for treating a variety of problems either alone or in conjunction with other therapies. Overeating has been extensively studied using controlled trials (Abrahamson 1977), while smoking (Raw 1978), studying (Goldiamond 1965), and a number of other problems (Rimm and Masters 1979) have all been treated with self-control procedures. The evidence suggests that this is a promising approach (Mahoney and Arnkoff 1978).

Biofeedback

In biofeedback the subject is supplied with information about the state of some psysiological function of his body. The provision of this information, which may be accompanied by an incentive, may help the individual to gain voluntary control over an involuntary response. Since the introduction of biofeedback in the late 1960s, attempts have been made to treat many disorders and reviews have been given by Blanchard and Epstein (1977), Olton and Noonberg (1980), and Yates (1980), although much of the literature consists of single case reports.

The main application of biofeedback to psychiatric disorders has been in the treatment of generalized anxiety and tension. The underlying assumption is that if patients can be taught to reduce their physiological arousal, the psychological component of anxiety will also be diminished. A further assumption is that teaching the person to reduce activity in one measure of his physiological arousal will result in the generalized reduction of activity in other physiological systems, but although Yates (1980) has questioned the validity of both these assumptions, the beneficial effects of biofeedback training for generalized anxiety seem reasonably clear. The majority of experiments train subjects to reduce the activity in their occipitofrontalis muscles by providing auditory feedback in proportion to the amount of electrical activity present in the muscle. Subjects given feedback training show larger decrements in frontalis muscle activity than do control subjects, and subjective anxiety is also reduced.

However, there appears to be no difference between the effects of feedback training and general relaxation treatments of the type described by Bernstein and Borkovec (1973), and the changes produced usually return to pretreatment levels within 3–6 months (Canter et al. 1975; Townsend et al. 1975; Lavallée et al. 1977; Leboeuf and Lodge 1980). It seems reasonable to conclude that biofeedback is no more effective in treating anxiety than simpler relaxation techniques and that both treatments have a short-term effect.

Headache is widespread in general and psychiatric populations (Philips 1977; Philips and Hunter 1981) and biofeedback treatments have been applied to both migraine and tension headaches. Controlled trials indicate that although various forms of biofeedback can be effective, these are not superior to a general relaxation technique (Blanchard et al. 1978, 1979; Beaty and Haynes 1979; Kewman and Roberts 1980).

Electromyographic feedback has been shown to be an effective treatment for a variety of muscular dysfunctions associated with injury to the CNS and peripheral nerve injury. Brudny et al. (1976) reported some success in the treatment of the majority of 114 patients with a variety of disorders including hemiparesis, quadriplegia, secondary quadriceps muscle atrophy, and peripheral nerve injury. In each case appropriate target muscles were selected and feedback was provided to decrease spasticity during movement, and increase the strength and contraction of the affected muscle. Korein and Brudny (1976) have also reported a series of patients with spasmodic torticollis treated with biofeedback, and Basmajian et al. (1975, 1977) have summarized the results of their work with patients suffering from foot drop, impaired hand function and shoulder subluxation. Biofeedback was claimed to be useful in the majority of cases.

Other applications of biofeedback include the treatment of cardiac arrhythmias (Engel and Bleecker 1974), rectal incontinence attributed to physical causes (Engel et al. 1974) and epilepsy (Seifert and Lubar 1975; Lubar 1977; Sterman 1977; Sterman and MacDonald 1978; Kuhlman and Kaplan 1979).

THE COMPARATIVE EFFICACY OF BEHAVIOUR THERAPY

In judging the efficacy of behaviour therapy one must consider three distinct but interrelated questions: Is the treatment effective? Is it more effective than other specified treatments? and What aspects of the treatment contribute to its effectiveness? The second of these questions has provoked many opinions on the efficacy of behaviour therapy in relation to a variety of psychotherapies, including the claim that psychotherapy was no more effective than no formal psychological treatment (Eysenck 1952, 1960), and that behaviour therapy was effective and necessarily superior to psychotherapy (Kazdin 1979). These two propositions have been debated extensively (Bergin 1971; Rachman 1971;

Bergin and Lambert 1978; Kazdin and Wilson 1978; Shapiro 1980) and three recent publications, outlined below, represent different approaches to the investigation of therapeutic effectiveness.

Sloane et al. (1975) reported the effects of behaviour therapy and psychotherapy in comparison with the outcome of an untreated control group. This study employed highly experienced therapists, recruited patients who were attending a psychiatric outpatient clinic (who were randomly allocated to the treatment groups), and monitored the therapies to ensure that the differences between the forms of treatment were real and maintained. The results indicated that therapy was effective, although the non-treatment group made substantial gains. There was little difference between behaviour therapy and psychotherapy.

A second approach to the evaluation of effectiveness is exemplified by Smith and Glass (1977), who combined data from 375 studies, including analogue studies, in which psychological treatment had been compared with no treatment for a control group. Variations in factors such as the duration of treatment, outcome measures, and type of patient/client, were accounted for by statistical methods. Smith and Glass's conclusion was that, on average, treated individuals showed more improvement than those who remained untreated. Behaviour therapy and psychotherapy differed only marginally, with behaviour therapy having the slightly better outcome.

A third approach to the study of effectiveness is the 'box score' analysis of Luborsky et al. (1975), who reviewed 19 comparisons of psychotherapy with behaviour therapy. In 13 of the studies there was no difference in outcome for the two treatments, while all the remaining six had better outcomes for behaviour therapy.

These approaches have all attracted criticism (Eysenck 1978; Kazdin and Wilson 1978) which has drawn attention to three main methodological difficulties:

(1) *The subject samples are often heterogeneous.* In a study of phobics there may be object and animal phobics, social phobics and agoraphobics; see, for example, Gillan and Rachman (1974). It should not be assumed that identical psychological processes underlie these disorders, or that they will respond to the same aspects of treatment.

(2) *'Behaviour therapy' and 'psychotherapy' are heterogeneous groups of treatment.* Keisler (1966) has pointed out that therapy uniformity is a myth, although there are a number of treatments collectively known as 'behaviour therapy' which share a number of common assumptions. (The same point is valid for 'psychotherapy'.) The main problems arising from such global comparisons of behaviour therapy with psychotherapy are that particular treatments cannot be evaluated for their effectiveness, and when many treatments are included together in a 'package' they may include components which have competing effects.

(3) *They are difficulties in measuring outcome.* A single outcome measure, which correlates highly with all other measures, is unlikely to be forthcoming, and there is a lack of correlation between measures. This suggests that even a relatively circumscribed psychological problem such as a phobia is an elaborate construct with a number of features, such as psychological arousal and avoidance behaviour, which covary imperfectly (Lang 1969) and require several methods of measuring outcome. One consequence of this strategy is that a complex pattern of outcome data will inevitably result, and the distillation of this into an improved–unimproved–worse dimension can be misleading.

The main method of assessment in clinical trials has been by ratings made by trained assessors following an interview with the subject (Sloane et al. 1975). However, evidence from other areas of psychology indicates that interviews and self-reports of behaviour have low correlations with actual performance (Mischel 1968; Vernon 1969; Wiggins 1973). In an attempt to overcome the limitations of these assessment methods, there has been extensive use of direct observation of the target behaviour under simulated conditions, and of uniform procedures for the evaluation of behaviour therapy techniques such as behaviour avoidance tests (BAT) for phobias and compulsions, and role play tests for social problems. It is, however, unwarranted to assume that they have high predictive validities for real life conditions (Bernstein and Neitzel 1977; Bellack et al. 1978; Emmelkamp 1979). In interpreting test scores, it is wise to bear in mind Vernon's (1970, p. 213) stricture that 'a test measures only itself, but it is valid insofar as it can be shown to correlate with other observable behaviour'.

The above methodological problems are germane to all outcome studies and a further criticism has been made of the analyses of Luborsky et al. (1975) and Smith and Glass (1977); it has been argued that combining data from studies with widely differing levels of methodological sophistication is a dubious strategy (Eysenck 1978; Kazdin and Wilson 1978). In partial defence of this criticism it should be pointed out that Luborsky et al. (1975) and Smith and Glass (1977) did attempt to allow for the differences between studies, and Smith and Glass (1978) reported that the quality of the experiments did not seem to markedly affect the results, as the same trends emerged irrespective of whether the data base was good, bad or indifferent with respect to methodological sophistication.

In summary, there is a growing consensus of opinion that general questions regarding the efficacy of behaviour therapy and psychotherapy need to be replaced by more specific questions which ask 'What specific benefits accrue from a specific treatment given to a specific population?'

References

ABRAHAMSON, E.E. (1977) Behavioural approaches to weight control. *Behav. Res. Ther.*, **15**, 355.

ADAMS, H.E. & STURGIS, E.T. (1977) Status of behavioural reorientation techniques in the modification of homosexuality: a review. *Psychol. Bull.*, **84**, 1171.

ARGYLE, M. (1969) *Social interaction*. London: Methuen.
ARGYLE, M., BRYANT, B. & TROWER, P. (1974) Social skills training and psychotherapy: a comparative study *Psychol. Med.*, **4**, 435.
ASHRAM, B. & DONNER, L. (1968) Covert sensitization with alcoholics: a controlled replication. *Behav. Res. Ther.*, **6**, 7.
AYLLON, T. & AZRIN, N.H. (1968) *A token economy: A motivational system for therapy and rehabilitation*. New York: Appleton-Century-Crofts.
AYLLON, T. & HAUGHTON, E. (1964) Modification of symptomatic verbal behaviour of mental patients. *Behav. Res. Ther.*, **2**, 87.
AYLLON, T. & MICHAEL, J. (1959) The psychiatric nurse as a behavioural engineer. *J. exp. Analysis Behav.*, **2**, 323.
AYLLON, T., GARBER, S. & PISOR, K. (1975) The elimination of discipline problems through a combined school–home motivational system. *Behav. Ther.*, **6**, 616.
BANDURA, A. (1969) *Principles of Behaviour Modification*. New York: Rinehart and Winston.
BANDURA, A. (1977) Self efficacy: Toward a unifying theory of behaviour change. *Psychol. Rev.*, **84**, 191.
BANDURA, A., ADAMS, N.E. & BEYER, J. (1977) Cognitive processes mediating behavioural change. *J. Personality Soc. Psychol.*, **35**, 125.
BARLOW, D.H., LEITENBERG, H. & AGRAS, W.S. (1969) Experimental control of sexual deviation through manipulation of the noxious scene in covert sensitization. *J. abnorm. Psychol.*, **74**, 596.
BASMAJIAN, J.V., KULKULKA, C.G., NARAYAN, M.C. & TAKEBE, K. (1975) Biofeedback treatment of foot-drop after stroke compared with standard rehabilitation techniques, Part 1 Effects on voluntary control and strength. *Arch. phys. Med. Rehabil.*, **56**, 231.
BASMAJIAN, J.V., REGENOS, E.M. & BAKER, M.P. (1977) Rehabilitating stroke patients with biofeedback. *Geriatrics*, **32**, 85.
BEATY, E.T. & HAYNES, S.N. (1979) Behavioural intervention with muscle-contraction headache. A review. *Psychosom. Med.*, **41**, 165.
BEECH, H.R. & VAUGHAN, M. (1978) *Behavioural Treatment of Obsessional States*. Chichester: Wiley.
BELLACK, S.D., HERSEN, M. & TURNER, S.M. (1976) Generalization effects of social skills training in chronic schizophrenics. *Behav. Res. Ther.*, **14**, 391.
BELLACK, A.S., HERSEN, M. & TURNER, S.M. (1978) Validity of role play tests. Are they valid? *Behav. Ther.*, **9**, 448.
BERGIN, A.E. (1971) The evaluation of therapeutic outcome. In: *Handbook of Psychotherapy and Behaviour Change*, ed. Bergin, A.E. & Garfield, S.L., New York: Wiley.
BERGIN, A.E. & LAMBERT, M.J. (1978) The evaluation of therapeutic outcome. In: *Handbook of Psychotherapy and Behaviour Change: An Empirical Analysis*, ed. Garfield, S.L. & Bergin, A.E., 2nd ed. New York: Wiley.
BERNSTEIN, D.A. & BORKOVEC, T.D. (1973) *Progressive Relaxation Training*. Champaign: Research Press.
BERNSTEIN, D.A. & NIETZEL, M.T. (1977) Demand characteristics in behaviour modification. The natural history of a nuisance. *Prog. Behav. Mod.*, **4**, 119.
BLAKEMORE, C.B., THORPE, J.G., BARKER, J.C., CONWAY, C.G. & LAVIN, N.I. (1963) The application of faradic aversion conditioning in a case of transvestism. *Behav. Res. Ther.*, **1**, 29.
BLANCHARD, E.B., AHLES, T.A. & SHAW, E.R. (1979) Behavioural treatment of headaches. *Prog. Behav. Mod.*, **8**, 207.
BLANCHARD, E.B. & EPSTEIN, L.H. (1977) The clinical usefulness of biofeedback. *Prog. Behav. Mod.*, **4**, 163.
BLANCHARD, E.B., THEOBALD, D.E., WILLIAMSON, D.A., SILVER, B.V. & BROWN, D.A. (1978) Temperature biofeedback in the treatment of migraine headaches. *Archs gen. Psychiat.*, **35**, 581.
BLINDER, B.J., FREEMAN, D.M. & STUNKARD, A.J. (1970) Behaviour therapy of anorexia nervosa: Effectiveness of activity as a reinforcer of weight gain. *Am. J. Psychiat.*, **126**, 1093.
BRADY, J.P. & RIEGER, W. (1975) Behavioural treatment of anorexia nervosa. In: *Applications of Behaviour Modification*, ed. Thompson, T. & Dockens, W. London: Academic Press.
BRAUKMAN, C.J. & FIXEN, D.L. (1975) Behaviour modification with delinquents. *Prog. Behav. Mod.*, **1**, 191.
BROMET, E. & MOOS, R.H. (1977) Environmental resources and the post treatment functioning of alcoholic patients. *J. Health Soc. Behav.*, **18**, 326.

BROMET, E., MOOS, R., BLISS, F. & WUTHMAN, C. (1977) Post treatment functioning of alcohol patients: Its relation to program participation. *J. consult. clin. Psychol.*, **45**, 829.

BRUDNY, J., KOREIN, J., GRYNBAUM, B.B., FRIEDMAN, L.W., WEINSTEIN, S., SACHA-FRANKEL, G. & BELANDRES, P.V. (1976) EMG feedback therapy: Review of treatment of 114 patients. *Archs phys. Med. Rehabil.*, **57**, 55.

CANTER, A., KONDO, C.Y. & KNOTT, J.R. (1975) A comparison of EMG feedback and progressive muscle relaxation training in anxiety neurosis. *Br. J. Psychiat.*, **127**, 470.

CARR, E.G. (1977) The motivation of self-injurious behaviour: A review of some hypotheses. *Psychol. Bull.*, **84**, 800.

CAUTELA, J.R. (1967) Covert sensitization. *Psychol. Rep.*, **20**, 459.

CAUTELA, J.R. (1973) Covert processes and behaviour modification. *J. nerv. ment. Dis.*, **157**, 27.

CIMINERO, A.R., NELSON, R.O. & LIPINSKI, D.P. (1977) Self monitoring procedures. In: *Handbook of Behavioural Assessment*, ed. Ciminero, A.R., Calhoun, K.S. & Adams, H.E. New York: Wiley.

CONNOLLY, J., HALLAM, R.S. & MARKS, I.M. (1976) Selective association of fainting with blood-injury-illness fear. *Behav. Ther.*, **7**, 8.

DANAHER, B.G. (1974) Theoretical foundations and clinical applications of the Premack principle: review and critique. *Behav. Ther.*, **5**, 307.

EMMELKAMP, P.M.G. (1979) The behavioural study of clinical phobias. *Prog. Behav. Mod.*, **8**, 55.

EMRICK, C.D. (1975) A review of psychologically oriented treatment of alcoholism. II The relative effectiveness of different treatment approaches and the effectiveness of treatment versus no-treatment. *J. Stud. Alcohol*, **36**, 88.

ENGEL, B.T. & BLEECKER, E.R. (1974) Application of operant conditioning techniques to the control of the cardiac arrhythmias. In: *Contemporary Trends in Cardiovascular Psychophysiology*, ed. Obrist, P. et al. Chicago: Aldine Press.

ENGEL, B.T., NIKOOMANESH, P. & SCHUSTER, M.M. (1974) Operant conditioning of rectosphincteric responses in the treatment of rectal incontinence. *New Eng. J. Med.*, **290**, 646.

ERWIN, E. (1978) *Behaviour Therapy: Scientific, Philosophical and Moral Foundations*. Cambridge: Cambridge University Press.

EVANS, I.M. (1973) The logical requirements for explanations of systematic desensitization. *Behav. Ther.*, **4**, 506.

EYSENCK, H.J. (1952) The effects of psychotherapy: An evaluation. *J. consult. Psychol.*, **16**, 319.

EYSENCK, H.J. (1960) The effects of psychotherapy. In: *Handbook of Abnormal Psychology*, ed. Eysenck, H.J. London: Pitman Books.

EYSENCK, H. (1978) An exercise in mega-silliness. *Am. Psychol.*, **33**, 517.

FELDMAN, M.P. & MACCULLOCH, M.J. (1971) *Homosexual Behaviour: Therapy and Assessment*. Oxford: Pergamon Press.

FOA, E.B. & STEKETEE, G.S. (1979) Obsessive–compulsives: Conceptual issues and treatment interventions. *Prog. Behav. Mod.*, **8**, 1.

FOA, E., STEKETEE, G. & MILBY, J. (1980) Differential effects of exposive and response prevention in obsessive–compulsive washers. *J. consult. clin. Psychol.*, **48**, 71.

FOA, E.B., STEKETEE, G., TURNER, R.M. & FISCHER, S.C. (1980) Effects of imaginal exposure to feared disasters in obsessive–compulsive checkers. *Behav. Res. Ther.*, **18**, 449.

FORDYCE, W.F. (1976) *Behavioural Methods for Chronic Pain and Illness*. St. Louis: Mosby.

FRASER, D., ANDERSON, J. & GRIME, J. (1981) An analysis of the progressive development of vocal responses in a mute schizophrenic patient. *Behav. Psychother.*, **9**, 2.

GELDER, M.G., BANCROFT, J.H., GATH, D.H., JOHNSON, D.W., MATHEWS, A.M. & SHAW, P.M. (1973) Specific and non-specific factors in behaviour therapy. *Br. J. Psychiat.*, **123**, 445.

GILLAN, P. & RACHMAN, S. (1974) An experimental investigation of desensitization in phobic patients. *Br. J. Psychiat.*, **124**, 392.

GOLDIAMOND, I. (1965) Self control procedures in personal behaviour problems. *Psychol. Rep.*, **17**, 851.

GOTTMAN, J. & MARKMAN, H.J. (1978) Experimental designs in psychotherapy research. In: *Handbook of Psychotherapy & Behaviour Change*, ed. Garfield, S.L. & Bergin, A.E., 2nd ed. Chichester: Wiley.

HALL, J.N., BAKER, R.D. & HUTCHINSON, K. (1977) A controlled evaluation of token economy procedures with chronic schizophrenic patients. *Behav. Res. Ther.*, **15**, 261.

HALLAM, R. & RACHMAN, S. (1972) Theoretical problems of aversion therapy. *Behav. Res. Ther.*, **10**, 341.

HALLAM, R.S. & RACHMAN, S. (1976) Current status of aversion therapy. *Prog. Behav. Mod.*, **2**, 179.

HARRIS, S.L. & ERSNER-HERSHFIELD, R. (1978) Behavioural suppression of seriously disruptive behaviour in psychotic and retarded patients. A review of punishment and its alternatives. *Psychol. Bull.*, **85**, 1352.

HENDERSON, S., BYRNE, D.G., DUNCAN-JONES, P., ADCOCK, S., SCOTT, R. & STEELE, G.P. (1978) Social bonds in the epidemiology of neurosis: A preliminary communication. *Br. J. Psychiat.*, **132**, 463.

HERSEN, M. (1972) Nightmare behaviour: a review. *Psychol. Bull.*, **73**, 37.

HERSEN, M. & BELLACK, A.S. (1976) Social skills training for chronic psychiatric patients: Rationale, research findings and future directions. *Compreh. Psychiat.*, **17**, 559.

HUXLEY, P.J., GOLDBERG, D.P., MAGUIRE, G.P. & KINCEY, J.A. (1979) The prediction of the course of minor psychiatric disorders. *Br. J. Psychiat.*, **135**, 535.

JANDA, L.H. & RIMM, D.C. (1972) Covert sensitization in the treatment of obesity. *J. abnorm. Psychol.*, **80**, 37.

JANNOUN, L., MUNBY, M., CATALAN, J. & GELDER, M. (1980) A home-based treatment program for agoraphobia: replication and controlled evaluation. *Behav. Ther.*, **11**, 294.

JOSIASSEN, R.C., FANTUZZO, J. & ROSEN, A.C. (1980) Treatment of pedophilia using multistage aversion therapy and social skills training. *J. Behav. Ther. Exp. Psychiat.*, **11**, 55.

KAZDIN, A.E. (1974a) Covert modeling, model similarity and reduction of avoidance behaviour. *Behav. Ther.*, **5**, 325.

KAZDIN, A.E. (1974b) The effect of model identity and fear relevant similarity on covert modeling. *Behav. Ther.*, **5**, 624.

KAZDIN, A.E. (1974c) Effects of covert modeling and model reinforcement on assertive behaviour. *J. abnorm. Psychol.*, **83**, 240.

KAZDIN, A.E. (1974d) Self monitoring and behaviour change. In: *Self Control: Power to the Person*, ed. Mahoney, M.J. & Thoresen, C.E. Monterey: Brooks-Cole.

KAZDIN, A.E. (1977) *The Token Economy: A Review and Evaluation*. London: Plenum Press.

KAZDIN, A.E. (1978) *History of Behaviour Modification: Experimental Foundations of Contemporary Research*. Baltimore: University Park Press.

KAZDIN, A.E. (1979) Fictions, factions and functions of behaviour therapy. *Behav. Ther.*, **10**, 629.

KAZDIN, A.E. (1980) Covert and overt rehearsal and elaboration during treatment in the development of assertive behaviour. *Behav. Res. Ther.*, **18**, 191.

KAZDIN, A.E. & ROGERS, T. (1978) On paradigms and recycled ideologies: analogue research revisited. *Cognitive Ther. Res.*, **2**, 105.

KAZDIN, A.E. & SMITH, G.A. (1979) Covert conditioning: a review and evaluation. *Adv. Behav. Res. Ther.*, **2**, 57.

KAZDIN, A.E. & WILCOXON, L.A. (1976) Systematic desensitization and nonspecific treatment effects: a methodological evaluation. *Psychol. Bull.*, **83**, 729.

KAZDIN, A. & WILSON, G.T. (1978) *Evaluation of Behaviour Therapy*. Massachusetts: Ballinger.

KEISLER, D.J. (1966) Some myths of psychotherapy research and the search for a paradigm. *Psychol. Bull.*, **65**, 110.

KEWMAN, D. & ROBERTS, A.H. (1980) Skin temperature biofeedback and migraine headaches: a double-blind study. *Biofeedback and Self-Regul.*, **5**, 327.

KORITREN, J. & BRUDNY, J. (1976) Integrated EMG feedback in the management of spasmodic torticollis and focal dystonia: A prospective study of 80 patients. In: *The Basal Ganglia*, ed. Yahr, M.D. New York: Raven Press.

KUHLMAN, W.N. & KAPLAN, B.N. (1979) Clinical applications of EEG biofeedback training. In: *Clinical Applications of Biofeedback: Appraisal and Status*, ed. Gatchel, R.J. and Price, K.P. New York: Pergamon Press.

LANG, P.J. (1969) Fear reduction and fear behaviour: problems in treating a construct. In: *Research in Psychotherapy*, ed. Schlein, J.M. Washington D.C.: American Psychological Association.

LAVALLÉE, Y.-J., LAMONTAGUE, Y., PINARD, G., ANNABLE, L. & TÉTREAULT, L. (1977) Effects of EMG feedback, diazepam and their combination on chronic anxiety. *J. psychosom. Res.*, **21**, 65.

LEBOEUF, A. & LODGE, J. (1980) A comparison of frontalis EMG biofeedback training and progressive relaxation in the treatment of chronic anxiety *Br. J. Psychiat.*, **137**, 279.

LEVIS, D.J. & HARE, N. (1977) A review of the theoretical support for the extinction approach of implosive (flooding) therapy. *Prog. Behav. Mod.*, **4**, 300.

LICK, J. & BOOTZIN, R. (1975) Expectancy factors in the treatment of fear: Methodological and theoretical issues. *Psychol. Bull.*, **82**, 917.

LIDDLE, A. & LYONS, M. (1978) Thunderstorm phobias. *Behav. Res. Ther.*, **16**, 306.

LITTLE, L.M. & CURRAN, J.P. (1978) Covert sensitization: A clinical procedure in need of some explanations. *Psychol. Bull.*, **85**, 513.

LUBAR, J.F. (1977) Electroencephalographic biofeedback methodology and the management of epilepsy. *Pavlovian J. Biol. Sci.*, **12**, 147.

LUBORSKY, L., SINGER, B. & LUBORSKY, L. (1975) Comparative studies of Psychotherapies: Is it true that 'everyone has won and all must have prizes'? *Archs gen. Psychiat.*, **32**, 995.

MAHONEY, M.J. & ARNKOFF, D.B.(1978) Cognitive and self control therapies. In: *Handbook of Psychotherapy and Behaviour Change: An Empirical Analysis*, ed. Garfield, S.L. & Bergin, A.E., 2nd ed. New York: Wiley.

MALETSKY, B.M. (1980) Self-referred versus court-referred sexually deviant patients: success with assisted covert sensitization. *Behav. Ther.*, **11**, 306.

MALETSKY, B.M. & GEORGE, F.S. (1973) The treatment of homosexuality by 'assisted' covert sensitization. *Behav. Res. Ther.*, **11**, 655.

MARKS, I. (1975) Behavioural treatments of phobic and obsessive compulsive disorders: A critical appraisal. *Prog. Behav. Mod.*, **1**, 66.

MARKS, I. (1978) Behavioural psychotherapy of adult neurosis. In: *Handbook of Psychotherapy and Behaviour Change: An Empirical Analysis*, eds. Garfield, S.L. & Bergin, A.E., 2nd ed. Chichester: Wiley.

MARKS, I. & GELDER, M.G. (1967) Transvestism and fetishism: A clinical and psychological change during faradic aversion. *Br. J. Psychiat.*, **113**, 711.

MARKS, I.,HODGSON, R. & RACHMAN, S. (1975) Treatment of chronic obsessive–compulsive neurosis by in vivo exposure. *Br. J. Psychiat.*, **127**, 349.

MARSHALL, W.L., GAUTHIER, J. & GORDON, A. (1979) The current status of flooding therapy. *Prog. Behav. Mod.*, **7**, 205.

MARZILLIER, J.S., LAMBERT, C. & KELLETT, J. (1976) A controlled evaluation of systematic desensitization and social skills training for socially inadequate psychiatric patients. *Behav. Res. Ther.*, **14**, 225.

MATHEWS, A.M. (1978) Fear reduction research and clinical phobias. *Psychol. Bull.*, **85**, 390.

MATHEWS, A., TEASDALE, J., MUNBY, M., JOHNSTON, D. & SHAW, P. (1977) A home based treatment program for agoraphobia. *Behav. Ther.*, **8**, 915.

MCCONAGHY, N. (1977) Behavioural treatment of homosexuality. *Prog. Behav. Mod.*, **5**, 310.

MCFALL, R.M. & HAMMEN, C.L. (1970) Motivation, structure and self-monitoring: the role of non-specific factors in smoking reduction. *J. consult. clin. Psychol.*, **35**, 135.

MEICHENBAUM, D. (1971) Examination of model characteristics in reducing avoidance behaviour. *J. Personality Soc. Psychol.*, **17**, 298.

MEYER, V., LEVY, R. & SCHNURER, A. (1974) The behavioural treatment of obsessive–compulsive disorder. In: *Obsessional States*, ed. Beech, H.R. London: Methuen.

MILLER, P.M., HERSEN, P., EISLER, R.M. & HEMPHILL, D.P. (1973) Electrical aversion therapy with alcoholics: An analogue study. *Behav. Res. Ther.*, **11**, 491.

MILLS, H., AGRAS, S., BARLOW, D. & MILLS, J. (1973) Compulsive rituals treated by response prevention. *Archs gen. Psychiat.*, **28**, 524.

MINEKA, S. (1979) The role of fear in theories of avoidance learning, flooding, and extinction. *Psychol. Bull.*, **86**, 985.

MISCHEL, W. (1968) *Personality and Assessment.* New York: Wiley.

MOSTOFSKY, D.I. & BALASCHAK, B.A. (1977) Psychobiological control of seizures. *Psychol. Bull.*, **84**, 723.

NELSON, R.O. (1977) Assessment and therapeutic functions of self-monitoring. *Prog. Behav. Mod.*, **5**, 264.

OLTON, D.S. & NOONBERG, A.R. (1980) *Biofeedback: Clinical Applications in Behavioural Medicine.* Englewood Cliffs: Prentice-Hall.

PARKINSON, L. & RACHMAN, S. (1980) Are intrusive thoughts subject to habituation? *Behav. Res. Ther.*, **18**, 409.

PERCELL, L.P., BERWICK, P.T. & BEIGEL, A. (1974) The effects of assertive training on self concept and anxiety. *Archs gen. Psychiat.*, **31**, 502.

PHILIPS, C (1977) Headache in general practice. *Headache*, **16**, 322.

PHILIPS, C. & HUNTER, M. (1981) Headache in a psychiatric population. *J. nerv. ment. Dis.*, **170**, 34.

RACHMAN, S. (1966) Studies in desensitization II: Flooding. *Behav. Res. Ther.*, **4**, 1.

RACHMAN, S. (1968) The role of muscular relaxation in desensitization therapy. *Behav. Res. Ther.*, **6**, 159.

RACHMAN, S. (1971) *The Effects of Psychotherapy*. Oxford: Pergamon Press.

RACHMAN, S. (1976a) The passing of the two stage theory of fear and avoidance: fresh possibilities. *Behav. Res. Ther.*, **14**, 125.

RACHMAN, S.J. (1976b) Observational learning and therapeutic modelling. In: *Theoretical and Experimental Bases of Behaviour Therapies*, ed. Feldman, P. & Broadhurst, A. Chichester: Wiley.

RACHMAN, S., COBB, J., GREY, S., McDONALD, B., MAWSON, D., SARTORY, G. & STERN, R. (1979) The behavioural treatment of obsessional–compulsive disorders, with and without clomipramine. *Behav. Res. Ther.*, **17**, 467.

RACHMAN, S. & DE SILVA, P. (1978) Abnormal and normal obsessions. *Behav. Res. Ther.*, **16**, 233.

RACHMAN, S.J. & HODGSON, R.J. (1980) *Obsessions and Compulsions*. Englewood Cliffs: Prentice-Hall.

RACHMAN, S. & TEASDALE, J. (1969a) Aversion Therapy: An appraisal. In: *Behaviour Therapy: Appraisal and Status*, ed. Franks, C.M. New York: McGraw-Hill.

RACHMAN, S. & TEASDALE, J. (1969b) *Aversion Therapy and Behaviour Disorders*. London: Routledge and Kegan Paul.

RAW, M. (1978) The treatment of cigarette dependence. In: *Research Advances in Alcohol and Drug Problems*, ed. Israel, Y., Glaser, F.B., Kalant, H., Popham, R.E., Schmidt, W. & Smart, R.G., Vol. 4. New York: Plenum.

RAYMOND, M. & O'KEEFE, K. (1965) A case of pin-up fetishism treated by aversion conditioning *Br. J. Psychiat.*, **111**, 579.

REKERS, G.A., YATES, C.E., WILLIS, T.J., ROSEN, A.C. & TAUBMAN, M. (1976) Childhood gender identity change: operant control over sex-typed play and mannerisms. *J Behav. Ther. Exp. Psychiat.*, **7**, 51.

RIMM, D.C. & MASTERS, J.C. (1979) *Behaviour Therapy: Techniques and Empirical Findings*, 2nd ed. New York: Academic Press.

RISLEY, T.R. (1968) The effects and side effects of punishing autistic behaviours of a deviant child. *J. Appl. Behav. Anal.*, **1**, 21.

ROOTH, F.G. & MARKS, I.M. (1974) Persistent exhibitionism: short term response to aversion, self regulation, and relaxation treatments. *Archs Sexual Behav.*, **3**, 227.

ROPER, G., RACHMAN, S. & MARKS, I. (1975) Passive and participant modelling in exposure treatment of obsessive–compulsive neurotics. *Behav. Res. Ther.*, **13**, 271.

ROSEN, G.M. (1976) Subjects' initial therapeutic expectancies and subjects' awareness of therapeutic goals in systematic desensitization: a review. *Behav. Ther.*, **7**, 14.

ROSENTHAL, T.L. & BANDURA, A. (1978) Psychological modeling: theory and practice. In: *Handbook of Psychotherapy and Behaviour Change: An Empirical Analysis*, ed. Garfield, S.L. & Bergin, A.E. Chichester: Wiley.

ROSENTHAL, T.L. & ZIMMERMAN, B.J. (1978) *Social Learning and Cognition*. New York: Academic Press.

RUSSELL, M.A.H., ARMSTRONG, E. & PATEL, U.A. (1976) Temporal contiguity in electric aversion therapy for cigarette smoking. *Behav. Res. Ther.*, **14**, 103.

SEIFERT, A.R. & LUBAR, J.F. (1975) Reduction of epileptic seizures through EEG biofeedback training. *Biol. Psychol.*, **3**, 157.

SHAPIRO, M.B. (1966) The single case in clinical-psychological research. *J. gen. Psychol.*, **74**, 3.

SHAPIRO, M.B. (1975) The single variable approach in assessing the intensity of feeling of depression. *Eur. J. Behav. Anal. Mod.*, **1**, 62.

SHAPIRO, D.A. (1980) Science and psychotherapy: the state of the art. *Br. J. med. Psychol.*, **53**, 1.

SHEPHERD, G.W. (1978) Social skills training: the generalization problem—some further data. *Behav. Res. Ther.*, **16**, 287.

SHEPHERD, G.W. (1981) Social functioning and social skills. Unpublished manuscript. Dept. of Psychology, Institute of Psychiatry.

SHIPLEY, R.H. & BOUDEWYNS, P.A. (1980) Flooding and implosive therapy: are they harmful? *Behav. Ther.*, **11**, 503.

SINGH, N.N., DAWSON, M.J. & GREGORY, P.R. (1980) Suppression of chronic hyperventilation using response-contingent aromatic ammonia. *Behav. Ther.*, **11**, 561.

SIPICH, J.F., RUSSELL, R.K. & TOBIAS, L.L. (1974) A comparison of covert sensitization and 'non-specific' treatment in the modification of smoking behaviour. *J. Behav. Ther. Exp. Psychiat.*, **5**, 201.

SKINNER, B.F. (1953) *Science and Human Behaviour.* New York: Macmillan.

SLOANE, R.B., STAPLES, F.R., CRISTOL, A.H., YORKSTON, N.J. & WHIPPLE, K. (1975) *Psychotherapy Versus Behaviour Therapy.* Cambridge, Mass.: Harvard University Press.

SMITH, M.L. & GLASS, G.V. (1977) Meta analysis of psychotherapy outcome studies. *Am. Psychol.*, **32**, 752.

SMITH, ML. & GLASS, G.V. (1978) Reply to Eysenck. *Am. Psychol.*, **33**, 517.

SOLYMON, L., SHUGAR, R., BRYNTWICK, S. & SOLYMON, C. (1973) Treatment of fear of flying. *Am. J. Psychiat.*, **4**, 423.

STAMPFL, T.G. & LEVIS, D.J. (1967) Essentials of implosive therapy: A learning theory based psychodynamic behavioural therapy. *J. abnorm. Psychol.*, **72**, 496.

STAMPFL, T.G. &LEVIS, D.J. (1968) Implosive therapy—a behavioural therapy? *Behav. Res. Ther.*, **6**, 31.

STERMAN, M.B. (1977) Sensorimotor EEG operant conditioning: experimental and clinical effects. *Pavlov. J. Biol. Sci.*, **12**, 63.

STERMAN, M.B. & MACDONALD, L.R.(1978) Effects of EEG feedback training on seizure incidence in poorly controlled epileptics. *Epilepsia*, **19**, 207.

STERN, R.S., LIPSEDGE, M.S. & MARKS, I.M. (1975) Obsessive ruminations: a controlled trial of a thought-stopping technique. *Behav. Res. Ther.*, **11**, 659.

STERN, R.S. & MARKS, I.M. (1975) A comparison of brief and prolonged flooding in agoraphobics. *Archs gen. Psychiat.*, **28**, 270.

SWANN, VAN BUSKIRK, S. (1977) A two-phase perspective on the treatment of anorexia nervosa. *Psychol. Bull.*, **84**, 529.

TOWNSEND, R.E., HOUSE, J.F. & ADDARIO, D.A. (1975) A comparison of biofeedback-mediated relaxation and group therapy in the treatment of chronic anxiety. *Am. J. Psychiat.*, **132**, 598.

TWENTYMAN, C.T. & ZIMERING, R.T. (1979) Behavioural training of social skills: A critical review. *Prog. Behav. Mod.*, **7**, 319.

VERNON, P.E. (1969) *Personality Assessment: A Critical Survey.* London: Methuen.

VOGLER, R.C., LUNDE, S.E., JOHNSON, G.R. & MARTIN, P.L. (1970) Electrical aversion conditioning with chronic alcoholics. *J. consult. clin. Psychol.*, **34**, 302.

WATTS, F. (1979) The habituation model of systematic desensitization. *Psychol. Bull.*, **86**, 627.

WIGGINS, J.S. (1973) *Personality and Prediction: Principles of Personality Assessment.* Reading, Massachusetts: Addison-Wesley Pub. Co.

WOLPE, J. (1958) *Psychotherapy by Reciprocal Inhibition.* Stanford: Stanford University Press.

WOLPE, J. (1969) *The Practice of Behaviour Therapy.* New York: Pergamon.

YATES, A.J. (1980) *Biofeedback and the Modification of Behaviour.* New York: Plenum Press.

ZIGLER, E. & PHILIPS, L. (1960) Social effectiveness and symptomatic behaviours. *J. abnorm. Psychol.*, **61**, 231.

ZIGLER, E. & PHILIPS, L. (1961) Social competence and outcome in psychiatric disorder. *J. abnorm. Psychol.*, **63**, 264.

Supplementary Bibliography

BECK, A.T. (1976) *Cognitive Therapy and the Emotional Disorders.* New York: International Universities Press.

BREHM, S.S. (1976) *The Application of Social Psychology to Clinical Practice.* New York: Wiley.

ELLIS, A. & GRIEGER, R. (1977) *Handbook of Rational–Emotive Therapy.* New York: Springer-Verlag.

FOREYT, J.P. & RATHJEN, D.P. (1978) *Cognitive Behaviour Therapy.* New York: Plenum.

GOLDFRIED, M.R. & DAVISON, G.C. (1976) *Clinical Behaviour Therapy.* New York: Holt.

HAYNES, S.N. (1978) *Principles of Behavioural Assessment.* New York: Gardner Press.

JACOBSON, N.S. (1979) Behavioural treatments for marital discord: A critical appraisal. *Prog. Behav. Mod.*, **8**, 169.

LANYON, R.I. (1978) Behavioural approaches to stuttering. *Prog. Behav. Mod.*, **6**, 48.

MAHONEY, M.J. (1974) *Cognition and Behaviour Modification.* Cambridge, Massachusetts: Ballinger.

MARKS, I.M. (1976) Management of sexual disorders. In: *Handbook of Behaviour Modification and Behaviour Therapy*, ed. Leitenberg, H. Englewood Cliffs: Prentice Hall.

MASH, E.J., HANDY, L.C. & HAMERLYNCK, L.A.(1976) *Behaviour Modification Approaches to Parenting*. New York: Brunner/Mazel.

PATTERSON, G.R., WEISS, R.L. & HOPS, H. (1976) Training of marital skills: some problems and concepts. In: *Handbook of Behaviour Modification and Behaviour Therapy*, ed. Leitenberg, H. Englewood Cliffs: Prentice-Hall.

REHM, L.P. (1981) *Behaviour Therapy for Depression*, ed. Rehm, L.P. New York: Academic Press.

11

Social Treatments in Psychiatry

G.E. Berrios

INTRODUCTION

Psychiatric disorder and its maladaptive consequences can be corrected by physical, psychological and social means. The last refers to modification of those aspects of social context which are relevant to behavioural change. These include both the relationships of the patient to others and to his physical environment.

There are many modificatory techniques which have developed from both empirical and theoretical sources; for example, the age-old view that work is good for the soul has been incorporated into clinical practice, and learning theory has also been applied to the shaping of specific behaviours as in the case of 'token system' programmes.

In general, rehabilitation programmes last for several months, and it is hoped that the resultant adaptive behaviours will continue after treatment to create a positive spiral of social success. The factors which maintain these new behaviours are influenced not only by the chronicity of the original psychiatric illness but also by the availability of community resources.

Ideally, social therapy must be individualized, but in practice this is not always possible, and 'therapeutic milieus' have been organized which try to cater for groups of patients who have suffered from similar disorders (e.g. the schizophrenias). This approach is not always satisfactory, as some maladaptive behaviours which prevent rehabilitation may be due to a variety of personality factors which have become more overt as a result of an underlying psychotic illness. Thus, a variety of handicaps may not be adequately managed by interventions aimed at a group of patients.

The mechanisms underlying the efficacy of some forms of social therapy are unclear. In general, they have been thought to consist largely of 'social processes', but insufficient attention has been given to the psychological mechanisms by which patients perceive the interventions which may lead to social change. A severe psychosis may bring in its wake cognitive dysfunction which will distort the patient's perception and interpretation of 'normal' social interactions, and it cannot be assumed that only if sufficient 'social pressure' is brought to bear on the patient, the psychotic symptoms (or defect state) can be overcome.

The increasing awareness of the disadvantages of institutionalization has led to therapeutic and political advance, but the potential positive attributes of the psychiatric hospital must not be forgotten (Barton 1959; Ochberg et al. 1972). The question, 'How can one prevent institutions from creating symptoms?' should be followed by, 'Which symptoms are due to institutionalization and which to the physical and psychological concomitants of the patient's underlying condition?' Low intelligence, poor education, and physical disability have, not surprisingly, been found to predispose an individual to institutional life (Liberakis 1981).

Some forms of social therapies have been particularly concerned with sponsoring a particular view of mental illness and occasionally have taken an antimedical stance. However, the medical approach to the most severe forms of psychiatric disorder led to the development of treatments which have included the social dimension. Of course, 'psychiatric disorder' encompasses a wide variety of conditions, and although the concept of 'illness requiring treatment by doctors' is often appropriate, in varying degrees, psychiatrists are also expected to provide a service for some individuals whose presenting disturbance seems mainly due to social and environmental factors.

Detailed analysis of the obstacles preventing rehabilitation of psychiatric patients has led to the identification of both primary and secondary handicaps. Different treatment approaches have been developed for the range of handicaps which are commonly encountered, and these have mainly been applied in mental hospitals, where workshops and industrial therapy units have encouraged patients to relearn the skills necessary for adequate functioning in society, or to maximize their potential in the institution. Such facilities must provide protection and allow a certain level of dependence, while providing a sufficient challenge to bring out hidden potential (Early and Magnus 1968). Of course, the nature of the goals of rehabilitation must take into account the prevailing social conditions; it is unrealistic to set goals of employment outside hospital if society is unable, or unwilling, to absorb the retrained individual.

Most of our knowledge with regard to the rehabilitation of psychiatric patients has been based on experience with individuals suffering from the schizophrenias, and the Royal College of Psychiatrists' report on Rehabilitation (1980) put great emphasis on the management of postschizophrenic defect states. It concluded that patients with 'milder affective and neurotic symptoms' require separate attention.

There has been a tendency to confuse rehabilitation, community psychiatry and social psychiatry. Rehabilitation involves a set of practical techniques for the modification of maladaptive social behaviours (Lewis 1955), while community psychiatry refers to the practice of psychiatry outside the hospital, and the involvement of members of society (including various organisations) in this process (Bennett 1978; Berrios 1980; Bender 1979; Levine 1981). Social psychiatry (Arthur 1971; Carleton and Mahlendorf 1979) consists of a rather complex set of theoretical views and various observations related to the social aetiology of psychiatric disorders, their epidemiology, and their social impact.

The role of the traditional psychiatric hospital in rehabilitation has caused some debate, and enthusiasm for community psychiatry has contributed to some unrealistic claims that the psychiatric hospital has outlived its usefulness (Müller 1982). Many of the new 'long-stay' patients suffer severe psychoses which are determined largely by biological rather than social factors (Goldberg 1974), and many of these patients could not survive outside an institution or some form of sheltered and supervised environment. If no finances are available to create hostels and sheltered occupational facilities, a humane hospital community is still required in addition to the 'acute' (i.e. short-stay) provisions (Majastre 1972).

With regard to the creation of a therapeutic social milieu in an institution, a balance has to be struck between encouraging a positive and supportive community spirit (by attending to group processes and interactions), and a consideration of each patient's individual problems. Both approaches must be combined, but an exaggerated emphasis on the group or community aspects of the unit may not pay sufficient attention to individual needs. Stevens (1973) has stated that 'socially isolated chronic schizophrenic patients should not be placed in therapeutic communities which produce role expectations which the patient cannot meet'. Thus, the individual assessment of handicap, the rational use of medical diagnosis and treatment, and the acceptance of profound psychological differences and needs in each patient is crucial. For example, it is important to know the price which patients may have to pay in terms of subjective distress, for 'living in the community', when this means living in a hostel or boarding house with little or no social stimulation from a neighbourhood which may want nothing to do with them. It is also important to know to what extent overt rehabilitation (e.g. the ability to 'survive' in a hostel) leads to the development of a subjective ability to obtain satisfaction from life. It may be that in terms of subjective experience, living in a hospital ward which provides abundant social stimulation is more satisfying than an anonymous and empty life outside the institution (Lehmann et al. 1982).

PRINCIPLES AND TECHNIQUES OF REHABILITATION

Introduction

Rehabilitation has been defined as 'the process of restoring a handicapped person, if not to the level of function and the same position which he had achieved before the onset of the illness, then at least to a situation in which he can make use of his residual capacities within as normal as possible a social context' (Wing 1959). The 'handicapped person' is in need of help because of a degree of 'social disablement' which has been defined as 'the state of an individual who is unable to perform socially up to the standards expected by himself or herself, by people important to him or her and by society in general'. Both medical and social components of disablement must be recognized, and exclusively medical or social 'models' are inadequate to describe, explain, or help, psychiatric disabilities. These above definitions indicate the basic principles underlying rehabilitation, which are to identify and assess the handicap, to design and implement individual rehabilitation programmes, and to assess outcome (Wing and Morris 1981; Talbott 1978).

Identification and Assessment of Handicap

The psychiatrically ill patient exhibits a number of deficiencies in psychological and physical function. Some of these are a direct result of his illness, others are derived from an interaction between illness and premorbid personality, and some stem from the patient's own reaction (and society's reaction) to his illness. These so-called primary and secondary handicaps (Wing 1959) are often difficult to distinguish and their combination may lead to a progressive decline in the patient's performance even after the primary condition has been stabilized or successfully treated (Goldberg 1974). Primary handicaps refer to those symptoms of the disease that tend to produce relevant disability. For example, anhedonia, shortened attention span and alogia are primary to some schizophrenic states and do not result from 'psychological' responses to particular conflicts (Andreasen and Olsen 1982).

However, the presence of a symptom does not necessarily lead to the development of a handicap, which is determined by the interaction between the functional disturbance and a given social need. For example, auditory hallucinations or marked delusions only produce social handicap if they control or interfere with everyday behaviour, and patients who experience severe symptomatology are often able to function surprisingly well in the community. From this interactional definition of 'handicap' it follows that the nature and demands of the social environment are of crucial importance in the development and perpetuation of handicaps. The International Pilot Study of Schizophrenia (Carpenter et al. 1973) reported that outcome appeared better in Nigeria than in Denmark, and this may be partly explained by differences in social demands.

As a result of primary handicaps, patients may develop secondary phenomena such as anxiety or depressed moods. These symptoms may come to occupy the centre of the stage, when they amplify the intensity of any residual primary handicap, and lead to incapacity, and loss of self-confidence.

Aspects of both primary and secondary handicaps are to a certain extent modulated by the 'pathoplastic' effect of the patient's premorbid intellect, personality and social competence. Thus, assessment must try to identify premorbid assets (or deficiencies), which are likely to be less amenable to a programme of rehabilitation (Wing 1963).

Whether handicaps are premorbid, primary or secondary, they must be carefully described, and, if possible, measured. However, an assessment of various aspects of cognitive function by a clinical psychologist is often of little value because the patient's residual capacity may be concealed by symptoms or the effects of medication, while paranoid, catatonic or severely retarded patients may be untestable (Klein and Spohn 1964; Orme 1970). Thus, clinical psychologists often prefer to assess behavioural characteristics (Griffiths et al. 1974). Griffiths (1974) reported that early assessment of motivation, self-confidence and the patient's view of the presence and extent of handicap, was able to predict work status 17 months later.

It is often useful to assess the patient's capabilities in settings which provide a range of tasks including industrial, domestic and clerical work. This can be achieved by admitting the patient to a Rehabilitation Assessment unit for a period of 2 weeks (Mahmood 1979). In the Tooting Bec unit described by Mahmood, each patient's work was rated by the staff by means of three standardized assessment techniques (Griffiths 1973; Mahmood 1978; Watts 1978). The tasks provided included cooking, cleaning, the use of household appliances (e.g. washing and sewing machines), and clerical tasks. In addition, cognitive functions were assessed, if possible, and a full psychiatric history was obtained. An individualized rehabilitation programme could then be drawn up for each patient. This unit assessed 162 patients during its first 6 months, and 30% were referred for further 'industrial therapy', involving simple manufacturing or processing tasks. Another 30% were considered suitable for other forms of occupational therapy, while 5% went on to receive day care. Another 5% took up some form of hospital employment. Twenty per cent were deemed 'unsuitable' for the assessment procedure (either because they were too ill or refused to attend the unit), and 10% did not complete assessment on account of their active symptomatology.

Ruesch et al. (1972) designed a rating scale to measure 'social disability' which was standardized in a group 100 patients with both physical and psychiatric handicap. This scale is a useful instrument for research purposes but is probably too complex for everyday use.

Apart from the assessment of handicap, it is essential to determine the degree of social support which is available to the patient (Dean and Lin 1977). A number of scales to measure social support, defined as 'support accessible to an individual through social ties to other individuals, groups and the larger community', have been developed (Lin et al. 1981), although their value in relation to outcome prediction is unclear. However, there is some evidence that the presence of adequate social support is an indicator of positive outcome; for example, former patients rise to a higher level of performance when returning to a home where they were the 'bread winners' than when returning to live with their parents (Freeman and Simmons 1963). Of course, single marital state, and returning to the parental home may have simply reflected an early onset of severe illness.

Design of an Individual Rehabilitation Programme

Following the assessment, the rehabilitation team must organize a programme which will attempt to reduce deficits and enhance assets, bearing in mind the general principle that intervention must be directed to as many aspects of disability as possible (Goldberg 1974; Shepherd 1980).

Principles. The design of an individualized rehabilitation programme is based on a number of principles; there must be a clear knowledge of the patient's deficits and assets; an optimal level of stimulation avoids both under- and over-arousal; a controlled social environment is required; and a member of the rehabilitation team should be appointed as the 'key person' for each patient, so that a one-to-one relationship can be developed. Setting goals must involve flexibility and realism, as rehabilitation can often do no more than maintain the patient at a precarious level of functioning; each patient must be reassessed at regular intervals, and gradually increasing demands should be made, within the limits of his capabilities. Also, the minimum amount of support should be given, to prevent the patient from developing an unnecessary degree of dependence.

Each patient's programme includes a statement of the goals (short- and long-term), recommended activities (which can be categorized as predominant or secondary), and a time-table which is given to the patient. The degree of regimentation which is appropriate will vary considerably, but certain activities (e.g. industrial therapy) must be carried out at certain times and the teaching of various skills is also determined by staff time and resources. Also, the various routines of daily life such as getting up, washing and preparing meals, must be carried out in response to certain time cues. The time-table should clearly separate work time from leisure time, as many patients, whose lives have become empty and disorganized, have forgotten this distinction.

The predominant activity which is to be encouraged may help to reduce handicap or to enhance assets; for example, industrial therapy, one of the most popular predominant activities, is often used both as a way of encouraging work habits and skills, and of providing the patient with a framework in which other treatments, such as social skills training and psychotherapy, may be offered.

Industrial therapy units. Since the inception of the MRC Social Psychiatry Unit Experimental Workshop (Baker 1956) and the Piercy Report (1956), the UK Ministry of Health has considered that sheltered work is an essential ingredient of rehabilitation and that, ideally, hours, pay and working conditions should be similar to those in industry. Most psychiatric hospitals in the UK have developed some form of industrial therapy (Wansbrough and Miles 1968), and Bennett and Wing (1963) have listed five different functions of hospital workshops: occupation, education, treatment, assessment and research. These functions are complementary; for example, satisfactory prediction of employability can only be made when a patient's work performance is directly observed (Watts 1978). If adequately rehabilitated, former patients with chronic, severe handicaps can perform well in 'open' jobs, although in a recent study frequency of absenteeism was shown to be higher than among other employees (Wansbrough et al. 1979).

Working premises must be attractive and suitable, the standard of work must be kept high, and units must not become dependent on one patient or a group of patients for the completion of any particular job. Holidays are essential, and other rehabilitation needs must be considered (Morgan 1973). Cognitive handicaps must be borne in mind when tasks are assigned; for example, chronic schizophrenic patients often have impaired concentration. Such individuals should undertake jobs that can be rapidly completed so that the patient can obtain the satisfaction of achievement (Wadsworth et al. 1962). Diagnosis or intelligence do not seem to be good predictors of capacity to work (Griffiths 1973), although O'Connor and Rawnsley (1959) found that chronic paranoid patients 'will respond better to a regime in which socially rewarding experiences are made available, but not thrust upon them'.

Social skills training. This is often a 'secondary activity' in a patient's rehabilitation programme and lack of social competence is a common correlate of psychiatric disorder. Whatever its origin, such a lack engenders feelings of inadequacy, isolation and rejection, which compound distress and resentment, thus perpetuating social dysfunction. Efforts at rehabilitation are often hindered by the patient's inability to interact freely in the Industrial Therapy Unit, when the teaching of social skills may be of particular value (Ziegler and Phillips 1961).

For patients with chronic schizophrenia, social skills training is often indicated. However, it should be remembered that social withdrawal may sometimes be providing a protective function, as a high 'expressed-emotion environment' may increase the probability of relapse (Vaughn and Leff 1976). Lack of social competence may result from a number of factors such as coexistence of approach and avoidance, severe disturbance of mood or motivation, difficulty in expressing emotion, and lack of cognitive skills (Trower et al. 1978).

Lack of social competence may generate anxiety when the patient is placed in certain situations. Avoidance and social withdrawal often follow, but these maladaptive behaviours do not always serve to reduce the patient's discomfort (Wolpe 1969). However, attempts to reduce social anxiety in schizophrenic patients by systematic desensitization have been unsuccessful (Serber and Nelson 1971). Other reports have suggested that 'assertive training' is more useful for the promotion of social skills (Hersen and Bellack 1976).

Social skills training can be offered individually or in groups. The latter seem to have certain advantages, as they constitute ready-made social situations in which participants can interact, while groups are also economical in terms of the therapist's time. The selection of patients is crucial, as a great deal of modelling can occur in groups; excessively anxious patients, and those who repeatedly exhibit disruptive behaviour, should usually be excluded.

Social skills groups must have a clear routine which includes a stable setting, continuity of therapist, revision of previous sessions, and a single 'skill theme' dealt with in each meeting. Sessions should also involve demonstration, imitation, practice, shaping, guidance and realistic homework assignments (Goldstein et al. 1976). Common skills included in training are introductory skills (salutation etc.); observational skills (e.g. self-monitoring); recognition of emotions and attitudes; listening skills; speaking skills (e.g. verbal accuracy); and bodily movement skills (e.g. interactions, gaze exchange, timing, turn taking). Once such skills have been mastered, higher level social routines can then be organized (Trower et al. 1978).

It is hoped that improvement in the group setting will transfer to other social situations, and generalization can be facilitated by a number of strategies. These include making the treatment setting as realistic as possible, or by organizing outdoor excursions where natural situations will abound (Shepherd 1977).

Occupational therapy. The old emphasis on certain traditional tasks, such as basket making, has disappeared to the point that this kind of activity is often no longer available, despite a continuing need in a minority of patients (MacDonald 1970). Instead, music, art therapy, group psychotherapy, relaxation techniques, social skills training and drama therapy are now the central forms of occupational provision in the context of psychiatric disorder. Assessment (both in hospital and at home), has become one of the functions of the occupational therapist. Once handicaps have been identified, occupational therapists may also provide facilities for the patient to practice certain crafts which help to improve cognitive or practical performance. It is possible that a sensible balance between the old and the new occupational therapy techniques would provide the most effective use of this scarce resource.

Token systems. Since the original study by Ayllon and Azrin (1965) token systems have been considered by some as the treatment of choice for chronic behaviour disorder in institutionalized schizophrenic patients (McReynolds and Coleman 1972), and one study reported that 'token systems left schizophrenic symptomatology largely unaffected but were able to promote the skills and interests which enable patients to cope with their illness and live fuller lives'

(Baker and Hall 1975). In addition, these procedures have been recommended for inclusion in the management of certain short-stay patients (Crowley 1975). Token systems are complex sets of procedures which involve the staff giving the patients tokens (such as plastic counters) as rewards for desired behaviour. The tokens are subsequently 'cashed in' for rewards such as material possessions, but it is difficult to separate the effect of the tokens from factors such as increased staff attention and interest. Thus outcome studies must take into account variables related to the patients and the staff, as well as to the programme itself. Sex, age, diagnosis, disability and non-responsiveness to treatment are amongst the more important patient variables (Gripp and Magaro 1974), while the training, attitudes, morale and number of the staff also seem to influence outcome. Important variables which are related to the programme itself include the degree of attention to group processes at the expense of giving the patients individual attention, the goals of management, form of the tokens and the variety of back-up reinforcers. Token systems can present ethical problems, and have been criticized as sometimes depriving patients of their 'basic rights' (Tennent and Marshall 1974).

Implementation of Rehabilitation

The setting. The resources of a rehabilitation centre may include in-patients' hostels, supervised houses, workshops both in and out of hospital, day hospitals and day centres in the community. Ideally, accommodation, occupation and social support should not all be provided by the same institution as this encourages the disadvantages of the so-called total institution (Goffman 1961; Shepherd 1981).

One way of disengaging accommodation, occupation and social support is by providing day care, which separates accommodation from occupation, and divides social support between the two (Shepherd 1981). However, in-patient units in psychiatric hospitals are still required to provide 'asylum' and care for a particular group of severely handicapped patients, who have been called the 'new long stay', (i.e. those who have been resident from 1 to 5 years). Such patients are still accumulating, in spite of 'new methods of treatment and greater understanding of the effect of social environments' (Mann and Cree 1975). Even for such individuals, the use of hostels has been studied as an alternative to living in psychiatric hospitals (Hewett and Ryan 1975) and, more recently, a new kind of intensive hostel–ward has been designed for new long stay patients; the early results are encouraging (Bennett 1980).

Emphasis on 'community care' has also led to studies of the effects of varying the duration of hospital admissions (Glick et al. 1974; Hirsch et al. 1979). However, if there is inadequate provision of day centres, social workers, community services and out-patient clinics, early discharge often involves forcing the patient out of hospital into a less therapeutic environment.

The role of the therapeutic community. Much has been written on the achievements of the therapeutic community approach (Jensen 1980), and there is no doubt that this has fulfilled an important role in the evolution of the psychiatric hospital. Also, most psychiatric services have incorporated certain of its principles such as a recognition of the invaluable role of all the disciplines partaking in the care of the mentally ill, encouraging consultation of both staff and patients in the decision making, and the utilization of the therapeutic potential of group processes (Clark 1974). However, an undue emphasis on group meetings, free emotional expression and the reduction of staff authority has, at times, led to undesirable consequences (Zeitlyn 1967). These may include a persistently dirty and untidy environment and, on the part of the staff, a retreat from professionalism in their attempt to counter the undesirable effects of rigid authoritarianism.

Recently, attempts have been made to introduce a research dimension into the workings of the therapeutic community (Braff et al. 1979). Therapist variables such as warmth and empathy are crucial to successful outcome in psychotherapy, and similar personality characteristics are desirable in those involved in rehabilitation. Staff training and morale are also important, in that the slower tempo of recovery in severely handicapped patients (or the lack of it) may easily create frustration and boredom (Shepherd 1981). Organizational strategies such as periodic breaks and rotations for staff, designating particular members of the staff as key persons for specific patients, and involving all members of the team in assessment, decision making and management, are crucial for staff morale.

Administration. Knowledge of the administration and financial context in which rehabilitation takes place is also important (Rollin 1981); 'even if there were an adequate number of staff, adequately trained, with adequate resources ...it would still be essential to create effective mechanisms of co-ordination between them to provide a comprehensive, integrated and responsible rehabilitation service...' (Royal College of Psychiatrists' Report 1980). The Royal College of Psychiatrists has recommended the establishment of a District Multidisciplinary Rehabilitation Committee, which should include all relevant statutory and voluntary bodies, together with the appointment of a coordinator, whose function would be to arrange individual programmes of rehabilitation. Whatever coordinating mechanism will finally emerge, it is clear that 'for the 1980s there cannot be a single joint approach to psychiatric community care. A variety of approaches is needed at different levels...' (Jefferys 1979; Mollica 1980).

Assessment of Outcome

Crude measures of positive outcome such as recidivism and after-discharge employment may be of some value (Anthony et al. 1972). Recidivism has been defined as an inability to remain out of the hospital after treatment and discharge, and a recent analysis of 41 studies of patients who had undergone a programme of rehabilitation has shown that the incidence of recidivism after 1 year gradually increased as the follow-up period lengthened.

Employment is the other outcome criterion which can be readily used to assess the results of rehabilitation; a patient can be considered employed if he has either worked full-time throughout the period of follow-up, or is employed at the follow-up date. According to this definition, various studies on 'rehabilitated' patients have shown a postdischarge employment rate of between 10 and 40% (Wolkon et al. 1971; Lamb and Goertzel 1972; Cooper 1979).

However, recidivism and employment may not be sensitive enough to measure certain effects of rehabilitation, and it is not appropriate to consider these measures as 'either/or' categories. Thus scales can be constructed to identify degrees of recidivism and unemployment (Walker 1972). Also, improvement in specific aspects of performance may be disguised by assessment techniques which summate various measures. Thus physical, emotional and intellectual skills, as utilized in various social settings, should be analysed separately (Anthony et al. 1977). Another measurement of outcome may involve rating the degree of contact with various social agencies, and subjective 'quality of life' is a further important indicator of positive outcome which has been neglected. Anthony et al. (1978) have suggested that all rehabilitation practitioners must be trained in evaluation skills if our techniques are to be improved.

References

ANDREASEN, N.C. & OLSEN, S. (1982) Negative v. positive schizophrenia. *Archs gen. Psychiat.*, **39**, 789.

ANTHONY, W.A., BUELL, G.J., CHARRAT, S. & ALTHOFF, M.E. (1972) The efficacy of psychiatric rehabilitation. *Psychol. Bull.*, **78**, 447.

ANTHONY, W.A., COHEN, M.R. & VITALO, R. (1978) The measurement of rehabilitation outcome. *Schizophrenia Bull.*, **4**, 365.

ANTHONY, W.A., PIERCE, R.M. & COHEN, M.R. (1977) *Psychiatric Rehabilitation Practice: The Skills of Rehabilitation Programming, Book 2.* Amherst, Mass.: Carkhuff Institute of Human Technology.

ARTHUR, R.J. (1971) *An Introduction to Social Psychiatry.* Harmondsworth: Penguin Books.

AYLLON, T. & AZRIN, N.H. (1965) The measurement and reinforcement of behaviour of psychotics. *J. exp. Analysis Behav.*, **8**, 357.

BAKER, A.A. (1956) Factory in a hospital. *Lancet*, **i**, 278.

BAKER, R. & HALL, J. (1975) *A controlled study of a token economy.* (Paper presented to the Annual Conference of the British Association for Behavioural Psychotherapy, York)

BARTON, R. (1959) *Institutional Neurosis.* Bristol: John Wright.

BENDER, M.P. (1979) Community psychology, when? *Bull. Br. psychol. Soc.*, **32**, 6.

BENNETT, D. (1978) Community psychiatry. *Br. J. Psychiat.*, **132**, 209.

BENNETT, D. (1980) The chronic psychiatric patient today. *J. Roy. Soc. Med.*, **73**, 301.

BENNETT, D.H. & WING, J.K. (1963) Sheltered workshops for the psychiatrically handicapped. In: *Trends in the Mental Health Services*, ed. Freeman, J. & Farndale, J. Oxford: Pergamon Press.

BERRIOS, G.E. (1980) Community psychiatry and the crisis intervention team. *Prog. Psychopharmacol.*, **4**, 83.

BRAFF, D.L., BACHMAN, J., GLICK, I.D. & JONES, R. (1979) The therapeutic community as a research ward. Myths and facts. *Archs gen. Psychiat.*, **36**, 355.

CARLETON, J.L. & MAHLENDORF, V.R. (eds.) (1979) *Dimensions of Social Psychiatry*. Princeton: Science Press.

CARPENTER, W.T., STRAUSS, J.S. & BARTKO, J.J. (1973) Flexible system for the diagnosis of schizophrenia: Report from the W.H.O. International Pilot Study of Schizophrenia. *Science*, **182**, 1275.

CLARK, D.H. (1974) *Social Therapy in Psychiatry*. London: Pelican Books.

COOPER, P. (1979) Employment problems and prospects for chronic patients. In: *New Methods of Mental Health Care*, Meacher, M., Ed. Oxford: Pergamon Press.

CROWLEY, T.J. (1975) Token Programme in an Acute Psychiatric Hospital. *Am. J. Psychiat.*, **132**, 523.

DEAN, A. & LIN, N. (1977) The stress-buffering role of social support. *J. nerv. ment. Dis.*, **166**, 7.

EARLY, D. & MAGNUS, R.V. (1968) Industrial therapy organizations 1960–1965. *Br. J. Psychiat.*, **114**, 335.

FREEMAN, H.E. & SIMMONS, O.G. (1963) *The Mental Patient Comes Home*. New York: John Wiley.

GLICK, I.D., HARGREAVES, W.A. & GOLDFIELD, M.D. (1974) Short vs. Long Hospitalization. *Archs gen. Psychiat.*, **30**, 363.

GOFFMAN, E. (1961) *Asylums*. London: Pelican Books.

GOLDBERG, D. (1974) Principles of rehabilitation. *Compreh. Psychiat.*, **15**, 237.

GOLDSTEIN, A.P., SPRAFKIN, R.P. & GERSHAW, N.J. (1976) *Skill Training for Community Living*. Oxford: Pergamon Press.

GRIFFITHS, R.D.P. (1973) A standardized assessment of work behaviour of psychiatric patients. *Br. J. Psychiat.*, **123**, 403.

GRIFFITHS, R.D.P. (1974) Rehabilitation of chronic psychotic patients. *Psychol. Med.*, **4**, 316.

GRIFFITHS, R.D.P., HODGSON, R. & HALLAM, R. (1974) Structured interview for the assessment of work-related attitudes in psychiatric patients: preliminary findings. *Psychol. Med.*, **4**, 326.

GRIPP, R.F. & MAGARO, P.A. (1974) The token economy programme in the psychiatric hospital: a review and analysis. *Behav. Res. Ther.*, **12**, 205.

HERSEN, M. & BELLACK, A.S. (1976) Social skills training for chronic psychiatric patients: rationale, research findings and future directions. *Compreh. Psychiat.*, **17**, 559.

HEWETT, S.N. & RYAN, P. (1975) Alternatives to living in psychiatric hospitals. *Br. J. Hosp. Med.*, **17**, 65.

HIRSCH, S.R., PLATT, S., KNIGHTS, A. & WEYMAN, A. (1979) Shortening hospital stay for psychiatric care: effect on patients and their families. *Brit. med. J.*, **1**, 442.

JEFFREYS, P.M. (1979) Joint approaches to community care. In: *New Methods of Mental Health Care*, ed. Meacher, M., pp. 15–32. Oxford: Pergamon Press.

JENSEN, E., ed. (1980) *The Therapeutic Community*. London: Croom Helm.

KLEIN, E.B. & SPOHN, H.E. (1964) Behaviour dimensions of chronic schizophrenia. *Psychol. Rep.*, **11**, 773.

LEHMAN, A.F., WARD, N.C. & LINN, L.S. (1982) Chronic mental patients: the quality of life issue. *Am. J. Psychiat.*, **139**, 1271.

LEVINE, M. (1981). *The History and Politics of Community Mental Health*. New York: Oxford University Press.

LEWIS, A.J. (1955) *'Rehabilitation Programmes in England'. Elements of a Community Mental Health Programme*. N.Y. Millbank Memorial Fund.

LIBERAKIS, E.A. (1981) Factors Predisposing to Institutionalism. *Acta. psychiat. neurol. scand.*, **63**, 356.

LIN, N., DEAN, A. & ENSEL, W.M. (1981) Social support scales: a methodological note. *Schizophrenia Bull.*, **7**, 73.

MACDONALD, E. (1970) *Occupational Therapy in Rehabilitation*. London: Baillière Tindall.

MAHMOOD, Z. (1978) An objective application of the Lowenfeld mosaic test in work rehabilitation of psychiatric patients. *Br. J. Proj. Psychol.*, **23**, 31.

MAHMOOD, Z. (1979) The work of a rehabilitation assessment unit. *Bull. Br. psychol. Soc.*, **32**, 168.

MAJASTRE, J.-O. (1972) *L'introduction du changement dans un hôpital psychiatrique public*. Paris: Máspero.

MANN, S. & CREE, W. (1975) The 'New Long Stay' in Mental Hospitals. *Br. J. hosp. Med.*, **17**, 56.

MCREYNOLDS, W.T.I. & COLEMAN, J. (1972) Token economy: patient and staff changes. *Behav. Res. Ther.*, **10**, 29.

MOLLICA, R.F. (1980) Community mental health centres. An American response to Kathleen Jones J. *R. Soc. Med.*, **73**, 863.

MORGAN, R. (1974) Industrial therapy. *Brit. J. Hosp. Med.*, **8**, 231.

MÜLLER, C. (1982) *Les institutions psychiatriques, possibilités et limites*. Berlin: Springer.

OCHBERG, F.M. ZARCONE, V. & HAMBURG, D.A. (1972) Symposium on Institutionalism. *Compreh. Psychiat.*, **13**, 91.

O'CONNOR, N.N. & RAWNSLEY, K. (1959) Incentives with paranoid and non-paranoid schizophrenics in a workshop. *Br. J. med. Psychol.*, **32**, 133.

ORME, J.E. (1970) Long-stay psychiatric patients. In: *The Psychological Assessment of Mental and Physical Handicaps*, ed. Mittler, P., p. 237. London: Methuen and Co.

PIERCY REPORT (1956) Report of the Committee of Enquiry on the Rehabilitation Training and Resettlement of Disabled Persons. London: HMSO.

ROLLIN, H. (1981) Changing face of administration of mental hospitals. *J. R. Soc. Med.*, **74**, 641.

RUESCH, J., JOSPE, S., PETERSON, H.W. & IMBRAN, S. (1972) Measurement of social disability. *Compreh. Psychiat.*, **13**, 507.

SERBER, M. & NELSON, P. (1971) The ineffectiveness of systematic desensitization and assertive training in hospitalized schizophrenics. *J. behav. Ther. exp. Psych.*, **2**, 107.

SHEPHERD, G. (1977) Social Skills Training: The Generalization Problem. *Behav. Ther.*, **8**, 1008.

SHEPHERD, G. (1980) Planning the rehabilitation of the individual. In: *Principles of Psychiatric Rehabilitation*, ed. Watts, F.N. & Bennett, D. New York: John Wiley.

SHEPHERD, G. (1981) *The Function and Organization of Day Hospitals*. (Paper presented to the Italian Congress on 'Medicina Preventiva' in June 1981 in Rome.)

STEVENS, B.C. (1973) Evaluation of rehabilitation for psychotic patients in the community. *Acta. psychiat. scand.*, **49**, 169.

TALBOTT, J.A. (1978) *The Chronic Mental Patient. Problems, Solutions and Recommendations for a Public Policy*. Washington: American Psychiatric Association.

TENNENT, R.G. & MARSHALL, J.R. (1974) The token economy. *Br. J. hosp. Med.*, **17**, 89.

TROWER, P., BRYANT, B. & ARGYLE, M. (1978) *Social Skills and Mental Health*. London: Methuen and Co.

VAUGHN, C.E. & LEFF, J.P. (1976) The influence of family and social factors on the course of psychiatric illness: a comparison of schizophrenics and depressed neurotic patients. *Br. J. Psychiat.*, **129**, 125.

WADSWORTH, W., WELLS, B.W.P. & SCOTT, R.F. (1962). A comparative study of chronic schizophrenics and normal subjects on a work task involving sequential operations. *J. ment. Sci.*, **108**, 309.

WALKER, R. (1972) The Brockton Social Adjustment (BSA) Scale. *Dis. Nerv. System*, **33**, 542.

WANSBROUGH, N., COOPER, P. & MITCHELL, B. (1979) The employment patterns of former psychiatric patients. In: *New Methods of Mental Health Care*, ed. Meacher, M., p. 171. Oxford: Pergamon Press.

WANSBROUGH, N. & MILES, A. (1968) *Industrial Therapy in Psychiatric Hospitals*. London: King Edward's Hospital Fund for London.

WATTS, F.M. (1978) A Study of Work Behaviour in a Psychiatric Rehabilitation Unit. *Br. J. soc. clin. Psychol.*, **17**, 85.

WING, J.K. (1959) *Experimental and Clinical Studies of Chronic Schizophrenia*. Ph.D. Thesis, University of London.

WING, J.K. (1963) Rehabilitation of psychiatric patients. *Br. J. Psychiat.*, **109**, 635.

WING, J.K. & MORRIS, B. (eds) (1981) *Handbook of Psychiatric Rehabilitation Practice*. Oxford: Oxford University Press.

WOLKON, G.H., KARMEN, M. & TANAKA, H.T. (1971) Evaluation of a social rehabilitation programme for recently released psychiatric patients. *Community Ment. Health J.*, **7**, 312.

WOLPE, J. (1969) *The Practice of Behaviour Therapy*. Oxford: Pergamon Press.

ZEITLYN, B. (1967) The therapeutic community: fact or fantasy? *Br. J. Psychiat.*, **113**, 1083.

ZIEGLER, E. & PHILLIPS, L. (1961) Social competence and outcome in psychiatric disorder. *J. abnorm. soc. Psychol.*, **63**, 264.

12

Miscellaneous Treatments

T.R.E. Barnes

INTRODUCTION

'One of the reasons for the popularity of secret remedies is their secrecy. It is a case in which the old saying "*Omne ignotum pro magnifico*" applies.' (BMA Publication, 1909).

The five treatments discussed below occupy the periphery of psychiatric practice and, although not truly secret, have an air of mystery; their modes of action are obscure and their benefits uncertain. This chapter will attempt to evaluate the evidence for their therapeutic efficacy.

TRANSCENDENTAL MEDITATION IN ANXIETY

Transcendental meditation (TM) has been publicized in Western countries since the 1960s by the Maharishi Mahesh Yogi, and found favour with many young people of a generation which vigorously questioned the values of western societies. As West (1975) has pointed out, TM incorporated the ingredients of a 'successful non-professional teaching enterprise', including a mystifying theoretical background, and a charismatic leader. In addition it offered a technique for attaining bodily relaxation and a sense of well-being. It was claimed that after regular periods of meditation for even a few months the individual became more resilient to the stresses of life, worked with increased efficiency and was less likely to be dependent on drink, drugs or tobacco. Later research purported to show that TM improved reaction time (Appelle and Oswald 1974), intelligence (Tjoa 1975), hypertension (Benson and Wallace 1972; Blackwell et al. 1976), asthma (Wilson et al. 1975) and a variety of other conditions.

Recent findings have challenged some of these claims. Pollack et al. (1977) used TM in hypertension with disappointing results, and Anderson's attempts (1977) to treat heroin abuse were also unsuccessful. The claim that TM increased creativity (MacCallum 1977) was not supported by a controlled study

(Domino 1977). Even the assertion that TM is a unique state of consciousness (Banquet et al. 1977) has been challenged by the finding that sleep may constitute a considerable proportion of the time spent in meditating (Younger et al. 1975; Fenwick et al. 1977).

TM is accompanied by a number of physiological changes. There is a fall in oxygen consumption, metabolic rate, cardiac output, blood lactate, respiratory rate and pulse (Wallace and Benson 1972). Also, galvanic skin resistance rises to a relatively steady state, and increased alpha activity, apparently synchronized over the surface of the cortex is shown by the EEG (Banquet 1973; Glueck and Stroebel 1975). However these physiological changes may not be specific to TM, as they have been reported in other low arousal states (Benson et al. 1974; Benson 1975).

The physiological concomitants of TM can be contrasted with those of anxiety, and clinical trials have reported that TM is associated with a reduction in trait anxiety, i.e. anxiety in response to a standard stimulus (Orme-Johnson et al. 1973; Hjelle 1974; Lazar et al. 1977; Davies 1977). Such studies have been criticized on methodological grounds, initially by Smith (1975) and later by Zuroff and Schwartz (1978); many of these studies did not follow up their subjects and involved self-selected meditators. Zuroff and Schwarz felt that too much reliance had been placed on subjective reports, controlled studies did not randomize the assignment of subjects to the treatment and control groups, and 'placebo' treatments to control for non-specific effects of TM were inadequate. Unfortunately adequate placebo treatments are difficult to design; TM novices are usually trained by convinced meditators whose commitment is likely to influence outcome, while a plausible and apparently logical rationale is provided based on a vast body of literature which purports to be based on orthodox scientific theory. These aspects of the ambience of TM cannot be easily simulated to provide a controlled investigation. However, Smith (1976) attempted a comparison of TM, no treatment, and a placebo treatment which involved regularly sitting quietly with an expectation of benefit. The subjects had all volunteered for a free treatment for reduction of anxiety. There was no significant outcome difference between the treatment groups but both improved significantly more than the no-treatment group. Smith concluded that the crucial therapeutic ingredient in TM was a combination of sitting quietly and the expectation of benefit. Zuroff and Schwarz (1978) carried out a similar study which used muscle relaxation as the placebo. Thus their subjects were exposed for a 9-week period to one of the following: TM, no treatment or muscle relaxation training. Trait anxiety was greatly reduced in all three groups, and, on one self-report measure, the TM subjects reported a decline in anxiety. Zuroff and Schwarz (1980) followed up their subjects after 2 years and found that only a small group (15–20%) continued to derive satisfaction from the regular practice of TM. However, this high drop-out rate may have been partially due to the tendency for anxious individuals to 'find it difficult to persevere with the technique on a regular basis because they lack the necessary self discipline' (Kelly 1980).

In another controlled study Raskin et al. (1980) evaluated TM in chronic anxiety and compared it with two forms of relaxation therapy over a 6-week period. One of the relaxation treatments incorporated an electromyographic feedback technique which both induced and demonstrated the reduction in muscle tone. Although subjects were recruited by advertisement, only those volunteers who satisfied criteria for anxiety neurosis were included. A reduction in anxiety scores was shown in the three groups but neither TM nor the muscle biofeedback technique proved more effective than the other form of relaxation therapy. Patients were followed up for an average of 9 months and, in contrast to the findings of Zuroff and Schwarz (1980), not only was improvement generally maintained but most subjects, including those who practised TM, continued regular treatment practice 'at least 2 or 3 times per week'.

Thus TM does not seem superior to muscle relaxation training in the treatment of chronic anxiety. Zuroff and Schwarz (1980) concluded that TM was 'far less effective and satisfying than its proponents claim'. However, anxious patients who have not found relief with routine treatments and who express a positive interest in TM should probably be encouraged, as the higher their expectation of benefit, the greater the likelihood that the technique will be helpful. This conclusion should not be considered as an endorsement of the Maharishi's organization, whose promotional literature claims that TM can lead to levitation, and includes pictures of TM enthusiasts sitting in miraculous suspension several inches from the ground.

SLEEP DEPRIVATION IN DEPRESSION

Total Sleep Deprivation (TSD)

This is the first of two treatment techniques which have been investigated, and involves keeping the patient awake all night. Schulte (1971) noted that three depressed patients felt noticeably better after missing a night's sleep, and Pflug and Tölle (1971) followed up this observation with a therapeutic trial, comparing in-patients with 'endogenous' or 'neurotic' depression with normal subjects. The patients with endogenous depression all responded favourably, although the improvement only lasted a few days, while those with neurotic depression were mostly unaffected or slightly worse. The normal subjects complained of general malaise, headache and 'other vegetative symptoms'. These findings have been generally confirmed in subsequent studies in which approximately 30% of individuals with endogenous depression consistently showed a marked but relatively transient improvement lasting 1 or 2 days (Larsen et al. 1976; Bhanji and Roy 1975; Post et al. 1976; Svendsen 1976; Matussek et al. 1974; Voss and Kind 1974; Van den Burg and Van den

Hoofdakker 1975; Cole and Müller 1976; Gerner et al. 1979). Also, other studies of depressed individuals who did not show an improvement with this procedure (non-responders), and normal subjects deprived of a night's sleep, reported an increase in tension, confusion, hostility, anxiety, depression and, not surprisingly, tiredness (Cutler and Cohen 1979; Bhanji and Roy 1975; Post et al.1976). However, in many of these studies the patients had been receiving antidepressant medication which had been withdrawn at various times in relation to the sleep deprivation, i.e. 24 h to 10 days. This may have affected the results (Pflug and Tölle 1971; Post et al. 1976), as drug withdrawal may have induced adverse withdrawal symptoms, including a rebound increase in rapid eye movement (REM) sleep. Also, the explanation given to patients when medication was stopped, together with their expectations of further treatment, are additional variables which may have affected the results. The therapeutic effect of TSD appeared to be independent of sex, age, response to antidepressant treatment administered during previous depressive episodes, and classification into unipolar and bipolar illness (Larsen et al. 1976; Schilgen and Tölle 1980).

Bhanji and Roy (1975) maintained antidepressant medication in most of their patients throughout the duration of their trial. TSD was carried out, at the rate of 1 night per week, for between 1 and 14 treatments. There was no evidence of a relationship between number of treatments and outcome, but the effects may have been obscured by the effects of concurrent drug treatment. Other studies administered a series of TSD sessions and reported prolonged remissions without further treatment (Svendsen 1976; Larsen et al. 1976; Cole and Müller 1976; Van Scheyen 1975). Thus, although repeated TSD appears to be more efficient than a single treatment, follow-up information is scanty.

Schilgen and Tölle (1980) modified the TSD procedure as a result of their hypothesis that a therapeutic effect would occur when depressed patients were kept awake for the second half of the night. Coincidentally, Cutler and Cohen (1979) observed that normal subjects, staying awake all night, experienced euphoria, became more talkative and showed increased social interaction and activity during the same period, i.e. between 4.30 A.M. and 6.00 A.M. Schilgen and Tölle reported that this partial sleep deprivation was more acceptable to patients and was as effective as TSD, producing an improvement in depressive symptoms following one treatment. However, outcome was variable; the therapeutic effect usually subsided within several days, and, in some cases, after 24 h.

The mode of action of sleep deprivation remains unknown, although Pflug and Tölle (1971) suggested that this procedure involved a 'direct physiological attack' on circadian rhythms. Biochemical investigation of sleep deprivation has been limited to monitoring urinary and CSF amine metabolites. Matussek et al. (1974) found increased urinary noradrenaline and VMA following sleep deprivation in responders but not in non-responders. Post et al. (1976) reported no major changes in CSF amine metabolites following sleep deprivation but did note that methoxyhydroxyphenylglycol (MHPG) in CSF tended to decrease in responders and increase in non-responders. In another study, Kvist and Kirkegaard (1980) claimed to have identified a method for the prediction of a sustained response to TSD. Twenty-eight patients with endogenous depression were treated with 1 night's sleep deprivation; in eight patients an initial remission was obtained although five of these soon relapsed. A thyrotrophin-releasing hormone (TRH) stimulating test was performed before and after the treatment, and an increase of the peak plasma levels of thyrotropin (TSH) to over 2 µU/ml seemed to be associated with a favourable outcome. A correct prediction was made for all the responders, and peak TSH levels discriminated the early relapsers from those who maintained their improvement. Only two of the non-responders had a maximal TSH response over 2 µU/ml.

REM Sleep Deprivation

The second sleep deprivation treatment technique involves selective REM sleep deprivation. In this procedure, sleep is monitored electroencephalographically throughout the night, and the patients are awakened at the onset of each REM episode. As in TSD, the antidepressant effect is more marked in patients with endogenous than neurotic depression. Unlike TSD, REM deprivation can easily be evaluated by a double-blind trial using non-REM sleep awakenings as a control therapy. In such a trial, Vogel et al. (1975) reported a significant therapeutic effect for the procedure, and 50% of the endogenously depressed patients improved sufficiently to allow hospital discharge. Treatment was administered on consecutive nights until the patient had 30 awakenings in a single night or until the end of 6 nights. Patients were then allowed an uninterrupted night's sleep before the procedure began again.

Pilot studies (Vogel and Traub 1968a,b) on REM deprivation suggested that the technique was only therapeutic if 'REM pressure' built up, i.e. if, following cessation of the procedure, there was a 'rebound' increase in REM sleep. Vogel has suggested that the therapeutic action of antidepressant drugs is directly related to their REM suppressing properties (Vogel 1975). It was found (Vogel et al. 1975) that endogenously depressed patients who were unresponsive to REM sleep deprivation also tended to be unresponsive to further treatment with antidepressant drugs. This result was considered to be consistent with the idea that both treatments act via a similar mechanism. In addition, non-responders to REM sleep deprivation did benefit from ECT, which is an antidepressant treatment that does not suppress REM sleep (Vogel et al. 1975). However, Kvist and Kirkegaard (1980) reported that 6 out of 11 non-responders to sleep deprivation subsequently responded to antidepressant drugs, but although this finding appears to contradict Vogel's results, the studies are not strictly comparable, as Kvist and Kirkegaard's patients received TSD and Vogel's patients received specific REM deprivation.

One objection to Vogel's theory is that many drugs are known to suppress REM sleep but fail to function as antidepressants. Vogel has countered this criticism by stating that a drug can only act as an antidepressant if it is capable of reducing and maintaining REM sleep at or below a critical threshold level of 10% of total sleep time, with the subsequent accumulation of REM pressure. He has assembled evidence from a variety of studies to support his claim that only monoamine oxidase inhibitors and certain tricyclic antidepressants fulfil these criteria. However, doxepin, iprindole and trimipramine do not suppress REM sleep to any significant degree (Dunleavy et al. 1972) and would appear to be exceptions to the rule.

Unfortunately, a regimen of REM sleep deprivation which is carried out for several consecutive nights, is taxing for patients and therapists. Schilgen and Tölle (1980) commented that REM deprivation 'is a very elaborate method in which personnel and apparatus are concerned and will hardly become a generally used method of treatment'. However, although TSD is a less complicated procedure, and was first described over 10 years ago, it has also failed to achieve popularity, mainly because the therapeutic benefit is not usually sustained. The procedure has been considered as a clinical curiosity which is unsuitable as a routine therapy. It has not been exploited either as a diagnostic aid (Letemendia et al. 1981) or as a simple technique for producing rapid affective change. However, sleep deprivation consistently produces responders and non-responders amongst endogenously depressed patients, implying a heterogeneous disorder with subgroups that neuroendocrine tests might be able to identify. This is an area worthy of further study.

HYPNOSIS

So far no one has succeeded in specifying generally acceptable objective criteria for the hypnotic trance, but descriptive definitions are useful. Mellett (1980) modified Orne's definition (1973), and stated that 'hypnosis is an unusual (or altered) state of consciousness in which distortions of perception (possibly including those of place and time) occur as uncritical responses of the subject to notions from an objective source (usually the hypnotist) or a subjective source (his own memory) or both'. There is marked individual variation in susceptibility to hypnosis (Spiegel 1975). Bowers (1979) postulates that this depends on the subject's capacity to register information which is not consciously perceived.

Hilgard (1979) identified four kinds of psychological phenomena that occur during the trance state:

(1) Increased suggestibility. This extends to posthypnotic suggestion; subjects out of the trance state may unconsciously comply with an instruction given

to them during hypnosis, often acting in the suggested manner in response to a previously specified signal.

(2) Enhanced imagery and imagination, which may involve fantasy or visual memories from the past. Patients may be 'regressed' to events of earlier years, childhood, and presumably fantasized previous incarnations (O'Hara 1980).

(3) Subsidence of the planning function or, as Spiegel (1975) described it, 'abandonment of executive control', to the therapist.

(4) Reduction in reality testing. Distortions of reality are accepted uncritically in a state of what Orne calls 'trance logic'.

Hilgard noted these aspects of hypnosis as indicants of the trance state which are sufficient to assure both the subject and the hypnotist that hypnosis has been induced. However, it seems that they are also the features of this altered state of consciousness that allow it to be exploited for therapeutic effect. Hypnosis has been advocated as a therapy in its own right, and also as an adjunct to psychotherapy, psychoanalysis, or behavioural therapy techniques. Theoretically, the clinical applications in psychiatry are widespread, and Waxman (1980) considered that hypnosis has a treatment role in neurotic conditions (including neurotic depression), personality problems and psychosexual disorders. However, in practice, hypnosis is not a routine treatment in UK psychiatry.

There appear to be two basic treatment strategies for the use of hypnosis: hypnotic desensitization and hypnotic suggestion. Desensitization may be assisted by the development of powerful sensory images during hypnosis; for example, phobic patients can be exposed, in imagination, to severe anxiety-producing stimuli, using a graded hierarchy. The use of hypnosis may, in theory, be an adjunct to certain forms of psychotherapy, as recalling and reliving early experiences in an hypnotic trance may allow patients to confront early traumatic experiences. Under hypnosis the patient may be able to tolerate the memory without the adverse effects with which it had been previously associated (Waxman 1980). Some of the material to which the patient can be exposed may have been previously repressed, so that it became unavailable to conscious awareness and, as this is uncovered in the hypnotic state, the patient may show abreaction. This can be helpful in itself, but this procedure is not likely to be therapeutic unless the traumatic events are few and well circumscribed.

The second strategy for the use of hypnosis involves hypnotic suggestion. Although Waxman (1980) considered that symptom removal by direct suggestion during hypnosis is rarely therapeutic, Smith (1978) described two situations, associated with hysterical conversion symptoms, where this may be attempted. Firstly, when a patient presents with deafness, mutism or amnesia of hysterial origin, hypnotic suggestion may be used to initiate communication with the patient, and secondly, if hysterical conversion symptoms are well-entrenched, hypnosis can offer a suitable intervention which allows the patient to unconsciously discard the symptoms without 'loss of face'. However, Smith also pointed out that the same effect may result from 'relaxation without hypnosis, an X-ray photograph, massage and physiotherapy, short-wave diathermy, manipulation, nasty medicine, nice medicine, or a well-judged talk with a respected family doctor'. The therapeutic effect of hypnosis in this situation does not readily lend itself to scientific evaluation.

Hypnosis and Sexual Dysfunction

Jehu (1979) described three ways in which hypnosis may be employed in the treatment of sexual dysfunction. The first involves the investigation, recall and abreaction of traumatic sexual experiences. Secondly, hypnotically induced relaxation may be used to alleviate anxiety in desensitization procedures; for example, Fuchs et al. (1978) reported the benefits of 'hypnodesensitisation therapy' and vaginal dilators in 34 women with vaginismus. The 31 who completed therapy were symptom-free, and a 1- to 5-year follow-up revealed that normal sexual adjustment was maintained. However, the specific contribution of hypnosis to the success of the therapy is hard to evaluate, as the use of graded dilators alone can be an effective treatment for this condition. Other studies have combined hypnosis with behavioural techniques and the results are, similarly, difficult to interpret (Astrup 1974; Fabbri 1976; Nuland 1978). The third possible application of hypnosis to treatment of sexual dysfunction involves the use of suggestion to promote sexual responses.

Opinions differ on the value of these procedures, and patients' attitudes to therapy may be especially relevant (Lazarus 1973). Bernstein and Borkovec (1973) preferred progressive relaxation techniques, pointing out that hypnosis often has undesirable connotations for patients. Caution is recommended, especially in the selection of cases, as the procedure has its dangers (Koadlow 1979). Patients may misinterpret or distort suggestions made by the therapist during hypnosis, or intense erotic transference may develop. Reckless and Geiger (1978) warned that hypnosis in sex therapy should be practised 'only by skilled individuals who can combine the knowledge of hypnotic therapy with conventional psychotherapeutic skills'.

Hypnosis and Smoking

In 1971, Johnston and Donoghue reviewed all the studies on the modification of smoking behaviour by hypnosis that had accumulated during the previous decade. No doubt some of these had been precipitated by the increasing awareness of the dangers of cigarette smoking (Royal College of Physicians Report 1962). Johnston and Donoghue criticized the available literature on methodological grounds, considering that most reports were 'primarily anecdotal' and rarely in the form of a controlled study. The principal treatment approach had been the establishment of an aversion to smoking and cigarettes by hypnotic suggestion, although this was usually carried out in combination with other therapeutic techniques. The conclusion was that 'most authors claim success but their procedures cannot be reproduced'.

In 1970 Spiegel published two papers reporting on a 'single 45-minute treatment of psychotherapy reinforced by hypnosis', to stop smoking (Spiegel 1970a,b). The treatment method involved taking a smoking history followed by the induction of a hypnotic trance. In this 'receptive state of concentration' the subject concentrated on the following three injunctions:

(1) For your body smoking is a poison.
(2) You need your body to live.
(3) You owe your body this respect and protection.

The subject was then taught self-hypnosis and instructed to repeat the procedure on his own, ten times a day. Six hundred and fifteen smokers, most of whom had failed to give up smoking following previous therapy, were treated in this way. Six-month follow-up information was available on only 271 (44%) subjects and, of these, 121 had given up smoking completely and a similar number had reduced their smoking to some extent.

Berkowitz et al. (1979) carried out a replication study using this single-treatment method on 40 smokers. At a follow-up after 6 months, complete abstinence was found in 25% of those who could be contacted; this result was similar to that of Spiegel's study. However, although these results are impressive, they do not provide convincing evidence that hypnosis has a major treatment role in this area. Berkowitz et al. concluded that 'further studies that include non-treatment control groups are needed to validate the effects of the hypnotic treatment method'. Even more informative would be a study that included, as a control therapy, all the procedures in the single-treatment session except for the induction of a hypnotic trance.

ACUPUNCTURE

'That acupuncture is a system of cardinal importance in the history of Chinese medicine is not disputed by anyone, but its actual value in objective terms remained until recently, and to some extent still remains, the subject of great differences of opinion' (Lu and Needham 1980). In 1980 an article in *The Guardian* newspaper quoted the Chairman of the British Association of Acupuncturists as saying, 'We reckon to cure 80–90% of drug addicts, 70% of alcoholics, 60% of smokers and 40% of slimmers'.

Acupuncture has been used in Chinese medicine for at least 2000 years but no strong historical precedent for its application to the relief of mental illness seems to have been established. Lu and Needham (1980) listed the conditions traditionally treated by this method and psychiatric problems were not mentioned. Acupuncture is certainly used in both psychotic and neurotic disorders in China today but, according to reports from recent visitors, usually in association with other treatments, principally psychotherapy, group therapy, drugs and herbs (Mann 1972; Ratnavale 1973; Taipale and Taipale 1973; Kaada et al. 1974; Walls et al. 1975).

There are different methods of acupuncture, including manual rotation of the needles and the application of low- or high-frequency electrical stimulation (Editorial 1981). There is evidence that low-frequency electroacupuncture produces analgesia in animals and man and that this effect can be antagonized by the opiate-receptor-blocking drug naloxone (Pomeranz and Chiu 1976; Cheng et al. 1979; Abbate et al. 1980; Clement-Jones et al. 1980). However, this drug has no effect on analgesia induced by high-frequency electroacupuncture. It appears that low-frequency electroacupuncture can release β-endorphin, perhaps from certain neurones of the periaqueductal grey matter, while high-frequency stimulation may release *met*-enkephalin, the effects of which are not blocked by naloxone. However, as the relief of pain with a placebo and other psychological variables may be mediated by endogenous opioids, the specificity of the techniques of acupuncture remain to be determined.

The western literature contains a few anecdotal reports on the benefits of acupuncture in a mixture of psychiatric conditions (Kurland 1976; Shuaib and Haq 1977; Spinetti 1980). Only one double-blind trial, incorporating a controlled treatment of random needling (pseudo-acupuncture) has been published (Kane and DiScipio 1979), and it was claimed that the findings suggested that acupuncture could exert a therapeutic effect in schizophrenia. However, only three patients were involved.

There is no clear evidence for the use of acupuncture in psychiatric illness except for the relief of withdrawal symptoms in heroin addicts (see below). The effects of acupuncture on the endogenous opioids have established a tenuous link with the schizophrenias as the role of endorphins in this group of disorders has been the subject of much recent research and speculation (Usdin et al. 1979; Schachter 1981; Mackay 1981). There are two basic contradictory hypotheses. The first is that the schizophrenias are associated with too little endorphin activity. The predictions based on this premise are that the condition would be improved by the administration of synthetic β-endorphin and, possibly, by acupuncture. The second is that the schizophrenias are associated with excessive endorphin activity, so that the condition might be expected to improve following the administration of naloxone. Each of the hypotheses has attracted experimental support but results have often been equivocal (Pickar et al. 1981).

Acupuncture and Drug Withdrawal

As Chen (1977) has pointed out, the release of endogenous opioids with acupuncture provides a possible explanation for its beneficial effects in the management of some forms of drug addiction. Theoretically, the effects of opiate drug withdrawal might be ameliorated by the stimulation of increased endogenous opioid activity. The technique usually employed, involving electroacupuncture, was developed by Wen and Cheung (1973) for relief of the withdrawal symptoms of heroin addiction. In experiments on morphine-addicted mice, the electroacupuncture method was found to suppress withdrawal behaviours and increase 'opiate-like activity', probably due to β-endorphin in the brain (Ho et al. 1978). The technique was also reported to be effective in man (Patterson 1974; Tseung 1974; Bourne 1975; Tennant 1976; Shuaib 1976).

Clement-Jones et al. (1979) treated heroin withdrawal symptoms with electroacupuncture and found this was associated with an increase in CSF *met*-enkephalin. There was no change in β-endorphin levels but these had been elevated in both blood and CSF prior to acupuncture. These investigators reported that the clinical features of withdrawal were suppressed during therapy and concluded that *met*-enkephalin release was involved in the effective treatment of drug withdrawal with electroacupuncture.

HAEMODIALYSIS IN SCHIZOPHRENIA

The first description of haemodialysis as a treatment for schizophrenia was by Feer et al. (1960). Out of five cases of schizophrenia, three improved after only one or two treatments. Subsequently, Wagemaker and Cade (1977, 1978) and Wagemaker (1978) reported a dramatic reduction in symptoms in 10 out of 15 schizophrenic patients undergoing dialysis. Although these studies were uncontrolled, interest in this possible therapy was aroused.

Case reports of patients with both schizphrenia and renal failure undergoing haemodialysis, appeared in the literature. In two cases the mental state improved (Weddington 1977; Ferris 1977) but negative results were also reported (Levy 1977; Kroll et al. 1978). Later Port et al. (1978) conducted a survey of 50 such patients. Following haemodialysis, 40 patients were unchanged, eight had improved and two had become worse. The authors concluded that haemodialysis did not improve the clinical manifestations of schizophrenia, but clinical trials continued, and in 1980 Fogelson et al. calculated that 92 non-uraemic schizophrenic patients had received haemodialysis in 11 uncontrolled studies. Twenty-two patients (24%) had shown marked improvement, 21 (23%) had shown partial improvement, 47 (51%) had shown no change and two (2%) had become worse. Fogelson et al. suggested that much of the described improvement in negative symptoms might be attributable to the reduction or cessation of antipsychotic medication occurring during haemodialysis. Later the same year the first double-blind study appeared. Diaz-Buxo et al. (1980) subjected four chronic schizophrenic patients to both real haemodialysis and sham dialysis. Three failed to show any improvement at all, one patient demonstrated 'questionable improvement' but relapsed on continued haemodialysis.

In 1977 Wagemaker thought that a possible biochemical explanation for this treatment was that haemodialysis filtered out a toxic polypeptide from the bloodstream which the kidney would not normally remove. This substance was later claimed to be beta-leu^5-endorphin (Palmour et al. 1977; Cox et al. 1979) and this was reported to be present in excess in the dialysate from psychotic patients. These findings have not been confirmed and serious doubts about the chemical identification of this particular endorphin have been raised (Lewis et al. 1979; James and Hearn 1980). Port et al. (1978) and Kolff (1978) have also questioned the ability of haemodialysis effectively to remove this abnormal peptide.

References

ABBATE, D., SANTAMARIA, A., BRAMBILLA, A., PARERAI, A.E. & DiGIULIO, A.M. (1980) β-endorphin and electro-acupuncture. *Lancet*, **ii**, 1309.

ANDERSON, D.J. (1977) Transcendental meditation as an alternative to heroin abuse in servicemen. *Am. J. Psychiat.*, **134**, 1308.

APPELLE, S. & OSWALD, L.E. (1974) Simple reaction time as a function of alertness and prior mental activity. *Perceptual and Motor Skills*, **38**, 1263.

ASTRUP, C. (1974) Flooding therapy with hypnosis. *Behav. Ther.*, **5**, 704.

BANQUET, J.P. (1973) Spectral analysis of the EEG in meditation. *Electroenceph. clin. Neurophysiol.*, **35**, 143.

BANQUET, J.P., SAILHAN, M., CARETTE, F., HALOUT, S. & LUCIEN, M. (1977) EEG analysis of spontaneous and induced states of consciousness. In: *Scientific Research on the Transcendental Meditation Program*, ed. Orme-Johnsone, D.W. & Farrow, J.T., Collected Papers, vol. 1, pp. 165–172. MERU Press.

BENSON, H. (1975) *The Relaxation Response*. New York: Morrow.

BENSON, H., BEARY, J.F. & CAROL, M.P. (1974) The relaxation response. *Psychiatry*, **37**, 37.

BENSON, H. & WALLACE, R.K. (1972) Decreased blood pressure in hypertensive subjects who practiced meditation. *Circulation*, **45** and **46** (suppl. II), 516.

BERKOWITZ, B., ROSS-TOWNSEND, A. & KOHBERGER, R. (1979) Hypnotic treatment of smoking: the single-treatment method revisited. *Am. J. Psychiat.*, **136**, 83.

BERNSTEIN, D.A. & BORKOVEC, T.D. (1973) *Progressive relaxation training: a manual for the helping professions*. Champaign, Illinois: Research Press.

BHANJI, S. & ROY, G.A. (1975) The treatment of psychotic depression by sleep deprivation: a replication study. *Br. J. Psychiat.*, **127**, 222.

BLACKWELL, B., BLOOMFIELD, S., GARTSIDE, P., ROBINSON, A., HANENSON, I., MAGENHEIM, H., NIDLICH, S. & ZIGLER, R. (1976) Transcendental meditation in hypertension. Individual response patterns. *Lancet*, **i**, 223.

BOURNE, P.G. (1975) Non-pharmacological approaches to the treatment of drug abuse (and withdrawal symptoms). *Am. J. Chin. Med.*, **3**, 235.

BOWERS, K.S. (1979) Hypnosis and dissociation. In: *Consciousness: Brain, States of Awareness and Mysticism*, ed. Goleman, D. & Davidson, R.J., pp. 151–8. New York: Harper & Row.

BRITISH MEDICAL ASSOCIATION (1909) *Secret Remedies*. London: BMA.

CHEN, G.S. (1977) Enkephalin, drug addiction and acupuncture. *Am. J. Chin. Med.*, **5**, 25.

CHENG, R., POMERANZ, B. & YU, G. (1979) Dexamethasone partially reduces and 2% saline-treatment abolished electro-acupuncture analgesia: these findings implicate pituitary endorphins. *Life Sci.*, **24**, 1481.

CLEMENT-JONES, V., LOWRY, P.J., McLOUGHLIN, L., BESSER, G.M., REES, L.H. & WEN, H.L. (1979) Acupuncture in heroin addicts: changes in *met*-enkephalin and β-endorphin in blood and cerebrospinal fluid. *Lancet*, **ii**, 380.

CLEMENT-JONES, V., TOMLIN, S., REES, L.H., McLOUGHLIN, L., BESSER, G.M. & WEN, H.L. (1980) Increased β-endorphin but not *met*-enkephalin levels in human cerebrospinal fluid after acupuncture for recurrent pain. *Lancet*, **ii**, 946.

COLE, M.G. & MÜLLER, H.F. (1976) Sleep deprivation in the treatment of elderly depressed patients. *J. Am. geriat. Soc.*, **24**, 308.

COX, B.M., ROSS, M., GOLDSTEIN, A. & PALMOUR, R.M. (1979) Pharmacological characterisation of the *leu*[5] analogue of human β-endorphin. *Brain Res.*, **165**, 311.

CUTLER, N.R. & COHEN, H.B. (1979) The effect of one night's sleep loss on mood and memory in normal subjects. *Compreh. Psychiat.*, **20**, 61.

DAVIES, J. (1977) The transcendental meditation program and progressive relaxation: comparative effects on trait anxiety and self actualization. In: *Scientific Research on the Transcendental Meditation Program*. ed. Orme-Johnson, D.W. & Farrow, J.T., Collected Papers, vol. 1, pp. 449–52. MERU Press.

DIAZ-BUXO, J.A., CAUDLE, J.A., CHANDLER, J.T., FARMER, C.D. & HOLBROOK, W.D. (1980) Dialysis of schizophrenic patients: a double-blind study. *Am. J. Psychiat.*, **137**, 1220.

DOMINO, G. (1977) Transcendental meditation and creativity: an empirical investigation. *J. appl. Psychol.*, **62**, 358.

DUNLEAVY, D.L.F., BREZINOVA, V., OSWALD, I., MACLEAN, A.E. & TINGKER, M. (1972) Changes during weeks in effects of tricyclic drugs on the human sleeping brain. *Br. J. Psychiat.*, **120**, 663.

EDITORIAL, (1981) How does acupuncture work? *Br. med. J.*, **283**, 746.

FABBRI, R. (1976) Hypnosis or behaviour therapy: a coordinated approach to the treatment of sexual disorders. *Am. J. clin. Hypnosis*, **19**, 4.

FEER, H., THOELEN, H., MASSINI, M.A. & STAUB, H. (1960) Haemodialysis in schizophrenia. *Compreh. Psychiat.*, **1**, 338.

FENWICK, P.B., DONALDSON, S., GILLIS, L., BUSHMAN, J., FENTON, G.W., PERRY, I., TILSLEY, C. & SERAFINOWICZ, H. (1977) Metabolic and EEG changes during transcendental meditation; an explanation. *Biol. Psychol.* **5**, 101.

FERRIS, G.N. (1977) Can dialysis help the chronic schizophrenic? *Am. J. Psychiat.* (letter), **134**, 1310.

FOGELSON, D.L., MARDER, S.R. & VAN PUTTEN, T. (1980) Dialysis for schizophrenia: review of clinical trials and implications for further research. *Am. J. Psychiat.*, **137**, 605.

FUCHS, K., HOCH, H., PALDI, E., ABRAMOVICI, H., BRANDES, J.M., TIMOR-TRITSCH, I. & KLEINHAUS, M. (1978) Hypnodesensitization therapy of vaginismus: in vitro and in vivo methods. In: *Handbook of Sex Therapy*, ed. LoPiccolo, J. & LoPiccolo, L., pp. 261–70. New York: Plenum Press.

GERNER, R.H., POST, R.M., GILLIN, J.C. & BUNNEY, W.E. (1979) Biological and behavioural effects of one night's sleep deprivation in depressed patients and normals. *J. Psychiat. Res.*, **15**, 21.

GLUECK, B.C. & STROEBEL, C.F. (1975) Biofeedback and meditation in the treatment of psychiatric illness. *Compreh. Psychiat.*, **16**, 303.

THE GUARDIAN (December 12th 1980). Just twiddle your ear and you'll kick the habit, p. 9.

HILGARD, E.R. (1979) The hypnotic state. In: *Consciousness: Brain, States of Awareness and Mysticism*, ed. Goleman, D. & Davidson, R.J., pp. 147–150. New York: Harper and Row.

HJELLE, L.A. (1974) Transcendental meditation and psychological health. *Perceptual and Motor Skills*, **39**, 623.

HO, W.K.K., WEN, H.L., LAM, S. & MA, L. (1978) The influence of electroacupuncture on naloxone-induced morphine withdrawal in mice: elevation of brain opiate-like activity. *Eur. J. Pharmac.*, **49**, 197.

JAMES, N.M.C.I. & HEARN, M.T.W. (1980) Haemodialysis, endorphins and schizophrenia. *Am. J. Psychiat.*, **137**, 488.

JEHU, D. (1979) *Sexual Dysfunction*. Chichester: John Wiley and Sons.

JOHNSTON, E. & DONOGHUE, J.R. (1971) Hypnosis and smoking: a review of the literature. *Am. J. clin. Hypn.*, **13**, 265.

KAADA, B.R., HOEL, E., LESETH, K., NYGAARD-ØSTBY, B., SETEKLEIV, J. & STOVNER, J. (1974) Acupuncture analgesia in the People's Republic of China—with glimpses of other aspects of Chinese Medicine. *Tidsskr. norske Laegeforen*. **94**, 417.

KANE, J. & DiSCIPIO, W.J. (1979) Acupuncture treatment of schizophrenia: report on three cases. *Am. J. Psychiat.*, **136**, 297.

KELLY, D. (1980) *Anxiety and Emotions*. Springfield, Illinois: Charles C. Thomas.

KOADLOW, E. (1979) Contraindications and indications to the use of hypnosis in psychosexual dysfunction. *Aust. J. Clin. Exp. Hypnosis*, **7**, 253.

KOLFF, W.J. (1978) Dialysis of schizophrenics—weird and novel applications of dialysis, hemofiltration, hemoperfusion and peritoneal dialysis: witchcraft? *Artif. Organs*, **2**, 277.

KROLL, P.D., PORT, F.K. & SILK, K.R. (1978) Haemodialysis and schizophrenia: a negative report. *J. nerv. ment. Dis.*, **166**, 291.

KURLAND, H.D. (1976) ECT and ACU-EST in the treatment of depression. *Am. J. Chin. Med.*, **4**, 289.

KVIST, J. & KIRKEGAARD, C. (1980) Effect of repeated sleep deprivation on clinical symptoms and the TRH test in endogenous depression. *Acta psychiat. neurol. scand.*, **62**, 494.

LARSEN, J.K., LINDBERG, M.L. & SKOVGAARD, B. (1976) Sleep deprivation as treatment for endogenous depression. *Acta psychiat. neurol. scand.*, **54**, 167.

LAZAR, Z., FARWELL, L. & FARROW, J.T. (1977) The effects of the transcendental meditation program on anxiety, drug abuse, cigarette smoking and alcohol consumption. In: *Scientific Research on the Transcendental Meditation Program*, ed. Orme-Johnson, D.W. & Farrow, J.T., Collected Papers, vol. 1, pp. 524–35, MERU Press.

LAZARUS, A.A. (1973) 'Hypnosis' as a facilitator in behaviour therapy. *Int. J. clin. exp. Hypnosis*, **21**, 25.

LETEMENDIA, F.J.J., PROWSE, A. & SOUTHMAYD, S. (1981) Diagnostic use of sleep deprivation. *Br. J. Psychiat.* (letter), **138**, 352.

LEVY, N.B. (1977) Can dialysis help the chronic schizophrenic? *Am. J. Psychiat.* (letter), **134**, 1311.

LEWIS, R.V., GERBER, L.D., STEIN, S., STEPHEN, R.L., GROSSER, B.I., VELICK, S.F. & UDENFRIEND, S. (1979) On βH-leu^5-endorphin and schizophrenia. *Archs gen. Psychiat.*, **36**, 237.

LU, G-D. & NEEDHAM, J. (1980) *Celestial Lancets: A History and Rationale of Acupuncture and Moxa*. Cambridge: Cambridge University Press.

MACCALLUM, M.J. (1977) The transcendental meditation program and creativity. In: *Scientific Research on the Transcendental Meditation Program*, ed. Orme-Johnson, D.W. & Farrow, J.T., Collected Papers, vol. 1, pp. 410–414, MERU Press.

MACKAY, A.V.P. (1981) Endorphins and the psychiatrist. *Trends in Neurosci.*, **4**, 5.

MANN, F. (1972) *Acupuncture: The Ancient Chinese Art of Healing*, pp. 149–65. New York: Vintage Books.

MATUSSEK, N., ACKENHEIL, M., ATHEN, D., BECKMANN, H., BENKERT, O., DITTMER, T., HIPPIUS, H., LOOSEN, P., RÜTHER, E. & SCHELLER, M. (1974) Catecholamine metabolism under sleep deprivation therapy of improved and not improved depressed patients. *Pharmakopsychiatrie*, **7**, 108.

MELLETT, P. (1980) Current reviews on the psychophysiology of hypnosis. *Br. J. hosp. Med.*, **23**, 441.

NULAND, W. (1978) The use of hypnosis in psychic impotence. In: *Hypnosis At Its Bicentennial*, ed. Frankel, F.H. & Zamansky, H.S. New York: Plenum Press.

O'HARA, M. (1980) *New Hope Through Hypnotherapy*. Tunbridge Wells: Abacus Press.

ORME-JOHNSON, D.W., ARTHUR, G., FRANKLIN, L., O'CONNELL, J. & ZOLD, T. Transcendental meditation and drug abuse counselors. (1973) In: *The Psychobiology of Transcendental Meditation*, ed. Kanellakos, D.P. & Ferguson, P.C. Los Angeles: Maharishi International University Press.

ORNE, M.T. (1973) In: *Hypnosis: Research Developments and Perspectives*, eds. Fromm, E., Shor, R.E. London: Paul Elek Scientific Books.

PALMOUR, R.M., ERVIN, F.R., WAGEMAKER, M. & CADE, R. (1977. *Characterization of a peptide derived from the serum of psychiatric patients*. Paper presented at the Society for Neuroscience, Anaheim, California, Nov. 8.

PATTERSON, M.A. (1974) Electro-acupuncture in alcohol and drug addiction. *Clin. Med.*, **81**, 9.

PFLUG, B. & TÖLLE, R. (1971) Disturbance of the 24-hour rhythm in endogenous depression and the treatment of endogenous depression by sleep deprivation. *Int. Pharmacopsychiat.*, **6**, 187.

PICKAR, D., DAVIS, G.C., SCHULTZ, S.C., EXTEIN, I., WAGNER, R., NABER, C.H., GOLD, P.W., VAN KAMMEN, D.P., GOODWIN, F.K., WYATT, R.J., LI, C.H. & BUNNEY, W.E. (1981) Behavioural and biological effects of acute β-endorphin injection in schizophrenic and depressed patients. *Am. J. Psychiat.*, **138**, 160.

POLLACK, A.A., CASE, D.B., WEBER, M.A. & LARAGH, J.H. (1977) Limits of transcendental meditation in the treatment of essential hypertension. *Lancet*, **i**, 73.

POMERANZ, B. & CHIU, D. (1976) Naloxone blockade of acupuncture analgesia: endorphin implicated. *Life Sci.*, **19**, 1757.

PORT, F.K., KROLL, P.D. & SWARTZ, R.D. (1978) The effect of hemodialysis on schizophrenia: a survey of patients with renal failure. *Am. J. Psychiat.*, **135**, 743.

POST, R.M., KOTIN, J. & GOODWIN, F.K. (1976) Effects of sleep deprivation on mood and central amine metabolism in depressed patients. *Archs gen. Psychiat.*, **33**, 627.

RASKIN, M., BALI, L.R. & PEEKE, H.V. (1980) Muscle biofeedback and transcendental meditation. *Archs gen. Psychiat.*, **37**, 93.

RATNAVALE, D.N. (1973) Psychiatry in Shanghai, China: observations in 1973. *Am. J. Psychiat.*, **130**, 1082.

RECKLESS, J. & GEIGER, N. (1978) Impotence as a practical problem. In: *Handbook of Sex Therapy*, ed. LoPiccolo, J. & LoPiccolo, L. pp. 295–321. New York: Plenum Press.

ROYAL COLLEGE OF PHYSICIANS OF LONDON (1962) *Smoking and Health*. London: Pitman Books.

SCHACHTER, M. (1981) Enkephalins and endorphins. *Br. J. Hosp. Med.*, **25**, 128.

SCHILGEN, B. & TÖLLE, R. (1980) Partial sleep deprivation as therapy for depression. *Archs gen. Psychiatry*, **37**, 267.

SCHULTE, W. (1971) Zum problem der Provokation und Klupierung von melancholischen Phasen. *Schweizer. Arch. Neurol. Psychiat.*, **109**, 427.

SHUAIB, M. (1976) Acupuncture treatment of drug dependence in Pakistan. *Am. J. Chin. Med.*, **4**, 403.

SHUAIB, M. & HAQ, M.F. (1977) Electro-acupuncture treatment in psychiatry. *Am. J. Chin. Med.*, **5**, 85.

SMITH, J.C. (1975) Meditation as psychotherapy: a review of the literature. *Psychol. Bull.* **82**, 558.

SMITH, J.C. (1976) Psychotherapeutic effects of transcendental meditation with controls for expectation of relief and daily sitting. *J. consult. clin. Psychol.*, **44**, 630.

SMITH, A.C. (1978) Hysteria. In: *Current Themes in Psychiatry*, ed. Gaind, R.N. & Hudson, B.L., vol. 2, pp. 125–33. London: Macmillan.

SPIEGEL, H. (1970a) Termination of smoking by a single treatment. *Archs envir. hlth*, **20**, 736.

SPIEGEL, H. (1970b) A single-treatment method to stop smoking using ancillary self-hypnosis. *Int. J. clin. exp. Hypnosis*, **18**, 235.

SPIEGEL, H. (1975) Hypnosis: an adjunct to psychotherapy. In: *Comprehensive Textbook of Psychiatry*, ed. Freedman, A.M., Kaplan, H.I. & Sadock, B.J., 2nd ed., vol. 2, pp. 1843–1850. Baltimore: Williams and Wilkins.

SPINETTI, G. (1980) L'agopuntura nella terapia psichiatrica. *Minerva psichiat.*, **21**, 167.

SVENDSEN, K. (1976) Sleep deprivation therapy in depression. *Acta psychiat. neurol. scand.*, **54**, 184.

TAIPALE, V. & TAIPALE, I. (1973) 1. Chinese psychiatry: a visit to a Chinese mental hospital. *Archs gen. Psychiat.*, **29**, 313.

TENNANT, F.S. (1976) Outpatient heroin detoxication with acupuncture and staple puncture. *West. J. Med.*, **25**, 191.

TJOA, A. (1975) Meditation, neuroticism and intelligence: a follow-up. *Gedrag: Tijdschrift voor Psychologie*, **3**, 167.

TSEUNG, Y.K. (1974) Acupuncture for drug addiction. *Lancet*, **ii**, 839.

USDIN, E., BUNNEY, W.E. & KLINE, N.S. (1979) *Endorphins in Mental Health Research*, London: Macmillan.

VAN DEN BURG, W. & VAN DEN HOOFDAKKER, R.H. (1975) Total sleep deprivation in endogenous depression. *Archs gen. Psychiat.*, **32**, 1121.

VAN SCHEYEN, J.D. (1975) Slaap deprivatie bij de behandeling van unipolaire (endogene) vitale depressies. *Ned. Tijdschr. Geneesk.*, **121**, 564.

VOGEL, G.W., THURMOND, A., GIBBONS, P., SLOAN, K., BOYD, M. & WALKER, M. (1975) REM sleep reduction effects on depression syndromes. *Archs gen. Psychiat.*, **32**, 765.

VOGEL, G.W. (1975) A review of REM sleep deprivation. *Archs gen. Psychiat.*, **32**, 749.

VOGEL, G.W. & TRAUB, A.C. (1968a) The effect of REM deprivation on psychotically depressed patients. *Psychophysiol.*, **4**, 382.

VOGEL, G.W. & TRAUB, A.C. (1968b) Further studies on REM deprivation of depressed patients. *Psychophysiol.*, **5**, 239.

VOSS, A. & KIND, H. (1974) Ambulant Behandlung endogener Depression durch Schlafentzug. *Praxis*, **63**, 564.

WAGEMAKER, H. (1977) (letter) *Am. J. Psychiat.*, **134**, 1311.

WAGEMAKER, H. (1978) The effect of haemodialysis on fifteen chronic process schizophrenics. *Artif. Organs*, **2**, 205.

WAGEMAKER, H. & CADE, R. (1977) The use of haemodialysis in chronic schizophrenics. *Am. J. Psychiat.*, **134**, 684.

WAGEMAKER, H. & CADE, R. (1978) Haemodialysis in chronic schizophrenic patients. *Sth. Med. J.*, **71**, 1463.

WALLACE, R.K. & BENSON, H. (1972) The physiology of meditation. *Sci. Am.*, **226** (2), 85.

WALLS, P.D., WALLS, L.H. & LANGLEY, D.G. (1975) Psychiatric training and practice in the People's Republic of China. *Am. J. Psychiat.*, **132**, 121.

WAXMAN, D. (1980) Clinical applications of hypnosis in psychiatry. *Br. J. Hosp. Med.*, **23**, 456.

WEDDINGTON, W.W. (1977) Can dialysis help the chronic schizophrenic? (1977) (letter) *Am. J. Psychiat.*, **134**, 1310.

WEN, W.L. & CHEUNG, S.Y.C. (1973) Treatment of drug addiction by acupuncture and electrical stimulation. *Asian med. J.*, **9**, 138.

WEST, L.J. (1975) Transcendental meditation and other non-professional psychotherapies. In: *Comprehensive Textbook of Psychiatry*, ed. Freedman, A.M., Kaplan, H.I. & Sadock, B.J., 2nd ed., vol. 2, pp. 2561–7. Baltimore: Williams and Wilkins.

WILSON, A.F., HONSBERGER, R., CHIU, J.T. & NOVEY, H.S. (1975) Transcendental meditation and asthma. *Respiration*, **32**, 74.

YOUNGER, J., ADRIANCE, W. & BERGER, R.J. (1975) Sleep during transcendental meditation. *Percept. Mot. Skills*, **40**, 953.

ZUROFF, D.C. & SCHWARZ, J.C. (1978) Effects of transcendental meditation and muscle relaxation on trait anxiety, maladjustment, locus of control and drug use. *J. consult. clin. Psychol.*, **46**, 264.

ZUROFF, D.C. & SCHWARZ, J.C. (1980) Transcendental meditation versus muscle relaxation: a two-year follow-up of a controlled experiment. *Am. J. Psychiat.*, **137**, 1229.

PART TWO

Management

13

Management of Psychiatric Disorders Associated with Identifiable Somatic Disease

G.E. Berrios

INTRODUCTION

'Organic' disease (i.e. an identifiable change in somatic structure and/or function which is judged to be undesirable) and psychiatric disorder are often found together, and research suggests that this is not a chance association (Lipowski 1975; Hall et al. 1978). For example, in a general practice population Eastwood and Travelyan (1972) found that 49.2% of patients with psychiatric disorder had major physical illness, and that this was significantly higher than in non-psychiatric controls; also Shinozaki (1976) has found that deaths amongst psychiatric in-patients were higher than in a control population. The nature of any causal links has proved difficult to elucidate, but clinical observation suggests that at least five mechanisms may be found, acting alone or in combination.

Firstly, abnormal behaviour may result from organic brain or systemic pathology which involves structural changes to nerve cells or an identifiable process which affects neuronal functions. These psychiatric states constitute the organic psychiatric disorders 'proper', and the size of this group will be enlarged by further advances in medical science. Psychiatric symptoms of organic disease acquire diagnostic importance if they precede the other clinical signs (Hall et al. 1978), and may help with differential diagnosis provided that close attention is given to their descriptive phenomenology. For example, Kraepelin claimed that the psychiatric symptoms which accompany certain organic diseases are characterized by subtle clinical qualities, although Chaslin (1892) and Bonhoeffer (1910) considered organic psychiatric phenomena to be non-specific with regard to aetiology. Jaspers (1963) suggested a hierarchical view of diagnosis, according to which organic symptoms take precedence over other psychopathological manifestations. For example, 'schizophrenic' symptoms do not necessarily mean the presence of a schizophrenic illness if they are accompanied by a relevant neurological disorder (Schneider 1959; Davison and Bagley 1969).

A second possible mechanism to explain the association between somatic disease and psychiatric disorder considers the psychiatric complication to be a psychological 'reaction' (Starobinski 1977) to the physical disease (Lloyd 1977). For example, anxiety and depressive states may accompany a number of physical disorders (Kathol and Petty 1981). The causal link in these cases is assumed to be psychological in nature and analogous to that involved in grief reactions (Jacobs and Douglas 1979). However, in some cases, such as depression associated with occult neoplasm (Fras et al. 1967; Whitlock and Siskind 1979; Maguire 1981), unknown metabolic effects might play some aetiological role.

A third mechanism involving some form of non-conscious mental activity must sometimes be invoked to explain the presence of psychiatric symptoms when the above type of explanations do not apply. For example, reduced potency may occasionally be seen as a temporary complication of colostomy (Dlin et al. 1969) even when there is no evidence of damage to the nerves. Psychodynamic theories have been developed to conceptualize the internal processes affecting the subject's attitude to sexual potency and to suggest therapeutic techniques to bring them to conscious awareness.

The fourth mechanism postulates that psychiatric disorder may result from the direct or indirect social consequence of physical disease. Human resilience to different life events varies considerably, so that a patient may cope well with the personal impact of, for example, a mastectomy operation but become depressed later in response to sexual difficulties resulting from her husband's inability to adjust to her disfigurement.

The last mechanism involves iatrogenic psychiatric complications following pharmacological, surgical or psychological treatment of physical disease. For example, depression may follow antihypertensive medication (Bant 1978; Pottash et al. 1981; Tyrer 1981), confusional states can result from anticholinergic medication (Johnson et al. 1981) and psychiatric disorders may follow a number of surgical interventions (Morse and Litin 1969; Rubinstein and Thomas 1969; Davis and Beumont 1973; Parkes and Napier 1973; Nadelson 1976). This chapter will mainly deal with those psychiatric syndromes arising from the first mechanism which has been described.

CLASSIFICATION OF ORGANIC MENTAL DISORDERS

Organic states can be classified according to clinical features, aetiology and prognosis. I.C.D. 9 (1978) combines all three criteria and defines organic psychotic conditions (290–294) as 'syndromes in which there is impairment of orientation, memory, comprehension, calculation, learning capacity and judgement ... there may also be shallowness or lability of affect, or a more persistent disturbance of mood, lowering of ethical standards and exaggeration or emergence of personality traits, and diminished capacity for independent decision', i.e.:

290 - Senile and presenile organic psychotic conditions
291 - Alcoholic psychoses
292 - Drug psychoses
293 - Transient organic psychotic conditions
294 - Other organic psychotic conditions (chronic)

The American Diagnostic and Statistical Manual of Mental Disorders (DSM III, 1980) distinguishes between 'organic brain syndrome' and 'organic mental disorder'. The former refers to 'a constellation of psychological or behavioural signs and symptoms without reference to aetiology (e.g. delirium, dementia)'. The latter 'designates a particular organic brain syndrome in which the aetiology is known or presumed (e.g. alcoholic withdrawal delirium, multi-infarct dementia)'.

The organic brain syndromes of DSM III comprise:

(1) Delirium and dementia (in which the cognitive impairment is relatively global)

(2) Amnestic syndrome and organic hallucinations (which involve relatively selective impairments)

(3) Organic delusional syndrome and organic affective syndrome (which have features resembling schizophrenic or affective illness respectively)

(4) Organic personality syndrome

(5) Intoxication and withdrawal

(6) Atypical or mixed organic brain syndrome (this is the residual category)

Category 3 of the DSM III is a partial recognition of the group of states described by Wieck (1961) as 'transitional' or 'transitory' states ('*Durchgangssyndrom*') which refer to acute psychotic states of organic origin without clouding of consciousness.

PSYCHIATRIC DISORDERS IN THE GENERAL HOSPITAL

Psychiatrists working in general hospitals may be consulted by their medical colleagues about patients exhibiting acute psychiatric symptoms or showing intense distress in relation to their illness or social circumstances. This role for the psychiatrist is variously termed 'Consultation–liaison psychiatry' or 'general hospital psychiatry' (Hackett and Cassem 1978). 'Consultation' involves diagnosis and management, while 'liaison' refers to teaching, research and the public relations aspects of psychiatry. Some American writers feel that these activities should be inseparable (Lipowski 1975*b*). In fact, general hospital psychiatry is an amalgam of various activities and theoretical approaches, including the diagnosis and management of organic mental disorders, assessment of the psychological complications of physical disease, treatment of psychiatric emergencies, and analysis of persistent somatic complaints when organic pathology does not seem to exist.

General hospital psychiatry has been seen by some as the realization of cherished ideals for professional integration and as the fulfilment of a holistic view of disease which places mental illness in its proper context. However, general hospital psychiatric units often remain isolated from the rest of the hospital, for psychiatrists do not always manage to develop adequate links with their medical and surgical colleagues. Liaison is often unsatisfactory unless the psychiatrist becomes a member of the medical or surgical team and is in the position to influence the referral process. A common reason for referral is behavioural disturbance which disrupts the ward routine or the patient's medical treatment, and while this may be automatically assumed to be the result of primary psychiatric disorder, such disruptive behaviour may result from understandable interaction between the patient and his environment. For example, patients may behave obstructively to express resentment for not being given adequate information about the exact nature of their condition and its prognosis.

Another common reason for referral is to elicit any psychiatric disorder in patients with persistent physical symptoms and negative investigations. The inexperienced psychiatrist may prematurely accept the view that a series of negative investigations excludes the possibility of physical disease and that a psychiatric illness must be present. Not surprisingly, most patients who are told by their physician that all their symptoms are 'in the mind' and that they need a psychiatrist, become anxious, worried, depressed or angry, and it is easy for the psychiatrist to magnify or misinterpret these emotions and convert them into a psychiatric diagnosis. Psychiatric illness should only be diagnosed on the basis of positive symptoms, and if none are present the psychiatrist must not hesitate to say so. This is particularly important as, in a number of cases, such as those involving occult malignancy or endocrine disturbance, further investigations will, sooner or later, yield positive results.

Patients who present particular management difficulties are the very chronic attenders at medical or surgical clinics. Such individuals are often recognized by the thickness of their case notes, and present with such disorders as Briquet's syndrome, severe hypochondriacal or delusional states, panneurosis with multiple somatic complaints, or (rarely) the Munchausen syndrome. The role of the psychiatrist in such cases is to rescue the patient from overenthusiastic medical or surgical investigation and treatment. However, therapeutic success is rare.

A fourth common reason for psychiatric referral in the general hospital is that 'disposal' has become a problem, in particular if the patient is elderly, brain damaged or chronically infirm. At times, wishful thinking (or even deliberate misrepresentation) may lead neurosurgical colleagues to describe an apallic or vegetative state as a 'catatonic syndrome', a traumatic dementia as 'depression', or a fluent dysphasia as 'schizophrenia'. The psychiatrist must resist inappropriate demands for admission to a psychiatric hospital, but the suitability of a patient for psychiatric care should be assessed on the patient's need rather than on diagnosis. For example, whether a demented and physically infirm elderly patient is to be nursed in a geriatric or psychiatric ward will be partially determined by the degree of overt disruptive behaviour. Severely brain injured patients (even if they exhibit obvious 'behavioural disorder') often require intensive and specialized nursing of the kind that is not available in the average psychiatric hospital; furthermore, they may require specific and personalized rehabilitatory techniques which are only available in specialized 'brain damage units'. It is important to realize that brain-damaged patients often exhibit abnormal behaviour which may be inappropriately interpreted as malingering or hysteria. On the other hand, if psychiatric phenomena such as depression, obsessional behaviour, or phobias are present they must be vigorously treated if they hamper rehabilitation. However, it is rarely necessary for patients to be transferred to a psychiatric unit on account of such symptoms.

Other reasons for psychiatric referral include the assessment of requests for plastic surgery, and the management of chronic pain, sleep disorders, functional vomiting, eating disorders or tension headaches. Also, an opinion may be sought regarding the differential diagnosis of seizures, and mood disorder associated with a variety of diseases including multiple sclerosis, Crohn's disease, myasthenia gravis and Parkinson's disease. Renal units (Pritchard 1982) and clinical haematology (Clarke et al. 1982) may also require the help of a psychiatrist.

DEMENTIA

This disorder is considered in Chapter 24 (pp. 445–53).

DELIRIUM

Clinical Features

Delirium refers to a fluctuating cluster of behavioural and mental symptoms which are seen in direct temporal correlation with a number of neurological or systemic conditions (Lipowski 1980). Clouding of consciousness with disorientation (Berrios 1982) and perceptual, cognitive, emotional and behavioural disorder constitute its most important signs and symptoms.

The aetiology and speed of onset of the organic pathology influence the quality of the delirium. A prodromal period of irritability, anxiety, insomnia and/or nightmares often heralds the condition, and the impairment of consciousness may be preceded by reduced attention, 'absent-mindedness', or forgetfulness. The clouding of conciousness reflects a reduction in cerebral arousal and it is often possible to correlate the level of consciousness with EEG changes (Kiloh et al. 1972). In general, the degree of slowing of the EEG is a more reliable index of reduced arousal than the percentage of dominant rhythms. Disorientation and confusion tend to be worse towards the evening, and this may be related to circadian rhythms or to external factors such as sensory or sleep deprivation. Marked impairment of consciousness may be accompanied by speech hesitations, incoherence of thought and fragmentation of action of which there is little recollection after remission.

The sensory distortions and visual hallucinations that accompany delirium may be exacerbated by situations where there is perceptual ambiguity. These perceptual disturbances may result from a 'release' of subcortical activity, from a direct irritation of sensory pathways or, on occasions, from dreaming breaking through into consciousness (as seems to be the case in delirium tremens). Visual hallucinations tend to be fleeting and elementary. Some patients may retain insight and worry about the possibility of 'going mad', while others lose insight early and react to their visions with fear or pleasure. It is not clear what variables determine this differential response. Auditory and tactile hallucinations may also occur.

The content of the visual hallucination may occasionally indicate diagnosis or the localization of a brain lesion, but false positives and negatives abound. Hallucinations characterized by geometric patterns and elementary distortions seem more common in toxic and drug induced states, while formed visual hallucinations, such as faces or panoramic visions, are related to temporal and occipital lobe pathology (Hecaen and Albert 1979). Sometimes patients do not admit to having these experiences and their presence can only be surmised from their behaviour. On occasions, hallucinatory activity can be initiated or terminated by direct suggestion, by changes in the topic of conversation, or by other environmental modifications.

Illusions or hallucinations often impair the patient's hold on reality and the continuity of goal-directed behaviour. Efforts to make sense of chaotic experiences can result in delusional interpretation, uncertainty and persecutory ideas. Jumping out of the window or making a determined attack upon the staff may be the first indication of the existence of such phenomena.

The psychopathological symptomatology of delirium may be accompanied by physical manifestations such as tachycardia, fever, sweating, dilation of pupils, tremor, grand mal seizures, myoclonic jerks and ataxia. Some patients respond to their psychological and physical distress by withdrawing to their beds, hiding under the bed covers and looking perplexed and frightened. This state, sometimes called 'quiet delirium' is far more common than the 'excited form' which is described in most textbooks. It is also less often seen by psychiatrists. The most common reason of referral in cases of delirium is disruptive or antisocial behaviour.

Management

The management of delirium consists of the treatment of the causal disease and the psychiatric symptoms, together with basic nursing care. Three general points must be remembered in relation to medical treatment: in many cases management of the underlying condition is sufficient to cause the disappearance of the delirium; medical or surgical treatment may occasionally worsen the syndrome; while the cause of some deliria, for example, those resulting from severe brain injury, cannot be treated.

Most neurological or systemic conditions, if severe enough, may cause delirium, in particular head injury, cerebrovascular accident, hypertensive encephalopathy, epilepsy, meningitis, encephalitis, brain tumour, subdural haematoma and systemic conditions such as cardiovascular, respiratory, or endocrinological disorder, hepatic or renal failure, alcoholism, and withdrawal of certain drugs.

Factors that may determine the appearance of delirium in a particular individual are not always clear. The type and intensity of the physical illness are necessary but not sufficient causes, and personal factors such as old age, brain damage, chronic disease, habituation to drugs or alcohol, history of previous delirium or depression, preoperative insomnia, mental state before illness, or surgical intervention may be of relevance (Willi 1966; Morse and Litin 1969; Morse 1970; Varsamis 1978).

Adequate symptomatic management is important but the delirious patient must not be sedated unless it becomes mandatory due to severe disruptive behaviour, i.e. continually pulling out an intravenous drip or attempts at self-injury. Barbiturates or chloral hydrate should never be used, as they reduce arousal and thereby worsen behavioural problems, while benzodiazepines are indicated only in cases where anticonvulsant effects are also required. In general, a neuroleptic is the drug of choice. Phenothiazines, such as chlorpromazine (± 100 mg intramuscularly followed by 100 mg 4–6 hourly), often produce adequate sedation, but also hypotension, hypothermia, anticholinergic effects and excessive drowsiness. Thioridazine is slightly better in this respect. Haloperidol produces fewer of the above side effects and achieves tranquillization without undue sedation in excitement syndromes (Oldham 1976) A starting dose of 10 mg (intravenously or intramuscularly) can be followed by 10 mg 1–2 hourly until sedation has been achieved. Subsequently, a dose of up to 30 mg (or sometimes more) can be given orally twice a day. If extrapyramidal side effects are produced, they should be neutralized by procyclidine.

Many delirious patients respond to nursing care alone. The fluctuating nature of the syndrome provides lucid periods during which a relationship should be established with the patient, who should be nursed in a well-lit side-room and given a meaningful sensory input such as photographs of relatives or television. A specified nurse should spend as much time as possible with the patient, and repeatedly reassure him that he is not going mad, as his symptoms are temporary and result from his physical illness. If the availability of staff does not allow for this, relatives can be invited to help. If motor agitation is extreme, and the patient is in danger of hurting himself, he should be nursed on a mattress on the floor. Adequate toileting routines, monitoring of biological functions, hydration and sleep, and time-tabling of tranquillizing medication are all important, and also provide patients with external reference points.

On occasions, improvement of the underlying physical condition does not result in a remission of the delirious state. In such cases it may be appropriate to give ECT if the symptoms persist; two or three treatments are usually sufficient (Roth and Rosie 1953; Kramp and Bolwig 1981).

NEUROLOGICAL DISEASE AND PSYCHIATRY

Parkinson's Disease (Marsden and Fahn 1982)

James Parkinson (1817) did not include psychiatric symptoms in the definition of his syndrome; the cases he described exhibited sleep disorders, delirium-like periods and depression. However, since the late nineteenth century, psychopathological complications including personality disorder, neurotic symptoms (obsessions, compulsions, phobias and anxiety states), psychotic states (delusional depression and schizophrenia-like states) and dementia have been considered as common features of the disease (Serby 1980).

The most common psychiatric complications are depression (Robins 1976), dementia (Lieberman et al. 1978) and the psychological side effects of anticholinergic (Johnson et al. 1981) and L-DOPA medication (Mindham et al. 1976). Depression is not related to the degree of motor disability and may respond to antidepressant medication or ECT. There is some circumstantial evidence that the motor component of the disease may also improve temporarily after ECT, but it is not known whether this is a direct effect, or is mediated by the relief of depression (Yudofsky 1979). Manic states are very rare, although states of excitement may occur in the context of drug-induced delirium. Anticholinergic agents, and occasionally L-DOPA, may provoke a number of cognitive changes including drowsiness, lethargy, mild confusion and, less frequently, psychotic states or delirium (Johnson et al. 1981). Schizophrenia-like states have also been described (Hollister and Glazener 1961; Crow et al. 1976).

The reported incidence of 'dementia' in Parkinson's disease varies from 14% to 81%, which probably reflects differences in research methodology. The cognitive impairment is not correlated with the severity of the motor disability and no treatment exists for this complication. L-DOPA does not seem to affect the development of dementia (Editorial 1981).

Huntington's Chorea

Psychiatric complications can develop before, during and in the late stages of this disease (McHugh and Folstein 1977); personality disorders (Minsky and Guttman 1938), neurotic and psychotic symptoms (Garron 1973), and dementia (Caine et al. 1978) are commonly described.

The practical difficulty with the treatment of psychotic complications is that neuroleptics may worsen the chorea. This is unfortunate because paranoid and schizophrenia-like states are frequent complications (Roccatagliata 1979). Severe depressive syndromes may respond to ECT or antidepressants, and it has been claimed that sodium valproate can sometimes relieve the motor syndrome when given in the earlier stages of the disease (Shoulson et al. 1976). There is no treatment for the dementia syndrome. A great deal of social work support for the family may be required as severe social disruption is not uncommon (Dewhurst et al. 1970).

Huntington's chorea is a severe and rare disease. Prevention by genetic counselling and identification of carriers is therefore important. Tests for the latter have not yet been developed but minor behavioural disorders may occasionally help to identify those who will develop the disease and L-DOPA may precipitate chorea in those at genetic risk (Klawans et al. 1973). The value of this procedure has not yet been adequately studied.

Gilles de la Tourette Syndrome and Other Tic States

Genetic evidence supports the view that Gilles de la Tourette syndrome is caused by an organic dysfunction. Of the various therapeutic approaches, haloperidol and pimozide seem to be the most successful (Shapiro et al. 1978) and the appropriate dose must be determined by the severity of the condition, the age of the patient and the development of side effects. Fluctuations in the intensity of the syndrome make therapeutic outcome studies difficult as a number of affected patients tend to improve with time. When complicated by severe obsessional or compulsive phenomena, clomipramine should be prescribed. Depression and lethargy may also be found in association with the condition or its treatment, and the author has occasionally prescribed methylphenidate (5–10 mg twice daily). Surprisingly, this does not worsen the motor symptoms and may produce an improved mood state.

Tics are purposeless, stereotyped and repetitive jerky movements seen in otherwise healthy subjects, which may be worsened by emotional factors (Marsden 1977; Tibbetts 1981). The incidence of tics in children is about 12% and, in general, they have a good prognosis, although in a small minority the disorder will continue into adolescence and adulthood. In some of these patients maladaptive learning or the development of secondary gain will have contributed to the development of the disorder. Many methods of treatment have been used for tics, including behavioural techniques, biofeedback, suggestion, hypnotism, neuroleptics and even surgery. However, tics should be treated only if social functioning is very disrupted as some of the treatments may be worse than the disease.

Writer's cramp, blepharospasm and spasmodic torticollis are, in general, more disabling than tics and require closer attention. Psychological factors may sometimes be relevant but, in general, these states are probably of organic aetiology and may sometimes constitute partial forms of torsion dystonia (Roth 1980). Haloperidol (Mandell 1970), carbamezapine (Isgreen et al. 1976) and L-DOPA (Barbeau 1970) have been tried, with only modest results. Behavioural therapy methods have had limited success in writer's cramp (Liversedge and Sylvester 1955), while the use of relaxation techniques (Crisp and Moldolfsky 1960) and biofeedback (Bindman and Tibbetts 1977) have also been reported. Surgery can often be of some help in severe torticollis or retrocollis (Podinisky 1968).

Postconcussional Syndrome

This has also been called 'post-traumatic syndrome' (Kelly and Smith 1981) and 'accident neurosis' (Miller 1961). It is increasingly believed that the features of this syndrome have an organic basis (Taylor 1967; Kelly 1981), and it has been claimed that post-traumatic loss of consciousness and amnesia, however brief, almost always implies brain damage (Noseworthy et al. 1981). It has also been reported that return to work after the settlement of litigation does not occur as often as it was once believed, and that many patients return to work before any compensation is settled (Kelly and Smith 1981). In addition, the extent of social dysfunction in the brain-damaged is directly related to the severity of the head injury (Keshavan et al. 1981).

This new view of the postconcussional syndrome requires the psychiatrist to appreciate that psychotherapy or careful rehabilitation may not, after all, be sufficient (Editorial 1967). Symptoms such as headache, dizziness, lethargy, poor concentration, unreliable memory, insomnia, loss of libido and impotence may therefore require specific management, if this is available. Cerebral stimulants and L-DOPA may occasionally be tried when marked lethargy is present, while behavioural techniques and retraining may improve memory and concentration.

Improvement of the psychiatric symptoms in this syndrome may be the result of a number of factors such as reorganization or readaptation of neural pathways (Miller 1980*a*), relearning (Miller 1980*b*) and improvement of secondary or reactive mood disorder.

Multiple Sclerosis

This common demyelinating disease has many neurological and psychiatric manifestations. The neurological diagnosis is often uncertain during its early stages, when it may be considered as conversion hysteria, while later, there may be severe and widespread lesions leading to marked dementia (Koenig 1968). Most cases are between these extremes and the psychiatric complications result from a variety of mechanisms. On occasions, frontal lobe involvement may lead to euphoric disinhibited behaviour, and in the classic literature this inappropriate cheerfulness was considered as the main psychopathological complication (Cottrell and Wilson 1926). However, this has not been substantiated, and irritability and depression are common during the early stages of the disease (Surridge 1969). Other psychopathological symptoms include a tendency to develop hysterical conversions (Brain 1930) and, most importantly, the development of varying degrees of cognitive impairment (Jambor 1969).

For the psychiatrist, working closely with neurologists in the general hospital, the most common problem related to multiple sclerosis is the persistent depression which often interferes with rehabilitation. The depressive syndrome does not often respond to tricyclic antidepressants, but monoamine oxidase inhibitors induce some improvement. The usual pattern is for patients to become depressed as the physical complications begin to subside in response to the treatment with ACTH. This may be partly due to the effects of ACTH on mood. Vigorous social support, sexual counselling and practical advice with regard to structural alterations at home are also important. ECT may be of some benefit in some cases with marked suicidal tendency but, in the experience of the author, it may worsen the cognitive impairment.

Wilson's Disease

Wilson's disease is an inherited autosomal recessive abnormality in the hepatic excretion of copper, which results in toxic accumulation of the metal in the liver, brain and other organs (Walshe 1976). Various psychiatric disturbances may be evident early in the disease and include irritability, antisocial behaviour and neurotic phenomena, which can be superseded by psychotic states and schizophrenia-like syndromes (Beard 1959). Davison and Bagley (1969) have claimed that 'there is evidence to suggest that schizophrenia-like psychoses occur in association with Wilson's disease more frequently than chance expectation, and absence of genetic pre-disposition and progression to dementia confirm their organic basis'. Manic–depressive-like syndromes can also be seen, and occasionally bizarre behavioural disturbances occur which defy classification. Pharmacological reduction of the copper excess with penicillamine often leads to improvement of the psychiatric condition. Use of neuroleptics is limited by their extrapyramidal side effects. ECT may occasionally be used. Severe behavioural disturbance may occur in patients who become 'locked in', when they exhibit severe rigidity and anarthria without major cognitive impairment. In these cases it is crucial that ways are found (such as electronic gadgets) which allow the patient to communicate, or extreme frustration may engender antisocial behaviour. Insomnia is common and can be treated with benzodiazepines.

The Brain-Damaged Patient

The quality and duration of the psychiatric complications in brain-damaged patients vary according to the intensity, type and lateralization of the dysfunction (Jennett and Teasdale 1981; Ross and Rush 1981). Other factors which are relevant to the psychiatric sequelae are the type of onset and speed of progression of the injury, and the premorbid personality of the patient (Denecker 1960).

Head injury is the commonest cause of brain damage. Over 90% of deaths after severe head injury occur during the first 48 h (Carlsson et al. 1968), but modern resuscitatory techniques have led to the survival of severe cases with marked psychiatric sequelae. Duration of the post-traumatic amnesia is still the most commonly used index of severity, with less than 5 min being mild, and over 4 weeks extremely severe (Editorial 1961). In general it can be said that the most remarkable feature of the long-term course of patients with severe head injury is their capacity for recovery from both neurological and psychiatric deficits (Sisler 1978). Gradual improvement in cognitive function can go on for years but the mechanisms involved in this process are unknown; two explanations have been put forward: anatomical reorganization and functional adaptation (Miller 1980a), but as evidence for the former is limited in the adult (Levere 1975), it is likely that most of the recovery of psychological function occurs as a result of functional adaptation. On the basis of this hypothesis, a number of behavioural techniques can be used to train head injury patients to readapt (Miller 1980b).

Apart from specific psychological deficits involving attention, memory and perception, head injury patients may exhibit psychiatric symptoms such as panic attacks, phobias, depressions, obsessions, compulsions, hallucinations and delusions (Lishman 1973). Symptomatic treatment should be offered and may include antidepressant drugs, ECT, neuroleptics and behavioural techniques. Not infrequently the organic impairment releases hysterical symptoms which may complicate the picture and tempt the clinician to consider all the symptoms as hysterical.

Endocrinological Conditions and Psychiatry

Endocrinological disease is associated with an increased incidence of psychiatric complications (Smith et al. 1972; Sachar 1973; Beumont 1979), and it is assumed that brain dysfunction is the predominant mechanism involved (Ettigi and Brown 1978).

In general an organic disorder should be suspected when certain forms of affective disorder are found, for example, an atypical depressive syndrome with paranoid features, apathy or retardation which is unresponsive to treatment. Hyperthyroidism (Taylor 1975), hypothyroidism (Reed and Bland 1977), hyperparathyroidism (Gastewood et al. 1967), hypoparathyroidism (Fourman et al. 1967; Michie et al. 1971) and carcinoma of the pancreas (Fras et al. 1967) must be considered as possible diagnoses.

Panic attacks may occasionally be associated with phaeochromocytoma (Thomas et al. 1966), while a neurotic syndrome or uncharacteristic behaviour may be associated with insulinomas (Service et al. 1976) or functional hyperinsulinaemia (Marks and Rose 1965).

It is important to remember that the associated psychiatric syndrome may not improve even after successful treatment for the underlying endocrinopathy, so that active psychiatric treatment is often necessary. On the other hand, the psychiatric condition tends to remain resistant to therapy while the underlying condition persists.

Certain recognized disorders must be kept in mind; for example, surgical treatment for thyrotoxicosis may damage the vascular supply to the parathyroid and lead to a therapy-resistant form of 'irritable' depression which may improve on calcium therapy (Fourman et al. 1967). Cushing's syndrome is frequently observed to be associated with mental disorder, and Cohen (1982) found that 25% of a sample of 29 Cushing's patients suffered from depression, mainly those with a pituitary tumour. Depression seems to be the most common symptom (Carroll 1977), followed by an organic brain syndrome with varied involvement of memory and orientation (Whybrow and Hurwitz 1976). Steroid psychosis is yet another state of hypercortisolism which is associated with mental disorder. Hall et al. (1979) have found that psychotic reactions are more likely to develop when daily doses are in excess of 40 mg prednisone (or equivalent); that the most likely time of onset is 6 days after initiation of steroid therapy; that premorbid personality, previous psychiatric illness and history of previous steroid psychosis do not increase the likelihood of the patient developing an episode; that the most likely symptoms are anxiety, distractibility, pressure of speech, insomnia, depression, perplexity, auditory and visual

hallucinations, delusion, apathy and hypomania; and that tricyclic antidepressants worsen the condition. The phenothiazines are indicated in all cases. The
reported incidence of steroid psychosis varies according to the underlying
condition and dose of steroid, from 1.8% to 24% (Granville-Grossman 1971).
Popkin and McKenzie (1980) concluded that certain symptoms, such as
depressive and cognitive dysfunction, seem to be common to a number of
endocrinological disorders; that the therapeutic emphasis must always be on
the underlying endocrinopathy rather than on the psychiatric state; and that
treatment of the latter must wait until the endocrinological correction has taken
place.

Hypoglycaemia is another endocrinological state which may lead to temporary psychiatric disorder (Jefferson and Marshall 1981). The clinical manifestation of reduced blood glucose can be separated into two groups. Firstly,
palpitations, sweating, anxiety, tremor, weakness, and languor are associated
with a rapid decline in blood glucose, and secondly, headache, lightheadedness,
fatigue, lethargy, seizure, fugue-like states, episodic confusion and periods of
depersonalization. A number of these symptoms may lead to the diagnosis of
personality disorder or neurotic behaviour, and it is therefore important to
maintain a high level of suspicion when the behaviour is worse late in the
morning, as occurs in the reactive hypoglycaemias, or in episodes, as may occur
in the case of insulinomas. Treatment of the cause of the hypoglycaemia is
imperative.

Occasionally the association of psychiatric disorder and endocrinopathy may
be coincidental. In these cases the psychiatric condition will respond to
treatment independently of the endocrinological status.

Disorders of Fluid and Electrolyte Balance

These may result from disease or, on occasion, occur as a complication of
medication. A number of neuropsychiatric symptoms are associated with
disorders of sodium, potassium, calcium, phosphorus, magnesium, water or
acid–base balance (Baer 1973).

Sodium. Hypernatremia (i.e. when the serum concentration is above 150
mmol/litre) leads to central nervous system symptoms such as restlessness,
hyperactivity, depression of sensorium, disorientation, visual hallucinations,
tremor, muscle twitching and seizures (Logothetis 1966; Bruck et al. 1968;
Arieff and Guisado 1976). Hypernatremia may accompany such conditions as
diabetes insipidus, Cushing's syndrome, primary aldosteronism (Conn's syndrome) or accidental salt poisoning (e.g. due to the induction of vomiting in
subjects who have taken an overdose). The EEG may be normal but can show
slow activity or focal epileptic activity. The neuropsychiatric symptoms result
from a reduction of brain fluid, tissue shrinkage and secondary complications
such as damage to blood vessels and petechial haemorrhages. Correction of the

hypernatremia must take precedence, and be carried out gradually, as overenthusiastic water replenishment may lead to seizures.

Hyponatremia may be seen in oedematous states which may be due to congestive cardiac failure, hepatic cirrhosis, or the nephrotic syndrome. It can also be associated with the syndrome of inappropriate ADH secretion (Bartter and Schwarz 1967) and in compulsive water drinking (psychogenic polydipsia), which is sometimes encountered amongst the psychiatrically ill (Noonan and Ananth 1977). Serum levels of sodium under 130 mmol/litre may lead to anorexia, tiredness and dulled sensorium, while levels under 120 mmol/litre produce weakness, nausea, restlessness, confusion and delirium. Water intoxication shows similar symptoms, together with seizures, stupor, dysphasia, flapping tremor and coma. Psychotic patients who develop psychogenic polydipsia, when they drink large amounts of water, may soon develop water intoxication (Mendelson and Deza 1976; Noonan and Ananth 1977; Smith and Clark 1980). In these cases the increased intake may not be sufficient to explain the water intoxication syndrome, and it has been claimed that some of these patients also develop inappropriate secretion of antidiuretic hormone (ADH) (Raskind et al. 1972). This disorder consists of a continuous release of ADH unrelated to plasma osmolality, which leads to an expansion of extracellular fluid volume and to dilutional hyponatremia. Before treatment is offered to the psychotic patient with water intoxication, it is important to rule out inappropriate secretion of ADH.; its presence must be suspected when there is hyponatraemia in a patient with urine which is hypertonic relative to plasma. A complicating factor is that 'severe stress' may lead to a physiological release of ADH even in the presence of hypotonicity (Martin et al. 1977).

Potassium. Hyperkalaemia (i.e. when the serum level is over 5 mmol/litre) can be produced by excessive intake, impaired renal secretion and potassium shift from the intracellular compartments. Hyperkalaemia may produce atrial and ventricular fibrillation, cardiac arrest, heart block, general weakness, paraesthesiae, flaccid ascending paralysis, clouding of consciousness, confusion and dysarthria (Bull et al. 1953). Hypokalaemia (i.e. when the serum level is under 3 mmol/litre) is associated with gastrointestinal and renal loss, and intracellular shift. This is more likely to be seen in relation to psychiatric illness (e.g. in anorexia nervosa patients abusing laxatives), and is characterized by irritability, paraesthesiae, headache, dysphoric mood, weakness, 'depression', cognitive impairment, confusion and paralysis. Correction of the imbalance must be the priority of treatment.

Calcium. Hypercalcaemia leads to sedation, lack of energy, fatigue, irritability and memory deficit. This may be mistaken for affective disorder or early dementia, particularly in the elderly. Hypocalcaemia, on the other hand, is associated with increased neuromuscular irritability, anxiety and stuporous or catatonia-like states. The hyperventilation syndrome and its accompanying muscle spasm and paraesthesiae are related to a reduction of ionized calcium produced by the ensuing respiratory alkalosis.

Magnesium. Severe hypermagnesaemia produces lethargy, sedation and coma, while hypomagnesaemia is related to changes such as irritability, nervousness, restlessness, emotionality and a depressed mood. Tremors, hyperreflexia and athetoid movements can occasionally be seen.

Acid-balance disorder. Metabolic acidosis may be caused by renal disease, increased acid production or alkali loss, and leads to hyperventilation, fatigue, depression of consciousness, and anorexia. Metabolic alkalosis produces irritability, apathy, confusion and hypoventilation, and can be found in cases of volume depletion (such as occurs in the abuse of diuretics), in excessive alkali intake, or in potassium depletion.

Renal, Cardiovascular and Hepatic Disease and Psychiatry

Psychiatric symptoms can be seen in association with a number of failure syndromes in systemic disease. There is no identifiable pattern, and the most common are nonspecific feelings of malaise, lethargy, tiredness and headache which may resemble a depressive syndrome (Kathol and Petty 1981). In addition, typical confusional states or deliria can be seen. These stereotyped states develop in response to the severity and acuteness of the underlying condition. Occasionally the symptoms result from overmedication or from idiosyncratic responses to the treatment.

Renal disease. Renal failure may be defined as a reduction of kidney function to the point that it is no longer able to maintain chemical homeostasis. The psychiatric symptoms relate to the acuteness and severity of this state. The neuropsychiatric symptoms of uraemia include apathy, malaise, memory impairment, restlessness, stereotyped movements, insomnia, the restless-leg syndrome and decreased libido. In severe forms, so-called uraemic delirium can develop, with paranoid, demanding or negativistic behaviour, which may lead to confusion, visual hallucinations and muttering speech. Stupor and coma with generalized muscle twitching and convulsions are seen during the terminal stages. Schreiver (1959) described a patient who was given psychotherapy for a number of months to 'treat' a stereotyped movement of his knee which proved to be the first sign of renal failure.

Cardiovascular disease. A number of neuropsychiatric symptoms can be found in association with disease of the heart or its vessels, and worry about the illness, in particular myocardial infarction, may be of sufficient intensity to interfere with rehabilitation.

During the early stages of congestive cardiac failure the symptoms of paroxysmal nocturnal dyspnoea can be confused with nocturnal anxiety. Such impaired sleep may lead to diurnal mood disorder and tiredness. During severe congestive heart failure, patients often exhibit irritability, marked anxiety and temporary cognitive impairment with reduced concentration. Sedation with benzodiazepines must sometimes be considered.

Anxiety states, accompanied by an increased heart rate or palpitations, may, on occasion, be the patient's response to cardiac disorders, which include a number of arrhythmias. The engendered anxiety may itself trigger further palpitations by inducing atrial tachycardia. More severe disorders of rhythm (e.g. bradycardia or heart block), may lead to a reduction in cerebral circulation which may induce or worsen cognitive impairment (Abdon and Malmcrona 1975; Editorial 1977).

Anxiety states, accompanied by sweating and acute headache can be the only early manifestation of phaeochromocytoma (Deake and Ebough 1956; Mànger and Gifford 1977), and the fact that attacks may occur in certain situations, such as defaecation or sexual intercourse, can be misleading.

The cardiac myxoma is a benign, mostly atrial tumour (75% are in the left atrium), which produces various medical manifestations such as syncope, epileptiform seizures, coma, cyanosis, weakness, anaemia and weight loss; it can also produce psychiatric disorders such as 'episodic bizarre behaviour', and anxiety states (Greenwood 1968; Wenger 1970; Wharton 1977).

The psychiatrist can usefully be involved in the management of the psychopathological complications of common cardiovascular disorders such as myocardial infarction. Age may influence the symptomatology of this condition in that, in the elderly, up to 25% of coronary occlusions may be painless. Thus, medical attention is not usually sought at the time, and the presenting problems may be subsequent cardiac insufficiency or a confusional state.

Depression and anxiety may follow myocardial infarction (MI) and Kavanagh et al. (1975) found that about 34% of their sample were still depressed after 18 months. The tendency is relatively marked amongst the elderly (Peach and Pathy 1979), and one over-riding complication seems to be anxiety (Byrne 1979). The anxiety experienced by the MI patient tends to fluctuate between hospital admission and discharge, and marked fluctuations have been shown to predict poor rehabilitation outcome (Philip et al. 1979). Another common and potentially stress-inducing complication is sexual dysfunction after MI (Krop et al. 1971; McLane et al. 1980), and depression or anxiety may be secondary to this problem. The family of the patient who has had an MI may also develop anxiety and depression (Stern and Pascale 1979).

The identification of variables which might predict psychiatric outcome is not easy. If depression is apparent soon after the MI, this seems to predict a bad outcome (Stern et al. 1977), while the patient's occupation also seems to have some relevance, in that 'blue collar' workers develop more anxiety than their 'white collar' counterparts (Byrne 1980).

It has been argued that more attention should be paid to various aspects of rehabilitation following MI (Ross and Botha 1979; Billings 1980), and counselling, carried out by trained nurses, has been found to be of benefit (Naismith et al. 1979). In another study, behavioural treatment involving the teaching of relaxation training (in addition to counselling) was superior to counselling alone (Fielding 1980), and regulated physical exercise has also been found to be of benefit in terms of a number of physiological variables (Schlesinger and Barzilay 1980).

Gastrointestinal and hepatic disease in relation to psychiatry. McKeghey (1977) has classified the psychiatric complications associated with gastrointestinal disturbance under three headings: affective, cognitive and organic brain syndromes.

A depressed mood has been reported in association with carcinoma of the pancreas (Fras et al. 1967), and it is also a common accompaniment of the so-called posthepatitis syndrome when it tends to be refractory to conventional antidepressant therapy (Hall 1980). Depression can also follow inflammatory and chemical hepatitis (Read et al. 1967). Other conditions occasionally found in association with a depressive syndrome are ulcerative colitis, regional enteritis, cirrhosis, pernicious anaemia (Roos 1978), folic acid deficiency (Shulman 1979) and the carcinoid syndrome (Major et al. 1973).

Cognitive changes such as reduced concentration, memory impairment and confusion can be seen in hepatic encephalopathy and alcohol withdrawal, and may gradually develop into full-blown delirious or confusional states in direct proportion to the severity of the underlying pathology. Apart from hepatic encephalopathy, acute pancreatitis may lead to a number of neuropsychiatric complications such as memory deficit, agitation, disorientation and confabulation (Schuster 1980). However, a number of patients in this latter study were alcoholics.

References

ABDON, M.J. & MALMCRONA, R. (1975) High pacemaker implantation rate following 'cardiogenic neurology'. *Acta med. scand.*, **198**, 455.

ARIEFF, A.I. & GUISADO, R. (1976) Effects on the central nervous system of hypernatremic and hyponatremic states. *Kidney Int.*, **10**, 104.

BAER, L. (1973) Electrolyte metabolism in psychiatric disorders. In: *Biological Psychiatry*, ed. Mendes, J., pp. 199–234. Wiley, New York.

BANT, W.P. (1978) Antihypertensive drugs and depression: a reappraisal. *Psychol. Med.*, **1**, 275.

BARBEAU, A. (1970) Rationale for the use of L-DOPA in the torsion dystonias. *Neurology*, **20**, 96.

BARTTER, F.C. & SCHWARTZ, W.B. (1967) The syndrome of inappropriate water secretion of antidiuretic hormone. *Am. J. Med.*, **42**, 790.

BAUT, W.P. (1978) Antihypertensive drugs and depression: a reappraisal. *Psychol. Med.*, **8**, 275.

BEARD, A.W. (1959) The association of hepatolenticular degeneration with schizophrenia. *Acta. psychiat. neurol. scand.*, **34**, 411.

BERRIOS, G.E. (1982) Disorientation states and psychiatry. *Compreh. Psychiat.*, **23**, 479.

BEUMONT, P.J.V. (1979) The endocrinology of psychiatry. In: *Recent Advances in Clinical Psychiatry*, ed. Granville-Grossman, K. Vol. 3, pp. 185–224. Edinburgh: Churchill Livingstone.

BILLINGS, C.K. (1980) Management of psychological responses to myocardial infarction. *Southern med. J.*, **73**, 1367.

BINDMAN, E. & TIBBETTS, R.W. (1977). *Br. J. Psychiat.*, **131**, 143.

BONHOEFFER, K. (1910) *Die symptomatischen Psychosen*. Leipzig: Deuticke.

BRAIN, W.R. (1930) Critical review: disseminated sclerosis. *Q. Jl. Med.*, **23**, 343.

BRUCK, E., ABUL, G. & ACETO, T. (1968) Pathogenesis and pathophysiology of hypertonic dehydration with diarrhoea. *Am. J. Dis. Child.*, **115**, 122.

BULL, G.M., CARTER, A.B. & LOWE, K.G. (1953) Hyperpotassaemic paralysis. *Lancet*, **ii**, 60.

BYRNE, D.G. (1979) Anxiety as state and trait following survived myocardial infarction. *Br. J. Soc. Clin. Psychol.*, **18**, 417.

CAINE, E.D., HUNT, R.D., WEINGARTNER, H. & EBERT, M.H. (1978) Huntington's dementia. *Archs gen. Psychiat.*, **35**, 379.

CARLSSON, C.A., ESSEN, C. VON & LÖFGREN, J. (1968) Factors affecting the clinical course of patients with severe head injury. *J. Neurosurg.* **29**, 242.

CARROLL, B.J. (1977) Mood disturbance and pituitary-affected diseases. *Psychosom. Med.*, **39**, 54.

CHASLIN, P. (1892) La confusion mentale primitive. *Annal. Med. Psychol.*, **16**, 225.

CLARKE, M.G. et al. (1982) Psychiatric consultations in clinical haematology. *J. Royal Soc. Med.*, **75**, 613.

COHEN, S.I. (1982) Psychiatric aspects of Cushing's syndrome. *Br. J. Hosp. Med.*, **27**, 548.

COTTRELL, S.S. & WILSON,S.A.K. (1926) The affective symptomatology of disseminated sclerosis: a study of 100 cases. *J. Neurol. Psychopath.*, **7**, 1.

CRISP, A.H. & MOLDOFSKY, H. (1965) A psychosomatic study of writer's cramp. *Br. J. Psychiat.*, **111**, 841.

CROW, T.J., JOHNSTONE, E.C. & McCLELLAND, H.A. (1976) The coincidence of schizophrenia and parkinsonism: some neurochemical considerations. *Psychol. Med.*, **6**, 227.

DAVIS, H. & BEUMONT, P.J.V. (1973) Psychiatric aspects of laryngectomy. *S. Afr. med. J.*, **47**, 2192.

DAVISON, K. & BAGLEY, C.R. (1969) Schizophrenia-like psychoses associated with organic disorders of the central nervous system: a review of the literature. In: *Current Problems in Neuropsychiatry*, ed. Herrington, R.N. London: Royal Medico-Psychological Society.

DEAKE, F.R. & EBOUGH, E.G. (1956) Phaeochromocytoma and E.C.T. *Am. J. Psychiat.*, **113**, 295.

DENCKER, S.J. (1960) Closed head injury. *Archs gen. Psychiat.*, **2**, 569.

DEWHURST, K., OLIVER, J.E. & McKNIGHT, A.L. (1970) Socio-psychiatric consequences of Huntington's disease. *Br. J. Psychiat.*, **116**, 255.

DLIN, B.M., PERLMAN, A. & RINGOLD, E. (1969) Psychosexual response to ileostomy and colostomy. *Am. J. Psychiat.*, **126**, 374.

D.S.M. III (1980) *Diagnostic and Statistical Manual of Mental Disorders (Third Edition)*. Washington: American Psychiatric Association.

EASTWOOD, M.R. & TREVELYAN. M.H. (1972) Relationship between Physical and Psychiatric Disorder. *Psychol. Med.*, **2**, 363.

ECONOMO, C. VON 1931) *Encehalitis Lethargica*. London: Oxford University Press.

EDITORIAL (1961) The best yardstick we have. *Lancet*, **ii**, 1445.

EDITORIAL (1967) Post concussional syndrome. *Br. med. J.*, **iii**, 61.

EDITORIAL (1977) Cardiogenic dementia. *Lancet*, **i**, 27.

EDITORIAL (1981) Levodopa: long-term impact in Parkinson's disease. *Br. med. J.*, **i**, 417.

ETTIGI, P.G. & BROWN, G.M. (1978) Brain disorders associated with endocrine dysfunction. *Psychiat. Clin. North Amer.*, **1**, 117.

FIELDING, R. (1980) A note on behavioural treatment in the rehabilitation of myocardial infarction patients. *Br. J. Soc. Clin. Psychol.*, **19**, 157.

FOURMAN, P., DAVIS, R.H., RAWNSLEY, K. & JONES, K.H. (1967) Effect of calcium on mental symptoms in partial parathyroid insufficiency. *Lancet*, **ii**, 914.

FRAS, I., LITIU, E.M. & PEARSON, J.S. (1967) Comparison of psychiatric symptoms in carcinoma of the pancreas with those in some other intraabdominal neoplasms. *Am. J. Psychiat.*, **123**, 1553.

GARRON, D.G. (1973) Huntington's Chorea and Schizophrenia. In: *Advances in Neurology, Vol. 1*, ed. Barbeau, A. et al. New York: Raven Press.

GATEWOOD, J.W., ORGAN, C.H. & MEAD, B.T. (1975) Mental changes associated with hyperparathyroidism. *Am. J. Psychiat.*, **132**, 129.

GRANVILLE-GROSSMAN, K. (1971) *Recent Advances in Clinical Psychiatry*. London: J.R.A. Churchill.

GREENWOOD, W.F. (1968) Profile of atrial myxoma. *Am. J. Cardiol.*, **21**, 367.

HACKETT, T.P. & CASSEM, N.H. (1978) *Handbook of General Hospital Psychiatry*. St. Louis: Mosby.

HALL, R.C.W. (1980) Depression. In: *Psychiatric Presentations of Medical Illness*, ed. Hall, R.C.W. Leicester: M.T.P.

HALL, R.C.W. et al. (1978) Physical illness presenting as psychiatric disease. *Archs gen. Psychiat.*, **35**, 1315.

HALL, R.C.W., POPKIN, K.K., STICKNEY, S.K. & GARDNER, E.R. (1979) Presentation of the Steroid Psychoses. *J. nerv. ment. Dis.*, **167**, 229.

HECAEN, H. & ALBERT, M.L. (1979) *Human Neuropsychology*. New York: John Wiley.

HOLLISTER, L.E. & GLAZENER, F.S. (1961) Concurrent paralysis agitans and schizophrenia. *Dis. neur. Syst.*, **22**, 187.

I.C.D. 9 (1978) *Mental Disorders: Glossary and Guide to their Classification in Accordance with the Ninth Revision of the International Classification of Diseases*. Geneva: World Health Organization.

ISGREEN, W.P., FAHN, S., BARRETT, R.E. et al. (1976) Carbamezapine in torsion dystonia. In: *Dystonia. Advances in Neurology*, Vol. 14, ed. Eldridge, R. & Fahn, S. New York: Raven Press.

JACOBS, S. & DOUGLAS, L. (1979) Grief: A mediating process between a loss and illness. *Compreh. Psychiat.*, **20**, 165.

JAMBOR, J.K. (1969) Cognitive functioning in multiple sclerosis. *Br. J. Psychiat.*, **115**, 765.

JASPERS, K. (1963) *General Psychopathology*. Manchester: Manchester University Press.

JEFFERSON, J.W. & MARSHALL, J.R. (1981) *Neuropsychiatric Features of Medical Disorders*. New York: Plenum Medical.

JENNETT, B., SNOEK, J., BOND, M.R. & BROOKS, N. (1981). Disability after severe head injury: observations on the use of the Glasgow Outcome Scale. *J. Neurol. Neurosurg. Psychiat.*, **44**, 285.

JENNETT, B. & TEASDALE, G. (1981) *Management of Head Injuries*. Philadelphia: Davis.

JOHNSON, A.N., HOLLISTER, L.E. & BERGER, P.A. (1981) The anticholinergic intoxication syndrome. *J. clin. Psychiat.*, **42**, 313.

KATHOL, R.G. & PETTY, F. (1981) Relationship of depression to medical illness. *J. Affect. Dis.*, **3**, 111.

KAVANAGH, T., SHEPHERD, R.J. & TUCK, J.A. (1975) Depression after myocardial infarction. *C.M.A. Journal*, **113**, 27.

KELLY, R. (1981) The post traumatic syndrome. *J. R. Soc. Med.*, **74**, 242.

KELLY, R. & SMITH, B.N. (1981) Post traumatic syndrome: another myth discredited. *J. R. Soc. Med.*, **74**, 275.

KESHAVAN, M.S., CHANNABASAVANNA, S.M. & REDDY, G.N.N. (1981) Post-traumatic psychiatric disturbance: patterns and predictors of outcome. *Br. J. Psychiat.*, **138**, 157.

KILOH, L.G. et al. (1972) *Clinical Electroencephalography*, 3rd ed. London: Butterworths.

KLAWANS, H.L., PAULSON, G.W., RINGEL, S.P. & BARBEAU, A. (1973) The use of L-DOPA in the presymptomatic detection of Huntington's chorea. In: *Advances in Neurology Vol. 2*, ed. Barbeau, A. et al. New York: Raven Press.

KOENIG, H. (1968) Dementia associated with the benign form of multiple sclerosis. *Trans. Am. neurol. Ass.*, **93**, 227.

KRAMP, P. & BOLWIG, T.G. (1981) Electroconvulsive therapy in acute delirious states. *Compreh. Psychiat.*, **22**, 368.

KROP, H., HALL, D. & MEHTA, J. (1971) Sexual concerns after myocardial infarction. *Sex Disability*, **2**, 91.

LEVERE, (1975) Neural stability, sparing and behavioural recovery following brain damage. *Psychol. Rev.*, **82**, 344.

LIEBERMAN, A., CZIATOLOWSKI, M., KUPERSMITH, M. et al. (1978) Dementia in Parkinson's disease. *Ann. Neurol.*, **6**, 355.

LIPOWSKI, Z.J. (1975a) Psychiatry of Somatic Diseases: Epidemiology, Pathogenesis, Classification. *Compreh. Psychiat.*, **16**, 105.

LIPOWSKI, Z.J. (1975b) Consultation–liaison psychiatry: past, present and future. In: *Consultation–Liaison Psychiatry*, Ed. Pasnau, R.O. New York: Grune and Stratton.

LIPOWSKI, Z.J. (1980) Delirium. In: *Acute Brain Failure in Man*. Springfield, Illinois: Charles C. Thomas.

LISHMAN, W.A. (1973) The psychiatric sequelae of head injury: a review. *Psychol. Med.* **3**, 304.

LIVERSEDGE, L.A. & SYLVESTER, J.D. (1955) Conditioning techniques in the treatment of writer's cramp. *Lancet*, **i**, 1147.

LLOYD, G.G. (1977) Psychological reactions to physical illness. *Br. J. hosp. Med.*, **18**, 352.

LOGOTHETIS, J. (1966) Neurological effects of water and sodium disturbance. *Postgrad. med. J.*, **40**, 408.

MAGUIRE, P. (1981) Psychiatric aspects of malignant disease. *S.K. & F. Publications*, **4**, London: E.S.D.

MAJOR, L.E., BROWN, G.L. & WILSON, W.P. (1973) Carcinoid and psychiatric symptoms. *Sth. med. J.*, **66**, 787.

MANDELL, S. (1970) The Treatment of Dystonia with L-DOPA and Haloperidol. *Neurology*, **20**, 103.

MANGER, W.M. & GIFFORD, R.W. (1977) *Phaeochromocytoma*. Berlin, Heidelberg, New York: Springer-Verlag.

MARKS, E. & ROSE, F.C. (1965) *Hypoglycemia*. Oxford: Blackwell Scientific.

MARSDEN, C.D. & FAHN, S. (eds) (1982) *Movement Disorders*. London: Butterworths.

MARSDEN, C.D., TARSY, D. & BALDESSARINI, R.J. (1977) Spontaneous and drug-induced movement disorders in psychiatric patients. In: *Psychiatric Aspects of Neurological Disease*, ed. Benson, D.F. & Blumer, D. New York: Grune and Stratton.

MARTIN, J.B., REICHLIN, S. & BROWN, G.M. (1977) *Clinical Neuroendocrinology*, p. 74. Philadelphia: Davis.

McHUGH, P.R. & FOLSTEIN, M.F. (1977) Psychiatric syndromes of Huntington's chorea. In: *Psychiatric Aspects of Neurological Disease*, ed. Benson, D.F. and Blumer, D. New York: Grune and Stratton.

McKEGHEY, F.P. (1977) Psychiatric syndromes associated with gastrointestinal symptoms. *Clin. Gastroenterol.*, **6**, 675.

McLANE, M., KROP, H. & MEHTA, J. (1980) Psychosexual adjustment and counselling after myocardial infarction. *Ann. intern. Med.*, **92**, 514.

MENDELSON, W.B. & DEZA, P.C. (1976) Polydipsia, hyponatremia and seizures in psychotic patients. *J. nerv. ment. Dis.*, **162**, 140.

MICHIE, W., DUNCAN, T., HAMER-HODGES, D.W. et al. (1971) Mechanism of hypocalcaemia after thyroidectomy for thyrotoxicosis. *Lancet*, **i**, 508.

MILLER, E. (1980*a*) Psychological intervention in the management and rehabilitation of neuropsychological patients. *Behav. Res. Ther.*, **18**, 527.

MILLER, E. (1980*b*) The training characteristics of severely head-injured patients: a preliminary study. *J. Neurol. Neurosurg. Psychiat.*, **43**, 525.

MILLER, H. (1961) Accident neurosis. *Br. med. J.*, **ii**, 919.

MINDHAM, R.H.S., MARSDEN, C.D. & PARKES, J.D. (1976) Psychiatric symptoms during L-dopa therapy for Parkinson's disease and their relationship to physical disability. *Psychol. Med.*, **6**, 23.

MINSKY, L. & GUTTMAN, E. (1938) Huntington's chorea: a study of 34 families. *J. ment. Sci.*, **84**, 21.

MORSE, R.M. (1970) Postoperative delirium: a syndrome of multiple causation. *Psychosomatics*, **22**, 164.

MORSE, R.M. & LITIN, E.M. (1969) Postoperative delirium: a study of aetiological factors. *Am. J. Psychiat.*, **126**, 388.

NADELSON, T. (1976) The psychiatrist in the surgical intensive care unit. I—Postoperative delirium. *Archs gen. Psychiat.*, **111**, 113.

NAISMITH, L.D., ROBINSON, J.F., SHAW, G.B. & MACINTYRE, K.K.J. (1979) Psychological rehabilitation after myocardial infarction. *Br. Med. J.*, **i**, 439.

NOONAN, J.P.A. & ANANTH, J. (1977) Compulsive water drinking and water intoxication. *Compreh. Psychiat.*, **18**, 183.

NOSEWORTHY, J.H., MILLER, J., MURRAY, T.J. & REGAN, D. (1981) Auditory brain stem responses in postconcussion syndrome. *Arch. Neurol.*, **38**, 275.

OLDMAN, A.J.P. (1976) The rapid control of the acute patient by haloperidol. *Proc. R. Soc. Med.*, **69**, (suppl. 1), 23.

PARKES, C.M. & NAPIER, M.M. (1973) Psychiatric sequelae of amputation. *Br. J. hosp. Med.*, **4**, 610.

PEACH, H. & PATHY, J. (1979) Disability in the elderly after myocardial infarction. *J. R. Coll. Physicians*, **13**, 154.

PHILIP, A.E., CAY, E.L., VETTER, N.J. & STUCKEY, N.A. (1979) Short-term fluctuations in anxiety in patients with myocardial infarction. *J. psychosom. Res.*, **23**, 277.

PODINISKY, F. (1968) Torticollis. In: *Handbook of Clinical Neurology*, Vol. 6, ed. Vinken & Bruyn. Amsterdam: North Holland.

POPKIN, M.K. & MACKENZIE, T.B. (1980) Psychiatric presentation of endocrine dysfunction. In: *Psychiatric Presentation of Medical Illness*, ed. Hall, R.C.W., p. 139. Lancaster: M.T.P.

POTTASH, A.L.C., BLACK, H.R. & GOLD, M. (1981) Psychiatric complications of antihypertensive medications. *J. Nerv. ment. Dis.*, **169**, 430.

PRITCHARD, M. (1982) Psychological pressure in a renal unit. *Br. J. Hosp. Med.*, **27**, 512.

RASKIND, M.A., ORRUSTEIN, H. & CHRISTOPHER, T.G. (1972) Acute psychosis, increased water ingestion and inappropriate antidiuretic hormone secretion. *Am. J. Psychiat.*, **132**, 907.

READ, A.E., SHERLOCK, S., LAIDLOW, J. & WALKER, J.G. (1967) Neuropsychiatric syndromes associated with chronic liver disease and an extensive portalsystemic collateral circulation. *Q. Jl. Med.*, **36**, 135.

REED, K. & BLAND, R.C. (1977) Marked 'myxedema madness'. *Acta. psychiat. scand.*, **56**, 421.

ROBINS, A.H. (1976) Depression in patients with parkinsonism. *Br. J. Psychiat.*, **128**, 141.

ROCCATAGLIATA, G. (1979) *Psicosi e corea di Huntington*. Pisa: Pacini Editore.

ROOS, D. (1978) Neurological complications in patients with impaired vitamin B_{12} absorption following partial gastrectomy. *Acta psychiat. neurol. scand.*, **59**, (Suppl. 69), 1.

ROSS, E.D. & RUSH, A.J. (1981) Diagnosis and neuroanatomical correlates of depression in brain-damage patients. *Arch. gen. Psychiat.*, **38**, 1344.

ROSS, M.H. & BOTHA, H.P. (1979) Community participation in cardiac rehabilitation. *S. Afr. med. J.*, **ii**, 1126.

ROTH, M. & ROSIE, J.M. (1953) The use of E.C.T. in mental disease with clouding of consciousness. *J. ment. Sci.*, **99**, 103.

ROTH, M. (1980) Torsion dystonia, conversion hysteria and occupational groups. *Compreh. Psychiat.*, **21**, 292.

RUBINSTEIN, D. & THOMAS, J.K. (1969) Psychiatric findings in cardiotomy patients. *Am. J. Psychiat.*, **126**, 360.

SACHAR, E.J. (1973) Edocrine factors in psychopathological states. In: *Biological Psychiatry*, ed. Mendels, J., p. 175. New York: John Wiley.

SCHLESINGER, Z. & BARZILAY, J. (1980) Prolonged rehabilitation of patients after acute myocardial infarction and its effects on a complex of physiological variables. *Heart Lung*, **9**, 1038.

SCHNEIDER, K. (1959) *Clinical Psychopathology*. New York: Grune and Stratton.

SCHREIVER, G.E. (1959) Mental and personality changes in the uremic syndrome. *Med. Ann. Distr. Columbia*, **28**, 316.

SCHUSTER, M.M. (1980) Psychiatric manifestations of gastrointestinal disorders. In: *Psychiatric Presentatives of Medical Illness*, ed. Hall, R.C.W. Leicester: M.T.P.

SERBY, M. (1980) Psychiatric issues in Parkinson's disease. *Compreh. Psychiat.*, **21**, 317.

SERVICE, F.J. et al. (1976) Insulinoma. *Mayo Clinic Proc.*, **51**, 417.

SHAPIRO, A.K., SHAPIRO, E.S., BRUNN, R.D. & SWEET, R.D. (1978) *Gilles de la Tourette Syndrome*. New York: Raven Press.

SHINOZAKI, H. (1976) An epidemiological study of deaths of psychiatric inpatients. *Compreh. Psychiat.*, **17**, 425.

SHOULSON, I. et al. (1976) Huntington's disease: treatment with dipropylacetic acid and gamma aminobutyric acid. *Neurology*, **26**, 61.

SHULMAN, R. (1979) An overview of folic acid deficiency and psychiatric illness. In: *Folic Acid in Neurology, Psychiatry and Internal Medicine*, ed. Botez, M.I. and Reynolds, E.H. New York: Raven Press.

SISLER, G.C. (1978) Psychiatric disorder associated with head injury. *Psychiat. Clin. North Am.*, **1**, 137.

SMITH, C.K., BARISH, J., CORREA, J. & WILLIAMS, R.H. (1972) Psychiatric disturbances in endocrinological disease. *Psychosom. Med.*, **34**, 69.

SMITH, W.O. & CLARK, M.L. (1980) Self-induced water intoxication in schizophrenic patients. *Am. J. Psychiat.*, **137**, 1055.

STAROBINSKI, J. (1977) The word reaction: from physics to psychiatry. *Psychol. Med.*, **7**, 373.

STERN, M.J. & PASCALE, L. (1979) Psychological adaptation post-myocardial infarction: the spouse's dilemma. *J. psychosom. Res.*, **23**, 83.

STERN, M.J., PASCALE, L. & ACKERMAN, A. (1977) Life adjustment post-myocardial infarction. *Archs intern. Med.*, **137**, 1680.

SURRIDGE, D. (1969) An investigation into some psychiatric aspects of multiple sclerosis. *Br. J. Psychiat.*, **115**, 749.

TAYLOR, A.R. (1967) Post concussional sequelae. *Br. Med. J.*, **iii**, 67.

TAYLOR, J.W. (1975) Depression in thyrotoxicosis. *Am. J. Psychiat.*, **132**, 552.

THOMAS, J.E., ROOKE, E.D. & KVALE, W.F. (1966) The neurologists experience with phaeochromocytoma. *J. Am. med. Ass.*, **197**, 754.

TIBBETTS, R.W. (1981) Neuropsychiatric aspects of tics and spasms. *Br. J. Hosp. Med.*, **25**, 454.

TYRER, P.J. (1981) Drug-induced depression. *Prescribers' J.*, **21**, 237.

VARSAMIS, J. (1978) Clinical Management of Delirium. *Psychiat. Clin. North Am.*, **1**, 71.

WALSHE, J.K. (1976) Wilson's disease (hepatolenticular degeneration). In: *Handbook of Clinical Neurology Vol. 27*, ed. Vinken, P.J. et al. New York: American Elsevier.

WENGER, N.K. (1970) Tumours of the heart. In: *The Heart*, ed. Hurst, J.W. and Lague, R.B. New York: McGraw Hill.

WHARTON, R.N. (1977) Atrial myxoma masquerade. *Am. J. Psychiat.*, **134**, 1441.

WHITLOCK, F.A. & SISKIND, M. (1979) Depression and cancer: a follow-up study. *Psychol. Med.*, **9**, 747.

WHYBROW, P.C. & HURWITZ, T. (1976) Psychological disturbance associated with endocrine disease and hormone therapy. In: *Hormones, Behaviour and Psychopathology*, ed. Sachar, E.J. New York: Raven Press.

WIECK, H.H. (1961) Zur Klinischen Stellung des Durchgangs-syndroms. *Schweizer. Arch. Neurol. Psychiat.*, **88**, 409.

WILLI, J. (1966) In: *Akute psychische Begleiterscheinungen körperlicher Krankheiten*, ed. Bleuler, M. et al. Stuttgart: Theime.

YUDOFSKY, S.C. (1979) Parkinson's disease, depression and electroconvulsive therapy: a clinical and neurobiologic synthesis. *Compreh. Psychiat.*, **20**, 579.

14

Management of the Schizophrenias

G.E. Berrios

CLINICAL FEATURES

There are many definitions of the schizophrenias (Roth and McClelland 1979), including those with relatively restrictive diagnostic criteria which are coextensive with the concept of 'nuclear' schizophrenia. This assumes the presence of relatively strong hereditary factors, which may be related to the presence of a number of genetic markers such as defective eye tracking (Holzman and Levy 1977), HLA (Human leucocyte Antigen) subtypes (McGuffin et al. 1978) and a recognizable electrodermal curve (Venables 1981). It has been suggested that such patients can often be identified by the presence of certain so-called first rank symptoms (Schneider 1959), although their diagnostic significance is considerably reduced if mania or certain identifiable (i.e. organic) brain disorders are present. However, some authors have suggested that the minimum list of diagnostically relevant phenomena should include other signs such as the various kinds of abnormal thought processes known as 'formal thought disorder', and chronic multiple delusions and/or hallucinations (Roth and McClelland 1979).

A schizophrenic disorder consists of a variable number of the following phenomena in the absence of certain kinds of identifiable cerebral pathology (Davison and Bagley 1969) which are known to be associated with such signs and symptoms, and in the absence of any other recognized syndrome, such as mania, which may include such features (Brockington et al. 1978).

(1) The 'first rank' symptoms as described by Schneider (Mellor 1970); i.e. audible thoughts (the patient experiences hallucinatory voices speaking his thoughts aloud); two or more hallucinatory voices in disagreement or discussion; hallucinatory voices commenting on the patient; a feeling that hallucinatory bodily sensations are being imposed upon him by some external agency (somatic passivity); a feeling that thoughts are being taken from the patient's mind (thought withdrawal); a feeling that thoughts are not the patient's own, which is usually accompanied by a belief that they are being imposed by an

outside agency (thought insertion); a feeling that his thoughts are not contained but can be experienced by others (thought broadcasting); emotions, thoughts, impulses or actions which are experienced as being under outside control (passivity feelings); a perception (or thought) to which the patient assigns a delusional meaning (this process is known as delusional perception), which is not secondary to a pre-existing abnormal psychological phenomenon.

(2) Disorder of the form of thought processes (i.e. formal thought disorder), involving such phenomena as thought 'blocking', poverty of thought content, a reduced ability to think abstractly, distractibility, a lack of causal links, an imprecise use of words, overinclusion, and neologisms.

(3) Various phenomena which are not specific to schizophrenic syndromes:

(a) Hallucinations and/or delusions other than in (1).

(b) Mood disorders including 'blunting' of emotional responses, incongruity of affect, anxiety, perplexity, lack of motivation, and depression; lack of motivation, apathy and emotional blunting are examples of the so-called negative symptoms (Andreasen 1982).

(c) Abnormal overt behaviour including stupor, excitement, negativism, stereotypies, odd postures, and various non-specific bizarre acts.

(d) Impaired insight regarding the various problems associated with the disorder.

(e) Impairment of cognitive function. (This has been described mainly in patients with a severe, long-standing schizophrenic disorder.) (Johnstone et al. 1978).

The schizophrenias are considered by many to be a related group of disorders, as they show considerable variation with respect to the age of onset, the speed of development, the combination of the various signs and symptoms, response to treatment, degree of resolution of symptoms, and prognosis (Young and Meltzer 1980). Although various subtypes have been postulated, e.g. simple (mainly involving negative symptoms), hebephrenic (mainly involving formal thought disorder and mood changes), paranoid (mainly involving delusions and hallucinations), and catatonic (with predominant abnormal overt behaviour), many schizophrenic disorders cannot be categorized in this way, and during the course of an individual syndrome a change in the phenomenology may require a change in subtype classification.

Florid 'positive' features such as first rank symptoms, other delusions and hallucinations, disjointed thought processes, and abnormal overt behaviour are, in general, more responsive to neuroleptic medication than negative symptoms, but even a complete resolution of positive symptoms often leads to persistent negative features which hinder rehabilitation. In a small minority of patients, usually with both positive and negative features, the course is relentlessly progressive, showing little response to treatment; such individuals may need considerable care, sometimes as in-patients, for the rest of their lives while, at the other extreme, there is complete remission from all symptoms. Even if relapse occurs, such patients may again show complete remission. These differences in the course of schizophrenic disorders have led certain authors to postulate two main entities consisting of 'good prognosis' and 'defect' schizophrenia (Crow 1980; 1981), which could, however, represent different stages in the evolution of the same disease process (Mackay 1980). It has been claimed that a relatively poor outcome is associated with lack of precipitatory factors; low social class; single, separated, or divorced status; insidious onset; and lack of florid symptoms.

In many cases, there are early, non-specific features which precede clear evidence of illness. These include affective changes, hypochondriacal preoccupation, a degree of religious or philosophical rumination which interferes with normal activities, and progressive cognitive and social decline. Thus, the date of onset may be difficult to identify. The extent to which particular symptoms influence external behaviour is variable; for example, patients can experience intense delusions and hallucinations and yet still behave in a socially unremarkable manner.

MANAGEMENT

Diagnosis of Schizophrenic Disorders

Brockington et al. (1978) have compared ten definitions of 'schizophrenia' in respect of their reliability, concordance, and prediction of outcome, and one of the four relatively effective sets of criteria was that of Spitzer (1975). However, the clinician is less concerned with where to place the boundary of the schizophrenias than with the selection of the appropriate treatment methods for the individual patient, in particular whether or not to prescribe neuroleptic medication. In practice, if any of the commonly used sets of diagnostic criteria indicate a schizophrenic illness, a therapeutic trial with a neuroleptic is indicated, although these drugs may be ineffective, or of relatively limited value, especially when negative phenomena predominate. Factors other than the phenomenology must also be taken into account when making the diagnosis, including the nature and response to treatment of any previous psychiatric disorder, and any family history of a schizophrenia.

After taking a detailed history from the patient and a relative, the mental state examination should end, if possible, with a series of direct questions regarding the presence of the various phenomena associated with this group of disorders. However, it may be necessary to postpone the detailed examination of the mental state if this is likely to upset the patient. A thorough physical examination is then performed, even if there is a past history of schizophrenia, and the range of possible diagnoses is considered. Routine investigations usually include a blood count, ESR, VDRL, chest and skull X-ray and EEG. The differential diagnosis may include certain identifiable cerebral disorders (including drug-induced states, e.g. due to amphetamine and LSD, and certain epileptic phenomena), alcoholic hallucinosis, and manic–depressive psychosis, in particular mania (see Chapter 15). The absence of a disorder of consciousness cannot always be considered as crucial, as both false positives and negatives may occur. For example, a schizophrenic (or affective) psychosis occurring in the puerperium may be accompanied by confusion and disorientation (Berrios 1982b), while some schizophreniform psychoses resulting from identifiable cerebral pathology may occur in lucid consciousness. Early encephalitis is, perhaps, the most difficult disorder to eliminate, and the clinician must look out for any fluctuations in the level of consciousness, neurological signs, abnormalities in the EEG, or the presence of partial or generalized seizures. Drug-induced psychoses must always be suspected in young adults suffering from visual hallucinations. Sometimes, an obsessive–compulsive disorder without insight, or hallucinatory experiences in the setting of an hysterical dissociative state, may be mistaken for a schizophrenic illness.

The psychiatrist is often faced with difficulty in deciding whether an acute psychosis should be treated as a schizophrenic disorder (i.e. with neuroleptics other than the butyrophenones) or as a manic disorder (i.e. with haloperidol and lithium). This may be because the phenomenology may be non-specific and consonant with either diagnosis, or because there is a mixture of several first-rank schizophrenic phenomena together with some characteristically manic features. In the latter case, a diagnosis of schizo-affective disorder is often made, and although many of these syndromes are subsequently recognized as clearly schizophrenic or manic, it has been suggested that some of these patients suffer from a relatively distinct schizo-affective psychosis (Procci 1976). In practice, the clinician who is faced with such diagnostic difficulty may initially choose a neuroleptic such as haloperidol which is effective in both classes of disorder, or combine a phenothiazine (or thioxanthene) with haloperidol and/or lithium. Although a schizophrenic disorder can be wrongly diagnosed as mania, the reverse situation is more likely to occur. Thus, a psychotic patient who does not respond well to neuroleptics should be considered for a trial of lithium when mania is a possible diagnosis, or when an atypical schizophreniform presentation is coloured with affective features.

Management of Severe Schizophrenic Episodes

The patient with a severe schizophrenia usually benefits from early admission to hospital. An episode may occur de novo, or may be a relapse in the context of an ongoing disease, and the crisis which leads to a request for an urgent psychiatric assessment is often largely due to the results of the social consequence of the disorder. The patient may be admitted after an out-patient attendance or a domiciliary visit by the psychiatrist, or may be sent to the hospital by his general practitioner. Occasionally he may be brought by the police after being found in a public place exhibiting bizarre behaviour.

Often it is necessary for an uncooperative patient to be compulsorily detained and treated under the provision of an appropriate section of the Mental Health Act, but it should be remembered that, in practice, 'compulsory detention' for more than a few months often involves the patient living or working outside the hospital, even though the legal provision allows the psychiatrist to insist on treatment when this is appropriate and to intervene in a crisis. Agreement to detain and treat a patient compulsorily is usually present when a patient is floridly psychotic, but there may be differences of opinion between the psychiatrist, general medical practitioner, social worker and the patient's relatives. For example, this situation can arise with regard to those individuals with clear evidence of psychosis, perhaps with florid delusions and hallucinations, who, despite their disorder, maintain a precarious social adjustment, even though their lives have been severely affected. Some of these patients would show considerable improvement on depot neuroleptics, yet many are unwilling to cooperate. However, if no major crisis has arisen, the patient's family, social worker or general pratitioner may not be willing to follow the psychiatrist's advice that compulsory treatment is in the patient's best interests. Even if the general practitioner and social worker are agreed but the patient's family objects, it is usually prudent not to proceed with compulsory admission at once, even though this would be legally possible. It may be best to wait for the situation to deteriorate further, to a point at which the patient's family then agree that compulsory treatment is needed, as the long-term management of such patients in the face of determined opposition from the family is a situation to be avoided if at all possible. However, in rare cases, it may be appropriate to proceed with compulsory admission and treatment despite the family's objections.

Also, some patients with predominantly negative symptoms, which have led to a marked social decline, perhaps complicated by non-specific bizarre behaviour, petty crimes or alcoholism, may not fulfil the legal requirements for compulsory admission to hospital; no adequate provision is made for the care and support of such individuals in our society.

The initial primary objective of treatment must always be the reduction of the psychotic symptoms. This will help the patient to regain control of his social environment, and no purpose is served in 'allowing' the patient to 'work through' his psychosis, nor should the clinician attempt to interpret why the patient has 'chosen' to show psychotic symptoms. The psychotic patient no more selects his symptoms than the patient with encephalitis 'chooses' to be disorientated, although the content of the abnormal forms of mental experience will often be understandably shaped by the patient's personality and life situation. However, although 'insight-directed' psychotherapeutic techniques or exposure to emotionally charged group situations is contraindicated, the patient with an acute schizophrenia requires considerable supportive psychotherapeutic help, with reassurance and explanation.

Reduction in the intensity of the symptomatology is achieved by a combination of pharmacological management, supportive psychotherapy, and skilled nursing. Severely schizophrenic patients are often perplexed, bewildered, anxious or terrified by their experiences, and such reactions may, on occasions, lead to suicide (Planansky and Johnson 1971). Persistent reassurance concerning the pathological and temporary nature of certain psychotic experiences may be indicated, but argument about the truth of delusional beliefs should not be prolonged. A structured milieu in the hospital unit helps the patient regain a sense of reality, and should provide clean and tidy surroundings with staff members who are easily identifiable. This often gives the patient a clear sense of security and clear external reference points at a time when the boundaries between his internal and external world may be eroded by the disease. The provision of various occupational and social activities are also an important part of a milieu which is suitable for patients with a severe schizophrenic disorder, and such individuals may benefit from certain structured group activities such as relaxation exercises, art therapy, and certain kinds of group discussions which focus on the practical problems which arise in a hospital unit. However, if emotional arousal is likely in such meetings, either due to the patient's mental state or behaviour, or to the behaviour of other patients, these group activities must be avoided until sufficient improvement has taken place.

The use of neuroleptic medication during a severe schizophrenic episode is mandatory. Evidence in favour of a specific antipsychotic effect associated with the neuroleptic compounds is indisputable (Davis 1975; Davis et al. 1980), and it is therefore inaccurate to refer to these treatments as 'tranquillizers' or 'chemical straightjackets'. The available evidence suggests that, for groups of patients, there is not much difference between the efficacy of various neuroleptics, although it is usual to prescribe a sedative drug (e.g. chlorpromazine) in the presence of excitement, aggression or overactivity, to assist the process of nursing the patient during the severe episode. Conversely, a compound such as trifluoperazine may be the drug of first choice if the patient is apathetic and withdrawn. However, there is some evidence that schizophrenic retardation can respond to chlorpromazine (Goldberg et al. 1967). In practice, some patients appear to respond preferentially to a particular neuroleptic, but this cannot be predicted in a first episode. The initial choice of neuroleptic drug will depend on such factors as the need for sedation, the nature and severity of early side effects, and the history of response to drug treatment in any previous episodes. A phenothiazine or thioxanthene is usually the drug of first choice; there is less published evidence in support of the butyrophenones in schizophrenic disorders.

Initially a regimen of intramuscular injections of chlorpromazine may be appropriate if the patient's behaviour is very disturbed while, in the most severe cases, a combination of chlorpromazine and haloperidol may be suitable. The chlorpromazine can be given in the evening, while the haloperidol is administered during the day; this encourages night-time sleep without excessive day-time sedation. Less severely affected patients can be started on an oral preparation or, in some cases, on a depot injection of a neuroleptic, but it is usually best to start treatment with oral (or non-depot parenteral) medication which allows for greater initial flexibility of management; it may then be appropriate to substitute a depot preparation when symptoms begin to abate. A decision to start depot medication will be partly based on an estimate of the likely compliance of the patient with regard to his taking oral medication when he leaves hospital, and of the need for continuing medication after the maximum effect of medication has been obtained. (A minority of patients show little or no response to drugs.) Even if long-term prophylaxis is not indicated, it is usual to continue maintenance neuroleptic medication for at least 3–6 months after a severe episode which has apparently responded to pharmacological treatment, and as compliance in schizophrenic patients is generally poor, depot neuroleptics are to be preferred for maintenance therapy, although a minority can be relied upon to take their oral medication regularly.

An initial 'test dose' of a neuroleptic, particularly a depot preparation, is advisable. Relatively early side effects include dystonic reactions, Parkinsonian phenomena, and akathisia (see Chapter 2). Dystonic reactions require an intramuscular or intravenous antiparkinsonian agent, and these drugs also relieve parkinsonian side effects. However, although akathisia may respond to antiparkinsonian agents (Ayd 1975), many patients with this distressing restlessness do not improve to a significant extent with such treatment. In these cases, a benzodiazepine or a sedative phenothiazine such as chlorpromazine may provide some relief.

Other possible interventions in the management of a severe episode include ECT, anxiolytics (Jimerson et al. 1982), and the provision of social work support for the patient's family. ECT may be indicated when abnormalities of motor behaviour predominate (i.e. in 'catatonic' states), perhaps involving extreme excitement with violent or suicidal tendencies, or a stupor when the patient may sustain odd positions or refuse to eat or drink. Another indication for ECT is the presence of distressing or dangerous symptoms, such as auditory hallucinations instructing the patient to commit suicide, if they are relatively unresponsive to neuroleptics. Although ECT is rarely necessary in the management of the schizophrenias, it may lead to dramatic improvement in such cases.

Management of Chronic Schizophrenic Disorders

Although some schizophrenic disorders show complete remission and, even if they recur, have intervening symptom-free periods, the majority of schizophrenic patients exhibit a chronic disorder which can be defined as the presence of signs or symptoms for longer than an arbitrary period of 6 months.

Over the course of a chronic schizophrenic illness a patient may mainly attend an out-patient clinic or, in a small minority, may mainly require management as an in-patient. These two groups will be considered separately, although they cannot be clearly distinguished, as some patients receive roughly equal periods of in-patient and out-patient treatment. Also, over a period of years, the relative proportion of in-patient to out-patient management may change in either direction; for example, some of the most severely affected patients, who may require several years in hospital, may eventually become 'burned-out', in that their more florid treatment-resistant symptoms may abate. Thereafter, a further attempt can be made to rehabilitate the patient to living outside hospital with community support.

Schizophrenic patients who attend out-patient clinics include those with at least one previous admission to hospital with a severe episode which responded, completely or partially, to treatment, while others may have had a relatively mild disorder which did not require in-patient management. Schizophrenic out-patients usually attend every 1–2 months to be seen by the psychiatrist, but may also need additional interventions involving support outside the hospital, although, for some patients, out-patient review and treatment is all that is necessary.

Many patients with chronic schizophrenic disorders require help to combat a range of symptoms which can be considered under four main headings. Firstly, negative features of schizophrenia are often found; these are usually unresponsive to neuroleptic medication but may be alleviated by an attempt to modify the patient's social environment, together with a behavioural approach to encourage new learning. Secondly, after a course of neuroleptic treatment there may be residual schizophrenic features other than negative symptoms. The third edition of the Diagnostic and Statistical Manual (DSM III) has, in its category of 'residual type (295.6X)' of schizophrenia, described a combination of these first two categories of phenomena, characterized by absence of prominent psychotic features and 'emotional blunting, social withdrawal, eccentric behaviour, illogical thinking and loosening of associations'. Thirdly, the chronic schizophrenic patient may suffer from non-schizophrenic psychiatric disorders which have been precipitated or exacerbated by the psychosis or its sequelae. Examples include depression, anxiety, panic attacks, phobias, irritability, emotional lability and obsessive–compulsive phenomena. It is important to recognize such symptoms and not to assume that all the patient's symptoms and abnormal behaviour are the direct result of the schizophrenic disorder. Often these additional problems require treatment in their own right. Fourthly, side effects of neuroleptic treatment may contribute to the chronic schizophrenic's problems. Gardos and Cole (1976) have estimated that at least 40% of those schizophrenic out-patients who were reviewed required prophylactic neuroleptic medication to prevent relapse and, although a reduction or discontinuation of neuroleptic treatment may be possible if side effects are troublesome, this may provoke a recurrence of previous psychotic phenomena or an exacerbation of current symptoms. If it appears that a neuroleptic should be continued, specific treatment for certain side effects may have to be introduced.

The relatively early extrapyramidal side effects of the neuroleptics have been outlined previously (see also Chapter 2), and while they may occur during out-patient management, for example if a dose of neuroleptic is initiated or increased, the clinician who is monitoring the regular out-patient attender must pay particular attention to the recognition of the so-called amotivational response (Andrews 1973) and tardive dyskinesia.

The amotivational response to neuroleptics involves apathy and lethargy, but as these symptoms can also be negative features of schizophrenic disorders, it is often difficult to determine whether neuroleptic medication is a contributory factor. However, if a patient on a maintenance neuroleptic becomes increasingly apathetic, the discontinuation of the drug for a trial period may be indicated. Ayd (1975) has described apathy associated with akinesia in the initial stages of neuroleptic treatment and reported that depression could also be the result of neuroleptic treatment, both in the early stages and during chronic prophylactic administration. Ayd claimed that both the apathy and the depression responded to antiparkinsonian agents, and that there was a spontaneous resolution of the apathy after a few weeks. However, the value of antiparkinsonian medication in this respect is controversial.

The early recognition of tardive dyskinesia is important, and particular attention must be paid to any involuntary movements of the lower jaw, lips and tongue. Movements of the tongue can be the earliest sign, and the patient should be asked to open his mouth so that these can be investigated.

In addition, chronic neuroleptic medication can induce weight gain and sexual dysfunction. The latter can give rise to marital difficulties, and advice to both the patient and the spouse may then be required (Noonan et al. 1976).

Chronic schizophrenias in out-patient practice. Patients with chronic schizophrenic disorders are commonly seen in a psychiatric out-patient clinic for about half-an-hour every 4–6 weeks. The clinician must assess the current mental and physical state and social situation, evaluate any change since the last visit, review any medication, provide supportive psychotherapeutic help where appropriate, and coordinate other aspects of management.

It is commonly held that a schizophrenic disorder results from neurotransmitter dysfunction dependent on a genetic predisposition which may sometimes be precipitated or perpetuated by psychological and social variables (Strauss and Carpenter 1981). Thus the range of therapeutic interventions would be expected to include psychological and social factors; attempts have been made to categorize these so that they can be subjected to clinical investigation (Lader

1975; Leff 1976), and possible therapeutic interventions in chronic schizophrenic disorders include various forms of individual, family and group psychotherapy using supportive rather than insight-directed techniques (see Chapters 8 and 9); periods of in-patient admission during a crisis; and various forms of community support. The latter may involve visits to the patient and his family by a nurse or social worker, attendance at a day centre or sheltered workshop, advice and treatment based on behavioural principles by a clinical psychologist, and the provision of sheltered recreational and social activities at various times including evenings and weekends. Also, in urban areas, a 'drop-in' centre which is open for 24 h a day can provide immediate advice and support during a crisis, and thereby reduce the frequency of readmission to hospital. At times, compulsory drug treatment may be given on an out-patient basis, with the patient on 'extended leave' from the hospital. This arrangement is particularly suitable for patients who can remain outside hospital only if they receive regular depot medication, and who are otherwise unwilling to cooperate with this form of treatment.

Intensive psychotherapy based on psychoanalytic principles has been advocated for schizophrenic disorders by some psychiatrists (Fromm-Reichmann 1954; Sechehaye 1978; Benedetti 1980). However, such claims are based on uncontrolled studies and sometimes the signs and symptoms did not fulfil current diagnostic criteria. Beck et al. (1981) investigated the effects of relatively intensive psychotherapy in a group of 27 schizophrenic patients who were compared with 20 similar patients treated by other means, and there was no conclusive evidence of improved social functioning in the experimental group. In a recent review, Mosher and Keith (1979) concluded that there is no evidence in favour of the efficacy of intensive insight-directed psychotherapy during either the acute or chronic stage of a schizophrenic disorder.

Psychotherapeutic interventions include advice and encouragement, and should focus on practical solutions to current problems. A patient who still has some negative symptoms following the partial resolution of a severe episode may not be able to resume his previous level of responsibilities at work, and will need help to adjust to his reduced capabilities. Negative symptoms will also affect marital or family relationships, and interviews with some of the patient's relatives may also be beneficial. Other patients experience chronic delusions and hallucinations which are relatively 'well encapsulated', i.e. they are usually not apparent unless specific questions are asked. (These may have reduced in intensity as a result of neuroleptic treatment.) In such cases it is best not to discuss these psychotic phenomena at any length, although if these are influencing behaviour, the patient may accept advice as to how to act upon these experiences. As has been stated, the clinician should not engage in prolonged argument about delusional beliefs.

The findings that some high levels of expressed emotionality in the family group may be related to early relapse after discharge (Vaughn and Leff 1976), and that some schizophrenic patients do better in group or hostel accommodation than at home (Wing and Brown 1970), have provided some practical guidance for the management of chronic schizophrenic disorders. They have also given some support to the view that therapy of the natural group (i.e. the family) might sometimes reduce the frequency of relapse. 'Family therapy' can involve a wide range of techniques extending from intensive, formalized, insight-directed group meetings based on psychoanalytic principles, to less ambitious interventions when the psychiatrist, clinical psychologist or social worker asks those members of the family who are particularly involved with the patient to attend for a few sessions. The latter strategy is often valuable, and focusses on explanation, advice and support, although a family member may benefit from some insight if his defence mechanisms (see Chapter 9) have negative consequences for the patient, such as an overprotection which stifles initiative, or the setting of unrealistic goals.

The intensive, formalized methods of family therapy are sometimes based on unsubstantiated claims as to the role played by the family in the aetiology of a schizophrenic disorder (Bateson et al. 1956; Hirsch and Leff 1975), and there is no good evidence that this approach has yielded practical results in the treatment of the schizophrenias. Reduction of relapse rate and enhancement of social adjustment may, however, be associated with the more supportive forms of family therapy (Ro-Trock et al. 1977).

In their 1971 review, Bednar and Lawlis (1971) concluded that there was little evidence in favour of the various types of group psychotherapy in the management of acute schizophrenic disorders, although Mosher and Keith (1979) considered that there is room to suppose that groups using supportive techniques (see Chapter 9) can be useful in the rehabilitation of chronic schizophrenic patients. These authors reviewed the recent evidence which compared group psychotherapy with pharmacotherapy, group psychotherapy with psychological or social interventions, or which assessed the value of group therapy in the aftercare of schizophrenic patients following discharge from hospital. Only the studies of aftercare seemed to show some positive results, in that supportive group techniques were a means of helping the patient to resocialize and enhance his interpersonal skills.

The main facets of the patient's social environment may involve a job, a 'living group', and various social activities outside the home. As has been stated, a patient may not be able to regain his premorbid level of occupational ability, and appropriate advice should be given; the patient may have to be referred to a sheltered workshop if negative symptoms of schizophrenia are severe, as these can profoundly impair a capacity for sustained work, even though the patient may appear normal in other respects. With regard to the patient's living group, it has been clearly established that there is an optimal level of 'expressed emotion' in the household; too little stimulation (for example due to living alone) is not therapeutic, while an environment which makes excessive social demands, or involves frequent arguments and tension, is also to be avoided. Some patients require hostel accommodation, or a place in a 'group home' (i.e. a supervised house containing several patients). Several activities outside the home should be encouraged, and many psychiatric services organize evening recreational activities for those who require a relatively sheltered social environment. Some patients require a specific programme of rehabilitation as outlined in Chapter 11. It should be recognized that some chronic schizophrenic patients will never be able to remain outside an institution for any length of time without considerable and indefinite support involving such facilities as sheltered workshops, supervised hostels, day centres, social work visits, a community nursing service and access to support and advice when a crisis occurs in the evening or at night. These provisions are, in general, conspicuously inadequate, which may contribute to frequent readmissions to hospital in the course of some schizophrenic disorders. Although recent evidence seems to show that certain differences in the duration of hospital admissions did not correlate with several outcome variables (Glick et al. 1974; Hirsch et al. 1979), there is convincing evidence that a lack of community support is associated with a relatively high readmission rate. Mann and Cree (1976) considered that some of the younger patients who still require indefinite in-patient provision (i.e. the 'new long stay') could have been discharged if the appropriate facilities had been available.

Different individuals require various combinations and degrees of intervention, while the needs of the individual chronic patient will vary during the course of the illness. While community support should aim to maximize the patient's potential, an excessive degree of intervention may be counterproductive if this results in excessive dependence and the elimination of situations where initiative is required (Morgan 1974). Thus, flexibility is essential when determining the optimum level of community support, and this should be subject to regular review. Also the goals of management must not include improved performance if this is considered unrealistic; in such cases, the prevention of further deterioration may be just as important (Shepherd 1981).

Ideally, the responsibility for the management of some severely affected chronic schizophrenic patients should be shared between the psychiatric services and the 'community'. However, many people have ambivalent attitudes to chronic mental disorder, and even if there is verbal acceptance of the principles of community support, there may be active resistance in some neighbourhoods to the establishment of facilities such as a hostel or day centre. Thus, part of the psychiatrist's task is to try and modify such attitudes by taking part in educational activities which try and dispel exaggerated fears.

In-patient management of chronic schizophrenia. In the first years of a severe schizophrenic disorder, a few patients may spend most of their time as in-patients, while attempts are made to exert sufficient effects of medical, psychological and social treatments to enable the patient to live outside hospital. During this time the patient is usually managed in an admission ward which deals with the variety of psychiatric disorders requiring short-term, in-patient management. However, if it becomes clear that the patient will not be able to cope with living outside hospital for more than short periods of leave, a transfer to the part of the hospital which is designed for the care and rehabilitation of chronic, severe psychiatric disorder is indicated.

Thus, a psychiatric service must provide an active and caring community for 'long-stay' patients which can keep alive the assets which have been spared by the illness. Some of these patients may not have the potential to live and work outside hospital in the foreseeable future although, even in such cases, further rehabilitation may be possible if the illness eventually becomes burned-out. For such patients, the goals of rehabilitation may be relatively modest, such as an increasing participation in social and recreational activities in the hospital setting, but even if there is no sign of gradual improvement, the goal of the prevention of further deterioration must not be forgotten. In recent years it has been fashionable to consider that the discharge of any severely affected chronic patient from hospital to a boarding house or hostel represents a therapeutic advance. However many such individuals do not have adequate community support after discharge, and may deteriorate due to lack of sheltered occupation and social stimulation.

Although the 'therapeutic community' approach, with its emphasis on group meetings, is not appropriate in the management of severe schizophrenic episodes (see Chapter 9), group pressures can be utilized to shape attitudes and behaviour in long-stay hospital wards or day centres which cater for chronic schizophrenic disorders (Barton 1959; Almond 1975). Also, various behavioural strategies (see Chapters 10 and 11) have been successful in the management of chronic schizophrenic patients both in and out of hospital. These are more effective if the aim is to modify a relatively discrete aspect of behaviour (Baker 1975).

Aspects of the Pharmacological Management of the Schizophrenias

Optimal doses. An optimal neuroleptic dose regimen can be defined as that to which the largest number of a group of patients will respond, or the dose which combines a good therapeutic effect with minimal side effects in the individual patient. It must be specified for both oral and parenteral routes, and can be defined in grams per kilogram weight or in terms of plasma levels. In practice, standard dose regimens are derived from the mean amounts prescribed in studies which have been associated with an adequate therapeutic response (Davis and Garver 1978); however, the appropriate dose for the individual should be the lowest which is compatible with successful treatment or prophylaxis (Baldessarini and Davis 1980), and should be prescribed for the shortest possible period. As with most medical treatments, the potential gains have to be weighed against various side effects, so that the optimal dose will also depend on both these factors.

Dose of neuroleptic in severe schizophrenic disorders. The average starting dose of chlorpromazine in the treatment of a severe schizophrenic illness in hospital is between 300 and 500 mg daily, and is given in three or four doses. However, a larger daily dose of chlorpromazine is frequently indicated (for example up to 1000 mg daily), while 20–30 mg daily of trifluoperazine, or haloperidol up to 80 mg daily, are often prescribed during a severe episode.

The response to an increasing daily dose of chlorpromazine does not continue beyond a 'ceiling' of about 3000 mg (Davis and Garver 1978), while for fluphenazine the ceiling daily dose is about 30 mg (Quitkin et al. 1974), and for trifluoperazine about 60 mg (Wijsenbeek et al. 1974). However, despite the identification of these ceiling doses, correlations between oral dose (or plasma level) and therapeutic response are, in general, poor (Berrios 1982c).

Plasma levels of drug and active metabolites are determined by factors such as the rate of absorption from the gastrointestinal tract; initial metabolism in the liver; rate of metabolism; and type of predominant metabolic pathway in a given patient (Mackay et al. 1974; Phillipson et al. 1977). As there is considerable interpatient variation with respect to these and other relevant variables, there is a wide scatter in the plasma levels of a group of patients after a given dose (Davis et al. 1978). Other factors which may influence the therapeutic effects of a particular dose include a possible dose-dependent paradoxical reversal of dopamine receptor response, and an unacceptable intensification of side effects.

The apparent lower limit of the range of effective daily doses may be misleadingly lowered by spontaneous remissions and placebo responses; however, it should be noted that plasma levels due to depot medication are much lower than those obtained for oral medication, yet are clearly effective (Tune et al. 1980).

The patient who is refractory to neuroleptic treatment. The 'refractory' patient is one whose positive symptoms would be expected to improve after neuroleptic treatment, but who does not respond to a standard treatment regimen given for at least 8 weeks (Berrios 1982c).

At this point, the psychiatrist must review the diagnosis; it may be that the schizophreniform syndrome is, in fact, a manic illness, or some other non-schizophrenic disorder. The second step is to determine whether the patient has taken the prescribed medication; even with in-patients, especially those with paranoid features, there is a default rate for oral medication of between 11% and 19% (Johnson 1977). Where it is suspected that a patient is concealing his tablets and disposing of them subsequently, it is advisable to administer the neuroleptic in fluid form (which is more difficult to retain in the mouth), or parenterally. If previous compliance is judged to have been satisfactory, the third step is to determine whether any concomitant medication is reducing the bioavailability of the neuroleptic; for example antacids can decrease absorption of phenothiazines (Baldessarini 1980), and antiparkinsonian agents may reduce stomach emptying and gut motility, thus interfering with absorption (Rivera-Calimlin et al. 1978). The fourth step is to consider possible pharmacokinetic impediments to adequate bioavailability; for example, some subjects metabolize chlorpromazine in the intestine (this effect may be more marked in patients on chronic treatment) while, in others, much of this drug may be trapped during its initial passage through the liver and excreted unchanged in the bile. Also, protein binding in the plasma can on occasions be increased in the presence of abnormal proteins such as α_1-acid glycoprotein (Editorial 1979). Estimation of plasma levels of the parent drug and of any active metabolites may help to identify such causes of resistance to treatment with neuroleptic drugs, but current methods usually measure general neuroleptic activity rather than the bioavailable free fraction. Determination of CSF levels of neuroleptics is of theoretical advantage, but its routine use is impractical. Estimation of salivary levels of neuroleptics has also been studied (May et al. 1978; Van Putten et al. 1980), but the technique is affected by difficulties in the collection of saliva, and its contamination from oral neuroleptic intake.

The fifth step in the consideration of possible reasons for non-response to neuroleptics, in patients whose plasma levels of the drug are adequate, is to look for pharmacodynamic reasons for the lack of efficacy. Physiological indices of central dopamine receptor blockade can be used to determine whether sufficient neuroleptic has crossed the blood–brain barrier; for example, since phenothiazines have an α-adrenergic receptor blocking activity (Richelson 1980), the presence of miosis can be used to indicate its presence in the brain. Thus Sakalis et al. (1972) have found a correlation between plasma level of neuroleptic and miotic response, which did not exhibit tolerance for at least the first 36 days of treatment. This correlation seems to hold even at relatively low plasma levels of neuroleptic (Smolen et al. 1975), so that serial examination of pupillar size under standard light conditions before and after treatment may be a useful method to investigate neuroleptic bioavailability (Domino 1979).

Another physiological index is the determination of plasma prolactin (Meltzer and Fang 1976; Wiles et al. 1976; Kolakowska et al. 1979; Fuente and Rosenbaum 1981), and it has been claimed that there is a positive correlation between the level of plasma prolactin and the antipsychotic response after neuroleptic administration (Kolakowska et al. 1979). A similar relationship has been reported for haloperidol in chronic schizophrenia (Rama Rao et al. 1980). Although Gruen et al. (1978) have claimed that the prolactin response reaches its maximum level following relatively low doses of neuroleptics, which may not be sufficient to exert a therapeutic effect, Kolakowska et al. (1981) have shown that, in patients receiving standard doses of a phenothiazine, prolactin levels increase further after a dose of haloperidol. This suggests that the prolactin elevation induced by routine neuroleptic treatment had not reached 'ceiling', although they also found that additional haloperidol did not increase plasma prolactin if patients were receiving very high daily doses of medication.

Even if such phenomena as miosis, elevation of plasma prolactin, reduction of plasma growth hormone and marked extrapyramidal symptoms indicate that the patient's dopamine (DA) receptors have been reached by the neuroleptic, non-response of positive schizophrenic phenomena to neuroleptics could be due to a dissociation between the effects on dopaminergic pathways related to these physiological indices (i.e. the tuberohypophyseal and nigrostriatal systems), and the effects on the mesocortical tract which may be related to the pathogenesis of the schizophrenias. The recent identification of various sub-types of DA receptor populations differentially associated with the dopa-minergic tracts may add credence to this view. For example, it has been claimed that while DA-2 receptors mediate the antipsychotic effect of neuroleptics, the DA-1 receptors, which are linked with cyclic AMP, do not (Snyder 1981).

The relative proportion of positive and negative symptoms in a particular schizophrenic disorder may be related to lack of response to neuroleptics, and Mackay (1980) has postulated that negative symptoms might be associated with reduced dopaminergic activity; if this was present, a worsening of these features would be expected after neuroleptic administration. However, the hypothesis that dopamine agonists (e.g. amphetamines or L-DOPA) may activate the chronic schizophrenic patient with predominantly negative symptoms has not yet been fulfilled (Gerlach and Lühdorf 1975; Kornetsky 1976).

In summary, if compliance is found to be satisfactory, the clinician faced with a patient who is refractory to neuroleptics can increase the dose, change to another neuroleptic, or change from oral administration to the regular injection of a depot preparation. High-dose depot medication (e.g. up to 250 mg weekly of fluphenazine enanthate) has been tried for some patients whose symptoms were refractory to ordinary doses. Dencker (1978a,b) reported 119 patients treated with such 'megadoses', and claimed that this group showed a reduced incidence of extrapyramidal side effects compared with patients on lower doses and that this regimen was apparently beneficial in some cases. However, other authors have reported decreased seizure threshold, the 'malignant syndrome' (i.e. hypertonicity, dyskinesia, pallor, pulmonary congestion, hyperpyrexia and confusion, which can be fatal), and local reactions such as abscesses. In routine practice, doses in excess of flupenthixol decanoate 200 mg every 2 weeks or fluphenazine decanoate 100 mg every 2 weeks are rarely prescribed. A standard dose every 3–4 weeks would be flupenthixol 40 mg, or fluphenazine 25 mg. Despite claims that the former is less sedative, there appears to be no good evidence of differences with regard to side effects. In older patients, much lower doses are usually appropriate, while even in non-elderly adults, a dose such as 20 mg of a depot preparation of flupenthixol every 4 weeks appears to have efficacy in some cases.

Even when remediable causes for non-response to standard or high doses of neuroleptics have been dealt with, a few schizophrenic patients do not respond to such medication. Some, who suffer from the most severe syndromes, will remain in the hospital to add to the new long stay patients (Mann and Cree 1976) who are, however, aetiologically heterogeneous (Golden et al. 1981).

Maintenance treatment. Maintenance treatment refers to the regular administration of neuroleptics (often in depot form, every 1–8 weeks) with the aim of preventing relapse or a worsening of any residual symptoms.

Maintenance drug therapy may be only one part of a management plan, although some patients do not require other interventions apart from a regular review. In groups of chronic schizophrenic patients, the available evidence leaves no doubt that maintenance treatment can reduce the number of relapses requiring hospital admission (Hogarty et al. 1974). For example, Hirsch et al. (1973) investigated the effect of fluphenazine decanoate and followed up a group of patients for 9 months. A 66% relapse rate was found amongst placebo patients, as compared with an 8% rate in the group who received active treatment. When a group of patients has been managed by the same psychiatrist for several years, it is possible to identify those who are almost certain to relapse after medication has been discontinued (usually within 6 months), and who require maintenance treatment for relatively long periods of at least several years. On the other hand, for most chronic schizophrenic disorders, the appropriate drug, dose and period of maintenance treatment are not easy to determine. Depot medication has been a major advance mainly because it improves compliance, although it may be refused (Ayd 1975; Freeman 1976; Johnson 1977). Also, some patients appear to respond to a depot but not to oral neuroleptics. Another possible advantage of depot preparations is that, for reasons unknown, they may be able to exert therapeutic effects at plasma levels which are far lower than those produced by oral medication (Curry et al. 1978; Tune et al. 1980). However it should be noted that an accumulation of these drugs in the brain may not be reflected in plasma levels. It has been reported that, after an injection of 25 mg fluphenazine decanoate, plasma levels of up to 10 nanograms/ml are usually reached during the first day, and that this is followed by a sharp fall to under 1 nanogram/ml. In contrast, a 25 mg injection of fluphenazine enanthate does not produce a sharp rise on the first day but tends to sustain a relatively high level for the first 7 days, while flupenthixol decanoate produce peak levels about 4–6 days after injection. Such peaks are probably responsible for the regular appearance of mild side effects which can occur after a relatively constant interval following each depot injection (Curry et al. 1979; Wiles and Gelder 1979). It has been suggested that such variations in the plasma levels of depot neuroleptics may be aetiologically important in the development of tardive dyskinesia (Nasrallah 1980), although there are contrary views (Wiles 1979). Many possible variables can influence the rate of absorption of depot preparations, including the site of injection (which should usually be the upper, outer quadrants of the buttocks), the volume and medium of the injection, the concentration of the drug and the degree of muscular exertion. Local toxic necrosis has been reported due to the deposition of crystals of fluspirilene, which is injected in an aqueous medium (McCreadie et al. 1974).

If a patient experiences transient side effects after a constant interval following each depot injection, the timing of the dose should take into account the patient's commitments. For example, the injection can be scheduled so that side effects occur at a weekend if they would otherwise interfere with his weekday occupation.

Depot maintenance medication can be administered by a centralized facility consisting of an out-patient clinic staffed by psychiatrist, a nurse and a social worker. For a patient who will not, or cannot, attend regularly, the nurse should be available to visit the patient at home, monitor his condition, and administer the injection. Such patients should also be reviewed regularly by the psychiatrist at least every 6 months. The supervision and review of depot maintenance treatment requires a high degree of professional skill, as frequent changes in dose may be indicated; for example an increase may be required when the patient is experiencing stressful life events, or the dose may need to be decreased gradually until the minimum effective dose for a particular patient is determined. This may only be found after more than one relapse, but at the first signs of a worsening of signs and symptoms, an increase in the dose may prevent further deterioration. The optimum duration of maintenance treatment varies, and this is difficult to determine except by experience with the individual patient. In general, regular attempts must be made to discontinue the medication; after one severe episode this might be appropriate after 6–9 months, while after several episodes, attempts may be made every 3–5 years. For some patients, who have relapsed several times within a few months of stopping maintenance treatment, this should be continued indefinitely, although even in such cases further attempts at discontinuation should usually be made, perhaps every 7–10 years. The available evidence clearly demonstrates, in groups of schizophrenic patients, the efficacy of maintenance therapy with most conventional neuroleptics, and several general conclusions can be drawn:

(1) There is not much difference between the prophylactic efficacy of the various established neuroleptics for groups of patients, provided that compliance is good and the dosage adequate. However, for individual patients, one preparation may have considerable advantages over another. For example, a change of fluphenazine decanoate to fluphenazine enanthate has been reported to produce a relapse, and vice versa (Ayd 1975). Further evidence is needed to evaluate the indications for fluspirilene.

(2) It is unclear what variables are relevant to the development of tardive dyskinesia apart from age and total dose.

(3) Drug holidays (i.e. various patterns of intermittent medication which reduce the mean weekly intake of active drug) do not seem to be accompanied by increased relapse rates (Prien et al. 1973), although some have claimed that they may be related to the precipitation of tardive dyskinesia (Nasrallah 1980).

(4) A combination of more than one neuroleptic does not seem superior to maintenance treatment with a single drug (Davis and Garver 1978).

(5) Combinations of neuroleptics and antidepressants can sometimes induce a worsening of symptoms (Casey et al. 1961), but may be tried when a depressive syndrome is present which is not secondary to the neuroleptic treatment (Siris et al. 1978; Prussoff et al. 1979). Ayd (1975) has advocated giving one dose of an antiparkinsonian agent intravenously to determine whether any depressive symptoms are a side effect of neuroleptic medication. He claimed that, if this is the case, an improvement would be expected within an hour. Also, a trial period without medication may be advisable if there is doubt as to the aetiology of lack of motivation or other depressive phenomena.

(6) Abrupt withdrawal from maintenance neuroleptics may precipitate symptoms such as nausea, restlessness, sweating, diarrhoea, rigidity, akathesia, tremor, tics and an increase in schizophrenic symptoms (Gardos et al. 1978).

(7) There is a consensus among clinicians that the chronic use of antiparkinsonian medication should not be routine practice (Gerlach et al. 1977; Johnson 1979), as it is possible that these drugs are associated with reduced absorption of oral neuroleptics, reduced plasma levels (Loga et al. 1975; Singh and Kay 1975; Simpson et al. 1980) and precipitation of tardive dyskinesia (Nasrallah 1980). However Hansen et al. (1979) have reported that plasma levels of perphenazine or its metabolites are not influenced by biperiden or orphenadrine. If extrapyramidal side effects persist, the first step must be to try to reduce the dose of neuroleptic. However, in certain cases, when the minimum effective dose is still associated with these side effects, routine antiparkinsonian medication may be prescribed, although this may not be needed continuously; some patients experience side effects only in the initial phase of the period between injections, when the duration of the regimen of antiparkinsonian medication can be restricted accordingly.

(8) The management of tardive dyskinesia (TD) presents many unsolved problems. Preventative measures include ensuring that maintenance treatment is only given to those who benefit; prescription of the minimum effective dose; and the identification of early signs of this complication. The initial signs may emerge only after a neuroleptic is reduced or discontinued.

When TD appears medication is not necessarily withdrawn if a patient has been shown to relapse regularly in the past, but in other patients, a gradual discontinuation of the drug is indicated. If a relapse of the schizophrenic disorder is precipitated, this may be treated by a drug such as thioridazine, which has been reported to be less likely to induce TD, but if compliance or response is poor, the original depot may have to be restarted. Sometimes

stopping the neuroleptic worsens the TD, although there may be no relapse of
the psychosis; in such cases, although gradual improvement may take place
over many months, the TD may be sufficiently severe for it to become necessary
to restart the neuroleptic despite the risk of producing an eventual worsening of
this side effect (Gardos and Cole 1976). However, if possible, neuroleptic
treatment should not be reinstituted. Various drugs including deanol and
sodium valproate have been used in an attempt to treat TD, but the results are
not encouraging, although it has been claimed that some patients benefit
(Linnoila et al. 1976). A benzodiazepine may provide some relief (see Chapter
2).

The Management of Specific Schizophrenic States

Simple schizophrenia. This term refers to an early insidious onset of negative
features of schizophrenia, accompanied by a decreasing social competence. In
addition, hypochondriacal, sexual and religious preoccupations are commonly
associated. Sometimes, the clinician may confuse this presentation of a schizophrenic disorder with 'adolescent crisis of identity' and delay pharmacological treatment, although neuroleptics usually have, at best, a limited effect when
negative symptoms predominate. The prognosis of such a syndrome is relatively
poor; nonetheless, pharmacological treatment must be tried, and rehabilitation
started.

Catatonic syndromes. Both catatonic stupor (Berrios 1981) and excitement
(Stauder 1934) can be life threatening, and electroconvulsive therapy (ECT) is
still the treatment of choice, as these syndromes may not respond sufficiently or
quickly to a neuroleptic. Catatonic excitement is, in general, more difficult to
manage but usually responds to a combination of ECT and chlorpromazine or
haloperidol. However, there are reports of rare, severe forms of excitement, the
so-called lethal catatonias, which may lead to death from exhaustion and
hyperthermia; it is possible that these cases are misdiagnosed forms of acute
encephalitis. The neuroleptic-induced 'malignant syndrome', which has been
previously described, may occasionally be confused with catatonic excitement
(Morris et al. 1980; Bourgeois and Tignol 1981).

The sodium amytal test can be helpful in the differential diagnosis of a stupor
(see Chapter 13).

Monosymptomatic psychoses. This term incorporates a number of syndromes
including that of 'delusional parasitosis', which is characterized by delusions of
infestation, often accompanied by tactile hallucinations (Berrios 1982*c*). The
relationship of this and other monosymptomatic psychoses with the rest of the
schizophrenias is uncertain, but pimozide and other neuroleptics have been
found to be of value in some of these syndromes (Riding and Munto 1975; Reilly
et al. 1978). Also, there are anecdotal reports that a monoamine oxidase

inhibitor can be effective. However, despite these claims, many of these patients do not respond to pharmacological treatment. Another disorder with a circumscribed delusion occurs in adolescents who express such beliefs that they emit a foul smell, or have facial features larger than normal (Pryse-Phillips, 1971). Such delusions are also found in older age groups and have attracted another label of 'dysmorphophobia' (Liberman 1974). Although at times this seems to be an understandable reaction in an individual with marked paranoid personality traits, some examples of this syndrome are often considered to be related to the schizophrenic or affective disorders: the same can be said of circumscribed delusional hypochondriasis.

Post-psychotic depression. Affective disorder involving depression and anxiety can be seen preceding (Conrad 1958), during (Shanfield et al. 1970) or following (McGlashan and Carpenter 1976) a schizophrenic illness. When a persistent depressive syndrome follows the remission of a severe schizophrenic episode (Gloperud and Depue 1979), the possible causes must be reviewed; depressive symptoms can be an integral part of acute or chronic schizophrenic disorder (Hirsch 1981), an understandable reaction to the sequelae of illness, or the result of the side effects of neuroleptic medication (Andrews 1973; Ayd 1975). If the depressive phenomena are severe, it may be appropriate to prescribe antidepressant medication, although in general the beneficial effects are limited. Nevertheless, an attempt must be made to treat depressive symptoms with all available methods, because of the risk of suicide. If antidepressants are prescribed, the patient must be regularly reviewed, as tricyclics can worsen or precipitate schizophrenic delusions and hallucinations (Siris et al. 1978).

Grafted schizophrenias. The mentally handicapped may develop schizophrenic illness (Reid 1976), which can be difficult to recognize due to the limited ability of the patient to communicate his experiences, and to non-specific behavioural disturbance resulting from the pathoplastic effects of the pre-existing condition (Corbett 1979). Neuroleptic medication is indicated (Snaith et al. 1979).

Schizophrenic-like states associated with organic and toxic factors. Amphetamine psychosis (Connell 1958; Janowsky and Risch 1979), cocaine psychosis (Post 1975) and alcoholic psychosis (Cutting 1978) may appear during or after the episode of abuse. The first step in management is to encourage the patient to stop consumption of the drug, and then neuroleptic treatment is instituted for varying periods. If, as in some cases of alcoholic hallucinosis, neuroleptic treatment is required for some time after withdrawal from alcohol, and especially if the patient will not stop drinking, a depot preparation may be indicated. Also community support is always necessary.

Schizophrenic-like psychoses can also be seen in the context of Huntington's chorea (Rosenbaum 1941), Wilson's Disease (Beard 1959), lupus erythematosis

(Fainglass et al. 1976), treatment with corticosteroids (Hall 1979), and other neurological or systemic conditions. In the author's experience, flupenthixol can be successful in the control of schizophrenic-like disorders in those suffering from hepatolenticular degeneration who are already taking penicillamine, and does not produce a worsening in rigidity or dysarthria. In Parkinson's disease, psychotic states may be more successfully managed with ECT than neuroleptics (Chapter 13), while the psychotic concomitants of collagen diseases such as Crohn's disease can also be difficult to manage with neuroleptics, due to an increased production of α_1-acid glycoprotein (Editorial 1979), which binds the neuroleptic and thus reduces bioavailability. In such cases, and in the psychoses resulting from the administration of corticosteroids, early ECT treatment is usually indicated. The schizophrenic-like state which can accompany temporal lobe epilepsy responds well to neuroleptics, and ECT is rarely needed (see Chapter 13). Hearing loss may be associated with the precipitation of some paranoid states in the elderly, and its correction may be relevant to their treatment (Editorial 1981).

Paranoid syndromes. These are a heterogeneous group of disorders in which delusions of persecution and/or grandiosity are predominant (Manschreck 1979), and many are generally accepted to be part of the schizophrenias. Paranoid schizophrenia has a predominance of relatively circumscribed delusions (usually persecutory) and hallucinations, and a relatively late onset, usually between the ages of 30 and 39 (Angst et al. 1973). There is less agreement about the nosological status of so-called paranoia (Kendler 1980) (which is similar to paranoid schizophrenia, but just involves persecutory and/or grandiose delusions), and of certain paranoid syndromes of late life which have been reported to be associated with social isolation and deafness. The syndrome of 'morbid jealousy', involving circumscribed delusions with the theme that the patient's spouse is being unfaithful may, in some cases, be a variant of paranoid schizophrenia or paranoia (Ey 1950). Some paranoid syndromes seem to be secondary to various conditions including identifiable cerebral disorder such as toxic states or dementia, an interaction between an individual with marked personality traits and his environment, or an affective disorder (Manschreck 1981).

The first step in management is diagnosis, and if the paranoid syndrome is secondary to another treatable disorder, the appropriate treatment is instituted; this may involve pharmacological treatment, social intervention to reduce isolation, or an attempt to modify excessive alcohol consumption. Although some patients with a paranoid schizophrenia or paranoia may benefit considerably from long-term treatment with depot neuroleptics, they are generally unwilling to accept such advice, and in many cases, because of their apparent normality at interview, compulsory treatment is not legally possible. Also, even if all aspects of the patient's social functioning are deteriorating rapidly and the psychiatrist feels that compulsory treatment is justified, the necessary agreement may not be forthcoming. However, when the patient's behaviour becomes sufficiently bizarre to convince all those concerned that intervention is essential, compulsory treatment with a depot neuroleptic can be instituted. Although the positive symptoms of some patients with paranoid schizophrenia show considerable or even complete remission, the delusions and hallucinations of many such patients merely become less intense over a period of several months. But even a modest remission can allow the patient to resume a degree of social integration outside hospital (Retterstöl 1970).

The morbid jealousy syndrome which, like paranoid states in general, is a heterogeneous group aetiologically, may sometimes respond to neuroleptics. However, the outlook is usually poor with regard to the delusion, although, in other respects, the patient's social adjustment may be unremarkable unless alcoholism is a complicating factor. If the spouse (usually a wife) is subject to repeated and severe physical violence, and the patient is unwilling to accept treatment or is unresponsive to treatment, separation may be the spouse's only way to avoid escalating violence and a possible fatal outcome.

As compliance is poor in most paranoid syndromes, depot medication is indicated when pharmacological treatment is appropriate, but in those patients who are compliant, trifluoperazine up to 30–40 mg daily is believed by many clinicians to be particularly valuable in these disorders. If a patient's medication can be supervised in hospital, or when the patient is prepared to cooperate (perhaps under supervision of a family member at home), then a trial with trifluoperazine is indicated. However, even if the patient responds to an oral neuroleptic while being supervised in hospital, a change to a depot preparation may need to be considered before discharge.

References

ALMOND, R. (1975) Issues in milieu therapy. *Schizophrenia Bull.*, **1**, 12.
ANDREASEN, N. (1982) Negative symptoms of schizophrenia. *Archs gen. Psychiat.*, **39**, 784.
ANDREWS, W.M. (1973) Long-acting tranquillizers and the amotivational syndrome in the treatment of schizophrenia. In: *Community Management of the Schizophrenic in Chemical Remission*, ed. King, E.H. Amsterdam: Excerpta Medica.
ANGST, J. et al. (1973) In: *Verlauf und Ausgang schizophrener Erkrankungen*, ed. Huber B. Stuttgart: Schattauer.
AYD, F.J. (1975) The depot fluphenazines: a reappraisal after 10 years' clinical experience. *Am. J. Psychiat.*, **132**, 791.
BAKER, R. (1975) Behavioural techniques in the treatment of schizophrenia. In: *New Perspectives in Schizophrenia*, ed. Forrest, A. & Affleck, J., pp. 215–41. Edinburgh: Churchill Livingstone.
BALDESSARINI, R.J. (1980) Drugs and the treatment of psychiatric disorders. In: *The Pharmacological Basis of Therapeutics*, ed. Goodman & Gilman, 6th ed. New York: MacMillan.
BALDESSARINI, R.J. & DAVIS, J.M. (1980) What is the best maintenance dose of neuroleptics in schizophrenia? *Psychiat. Res. Rep.*, **3**, 115.
BARTON, R. (1959) *Institutional Neurosis*. Bristol: John Wright.
BATESON, G. et al. (1956) Toward a theory of schizophrenia. *Behavl Sci.*, **1**, 251.
BEARD, A.W. (1959) The association of hepatolenticular degeneration with schizophrenia. *Acta psychiat. neurol. scand.*, **34**, 411.

BECK, J.C. et al. (1981) An empirical investigation of psychotherapy with schizophrenic patients. *Schizophrenic Bull.*, **7**, 241.

BEDNAR, R.L. & LAWLIS, G.F. (1971) Empirical research in group psychotherapy. In: *Handbook of Psychotherapy and Behaviour Change*, ed. Bergin, A.E. & Garfield, S.L. New York: John Wiley.

BENEDETTI, G. (1980) Individual psychotherapy of schizophrenia. *Schizophrenia Bull.*, **6**: 633.

BERRIOS, G.E. (1981) Stupor revisited. *Compreh. Psychiat.*, **22**, 466.

BERRIOS, G.E. (1982a) Tactile hallucinations. *J. Neurol. Neurosurg. Psychiat.*, **45**, 285.

BERRIOS, G.E. (1982b) Disorientation states and psychiatry. *Comp. Psychiat.*, **23**, 479.

BERRIOS, G.E. (1982c) Neuroleptic-refractory patients and their plasma levels. *L'Encephale*, **8**, 503.

BOURGEOIS, M. & TIGNOL, J. (1981) Hyperthermie et syndromes malins au cours des traitements neuroleptiques. *Encyclopédie Medico-Chirurgicale, Psychiatrie*, 37860B20, Paris: Ed. Techniques.

BROCKINGTON, I.F. & KENDELL, R.E., LEFF, J.P. (1978) Definitions of schizophrenia: concordance and prediction of outcome. *Psychol. Med.* **8**, 387.

BROCKINGTON, I.F. et al. (1980) Manic patients with schizophrenic or paranoid symptoms. *Psychol. Med.*, **10**, 73.

CASEY, J.F. et al. (1961) Combined drug therapy of chronic schizophrenics. Controlled evaluation of placebo, dextroamphetamine, imipramine, isocarboxazid and trifluoperazine added to maintenance doses of chlorpromazine. *Am. J. Psychiat.*, **117**, 997.

CONNELL, P.H. (1958) *Amphetamine Psychosis*. Maudsley Monograph 5. London: Oxford Univ. Press.

CONRAD, K. (1958) *Die beginnende Schizophrenie*. Stuttgart: Thieme.

CORBETT, J.A. (1979) Psychiatric morbidity and mental retardation. In: *Psychiatric Illness and Mental Handicap*, ed. James, F.E. & Snaith, R.P. London: Gaskell.

CROW, T.J. (1980) Positive and negative schizophrenic symptoms and the role of dopamine. *Br. J. Psychiat.*, **137**, 383.

CROW, T.J. (1981) Positive and negative schizophrenic symptoms and the role of dopamine. *Br. J. Psychiat.*, **139**, 251.

CURRY, S.H., ALTAMURA, A.C. & MONTGOMERY, S. (1979) Unwanted effects of fluphenazine enanthate and decanoate. *Lancet*, **i**, 331.

CURRY, S.H., WHELPTON, R., SCHEPPER, P.J. et al. (1978) Plasma-fluphenazine concentrations after injection of long-acting esters. *Lancet*, **i**, 1217.

CUTTING, J. (1978) A reappraisal of alcoholic psychoses. *Psychol. Med.*, **8**, 285.

DAVIS, J.M. (1975) Maintenance therapy in psychiatry 1. Schizophrenia. *Am. J. Psychiat.* **132**, 1237.

DAVIS, J.M. et al. (1978) Plasma levels of antipsychotic drugs and clinical response. In: *Psychopharmacology: A Generation of Progress*, ed. Lipton, K.A. et al. New York: Raven Press.

DAVIS, J.M. et al. (1980) Important issues in the drug treatment of schizophrenia. *Schizophrenia Bull.* **6**: 70.

DAVIS, J.M. & GARVER, D.L. (1978) Neuroleptics: clinical use in psychiatry. In: *Handbook of Psychopharmacology Vol. 10*, ed. Iversen, L.L. et al. New York: Plenum Press.

DAVISON, K. & BAGLEY, C.R. (1969) Schizophrenia-like psychoses associated with disorders of the central nervous system: a review of the literature. In: *Current Problems in Neuropsychiatry*, ed. Herrington, R.N. Kent: Headley Bros.

DENCKER, S.J., JOHANSSON, R., LUNDIN, L. & MALM, U. (1978a) High doses of fluphenazine enanthate in schizophrenia. *Acta psychiat. scand.*, **57**, 405.

DENCKER, S.J. (1978b) The safety of high-dose depot fluphenazine therapy. In: *Depot fluphenazines: Twelve Years' Experience*, ed. Ayd, F.J. Baltimore: Ayd Medical Communication.

DOMINO, E.F. (1979) Importance of blood levels of neuroleptics in the treatment of schizophrenia. In: *The Kinetics of Psychiatric Drugs*, ed. Schoolar, J.C. & Claghorn, J.C. New York: Brunner Mazel.

DSM III (1980) *Diagnostic and Statistical Manual of Mental Disorders*, 3rd ed. Washington, D.C: American Psychiatric Association.

EDITORIAL, (1979) Is drug binding to α_1-acid-glycoprotein clinically important? *Lancet*, **i**, 368.

EDITORIAL, (1981) Hearing loss and perceptual dysfunction in schizophrenia. *Lancet*, **ii**, 848.

EY, H. (1950) Jalousie morbide. In: *Études Psychiatriques*, Vol. 2, Étude 18. Paris: Desclée de Brouwer.

FAINGLASS, E.J., ARNETT, F.C., DORSCH, C.A. et al. (1976) Neuropsychiatric manifestations of systemic lupus erythematosus. *Medicine*, **55**, 323.

FREEMAN, H. (1976) Long-acting neuroleptics and their place in community mental health services in the United Kingdom: the Salford Experience. *Acta Psychiat. Belg.*, **76**, 786.

FROMM-REICHMANN, F. (1954) Psychotherapy of schizophrenia. *Am. J. Psychiat.*, **111**, 410.

FUENTE, de la, J.R. & ROSENBAUM, A.H. (1981) Prolactin in psychiatry. *Am. J. Psychiat.*, **138**, 1154.

GARDOS, G. et al. (1978) Withdrawal syndromes associated with antipsychotic drugs. *Am. J. Psychiat.*, **135**, 1321.

GARDOS, G. & COLE, J.O. (1976) Maintenance antipsychotic therapy: is the cure worse than the disease? *Am. J. Psychiat.*, **133**, 32.

GERLACH, J. et al. (1977) Antiparkinsonian agents and long-term neuroleptic treatment. *Acta psychiat. scand.*, **55**, 251.

GERLACH, J. & LÜDORF, K. (1975) The effect of L-DOPA on young patients with simple schizophrenia, treated with neuroleptic drugs. *Psychopharmacologia*, **44**, 105.

GLICK, I.D., HARGREAVES, W.A. & GOLDFIELD, M.D. (1974) Short vs. long hospitalization. *Archs gen. Psychiat.*, **30**, 262.

GLOPERUD, E. & DEPUE, R.A. (1979) Affective symptoms, schizophrenia and the conceptual ambiguity of post psychotic depression. *Schizophrenia Bull.*, **5**, 554.

GOLDBERG, S.C. et al. (1967) Prediction of improvement in schizophrenia under four phenothiazines. *Archs gen. Psychiat.*, **16**, 107.

GOLDEN, C.J. et al. (1981) Structural brain deficits in schizophrenia. *Archs gen. Psychiat.*, **33**, 1014.

GRUEN, P.H. et al. (1978) Relation of plasma prolactin to clinical response in schizophrenic patients. *Archs gen. Psychiat.*, **35**, 1222.

HALL, R.C.W. et al. (1979) Presentation of the steroid psychoses. *J. nerv. ment. Dis.*, **167**, 229.

HANSEN, L.B., ELLEY, J. & CHRISTENSEN, T.R. (1979) Plasma levels of perphenazine and its major metabolites during simultaneous treatment with anticholinergic drugs. *Br. J. Clin. Pharmacol.*, **7**, 75.

HIRSCH, S.R. (1981) Do neuroleptics cause depression in the schizophrenias? Paper presented at W.P.A. Meeting, New York.

HIRSCH, S.R. et al. (1973) Outpatients maintenance of chronic schizophrenic patients with long acting fluphenazine: double blind placebo trial. *Br. med. J.*, **i**, 633.

HIRSCH, S.R. & LEFF, J.P. (1975) *Abnormalities in Parents of Schizophrenics*. Institute of Psychiatry Maudsley Monograph No. 22. Oxford: Oxford University Press.

HIRSCH, S.R., PLATT, S., KNIGHTS, A. & WEYMAN, A. (1979) Shortening hospital stay for psychiatric care: effect on the patients and their families. *Br. med. J.*, **i**, 442.

HOGARTY, G.E. et al. (1974) The Collaborative Study Group: Drug and sociotherapy in the aftercare of schizophrenic patients II—Two years relapse rate. *Archs gen. Psychiat.*, **31**, 603.

HOLZMAN, P.S. & LEVY, D.L. (1977) Smooth pursuit eye movements and functional psychoses: a review. *Schizophrenia Bull.*, **3**, 15.

JANOWSKY, D.S. & RISCH, C. (1979) Amphetamine psychosis and psychotic symptoms. *Psychopharmacology*, **65**, 73.

JIMERSON, D.C. et al. (1982) Diazepam in schizophrenia. *Am. J. Psychiat.*, **139**, 489.

JOHNSON, D.A.W. (1977) Practical considerations in the use of depot-neuroleptics for the treatment of schizophrenia. *Br. J. hosp. Med.*, **17**, 546.

JOHNSON, D.A.W. (1979) Use of antiparkinsonian medication in patients treated with depot neuroleptics. In: *Neuroleptics and Schizophrenics*, ed. Simister, J.M. Luton: Lundbeck Publication.

JOHNSTONE, E.C. et al. (1978) The dementia of dementia praecox. *Acta psychiat. scand.*, **57**, 305.

KENDLER, K.S. (1980) The nosological validity of paranoia (simple delusional disorder). *Archs gen. Med.*, **37**, 699.

KOLAKOWSKA, T. et al. (1979) Clinical significance of plasma drug and prolactin levels during acute chlorpromazine treatment: a replication study. *Br. J. Psychiat.*, **135**, 352.

KOLAKOWSKA, T. et al. (1981) Plasma protein response to haloperidol challenge. *Br. J. Psychiat.*, **139**, 400.

KORNETSKY, C. (1976) Hyporesponsivity of chronic schizophrenic patients to Dextroamphetamine. *Archs gen. Psychiat.*, **33**, 1425.

LADER, M. (1975) *The Psychophysiology of Mental Illness*, pp. 157–187. London: Routledge & Kegan Paul.

LEFF, J. (1976) Assessment of psychiatric and social state. *Br. J. Clin. Pharmacol. (Suppl. 2)*, **3**, 385.

LIBERMAN, R. (1974) A propos des dysmorphophobies de l'adolescent. *Rev. Neuropsychiat.*, **22**, 695.

LINNOILA, M., VIUKARI, M. & HIETALA (1976) Effect of sodium valproate on tardive dyskinesia. *Br. J. Psychiat.*, **129**, 114.

LOGA, S., CURRY, S. & LADER, M. (1975) Interactions of orphenadrine and phenobarbitone with chlorpromazine: plasma concentrations and effects in man. *Br. J. Clin. Pharmacol.*, **2**, 197.

MACKAY, A.V.P. (1980) Positive and negative schizophrenic symptoms and the role of dopamine. *Br. J. Psychiat.*, **137**, 379.

MACKAY, A.V.P. et al. (1974) The relationship of plasma chlorpromazine and its hydroxy and sulphoxide metabolites in a large population of chronic schizophrenics. *Br. J. clin. Pharmacol.*, **1**, 425.

MANN, S.A. & CREE, W. (1976) [New] long stay psychiatric patients: a national sample survey of fifteen mental hospitals in England and Wales 1972/3. *Psychol. Med. 6:* 603.

MANSCHRECK, T.C. (1979) The assessment of paranoid features. *Compreh. Psychiat.*, **20**, 370.

MANSCHRECK, T.C. (1981) Paranoid behaviour. In: *Psychiatric Medicine Update, M.C.H. Review for Physicians*, ed. Manschreck, T.C., 65–76. Edinburgh: Churchill-Livingstone.

MAY, P.R. et al. (1978) Test dose response in schizophrenia. *Archs gen. Psychiat.*, **35**, 1091.

McCREADIE, R.G., KIERNAN, W.E.S., VENNER, R.M. & DENHOLM, R.B. (1979) Probable toxic necrosis after prolonged fluspirilene administration. *Br. med. J.*, **1**, 523.

McGLASHAN, T.H. & CARPENTER, W.T. (1976) Post-psychotic depression in schizophrenia. *Archs gen. Psychiat.*, **33**, 231.

McGUFFIN, P., FARMER, A.E. & RAJAH, S.M. (1978) Histocompatibility antigens and schizophrenia. *Br. J. Psychiat.*, **132**, 149.

MELLOR, C.S. (1970) First rank symptoms of schizophrenia. *Br. J. Psychiat.*, **117**, 15.

MELTZER, H.Y. & FANG, V.A. (1976) The effects of neuroleptics on serum prolactin in schizophrenic patients. *Archs gen. Psychiat.*, **33**, 279.

MORGAN, R. (1974) Industrial therapy. *Br. J. hosp. Med.*, **8**, 231.

MORRIS, H.H., McCORMICK, W.F. & REINARZ, J.A. (1980) Neuroleptic malignant syndrome. *Arch. Neurol.*, **37**, 462.

MOSHER, L.R. & KEITH, S.J. (1979) Research on the psychosocial treatment of schizophrenia: A summary report. *Am. J. Psychiat.*, **136**, 623.

NASRALLAH, H.A. (1980) Neuroleptic plasma levels and tardive dyskinesia: a possible link? *Schizophrenic Bull.*, **6**, 4.

NOONAN, J.P.H. et al. (1976) Sex and neuroleptic medication. *Psychiat. J. Univ. Ottawa*, **7**, 86.

PHILLIPSON, O.T. et al. (1977) Correlation between plasma chlorpromazine and its metabolites and clinical ratings in patients with acute relapse of schizophrenic and paranoid psychoses. *Br. J. Psychiat.*, **131**, 172.

PLANANSKY, K. & JOHNSON, R. (1971) The occurrence and characteristics of suicidal preoccupations and acts in schizophrenia. *Acta psychiat. scand.*, **47**, 473.

POST, R.M. (1975) Cocaine psychosis: a continuum model. *Am. J. Psychiat.*, **132**, 225.

PRIEN, R.F. et al. (1973) Intermittent pharmacotherapy in chronic schizophrenia. *Hosp. Community Psychiat.*, **24**, 317.

PROCCI, W.R. (1976) Schizo-affective psychosis: fact or fiction? *Archs gen. Psychiat.*, **33**, 1167.

PRUSSOFF, B.A. et al. (1979) Treatment of secondary depression in schizophrenia. *Archs gen. Psychiat.*, **36**, 569.

PRYSE-PHILLIPS, W. (1971) An olfactory reference syndrome. *Acta psychiat. scand.*, **47**, 484.

QUITKIN, F. et al. (1974) Very high dose vs. standard dosage fluphenazine in schizophrenia. *Archs gen. Psychiat.*, **32**, 1276.

RAMA RAO, V.A. et al. (1980) Clinical state plasma levels of haloperidol and prolactin: A correlation study in chronic schizophrenia. *Br. J. Psychiat.*, **137**, 518.

REID, A.H. (1976) Psychiatric disturbance in the mentally handicapped. *Proc. R. Soc. Med.*, **69**, 509.

REILLY, T.M., JOPLING, W.H. & BEARD, A.W. (1978) Successful treatment with pimozide of delusional parasitosis. *Br. J. Derm.* **98**, 457.

RETTERSTÖL, N. (1970) *Prognosis in Paranoid Psychoses.* Oslo: Universitets Forlaget.

RICHELSON, E. (1980) Neuroleptics and neurotransmitter receptors. *Psychiat. Ann.*, **10**, 459.

RIDING, J. & MUNRO, A. (1975) Pimozide in the treatment of monosymptomatic hypochondriacal psychosis. *Acta psychiat. scand.*, **52**, 23.

RIVERA-CALIMLIM, L. et al. (1978) Effects of mode of management on plasma chlorpromazine in psychiatric patients. *Clin. Pharmac. Ther.*, **14**, 978.

ROSENBAUM, D. (1941) Psychosis with Huntington's chorea. *Psychiat. Q.*, **15**, 93.

ROTH, M. & McCLELLAND, H. (1979) Problems of diagnosis and treatment in the borderlands of schizophrenia. In: *Neuroleptics and Schizophrenia*, ed. Simister, J.M., pp. 63–81. Luton: Luncbeck House.

RO-TROCK, G.K. et al. (1977) A family therapy outcome study in an in-patient setting. *Am. J. Orthopsychiat.*, **47**, 514.

SAKALIS, G. et al. (1972) Physiological and clinical effects of chlorpromazine and their relationship to plasma level. *Clin. Pharmac. Ther.*, **13**, 931.

SECHEHAYE, M.A. (1978) *Journal d'une schizophrène*. Paris: Presses Universitaires de France.

SCHNEIDER, K. (1959) *Clinical Psychopathology*. New York: Grune and Stratton.

SHANFIELD, S. et al. (1970) The schizophrenic patient and depressive symptomatology. *J. nerv. ment. Dis.*, **151**, 203.

SHEPHERD, G. (1981) The function and organization of day hospitals. *Italian Congress on Preventive Medicine, June 1981*.

SIMPSON, G.M. et al. (1980) Effect of antiparkinsonian medication on plasma levels of chlorpromazine. *Archs gen. Psychiat.*, **37**, 205.

SINGH, M.M. & KAY, S.R. (1975) A comparative study of haloperidol and chlorpromazine in terms of clinical effects and therapeutic reversal with benztropine in schizophrenia. Theoretical implications for potency differences among neuroleptics. *Psychopharmacologia*, **43**, 103.

SIRIS, S.G. et al. (1978) Use of antidepressant drugs in schizophrenia. *Archs gen. Psychiat.*, **35**, 1368.

SMOLEN, V.F. et al. (1975) Bioavailability analysis of chlorpromazine in humans from pupilometric data. *J. Pharmac. exp. Ther.*, **195**, 404.

SNAITH, R.P. et al. (1979) The drug treatment of mental illness and epilepsy in the mentally handicapped patient. In: *Psychiatric Illness and Mental Handicap*, ed. James, F.E. & Snaith, R.P. London: Gaskell.

SNYDER, S.H. (1981) Dopamine receptors, neuroleptics and schizophrenia. *Am. J. Psychiat.*, **138**, 460.

SPITZER, R., ENDICOTT, J. & ROBINS, E. (1975) *Research Diagnostic Criteria. Instrument NO. 58*. New York: New York State Psychiatric Institute.

STAUDER, K. (1934) Tödliche Katatonie. *Arch. Psychiat. NervKrankh.*, **102**, 614.

STRAUSS, J.S. & CARPENTER, W.T. (1981) *Schizophrenia*. New York: Plenum.

TUNE, L.E. et al. (1980) Low neuroleptic serum levels in patients receiving fluphenazine decanoate. *Am. J. Psychiat.*, **137**, 80.

VAN PUTTEN, T. et al. (1980) Plasma and saliva levels of chlorpromazine and subjective response. *Am. J. Psychiat.*, **137**, 1241.

VAUGHN, C.E. & LEFF, J.P. (1976) The influence of family and social factors on the course of schizophrenic illness: a comparison of schizophrenic and depressed neurotic patients. *Br. J. Psychiat.*, **129**, 125.

VENABLES, P.H. (1981) Psychophysiology of abnormal behaviour. *Br. med. Bull.*, **37**, 199.

WIJSENBEEK, H. et al. (1974) Trifluoperazine: A comparison between regular and high doses. *Psychopharmacologia*, **36**, 147.

WILES, D. (1979) Tardive dyskinesia and depot fluphenazine. *Br. J. Psychiat.*, **135**, 382.

WILES, D.H. et al. (1976) Clinical significance of plasma chlorpromazine levels I. Plasma levels of the drug, some of its metabolites and prolactin during acute treatment. *Psychol. Med.*, **6**, 407.

WILES, D.H. & GELDER, M.G. (1979) Plasma fluphenazine levels in radioimmunoassay in schizophrenic patients treated with depot injections of fluphenazine decanoate. *Br. J. Clin. Pharmacol.*, **8**, 565.

WING, J.K. & BROWN, G.W. (1970) *Institutionalism and Schizophrenia*. London: Cambridge University Press.

YOUNG, M.A. & MELTZER, H.Y. (1980) The relationship of demographic, clinical and outcome variables to neuroleptic treatment requirements. *Schizophrenia Bull.*, **6**, 88.

15

Management of Depression and Mania in Clinical Practice

DEPRESSION

Sir Martin Roth

Introduction

The literature that deals with the management of depressive syndromes conveys a misleading impression of polarized attitudes and practices in this field. Psychiatrists who have a special interest in pharmacological treatment do not treat depressed patients by prescribing drugs alone, while those who devote themselves to psychotherapeutic forms of management seldom permit patients to suffer from unremitting states of misery and hopelessness without recourse, where appropriate, to medication or an opinion from another colleague more familiar with biological treatments.

There is also general agreement that it is important to decide at the outset whether any form of medical treatment, in the strict sense of the term, is required; for a distinction has to be made between ordinary states of sadness, grief and disappointment on the one hand, and psychiatric disorder on the other. The evidence that there is a reasonably clear line of distinction is drawn from observations on the course and outcome of different types of mood disorder, and from pharmacological studies. Depressive states which can be understood in terms of response to adversity present with a relatively small span of 4–8 weeks. The psychiatrist should, of course, never refuse to give support in such cases, but this should focus on helping the individual to come to terms with his losses, defeats and difficulties by drawing upon his own emotional resources.

The clinician must realize that, when the nature and severity of a depressive syndrome is readily understandable as a reaction of the individual to stressful life events, the therapeutic potential for pharmacological treatment will usually prove relatively modest. The liberal prescription of antidepressant drugs in the management of mild and transient depressions has led to the wide dissemination of potentially dangerous substances, and has contributed to the rising tide

311

of self-poisoning and attempted suicide that has been witnessed in many countries in the past 25 years. Also, as many of these disorders are self-limiting, early initiation of formal or intensive psychotherapy may not only be premature, but may foster a state of dependence on the therapist, thus eroding the patient's confidence in his own ability to cope.

Diagnosis of Depressive Syndromes

Introduction. In the management of all depressive disorders account has to be taken of the presenting syndrome, any physical illness, the patient's personality, the quality of the premorbid and current pattern of adaptation, difficulties in interpersonal relationships, emotional conflicts, and sexual, familial or social problems that may have played a part in initiating symptoms, or may be active in their perpetuation. However, all causal factors, both essential and non-essential, do not merit the same weight and attention; for example, in a depressive syndrome in the context of bipolar affective disorder, biological factors are of over-riding importance, although personal, familial and social problems should not be neglected.

The rational treatment of a depressive syndrome demands, as an essential precondition, a categorical scheme for the classification of the signs and symptoms, an evaluation of a number of factors other than the depressive syndrome itself (such as personality, non-psychiatric illness, severity of any stressful life events, and previous level of adaptation), and a formulation of the likely aetiological factors. As will be described, there is persuasive evidence that, among the large and aetiologically heterogeneous group of individuals who present to doctors with a depressed mood, a minority suffer from one of several abnormalities of brain function which are qualitatively different from normality, and usually require a genetic predisposition for their development. During this chapter, such a hypothesized abnormality of brain function will be referred to as 'endogenous aetiology', and the presence of such a disorder can be inferred from the following factors:

(1) The nature of the signs and symptoms: i.e. if the disorder contains one or more of the features of the 'endogenous syndrome' which will be described. However, different elements of the endogenous syndrome carry varying diagnostic implications, and it should be noted that endogenous disorder may be present even though typical clinical features are inconspicuous.

(2) Aspects of the history of the depressive episode: i.e. if there is an apparent lack of sufficient environmental and personality factors which make the development of the syndrome understandable. (However the converse does not follow, as it seems that stressful life events may precipitate an endogenous pathogenic mechanism; thus the presence of adverse antecedent life events is of less diagnostic significance than their absence.)

(3) Certain features of the history of any previous episodes of affective disorder, i.e. if there have been previous depressive episodes with intervening symptom-free periods (especially if there were features of the endogenous depressive syndrome or if their development was not readily understandable); if previous episodes have apparently responded impressively to antidepressant drugs or ECT; or if there have been previous episodes of mania.

(4) A family history of affective disorder with the characteristics described in paragraph (3).

It should be noted that even if the aetiological formulation includes the presumption that endogenous disorder is present, an understandable reaction to stressful life events (which include the effects of the endogenous brain dysfunction itself), often makes a significant contribution to certain features of the syndrome. The relative importance of endogenous aetiology and psychosocial factors will therefore vary considerably between patients and, sometimes, between different episodes of depression in the same patient.

'Endogenous' (or 'autonomous') depression. A large body of evidence has accumulated in recent years to validate the qualitatively distinct character of this syndrome, although the number and composition of the features which coexist in individual patients show considerable variation, and there is no consensus as to the minimum number and characteristics of the criteria for the delineation of 'endogenous depression'. The endogenous syndrome includes psychomotor retardation, diurnal variation (worse in the morning), disturbed sleep with middle or late insomnia, qualitatively distinct form of depressive mood, and, more rarely, delusions with a depressive content (which may involve themes of hypochondriasis, guilt, or impending disaster), and (usually auditory) hallucinations. These features are of relatively high diagnostic significance compared with other aspects of the syndrome such as: excessive sleep; agitation; pessimistic, guilt-laden or nihilistic ideas which do not reach delusional proportions; decline of drive and sexual interest; loss of appetite and weight; blunting of pleasure; and suicidal thoughts or acts.

Such features do not necessarily imply a relatively severe depressive disorder. For patients with delusional and other 'psychotic' features represent only a small proportion of depressives in clinical practice. Amongst the remainder, many patients with the endogenous syndrome may be less severely ill both in terms of overt symptoms and subjective experience, than some individuals with a non-endogenous depressive syndrome.

As the status of endogenous depression is of crucial importance, an attempt will be made to summarize the evidence for its distinct character. Although the common association of non-endogenous features with endogenous depression creates a grey area between the endogenous and non-endogenous states, the presence of a cluster of endogenous features serves to establish the descriptive diagnosis, irrespective of any associated non-specific features, for there is a hierarchical principle, inherent in the Kraepelinian system, whereby the features of the endogenous syndrome have to be given priority in diagnosis. It is self-evident that the presence of a typical bipolar manic–depressive disorder is not called into question by concomitant neurotic symptoms, and the same line of reasoning applies when a unipolar endogenous depressive syndrome is present. This formulation is validated by experience in the management of these conditions, as when treatment for an endogenous depressive syndrome has been successful, the associated non-specific (or 'neurotic') symptoms will often fade or disappear, having been reactions to a very distressing condition. However, all the non-specific symptoms will not disappear if the patient's premorbid state was one of long-standing neuroticism.

Recent neuroendocrine investigations have provided a valuable biochemical adjunct to diagnosis in research studies. It has been known for many years that the plasma cortisol of some depressed patients is raised, and that there are associated changes in the circadian rhythm of cortisol secretion. More recently it has been shown that the activity of the hypothalamic–pituitary–adrenal axis can be assessed by monitoring the suppression of plasma cortisol following the administration of dexamethasone; for example, the work of Carroll et al. (1976, 1980) has shown that, in some depressed patients, a standard dose of 1 mg dexamethasone in the evening fails to exert its usual suppressive effect upon pituitary–adrenal activity. Early escape of plasma cortisol from a standard dose administered in this manner was found in more than 40% of patients with an endogenous syndrome. More recently a higher degree of sensitivity has been reported (Carroll 1982), and it seems that a positive test has an almost unequivocal significance. The dexamethasone suppression test (DST) tends to return to normal on recovery, and it has been recently claimed (Goldberg 1980) that those in whom abnormality persists are at special risk of relapse and should be kept on a maintenance course of tricyclic antidepressants. However this test is not routinely available. The DST also changes in parallel with the shift from depressive to manic illness (Carroll 1982), while the relatively high degree of specificity of the test is reflected by the fact that it is negative in non-endogenous depressive syndromes and in the schizophrenias. It is also of interest that patients with 'major depressive disorder' as identified by the 'Research Diagnostic Criteria' (RDC Criteria, Feighner et al. 1972) proved to be a more heterogeneous group in respect of the dexamethasone suppression test than did those clinically diagnosed as suffering from an endogenous syndrome. Schlesser et al. (1979) have published findings which suggest that resistance to dexamethasone suppression distinguishes three genetic subtypes of unipolar primary depressive disorders.

Another group of neuroendocrine investigations relates to administration of methylamphetamine. Checkley (1979) reported that patients with the syndrome of endogenous depression showed no increase in plasma cortisol after methylamphetamine administration, in contrast to those with non-endogenous depression or other psychiatric disorders, and he interpreted his findings as indicating that endogenous depressive patients have a specific central defect of α-adrenergic function.

Within the endogenous depressive group a distinction should also be made between cases with and without psychotic features, such as delusions, hallucinations and loss of insight. There is no reason to believe that these are genetically or aetiologically different, but there are certain differences in the treatment response and prognosis of psychotic cases to which reference will be made at a later stage.

The differentiation of unipolar endogenous depression and bipolar affective illness also has implications for diagnosis, treatment and prognosis. A depressive syndrome in a patient with a history of bipolar disorder tends to commence earlier and is more likely to be associated with psychomotor retardation, while Guze et al. (1975) found that a higher proportion of bipolar patients (53%) had delusions or hallucinations than unipolar cases (17%). A number of reports also describe unipolar patients as exhibiting more somatic symptoms, anxiety and agitation than bipolar cases. Also, some EEG differences have been reported, for example, involving the rate of augmentation of averaged evoked responses to light, with increasing intensity of stimulation (Buchsbaum et al. 1971). These are promising findings, but further observations will be required before the results can be applied in clinical practice. However, despite the validity of the unipolar/bipolar dichotomy in certain respects, unipolar depressions, with their poor defining criteria, are liable to become a repository for a heterogeneous group of disorders including anxiety and phobic states, and depressions in the setting of severe personality disorders (Roth and Barnes 1981). For such a group, the results of therapy and of scientific investigation would be expected to prove inconsistent.

Neurotic depression. Perhaps the most unexceptionable name for this heterogeneous group of disorders would be 'non-endogenous depressive syndrome', but 'neurotic depression' is clearer and simpler. These syndromes consist of a variable number of features such as: depressed mood, irritability, loss of interest, poor concentration, impaired motivation and energy, lack of enjoyment, reduced libido, preoccupation with current problems, anxiety, restlessness, sleep disturbance (usually difficulty in getting off to sleep with subsequent wakening and vivid dreams), poor appetite and moderate weight loss, various somatic complaints, a worsening of symptoms towards the end of the day, and thoughts of self-injury or suicide. A number of subdivisions have been suggested, and the one that is best validated is that of Paykel (Paykel 1972; Prusoff and Paykel 1977), who proposed three groups of non-endogenous non-psychotic depressions, comprising 'anxious depression', 'hostile depression', and depression in the setting of personality disorder. Some support for this distinction is that endogenous depressions responded best to amitriptyline while anxious depressions responded poorly both in the first and second study. It was, however, an unexpected finding that patients with anxious depressions fared worse than those with mood disorder in the setting of personality disorder.

It remains to be determined what relationship these three groups bear to the large number of other syndromes that have been defined with the aid of such terms as 'hysterical dysphoria', the 'self-pitying constellation' and 'characterological depression' among others. The question arises whether these are different disorders, or one and the same depressive syndrome in different personality settings. The need for more precise data on classification and treatment response is reflected by the finding of Akiskal et al. (1978) that all three suicides in their follow-up study of 100 'mild' depressive states had been drawn from the ranks of characterological depressives. Confusion may have been generated in this area by the failure to provide separate and independent specification for the presenting clinical syndrome and for the personality background.

The poor response of Paykel's cases of non-endogenous anxious depression to amitriptyline poses questions regarding the relationship between this group and the anxiety states. The line of demarcation is unclear and some workers doubt whether any valid distinction can be made. Yet there is evidence, both from investigations of clinical profiles and independent follow-up studies, that although symptoms may overlap, the anxiety and depressive syndromes can be differentiated (Gurney et al. 1972; Kerr et al. 1972; Roth et al. 1972; Schapira et al. 1972). In a recent enquiry (Mountjoy and Roth 1982), endogenous depressions were excluded and enquiries confined to non-endogenous depression, anxiety and phobic states. Eight rating scales for anxiety or depression (and one discriminating scale, the Newcastle anxiety depression scale) were submitted to multivariate analyses which were also undertaken in relation to the clinical findings recorded in the course of a structured interview. Once again, it proved possible to separate the depressive from the anxiety states. Certain implications for differential diagnosis and decisions about management may be deduced from these studies. If severe anxiety and tension with psychic and/or physical concomitants dominate the clinical picture, this argues in favour of an anxiety state which may be associated with such features as irritability, initial insomnia (perhaps followed by frequent waking), attacks of panic, signs of severe autonomic disturbance, or recurrent derealization. However, severe unremitting depression should be given precedence in diagnosis over all anxiety symptoms and treated accordingly.

The severity of illness does not provide a satisfactory basis for the classification or treatment of depressive syndromes. This was clearly reflected in the study of Akiskal et al. (1978) in which 100 patients with 'mild' depressive states were admitted to a prospective follow-up over a 4-year period. Of these patients, 18% developed bipolar disorder and 22% a unipolar disorder, while the majority of the remainder were considered to be suffering from depression in settings of alcoholism, sexual maladjustment, or anxiety, phobic, obsessional and hysterical neuroses. Thus, if depressive syndromes are classified on the basis of lack of severity, a heterogeneous group will be selected. The second lesson from this study is that the presence of prominent depressive symptoms does not automatically signify that the correct diagnosis is some form of depressive illness.

Schizoaffective disorder. The diagnostic problems posed by this group of disorders are complex and the literature conflicting (Brockington 1981). The subject cannot be fully reviewed here, but points which have a special bearing on therapy will be briefly considered.

When there is an adequate number of schizophrenic features to justify a diagnosis of schizophrenia in their own right, then this diagnosis would appear to be appropriate in the light of conventional clinical criteria. On the other hand, in the presence of a fully fledged picture of endogenous depression (or mania), with only one or perhaps two 'first-rank' schizophrenic symptoms, the term 'schizoaffective' has dubious validity as, in follow-up studies, the course of the disorder in such patients does not usually resemble that of affective disorder.

The Management of Depressive Illness

The discussion devoted to the diagnostic aspects draws its justification from the fact that the most important steps in the choice of appropriate interventions for a depressive syndrome are an accurate descriptive diagnosis, physical examination, certain routine screening tests and an aetiological formulation that takes full account of all relevant biological, familial, social, situational and personality factors. In arriving at a diagnostic formulation, the presence of life events which appear to be impressively related to the onset of symptoms does not deserve a great deal of weight. It certainly should not be permitted by itself to subdivide depressions into those with or without an endogenous disorder.

Admission to hospital. The clinician's first responsibility is to ensure that the patient does not lose his life in the course of a potentially reversible disorder. In deciding upon the need for in-patient or day-patient hospital treatment, he is guided by the type of depression, the complications encountered in previous attacks, age, assessment of suicidal risk, and the presence of concomitant features such as alcoholism and physical illness. Psychotic patients (i.e. those cases of an endogenous depressive syndrome with delusions and/or hallucinations) should always be treated in hospital, and so should all those who have made premeditated suicidal attempts in previous depressive episodes. Also, patients with recurrent suicidal urges elicited by the psychiatrist, or confided to a relative, or with a first attack of severe depression in late or middle life following a serious loss or some irremediable change in the patient's fortune, cannot be safely treated at home. Risk factors for suicide include living alone, male sex, previous suicidal attempts, and limited social contacts.

Alcoholism always magnifies the suicidal risk and all types of depression complicated by heavy drinking need to be treated under close supervision. This holds also for any chronic physical illness associated with depression, particularly in males, even when the disability is not particularly severe. A colouring of behaviour associated with hysterical personality disorder, in the form of self-dramatizing, importunate or manipulative behaviour, is liable to mask underlying depressive symptoms and lead to errors in diagnosis and management. When a diagnosis of 'hysteria' or 'hysterical personality' is made in a patient in whom hysterical symptoms or histrionic behaviour have developed with rapidity for the first time in middle and late life, it almost invariably proves to be incorrect. Endogenous depressive aetiology is one of the causes of such developments and this possibility should always be considered.

The great majority of people suffering from a severe depressive syndrome are prepared to enter hospital on an informal basis and settle there with a sense of security, feeling protected from their suicidal urges. However admission to hospital may entail considerable disruption within the family or some danger to employment if the patient is still at work. Only a small proportion of patients, who are usually psychotic and judged to be at high suicidal risk, require compulsory admission, while the majority of patients with relatively mild syndromes can be satisfactorily treated on an out-patient basis. Even in moderately severe cases, if the worst symptoms, including insomnia, can be brought under rapid control by medication, admission may be avoided and the patient may be able to continue at work. In some patients, electroconvulsive therapy (ECT) can be undertaken on an out-patient basis, although arrangements should always be made for the patient to spend a few hours under observation in a hospital ward, or a half day in a day hospital if one is available.

Psychiatric and physical evaluation. A comprehensive assessment must be undertaken in each patient who presents with depressive symptoms. This must include a careful history of the present illness, together with a systematic exploration of life events and stressful circumstances that may have contributed to its development. A history of previous disorder and a record of psychiatric illness in the family may provide valuable clues, and the developmental history should include a record of the patient's adaptation with regard to work, interpersonal relationships, sexual life and marriage. The premorbid personality should also be assessed. These are not merely rituals preordained by the tradition of psychiatric examination, as they serve to define the areas of vulnerability and the assets of the individual, and may shed light on the reasons for the adverse psychological effects of any relevant life events. A knowledge of the patient's assets is likely to prove important to treatment, after-care, and rehabilitation.

It may take some time to bring to light any relevant incidents, for they are liable to be obscured by denial, dissociation or a conscious and deliberate refusal to admit weakness. The first twinge of angina may have occurred a few months previously; there may have been an adverse verdict in an examination for life insurance; or the illness or death of a spouse or parent may have been more important for the patient's sense of security than had been realized or conceded. If a first episode of depression follows such events, it is frequently not very severe, but some individuals effect a silent exit by suicide soon after such changes in life situation (Kreitman 1977).

A full physical examination and routine screening tests are of particular importance. Patients with severe depressive symptoms contain a disproportionate number of those in middle and late stages of life and several enquiries have demonstrated that such patients show an excessive prevalence of physical disorder, particularly long-lasting illnesses that give rise to some measure of chronic restriction upon the patient's movements, activities, ambitions or life-style.

The incidence of somatic disease is relatively high in depressed men in comparison with depressed women, and the more proud the patient has been of his physical health, figure, virility, drive and energy, the more grave the emotional repercussions of physical illness seem to be.

In some cases, the presence of physical illness may be unknown to the patient; in a small minority of subjects, a depressive syndrome is the earliest harbinger of some occult somatic disease, perhaps a carcinoma. An excess mortality for cancer among groups of depressed individuals, as well as an increase in mortality overall, has been demonstrated in a number of studies (Kerr et al. 1969; Whitlock and Siskind 1979).

The presence of an occult physical illness should be particularly suspected in a syndrome of non-endogenous depression which has developed out of a relatively clear sky in an individual with a previously well-adjusted personality. In such cases, response to physical treatments is usually inadequate and transient, although a monoamine oxidase inhibitor may have beneficial effects. In cases with early cerebral disease or metabolic disturbance, clouding of consciousness may develop at an early stage of a course of ECT.

In some cases of frank organic disease, the depressive symptoms are variable and 'fragmented', in the sense that bizarre ideas of guilt, self-disparagement and nihilism may be seen in a setting of a relatively bland or labile affect. Even when progressive cerebral disease such as Alzheimer or multi-infarct dementia is present, depressive symptoms may respond relatively well to treatment in the short term.

Electro-convulsive therapy. In severely depressed patients who present a grave suicidal risk, particularly if delusions and/or hallucinations are present, it is rarely prudent to attempt treatment with antidepressant medication. Not only is it ineffective in severe cases, especially if psychotic features are present (Glassman et al. 1975; Bielski and Friedel 1976), but there is too long a latent period, of up to 4–6 weeks, even in cases with a good prognosis. The mental anguish endured by many such patients and the risks entailed will not allow a delay of this order and ECT is the treatment of choice in such cases. After a short period of 1 or 2 days of rest, in which an attempt is made to restore sleep and improve nutrition, therapy is commenced. ECT may also be the treatment of first choice in patients with less severe depression who have had previous episode which responded to ECT but not to antidepressants.

The majority of patients with bipolar and unipolar endogenous depressive syndromes and others in whom there is good evidence of endogenous aetiology, can be expected to respond favourably to ECT. Eighty-four per cent of those receiving this form of treatment in a 1965 Medical Research Council Trial improved after a 4-week treatment period as compared with 72% of those treated with imipramine, 38% with phenelzine, and 45% with placebo. Female patients responded better than males to ECT but the reverse pattern applied for antidepressant medication. However, the results with phenelzine probably understate the value of this form of treatment in depressive illness, as the drug was administered in inadequate doses and the criteria for entry into the trial recruited a patient population in which monoamine oxidase inhibitors are only rarely effective.

With very rare exceptions, ECT should be administered only with the aid of general anaesthesia and muscle relaxants. Under these conditions it is a very safe therapy. In a recent study of 200 000 treatments, one patient died during ECT and three within 72 h (Pippard and Ellam 1981). This has to be set against the expected mortality if the patients had remained untreated. ECT has been safely given to patients who have had previous myocardial infarction or cerebral infarcts, and to frail, elderly and debilitated patients. However a recent myocardial infarction (e.g. in the previous 2 months) is usually a contraindication, as is a recent cerebrovascular accident or a previous subarachnoid haemorrhage. Treatment should be administered only after any appropriate medical consultation has taken place, and a relatively experienced anaesthetist should be present when there is serious concomitant physical disease. There is evidence to suggest that unilateral ECT over the non-dominant hemisphere gives rise to less confusion, agitation, restlessness, disorientation for time and subjective memory impairment (D'Elia and Raotma 1975). However, for some patients, unilateral treatment may be less effective than the bilateral procedure, and a larger number of treatments may have to be administered. Hence in patients with typical endogenous presentations who fail to respond at all after five unilateral treatments, a change to treatment with a bilateral method is advisable. The relevant factors to be considered when deciding on unilateral or bilateral electrode placement are discussed in Chapter 6.

Unilateral therapy is the treatment of first choice in academic workers and in those whose lives demand a high level of intellectual activity. Obsessional and anxious individuals who can be expected from prior examination to respond with particular distress even to transient memory impairment should also be considered as particularly suitable for unilateral therapy.

The number of treatments administered has to be decided on an individual basis. In most cases of endogenous disorder, a course of six treatments will suffice but as many as 14 treatments may be needed in rare instances of exceptionally severe, long-standing depression. The average weekly frequency is two treatments, but in severe cases, three or four treatments may be given in the first week.

Following a course of ECT there may be amnestic gaps for the period during which treatment was being given, and some measure of impairment of short-term memory may continue for days or weeks in some cases. But it is rare for patients who have recovered or improved to complain of memory impairment 3–4 weeks after termination of treatment. It is also rare for those in whom treatment has succeeded to develop a fear and aversion for the procedure.

There are, however, patients who complain bitterly of markedly impaired memory, months and years after a course of ECT has been completed, although investigation with the aid of psychometric tests will rarely substantiate such claims. In most such cases, emotional difficulties or personality problems of long standing are associated. Clouding, with or without delirious features, lasting for hours or days during or after a short course of ECT is rare, even in elderly people. When it appears in the early stages of a course of treatment, the possibility of a concomitant disorder such as the early stage of dementia, an undetected neoplasm, some systemic disease, or a metabolic disorder, should be explored.

Tricyclic, tetracyclic and related compounds. A tricyclic antidepressant is usually the treatment of choice in depressed patients with evidence of endogenous aetiology unless the presence of severe psychotic symptoms and/or serious risk of suicide urgently require ECT. Tricyclic, tetracyclic and related drugs also seem to be of value in some patients with a neurotic syndrome but in such patients, the value of tricyclic and related drugs is more limited and uncertain, although a proportion of patients respond well.

The differences between the therapeutic effects of tricyclics are less marked than one would anticipate from the claims of pharmaceutical manufacturers and from the differential effects of the various compounds in blocking the uptake of noradrenaline as against 5-hydroxytryptamine. However, when insomnia or agitation is a particular problem, the drugs of first choice are amitriptyline or trimipramine, which have relatively marked sedative effects, although there is some evidence that pronounced anxiety and agitation are associated with a relatively poor response to tricyclics. On the other hand, when apathy and retardation are present, imipramine or protriptyline should be tried in the first instance. There is some evidence that clomipramine has some specific therapeutic action in cases of depression associated with obsessive –compulsive symptoms, while there is a rationale for using nomifensine as the drug of first choice for the depressive complications of parkinsonism, as it is a potent inhibitor of dopamine uptake. Mianserin is said to have relatively few anticholinergic and cardiotoxic effects, and to be relatively safe in overdosage. Thus, this drug may be prescribed for elderly patients and in those who present a suicidal risk, although evidence for the efficacy of tetracyclic compounds is, for the present, less impressive than that for the well-established tricyclic preparations. If treatment with mianserin or one of the newer tricyclics such as nomifensine should fail, a change to a well-established tricyclic may be indicated.

Patients often arrive in the psychiatric clinic after weeks or months of treatment on inadequate doses of tricyclic compounds. Precious time has often been lost, and pessimistic, guilt-laden subjects may be demoralized by the long period of failure. It is to be doubted on present evidence whether, in groups of patients with endogenous aetiology, any tricyclic compound has a clear advantage over the two best established ones, amitriptyline and imipramine. However, in the individual patient there are theoretical reasons for prescribing more than one tricyclic or tetracyclic, either in succession or together. This will be discussed further in the section on 'treatment-resistant' depressive syndromes.

Amitriptyline, which is often the tricyclic of first choice, should be commenced slowly with an initial dose of 25 mg increased every 3 or 4 days by 25 mg. If 150 mg daily (less in the elderly) can be given without serious side effects (at least half should be administered in the late evening), the dose is then increased further up to a maximum of 300 mg daily (less in the elderly), until slight anticholinergic side effects (accommodation difficulties and postural hypotension) make their appearance. An adequate trial of a tricyclic can be inferred if these side effects have been present, to a mild degree, for at least 4 weeks. If depressive symptoms start to improve, the dose can then be decreased until the above side effects are reduced or eliminated. The whole daily dose is administered at night by some therapists, but this does not suit everyone; some patients, the elderly in particular, fare better on divided doses, with about half given at night. Slow absorption preparations may reduce side effects associated with peak plasma levels, but there is no evidence that they are more effective.

Findings regarding the relation between plasma levels of parent drugs and metabolites and clinical response have proved contradictory but, in the case of nortriptyline, the view that commands most general acceptance is that there is a 'therapeutic window' between low and high levels, both of which are regarded as therapeutically ineffective. Thus, in some patients, a reduction of the dose of this drug, and perhaps of amitriptyline, which is metabolized to nortriptyline, may be beneficial.

Anticholinergic effects such as blurring of vision, dry mouth, increased sweating, urinary retention and the hazard of exacerbation of glaucoma are the commonest side effects. There is evidence that the anticholinergic effects are correlated with plasma levels in the case of nortriptyline (Åsberg et al. 1970). The drowsiness which is associated with some tricyclics renders driving hazardous, but it may decrease as treatment proceeds. Driving may then be cautiously resumed, at first under supervision. Alcohol tends markedly to aggravate drowsiness, and patients on antidepressants should be forbidden to drive after they have been drinking even when they are established on a stable maintenance dose. Convulsions will occasionally occur in the course of treatment with tricyclic compounds, probably through activation of a silent focus. The EEG need not be undertaken as a routine measure in all cases who are to receive antidepressive drugs but, with a history of attacks of unconsciousness, a record should be obtained. In the presence of specific epileptic abnormalities, tricyclics are probably best avoided unless the patient can be admitted for supervision until the dosage has reached the peak level and the decrease to a slightly lower dose has begun.

A full list of antidepressant drugs together with a description of their properties and main side effects appears in Chapter 3. However, brief reference will be made to some of the problems in treating elderly and middle-aged people with tricyclic compounds. Clouding of consciousness or delirium with hallucinations may develop as a result of central anticholinergic activity, and this calls for an immediate reduction in dosage. If this fails to control the complication, or if frequent nightmares continue, treatment should be abandoned, and the substitution of a tetracyclic compound may be indicated. The anticholinergic action of this class of drug is relatively weak, and they are less cardiotoxic than tricyclic compounds. Hypotension is particularly to be avoided in elderly subjects, and if tricyclic drugs, in particular clomipramine, are prescribed, they should be administered cautiously, starting with 10 mg twice or three times daily, which is increased by 10 mg every 3 days. If postural hypotension is manifest on small doses, treatment should be abandoned.

Although tricyclic compounds achieve their most striking successes in patients with endogenous aetiology, they also have a place in the treatment of some neurotic depressive states (Rowan et al. 1982). This may be because endogenous aetiology contributes to the disorder in those who respond, or because tricyclic antidepressants also have a beneficial effect on a depressed mood which is understandable in terms of the patient's personality and life experience. However, the proportion of favourable results in these disorders has proved to be inferior to that observed in the treatment of endogenous syndromes (Kiloh et al. 1962). Studies which have investigated the effects of psychotherapy alone or in combination with antidepressant drugs have provided useful guidelines for contemporary out-patient clinical practice, although it should be remembered that relatively mild depressive syndromes are aetiologically heterogeneous, and research in this area has been bedevilled by difficulty in delineating homogeneous groups.

Weissman (1979) has reviewed studies which compared the efficacy of psychotherapy and tricyclic antidepressants for relatively mild depressive syndromes, without features of the endogenous syndrome, which were treated in out-patient practice. Despite the methodological problems of the studies, it was concluded that psychotherapeutic intervention was better than no treatment, while several comparisons of antidepressant drugs with psychotherapy yielded equivocal results. Four studies which combined a tricyclic with psychotherapy claimed that there was an additive effect (Rush et al. 1977). Thus, psychotherapeutic interventions, including so-called cognitive therapy, which aims to restructure maladaptive cognitive themes such as a poor self-concept, offer an alternative or adjunct to drug treatment in many of the less severe depressions that predominate in an out-patient clientele. The psychiatrist should not prescribe an antidepressant in every case of depression which is formulated to be of a non-endogenous nature. In the management of many depressed patients, psychotherapeutic help may be the appropriate focus, perhaps in association with a hypnotic drug or intermittent anxiolytic medication. It should also be noted that in some neurotic depressive syndromes, tricyclics can intensify anxiety and give rise to side effects that may, for a time, increase distress. This may impair the patient's confidence in the therapist unless he has kept in close touch so as to be able to deal with such developments. If a tricyclic is prescribed in those with prominent anxiety, a sedative preparation with relatively few side effects, such as dothiepin, is indicated.

Monoamine oxidase inhibitors in depression. Although the verdict of a Medical Research Council trial in 1965 went against monoamine oxidase inhibitors (MAOIs) for the treatment of depression, there is reason to doubt whether such a conclusion was based on adequate evidence. In this study, dosage would be regarded as inadequate by present-day standards, and treatment was continued for only 4 weeks. Subsequent evidence suggests that MAOIs can be effective antidepressants, but clinical trials have been less frequently undertaken than in the case of tricyclic compounds (Morris and Beck 1974). However a number of controlled trials of phenelzine, which is the compound most often investigated, have indicated that this drug can be of benefit in some depressive disorders, usually in patients without features of the endogenous syndrome (Tyrer 1979), although there is some evidence to suggest that MAOI compounds can be effective in depressive syndromes both with and without endogenous aetiology. The older literature reported favourable results in what were called 'atypical' depressions (West and Dally 1959), but as some studies have reported favourable results in endogenous depressive syndromes (Pare and Sandler 1959), there is a strong indication for proceeding to a trial with an MAOI in depressions with presumed endogenous aetiology when a tricyclic or related substance has failed to elicit a response. It is particularly important to take this step in the treatment of a first episode of depression; if a course of ECT is instituted immediately after a failed trial of a tricyclic, the responsiveness of some patients with endogenous disorder to MAOIs may fail to come to light.

Also, there is evidence from a number of controlled trials that phenelzine can be of benefit in more than one type of affective disorder (Lipsedge et al. 1973; Tyrer et al. 1973; Mountjoy et al. 1977), and Tyrer concluded that phenelzine was more effective in anxiety neurosis, agoraphobia, anergic states and a mixture of anxiety with depression, than in neurotic depressive syndromes without conspicuous anxiety. Mountjoy et al. (1977) found that phenelzine produced significant improvement in some measures of anxiety in a population composed of patients with neurotic depressions, anxiety states and phobic neuroses.

In summary, the evidence suggests that MAOIs can often be of benefit in relatively mild depressive disorders, such as in those being treated in out-patient clinics (Shaw 1977), especially in patients in whom there is a mixture of anxiety and depression, with a predominance of the former. However, if an antidepressant is prescribed for subjects with persistent depression combined with anxiety, the drug of first choice remains a tricyclic compound. If it fails to elicit a response, a trial with an MAOI may then be justified. It is probable that some of the inconsistencies and uncertainties reflected in the literature on the treatment of affective disorders stem from the absence of a generally agreed classification in the difficult area of overlap between anxiety states and depressive disorders. In particular, there are no generally accepted rules as to which features should be given precedence, when anxiety and depression are combined. Zitrin et al. (1976) reported favourable results in the treatment of phobic patients with a tricyclic compound, but phobic features are not uncommon in depressive states, when they may sometimes be appropriately regarded as non-specific symptoms of the depressive disorder while, in phobic states proper, and in agoraphobia in particular, situational anxiety dominates the clinical picture. In these latter disorders it is preferable to start with a MAOI if pharmacotherapy is indicated.

In depressions where it is proposed to proceed from a course of treatment with a tricyclic or tetracyclic antidepressant to an MAOI, it is best to leave an interval of at least 10 days before commencing treatment with an MAOI, even though a shorter drug-free period proves safe and uneventful in the majority of cases.

Prophylactic antidepressant treatment. Prophylactic antidepressant drug treatment may need to be undertaken in order to reduce (or eliminate) the frequency or severity of recurrence of a unipolar depressive disorder with endogenous aetiology. Evidence that administration of tricyclics can exert a prophylactic effect comes from several sources (Mindham et al. 1973; Klerman et al. 1974), and the comprehensive review by Davis (1976) has established the value of such treatment beyond any reasonable doubt. This procedure is generally considered to be indicated when there are reasons to believe that there is an endogenous aetiological component to recurrent depressive episodes. However, there are no clear guidelines regarding the period for which the prescription of antidepressive medication should be sustained, and there is considerable scope for clinical judgment. Additional criteria for relatively long-term prophylactic treatment of affective disorders will be given in the subsequent section on treatment and prophylaxis with lithium carbonate.

In the case of patients who have made an indubitable response to pharmacological treatment of a severe episode of endogenous disorder, relatively short-term maintenance therapy over a period beyond the stage at which symptoms go into abeyance is usually desirable. But when episodes are separated by long intervals, maintenance treatment is not usually carried on beyond four months. After a variable period of 1–4 months it may be decided to reduce the dose to about 50–75 mg daily (less in the elderly) of amitriptyline or imipramine, or an equivalent amount of another compound. After treatment has eventually been discontinued, it should not be reinstituted until there is a recrudescence of symptoms, which may not occur for a number of years, if at all.

For other patients, treatment may have to be continued for longer periods, but when such a course is being considered, the history must be carefully reviewed to ascertain whether there is good evidence that a tricyclic compound had indeed exerted a therapeutic effect. In addition to recurrent depressive syndromes with an endogenous aetiological component, there is a group of patients with depression secondary to an obsessive–compulsive syndrome who benefit from long-term treatment with clomipramine. Also, some forms of chronic hypochondriasis appear to be helped by long-term medication with tricyclics.

In bipolar cases of affective disorder, i.e. with manic as well as depressive episodes, long-term treatment with tricyclics is generally contraindicated. Not only may attacks of mania or hypomania be precipitated, but there is some evidence that a maintenance tricyclic can exert a destabilizing effect and a shortening of intervals between bouts of illness (Wehr and Goodwin 1979). Thus, when a depressive phase of a bipolar disorder has responded to a tricyclic compound, prophylactic treatment should not be sustained for more than a few weeks.

Treatment with lithium carbonate. Despite claims that lithium is effective in the treatment of depressive phases in bipolar illness, this has not been established. However it is of value in the treatment not only of hypomanic or manic attacks, but of phases of 'mixed' psychosis consisting of a blend of manic and depressive features. These can give rise to considerable diagnostic difficulties, and some such patients may be initially diagnosed as suffering from a schizophrenic illness. However, a finding that often suggests the presence of an affective disorder is the failure of phenothiazines, even in high doses, to make a significant impression upon what is often a florid psychotic illness. In contrast, haloperidol combined with lithium will usually bring the disorder under control within a few days, although a proportion of such cases require ECT.

The decision to initiate prophylactic treatment with lithium carbonate is a serious one and should be rarely taken after a solitary attack of depression with endogenous features or of another form of manic–depressive illness. The condition may never recur or may not do so until several years have elapsed.

The prophylactic value of lithium for affective disorders of endogenous aetiology is now well authenticated (Davis 1976), and it reduces the frequency and severity of both depressive and manic phases of bipolar illness. Although this compound was, at first, employed only in bipolar manic–depressive illness, recent evidence has established that it is also effective in the prophylactic management of a substantial proportion of unipolar depressive disorders with endogenous aetiology, although the frequency of success is not as high as in bipolar cases or in recurrent unipolar manic disorders.

There is usually no indication for long-term lithium prophylaxis in cases of mild recurrent depressions that do not demand admission to hospital and respond to antidepressant drugs. This can also be said for some patients with mild hypomanic bouts of short duration. However if the individual in question carries high responsibility, when faulty judgements and decisions might have unfortunate or disastrous repercussions, prophylactic treatment for mild disorders may be indicated. In general, long-term prophylaxis should be confined to cases in which depression with endogenous aetiology (or mania, or mixed affective illness) has been of sufficient severity to cause significant disruption to the patient's life when at least one of the following criteria is met: there should have been at least two episodes in the preceding 2 years; the attacks of affective disorder have involved some suicidal risk or have threatened the livelihood, professional repute or social viability of the individual; a recurrence after even one episode would be particularly disruptive; or experience has shown that a patient is subject to severe episodes of depression or mania which cannot be brought rapidly under control.

Some therapists use a combination of lithium carbonate and tricyclic antidepressants in patients in whom the majority of severe attacks are depressive in character, but it has been claimed that this combination can destabilize mood in bipolar patients and it is probably inadvisable to employ it in unipolar cases also. If lithium in adequate doses fails in prophylaxis, its combination with a tricyclic compound may, if anything, prove even less successful.

Details of lithium carbonate administration have been described in Chapter

3. Before embarking on lithium prophylaxis renal function is assessed by physical examination, urea and electrolyte estimation, and urinanalysis, although renal impairment is not an absolute contraindication. Serum levels of about 1 mmol/litre used to be recommended as optimum, but it is now recognized that, for a high proportion of bipolar patients, lower serum levels of between 0.6 to 0.8 mmol/litre will suffice; many incapacitating side effects are averted on such a regimen.

The duration of prophylactic lithium treatment is unknown, but should certainly not be life-long in every case. The patient's condition should be regularly reviewed, and after a period of 3–4 years of total remission from attacks of affective disorder, the possibility of discontinuing the prophylactic regimen should be considered. Judgment as to the correct course to be adopted demands a judicious balance of pros and cons in the individual case. In some instances even a small chance of recrudescence will entail an unacceptable risk, while, in others, discontinuing treatment is the best course of action, provided the patient can be kept under regular observation.

Lithium may be effective in the rather ill-defined territory of schizoaffective disorder, so that in cases with a manic picture and one or two 'first-rank' symptoms of schizophrenia, lithium is well worth trying. Such cases are often merely atypical manic disorders, and the response to lithium alone or to a combination of lithium with a butyrophenone may make it possible to judge potential prophylactic efficacy. In contrast, lithium is unlikely to prove of value for patients exhibiting a wide span of schizophrenic symptomatology with depressive colouring. In recurrent atypical psychoses with a family history of bipolar or unipolar affective disorder, lithium is worth trying if the criteria which govern the use of lithium in prophylaxis are satisfied.

Treatment-resistant depressive syndromes. When a long-standing depressive syndrome with a presumed endogenous aetiological component has not responded to a tricyclic antidepressant and a subsequent course of up to 12–14 ECT sessions, the clinical diagnosis must be thoroughly re-evaluated. It may be that the mood disorder is an understandable reaction to events which are unknown to the clinician, in which case further psychological or social intervention may be indicated. Also, a further physical examination should be undertaken, perhaps with additional investigations. However, if endogenous disorder still seems likely, there are a number of pharmacological treatment options which are still available (Shaw 1977).

Firstly, the dose regimen of the previous course of a tricyclic antidepressant (or related compound) should be reviewed, as it is frequently found that the dose has been inadequate, or the patient did not comply with the clinician's instructions. In addition, it is known that for nortriptyline (which is a metabolite of amitriptyline as well as an antidepressant in its own right), other secondary amine tricyclics and, possibly, some other antidepressants or metabolites of antidepressants, there is a therapeutic window in which excessive doses are relatively ineffective. Thus, in some patients, a reduction of the dose of an antidepressant (e.g. nortriptyline, amitriptyline) may be effective, albeit rarely.

There are data pointing to the subdivision of depressive disorders with endogenous aetiology into two distinct subgroups, one related to reduced functional noradrenergic activity centrally, and the other to reduced serotonin (5 HT) activity. Their identification has been derived principally from the measurement of the urinary metabolite of noradrenaline (NA), 3-methoxy 4-hydroxyphenylglycol (MHPG), 50% of which is estimated to be of central origin, and CSF levels of the 5 HT metabolite 5-hydroxyindoleacetic acid (5 HIAA) which are thought to reflect central 5 HT turnover (Roth and Barnes 1981). It has been claimed that the subgroup of depressed patients with evidence of NA dysfunction has a relatively good response to antidepressants with potent noradrenaline reuptake inhibition properties, e.g. nomifensine, desipramine or imipramine, while depressive syndromes apparently related to 5 HT dysfunction may be more likely to respond to drugs which have a relatively potent effect on 5 HT reuptake inhibition, such as amitriptyline, clomipramine or zimelidine. However, although a trial of another antidepressant with a different pharmacological profile is often indicated in the management of treatment-resistant depressions of presumed endogenous aetiology, there is insufficient evidence to predict the outcome of such a strategy. Other possible treatment methods include the prescription of a monoamine oxidase inhibitor such as phenelzine or tranylcypromine, perhaps combined with L-tryptophan (e.g. 2 g three times daily) or a combination of two antidepressants which principally affect NA reuptake and 5 HT uptake respectively, e.g. maproptiline (about 80 mg daily—less in the elderly) and clomipramine (about 100 mg daily—less in the elderly), which also may be potentiated by being combined with L-tryptophan. Preliminary results from this 'broad-spectrum' strategy are said to be encouraging, but its efficacy remains to be clearly established. There has recently been renewed interest in bypassing the enterohepatic circulation by the intravenous administration of tricyclics and related compounds, but the value of this potentially dangerous procedure remains to be determined. Other possible combinations of antidepressants, such as a tricyclic with a monoamine oxidase inhibitor, are described in Chapter 3. It has also been claimed that flupenthixol (e.g. up to 6 mg a day, orally) has antidepressant properties, and that it may be of value in some 'treatment-resistant' cases.

If psychotic features (i.e. delusions, loss of insight or hallucinations) are present, a combination of a neuroleptic drug such as chlorpromazine with an antidepressant may be beneficial (this will also lead to an increase in tricyclic plasma levels; see Chapter 3), while it has been claimed that some non-psychotic treatment-resistant patients respond to dexamphetamine, e.g. 30 mg daily. Owing to the danger of misuse, and the legal restrictions regarding its prescription, this drug is rarely used. (Tranylcypromine has amphetamine-like actions, and is probably a more effective antidepressant than phenelzine.) Finally, there are anecdotal reports that lithium has apparently induced remission of symptoms in some treatment-resistant depressions.

If a patient has suffered severe and intractable depression for 5 years or more, one of the various types of modern and anatomically specific psychosurgical procedures should be considered, especially if marked tension and a high suicidal risk are present. Although this course should only be contemplated when all other interventions have been exhausted, it is probable that psycho-surgery has provided partial and even dramatic relief for some patients with long-standing and intractable depressive syndromes.

Psychotherapy. Where there is conclusive evidence of endogenous illness any attempt at intensive psychotherapy based on psychoanalytic theory or with a main aim of instilling insight is contraindicated. Such procedures can have the effect of intensifying self-disparaging introspection, thus exacerbating feelings of worthlessness and despair. In these cases, an attempt has to be made to penetrate the barrier created by such phenomena as psychomotor retardation, apathy, and persistent distressing thoughts, and to establish rapport with the patient. In cases when there is endogenous illness, reassurance that the illness is recoverable and an explanation of the manner in which morbid ideas are generated by mood disturbance may elicit no immediate response, but they are frequently recalled with gratitude after recovery. Adequate time spent in establishing rapport and gaining confidence will both ease distress and reap rewards when patients need to be persuaded to enter hospital, or to accept various forms of treatment.

It is not uncommon for resentment or animosity towards some close relation or a spouse to surge up during a depressive syndrome, particularly one with endogenous aetiology. Although the feelings of hostility and the rift which may develop in the course of a depression are rarely without some foundation, the problems of the relationship may be exaggerated out of all proportion to the real state of affairs. However, a seemingly ill-matched couple may, after the depressed partner has improved, successfully re-establish their relationship. Every effort should therefore be made to deter a depressed patient from taking important decisions either about marriage or other aspects of his life, particularly when there is clear evidence of endogenous disorder. After recovery, decisions which have been taken with regard to personal life are often regretted, but the effects may be irrevocable.

When at least part of a depressive syndrome is of a non-endogenous character, an attempt should be made to understand the relationship between the depressive disorder, the premorbid personality, the current life situation and the life events which seem to have been intimately associated with the commencement of symptoms. The character of the adverse situation which precedes the depression may suggest an 'Achilles' heel' with regard to the patient's personality, which has led to a disproportionately severe emotional response. A patient with a depressive syndrome may display his premorbid personality traits in an exaggerated or parodied form, and an understanding of the nature of the relationship between personality, any antecedent stress and the features of the depressive syndrome will do much to bring the main psychological problems into focus, and to define objectives for psychotherapy. Even in patients with indubitable endogenous illness, there is often a significant reactive component which in many cases is mainly due to the stress of the primary endogenous disorder.

An example of a vulnerable aspect of a patient's personality is shown by a woman who becomes depressed almost immediately after removal to a new home, as a result of the distance she has placed between herself and a parent who has been indispensable for her sense of security. Although she may have proved a competent housewife or mother, she may have been unable to take any decision with her mother's advice. Subsequently, such a patient is liable to a more severe depressive episode when her mother falls ill or dies.

The man whose depressive syndrome first appears following a physical illness will often have depended on physical fitness and physique for a sense of self-esteem, while the quest for high athletic achievement well into middle age or later is often associated with obsessional personality traits or long-standing fears of sudden death. In such individuals, a minor injury, a small myocardial infarction, a fleeting attack of anginal pain, or an experience which casts up the spectre of ageing, may be enough to precipitate a depressive disorder.

Some individuals become depressed when seemingly at the pinnacle of their success: for example, if a basically indecisive and anxious man is promoted to a post in which he can no longer be supported and advised by seniors who buttressed his fragile self-esteem. Faced with demands for which his old habits and assumptions are no longer adequate, he develops 'a promotion depression'.

In most of those who are recovering from depressive episode an endogenous , non-intensive, supportive forms of psychotherapy will suffice during the period of follow-up. However, recurrent endogenous depression, and bipolar manic —depressive illness in particular, may be associated with cumulative familial, social and personal problems, which may call for a great deal of psychotherapeutic endeavour with the individual and his family, with the involvement of a social worker. Indiscretions committed during a manic illness may prove humiliating or ruinous, causing serious damage to marriage and a professional career. Those who have cyclothymic tendencies between attacks of psychosis are liable to drink to excess, and this may contribute to the ever more florid nature of their psychoses which, in the manic phase, may be coloured by paranoid delusions and dangerously aggressive behaviour, without the alcoholic contribution to such disorders being suspected. A great deal of effort may have to be invested to assist the patient to come to terms with the painful and humiliating experiences of his illness, and to establish a planned and disciplined way of life that makes it possible for him to comply with the needs of maintenance treatment.

In depressions that occur in the setting of serious personality disorder, the limited objective of helping the individual over periods of crisis has to suffice in most cases, as intensive psychotherapy rarely makes any significant impression on the personality disorder as such. However, a minority of patients with depressive disorders of neurotic aetiology, with relatively moderate degrees of personality-related problems, and who seem strongly motivated, may be referred to a specialist in psychotherapy for assessment of their suitability for insight-directed psychotherapy on an individual or group basis.

MANIA

J.H. Dowson and Sir Martin Roth

Clinical Features and Differential Diagnosis

Mania, or its relatively mild forms known as hypomania, presents with a variable mixture of signs and symptoms, the most characteristic of which include overactivity, an elated mood with infectious jollity (which is, however, often associated with irritability), flight of ideas with pressure of speech, distractibility, bizarre behaviour with underlying grandiosity or arrogance, excessive spending, sexual disinhibition, delusions with a grandiose or persecutory content, reduced insight and poor sleep. Rarely, auditory hallucinations are present. The severity and nature of the symptoms may show sudden and frequent fluctuations, while in very severe cases patients may hardly sleep, and remain active throughout the day and night. Such behaviour, together with lack of food and drink, can lead to a life-threatening state of dehydration and exhaustion. However, at the other end of the scale, the diagnosis may not be readily apparent if the patient's abnormal behaviour merely involves phenomena such as increased but still productive activity, impaired judgement, or mild mood changes involving inappropriate optimism or a bland facetiousness. In some mild hypomanic syndromes there may be no clearly overt signs of overactivity or mood change, even though the patient behaves at times in a bizarre and uncharacteristic way, involving lack of social judgement and disinhibition. Although such behaviour constitutes a relatively mild form of this illness, it may have profound social consequences, as the patient is usually not perceived to be 'ill'.

There is persuasive evidence that, like depressions of endogenous aetiology, mania is due to an abnormality of brain function which is qualitatively distinct from normality, and which sometimes can be precipitated by life events or factors such as hormonal changes or drug administration. However mania can often develop out of a clear sky.

In some patients manic features are combined with schizophrenic phenomena. Wing and Nixon (1975) have pointed out that solitary Schneiderian 'first-rank' schizophrenic features in the context of a manic disorder do not warrant a diagnosis of schizophrenia but, at times, a blend of affective symptoms and schizophrenic-like features makes diagnosis difficult. For example, a manic syndrome may involve irritable, aggressive overactive behaviour with delusions of a persecutory kind (perhaps in which the patient believes he is being spied upon by special apparatus), together with auditory hallucinations or passivity feelings. A syndrome with such persecutory delusions has often attracted a diagnosis of schizophrenia but is more appropriately termed paranoid, or pseudo-schizophrenic, mania (Roth and Barnes 1981).

Brockington et al. (1980) have reported a series of 32 patients with schizoaffective mania; 21 received a final diagnosis of manic–depressive psychosis, six of schizophrenia, and five of 'disputed'. It is doubtful whether the presence of paranoid or grandiose delusions alone is ever inconsistent with a diagnosis of mania. It would seem from these findings that it is only among those patients with hallucinations and passivity phenomena in the setting of a manic picture that the outcome may sometimes approximate to that of a schizophrenic disorder, or to an intermediate position between the affective and schizophrenic psychoses. In routine practice, the danger lies in the denial of a therapeutic trial with lithium and haloperidol, alone or in combination, to patients with schizo–manic syndrome.

Management

The first step in management is diagnosis which, for the reasons outlined above, may present considerable problems in both mild and severe cases. Hypomania can present with a recent history of a succession of incidents involving uncharacteristic bizarre, disinhibited or irresponsible behaviour, but the patient may show no clear evidence of disorder at interview. In such cases insight is usually impaired, although the patient may be prepared to accept the psychiatrist's advice with regard to treatment. In more severe cases, a distinction from a schizophrenic illness or the controversial category of schizoaffective disorder may be difficult, and it is important to recognize a mixed manic–depressive syndrome, involving both depressive and manic features, as, in such cases, ECT should be considered at an earlier stage than if only manic phenomena are present. The process of diagnosis must also consider the possible presence of any identifiable somatic pathology, including the effects of prescribed or illicit drugs (Tyrer 1982).

Although some patients can be managed on an out-patient basis, day-patient or preferably in-patient treatment is usually essential for the more severe manic syndromes. As insight is usually poor, compulsory admission under an appropriate section of the Mental Health Act is often required. When a patient's behaviour is consistently and clearly abnormal, agreement for compulsory admission is usually present among the various professionals and the patient's relatives who are involved in this decision. However, when hypomanic behaviour is relatively mild and variable, and when the patient can appear 'normal' at interview despite a clear history of repeated bizarre and uncharacteristic activity, it can be difficult for the social worker, general medical practitioner, or the patient's relatives to substantiate a case for compulsory admission. However, in such cases patients may inflict irreparable harm to their marriage, job and social relationships, and perhaps amass large debts. Thus the psychiatrist must emphasize that the decision regarding compulsory admission must be based partly on the recent history of the patient's behaviour and not just on his demeanor at interview.

Treatment with haloperidol should be instituted as soon as possible. In mild cases, in a healthy non-elderly adult, an oral regimen of 3–20 mg daily in two doses may suffice, but in severe mania intramuscular haloperidol 10–30 mg may be given initially and 10 mg can be repeated every hour until the symptoms begin to abate. Blood pressure must be regularly monitored. Thereafter a twice-daily oral regimen can be substituted, usually within the range (for in-patients) of 40–100 mg daily. The oral regimen should initially be equivalent, in dose per 24 h, to the intramuscular dose during the initial treatment period, unless side effects or change in syndrome severity dictate otherwise. It should be remembered that the equivalent oral dose of haloperidol is about twice the intramuscular dose. Regular review of medication and flexibility of dose are essential, as the optimum dose regimen shows wide variation. Much lower doses than the above are usually appropriate in the elderly. It is probably not advisable to prescribe an antiparkinsonian agent routinely, but the patient must be carefully monitored for extrapyramidal symptoms and, if necessary, these should be treated without delay. In the case of acute dystonia, intravenous procyclidine is rapidly effective.

Some patients do not respond to haloperidol and, in such cases, several doses of intramuscular chlorpromazine at hourly intervals (e.g. 50–75 mg—less in the elderly) can be used for initial sedation; also, a late evening intramuscular or oral dose of chlorpromazine (e.g. 50 mg intramuscularly or 100 mg orally in a healthy non-elderly adult) can be combined with the regimen of haloperidol outlined above, if sleep is seriously impaired. It has been recommended that a test dose of chlorpromazine, 10 mg *i.m.*, should be given initially to exclude undue sensitivity (Shaw 1977), and that blood pressure should be carefully monitored, especially if regular doses are given.

As soon as the initial phase of treatment with intramuscular (or oral) neuroleptic is over, lithium carbonate should usually be added, although any contraindications must be borne in mind (see Chapter 3). This drug is an effective treatment for mania but usually takes about a week to exert significant effects. In some patients initial oral neuroleptic treatment can be combined with lithium from the outset, while lithium alone can be sufficient treatment for some mild hypomanic syndromes, if a delay in the therapeutic effect can be tolerated. In view of reports of an interaction between high doses of haloperidol and lithium, it is customary not to exceed 30 mg haloperidol a day when this combination is used. Thus in severe cases, when much larger doses of haloperidol are initially required, the start of lithium treatment should usually be delayed until the dose of haloperidol is reduced. However, in certain particularly severe cases there may be no alternative but to combine lithium with more than 30 mg haloperidol per day. The patient is established on a dose of lithium which produces blood levels (determined as described in Chapter 3) at the upper end of the therapeutic range, and when this has been achieved, an attempt can be made to reduce and then, if possible, discontinue, the neuroleptic medication. Benzodiazepines may also be useful, in addition to the other drugs, for particularly agitated and anxious patients.

ECT is a valuable treatment for those patients with severe mania who are relatively unresponsive to drug therapy, and is also indicated for some mixed states of mania and depression, when treatment of the manic component does not improve the depressive symptoms, which may even be exacerbated. However, in mild mixed affective states, lithium alone is often effective, perhaps combined with a benzodiazepine to reduce agitation and improve any sleep disorder. Although, as has been described, long-term prophylactic treatment of bipolar disorders with tricyclics is not recommended, these drugs are often required for the treatment of depressive episodes or mixed affective states in such patients.

Following the resolution of the manic episode, lithium treatment, with or without haloperidol, is usually continued for at least 1 month and, if lithium and haloperidol have been combined, an attempt can be made to reduce and discontinue the haloperidol before altering the dose of lithium. If relatively long-term prophylaxis is not indicated, all medication is gradually discontinued after a variable period of between 1 and 6 months; the main factors which have to be taken into account have already been considered in the section on the prophylaxis of depressive disorders. In some cases, relatively long-term prophylactic treatment with haloperidol alone (or in combination with lithium) should be considered, but lithium is usually the prophylactic drug of first choice. In rare cases, an oral or depot phenothiazine may be an adjunct to prophylactic treatment.

As described in Chapter 3, lithium should be avoided, if possible, in pregnancy or in women who are planning pregnancy. Breast-feeding is contraindicated. Patients on long-term lithium should be regularly reviewed by a psychiatric service, and blood lithium and creatinine should be regularly monitored. Thyroid function should be checked at yearly intervals. It is usual to attempt to wean patients off their lithium at intervals of about 2–4 years, but some patients require prophylactic treatment for considerably longer periods.

Finally, supportive psychotherapy and the regular involvement of a psychiatric social worker play an essential role in management of many manic patients, particularly those with relatively frequent recurrence of their disorder.

References

AKISKAL, H.S., BITAR, A.H., PUZANTIAN, V.R., ROSENTHAL, T.L. & WALKER, P.W. (1978) The nosological status of neurotic depression. *Archs gen. Psychiat.*, **35**, 756.

ÅSBERG, M., GRONHOLM, B., SJÖQUIST, F. & TUCK,D. (1970) Correlation of subjective side-effects with plasma concentrations of nortriptyline. *Br. med. J.*, **iv**, 18.

BIELSKI, R.J. & FRIEDEL, R.O. (1976) Prediction of tricyclic antidepressant response. A critical review. *Archs gen. Psychiat.*, **33**, 1479.

BROCKINGTON, I.F. (1981) The nosological status of schizoaffective psychosis. Paper presented at the 3rd International Congress of Biological Psychiatry.

BROCKINGTON, I.F., WAINWRIGHT, S. & KENDELL, R.E. (1980) Manic patients with schizophrenic and paranoid symptoms. *Psychol. Med.*, **10**, 73.

BUCHSBAUM, M., GOODWIN, F., MURPHY, D. & BORGE, G. (1971) A.E.R. in affective disorders. *Am. J. Psychiat.*, **128**, 19.

CARROLL, B.J., CURTIS, G.C. & MENDELS, J. (1976) Neuroendocrine regulation in depression. I and II. *Archs gen. Psychiat.*, **33**, 1039, 1051.

CARROLL, B.J., GREDEN, J.F. & FEINBERG, M. (1980) Neuroendocrine disturbances and the diagnosis and aetiology of endogenous depression. *Lancet*, **i**, 321.

CARROLL, B.J. (1982) The dexamethasone suppression test for melancholia. *Br. J. Psychiat.*, **140**, 292.

CHECKLEY, S.A. (1979) Corticosteroid and growth hormone responses to methylamphetamine in depressive illness. *Psychol. Med.*, **9**, 107.

DAVIS, J.M. (1976) Overview: maintenance therapy in psychiatry: II. Affective disorders. *Am. J. Psychiat.*, **133**, 1.

D'ELIA, G. & RAOTMA, H. (1975) Is unilateral ECT less effective than bilateral ECT. *Br. J. Psychiat.*, **126**, 83.

FEIGHNER, J.P., ROBINS, E., GUZE, S.B. et al. (1972) Diagnostic criteria for use in psychiatric research. *Archs gen. Psychiat.*, **26**, 57.

GLASSMAN, A., KANTOR, S.J. & SHOSTAK, M. (1975) Depression, delusions and drug response. *Am. J. Psychiat.*, **132**, 716.

GOLDBERG, I.K. (1980) Dexamethasone suppression test as indication of safe withdrawal of antidepressant therapy. *Lancet*, **i**, 376.

GURNEY, C., ROTH, M., GARSIDE, R.F., KERR, T.A. & SCHAPIRA, K. (1972) Studies in classification of affective disorders: the relationship between anxiety states and depressive states II. *Br. J. Psychiat.*, **121**, 162.

GUZE, S.B., WOODRUFF, R.A. & CLAYTON, P.J. (1975) The significance of psychotic affective disorders. *Archs gen. Psychiat.*, **32**, 1147.

KERR, T.A., ROTH, M., SCHAPIRA, K. & GURNEY, C. (1972) The assessment and prediction of outcome in affective disorders. *Br. J. Psychiat.*, **121**, 167.

KERR, T.A., SCHAPIRA, K. & ROTH, M. (1969). The relationship between premature death and affective disorders. *Br. J. Psychiat.*, **115**, 1277.

KILOH, L.G., BALL, J.R.B. & GARSIDE, R.F. (1962) Prognostic factors in treatment of depressive states with imipramine. *Br. med. J.*, **1**, 1225.

KLERMAN, G.L., DiMASCIO, A., WEISSMAN, M.M., PRUSOFF, B.A. & PAYKEL, E.S. (1974) Treatment of depression by drugs and psychotherapy. *Am. J. Psychiat.*, **131**, 186.

KREITMAN, N. (1977) In: *Parasuicide.* New York: John Wiley and Sons.

LIPSEDGE, B.S., HAJIOFF, J., HUGGINS, P., NAPIER, L., PEARCE, J. & PIKE, D.J., RICH, M. (1973) The management of severe agoraphobia: a comparison of iproniazid and systemic desensitization. *Psychopharmacologia*, **32**, 67.

MINDHAM, R.H.S., HOWLAND, C. & SHEPHERD, M. (1973) An evaluation of continuation therapy with tricyclic antidepressants in depressive illness. *Psychol. Med.*, **3**, 5.

MORRIS, J.B. & BECK, A.T. (1974) The efficacy of antidepressant drugs. *Archs gen. Psychiat.*, **30**, 667.

MOUNTJOY, C.Q. & ROTH, M. (1982) Studies in the relationship between depressive disorders and anxiety states: I. Rating Scales. II. Clinical Items. *J. Affect. Dis.* (In press.)

MOUNTJOY, C.Q., ROTH, M., GARSIDE, R.F. & LEITCH, I.M. (1977) A Clinical Trial of Phenelzine in Anxiety, Depressive and Phobic Neuroses. *Br. J. Psychiat.*, **131**, 486.

PARE, C.M.B. & SANDLER, M. (1959) A Clinical and biochemical study of a trial of iproniazid in the treatment of depression. *J. Neurol. Neurosurg. Psychiat.*, **22**, 247.

PAYKEL, E.S. (1972) Depressive typologies and response to amitriptyline. *Br. Psychiat.*, **120**, 147.

PIPPARD, J. & ELLAM, L. (1981) Electroconvulsive treatment in Great Britain, 1980. A report to the Royal College of Psychiatrists, London.

PRUSOFF, B.A. & PAYKEL, E.S. (1977) Typological prediction of responses to amitriptyline: a replication study. *Internat. Pharmacopsychiat.*, **12**, 153.

ROTH, M. & BARNES, T.R.E.B. (1981) The classification of affective disorders: a synthesis of old and new concepts. *Compreh. Psychiat.*, **22**, 54.

ROTH, M., GURNEY, C., GARSIDE, R.F. & KERR, T.A. (1972) Studies in the classification of affective disorders. The relationship between anxiety states and depressive illness. *Br. J. Psychiat.*, **121**, 147.

ROWAN, P.R., PAYKEL, E.S. & PARKER, R.R. (1982) Phenelzine and amitryptiline: effects on symptoms of neurotic depression. *Br. J. Psychiat.*, **140**, 475.

RUSH, A.J., BECK, A.T., KOVACS, M. & HOLLON, S. (1977) Comparative efficacy of cognitive therapy and pharmacotherapy in the treatment of depressed outpatients. *Cognitive Ther. Res.*, **1**, 17.

SCHAPIRA, K., ROTH, M., KERR, T.A. et al. (1972) The prognosis of affective disorders: The differentiation of anxiety states from depressive illness. *Br. J. Psychiat.*, **121**, 175.

SCHLESSER, M.A., WINOKUR, G. & SHERMAN, B.M. (1979) Genetic subtypes of unipolar primary depressive illness distinguished by hypothalmic–pituitary–adrenal axis activity. *Lancet*, **i**, 739.

SHAW, D.M. (1977) The practical management of affective disorders. *Br. J. Psychiat.*, **130**, 432.

TYRER, P. (1979) Clinical use of monoamine oxidase inhibitors. In: *Psychopharmacology of Affective Disorders*, ed. Paykel, E.S., Coppen, A., p. 159. Oxford: Oxford University Press.

TYRER, S.P. (1982) Mania: diagnosis and treatment. *Br. J. Hosp. Med.*, **28**, 67.

TYRER, P., CANDY, J. & KELLY, D. (1973) Phenelzine in phobic anxiety: a controlled trial. *Psychol. Med.*, **3**, 120.

WEHR, T.A. & GOODWIN, F.K. (1979) Rapid cycling in manic–depressives induced by tricyclic antidepressants. *Archs gen. Psychiat.*, **36**, 555.

WEISSMAN, M.M. (1979) The psychological treatment of depression. *Archs gen. Psychiat.*, **36**, 1261.

WEST, E.D. & DALLY, P.J. (1959) Effects of iproniazid in depressive syndromes. *Br. med. J.*, **1**, 1491.

WHITLOCK, F.A. & SISKIND, M. (1979) Depression and cancer: a follow-up Study. *Psychol. Med.*, **9**, 747.

WING, J. & NIXON, J. (1975) Discriminating symptoms in schizophrenia. *Archs gen. Psychiat.*, **32**, 853.

ZITRIN, C.M., KLEIN, D.F., LINDEMANN, C., TOBAK, P., ROCK, M., KAPLAN, J.H. & GANZ, V.H. (1976) Comparison of short-term treatment regimens in phobic patients: a preliminary report. In: *Evaluation of Psychological Therapies*, ed. Spitzer, R.L., Klein, D.F., Ch. 16, p. 233. Baltimore: Johns Hopkins University Press.

16

Management of Anxiety and Phobic States

C.Q. Mountjoy

THE NATURE OF THE SYNDROME

While anxiety may be found in any individual under stress, the use of the term 'anxiety state' (or neurosis) implies that the symptomatology appears to be out of proportion to any precipitating stress, or has been continued long beyond the time that would be normally expected. Anxiety symptoms have two components, psychic and somatic. Psychic anxiety includes a feeling of apprehension, fearfulness, tension or dread, and panic attacks may occur, in which the patient feels he is about to die. The symptoms of somatic anxiety include increased sweating, palpitations, diarrhoea, urgency and frequency of micturition, tension headaches, difficulty in swallowing, retching and muscular aches and pains. Additional symptoms such as difficulty in falling asleep, waking at night, impaired or increased appetite, a general feeling of fatigue and depressed mood are also frequently found. Hyperventilation may be a feature and the somatic effects of this behaviour may give rise to diagnosic difficulty.

Although there may be a general background of anxiety in a phobic state (or neurosis), the patient's principal complaint is of severe anxiety induced by particular objects or circumstances. These may be specific to one stimulus, or a small number of stimuli, as in animal phobias and some examples of fear of illness (although the specificity of an illness phobia is variable), or may involve a range of situations, as with agoraphobia and social phobia (Marks 1969). (Phobias which are appropriately classified as obsessive–compulsive phenomena will be considered in the next chapter.)

Many people have specific phobias, which have usually been established in early childhood, but these are usually of insufficient severity to require treatment. The majority of phobic patients seen in psychiatric practice present with agoraphobia. These individuals are usually female with premorbid overdependent and anxiety-prone personality traits. The onset may be sudden, and often occurs in a crowded place associated with a severe panic attack. The patient may be unable to travel any distance from her home unaccompanied, and often has a particular fear of crowded places such as supermarkets, buses or trains, although in some patients there is also fear of non-crowded public places. Other features may include avoidance, mood changes, depersonalization, derealization, claustrophobia and a fear of fainting, dying, or going mad. Patients often find devices for overcoming their fears such as arranging to do their shopping with their husband or children or by telephone.

The core of the 'social' phobia syndrome is usually a fear of being embarrassed in front of people who are known. The patient may also be unable to travel by bus or train for fear of meeting someone who is known and having to engage them in conversation, and there may be difficulty in speaking or eating in public, or using telephones when other people are in the room.

MANAGEMENT

Differential Diagnosis

The first step in management is diagnosis. The symptoms of anxiety may occur within the setting of virtually any other psychiatric disorder and to arrive at a diagnosis of an anxiety state it is necessary to exclude organic or functional psychoses, in particular thyrotoxicosis and an endogenous depressive syndrome, and to establish if there has been a definite change in the patient, with prominent symptoms of anxiety present from the start of the illness. Rare causes of episodic anxiety include phaeochromocytoma, epileptic disorders and mitral valve prolapse syndrome (Pariser et al. 1978). The symptoms of anxiety and depression frequently coexist (Roth et al. 1972; Prusoff and Klerman, 1974; Clancy et al. 1978) and it may be difficult to differentiate between a depressive syndrome and an anxiety phobic state (Hallam 1978). However, differentiation is possible in research studies (Gurney et al. 1972; Derogatis et al. 1972; Prusoff and Klerman 1974; Downing and Rickels 1974). A useful method for trying to determine whether one of the disorders is primary, is to determine whether the predominant feature at the start of the illness was depression or anxiety. In out-patient clinics and in general practice this may be difficult and, if there is doubt, the patient should be treated as having a depressive syndrome in the first instance (Johnstone et al. 1980).

Initial Management

A detailed history and assessment is required which should provide an indication of the patient's premorbid personality, current life situation, and recent or current stress. An attempt is then made to formulate any aetiological factors that can be identified.

Interest, concern, explanation, advice, an attempt to change aspects of the patient's environment, and reassurance are ingredients which should be part of the management of all patients with anxiety or phobic states, and in many instances form the most important therapeutic interventions. If particular conflicts or relationship difficulties are present, a more active psychotherapeutic approach may be needed, while referral to a specialist psychotherapist may be appropriate with a minority of patients. In addition, drug treatment, relaxation training, behaviour therapy and, in very rare instances, psychosurgery should be considered. Simple behavioural advice can be given by the general practitioner or psychiatrist, but referral to a clinical psychologist or other specialist in behavioural technique, is often required. Some patients with social phobias may benefit from psychotherapy in a group of individuals with similar problems.

Drug Treatments

Patients who are suffering from acute anxiety in relation to a specific stress may be helped by short-term sedation with a benzodiazepine and rest either at home or, in severe cases, by admission to hospital, especially if the stress arises from the home environment. If the anxiety is relatively persistent, regular treatment with benzodiazepines can be started. There are many benzodiazepines available with similar efficacy (Tyrer 1974); at times it may seem appropriate to choose one of the longer acting benzodiazepines because these tend to produce a more constant reduction in the level of anxiety, but shorter acting benzodiazepines often produce fewer side effects, especially in the elderly. A shorter-acting drug should also be used if a benzodiazepine is being used as a hypnotic or as a sedative for the immediate period before sleep.

As there is considerable variation in the amount of benzodiazepine required to modify anxiety, the patient should be given a small dose initially and be instructed to increase the dose over the course of the next few days until either the anxiety improves or side effects such as drowsiness, ataxia, or slurred speech are noticed. It is, of course, necessary to warn patients taking such drugs to be careful if they drive or come into contact with moving machinery. There is evidence that prolonged use of benzodiazepines is associated with a decreasing efficacy for the relief of anxiety, and that sudden withdrawal may give rise to symptoms similar to those of an anxiety state (Tyrer et al. 1981). However, this withdrawal syndrome subsides within a few days of stopping treatment. Because of these factors the patient should be advised that treatment with a benzodiazepine should last for no more than a few weeks, after which the dose will be gradually reduced. In the case of phobias, the patient should also be encouraged to face the feared situations when the anxiety has been partially alleviated. It is useful to suggest that the patient should take an extra dose of a benzodiazepine if anxiety is predictable in certain situations or if a panic attack develops and each patient should also be advised that they should attempt to remain in the feared situation until the symptoms of anxiety have diminished.

If the benzodiazepines are ineffective and a major component of the patient's anxiety consists of somatic (e.g. cardiac) symptoms of anxiety, the use of a β-blocker such as propranolol can be useful (Granville-Grossman and Turner 1966), but if this is inappropriate a monoamine oxidase inhibitor should be considered if further attempts at pharmacological control are indicated. There is quite good evidence of the value of these drugs for some patients with chronic anxiety, with or without phobias (Sargant and Dally 1962; Lipsedge et al. 1973; Tyrer et al. 1973; Robinson et al. 1973; Ravaris et al. 1976; Mountjoy et al. 1977) but the potential interaction of monoamine oxidase inhibitors with other drugs, and the warnings that must accompany their prescription, can make patients more anxious and unwilling to take their medication. Phenelzine is the monoamine oxidase inhibitor most frequently used in the UK, and although in the past there has been a tendency to confine the maximum daily dose to 45 mg, many patients fail to respond until they are receiving 60–90 mg per day. Therefore the dose of this drug should be increased to the maximum of 90 mg per day or until side effects become intolerable. The monoamine oxidase inhibitor tranylcypromine can be particularly useful for those anxious patients who are anergic and apathetic, presumably because of its additional amphetamine-like action. However habituation occurs to the latter effect.

Unfortunately it has not proved possible to predict which patients with anxiety and phobic states are likely to respond to monoamine oxidase inhibitors (Paykel et al. 1979; Mountjoy et al., 1980), and the duration of treatment with these drugs is difficult to estimate. Many patients relapse when the dosage is decreased and, although some patients are able to stop their medication altogether within 2–3 months and remain symptom-free, a number of patients appear to be helped by being maintained on monoamine oxidase inhibitors for many months or even years.

If none of these measures is satisfactory, small doses of phenothiazines are sometimes useful (Greenblatt and Shader 1974) though their beneficial effects must be set against the hazard of tardive dyskinesia. In general, phenothiazines should not be prescribed for anxiety states other than for short periods.

When a patient presents with a combination of an anxiety state and a depressive syndrome, a tricyclic antidepressant may be prescribed, especially if there is reason to believe that there is an underlying endogenous depressive illness. Even when the depressive syndrome does not contain the phenomena associated with endogenous illness and there is no other reason to suspect endogenous disorder, there is some evidence that a tricyclic antidepressant can have a beneficial effect on mood, although these effects are usually, at best, of modest clinical significance (Johnstone et al. 1980). However, there are reports that depressed patients can apparently have their symptoms of anxiety exacerbated when treated with tricyclics (Gurney et al. 1970; Rao and Coppen 1979). A number of studies have shown that some patients with anxiety and depression are improved with tricyclics, while others appear to respond to a monoamine oxidase inhibitor but, in the absence of evidence suggesting endogenous illness, there appears to be no way of predicting which patient with anxiety and depression will respond to which drug. An advantage of starting antidepressant treatment with a tricyclic is that it is possible to change relatively rapidly to a monoamine oxidase inhibitor if there is a failure of response, whereas a change of treatment from a monoamine oxidase inhibitor to a tricyclic calls for withdrawal of the monoamine oxidase inhibitor from the often deteriorating patient for a period of about 14 days before the tricyclics can be started. Most anxiety states, other than those which are an immediate response to severe stress, have been reported to carry a poor prognosis both in the response to treatment in the immediate episode and in terms of a subsequent relapse (Schapira et al. 1972; Noyes et al. 1980), and the results of drug treatment have not been particularly remarkable although many patients' symptoms can be alleviated. It should also be remembered that anxiety states and, to a lesser extent, phobic states, have a naturally fluctuating course, so that in many patients a spontaneous improvement is to be expected, whatever the intervention.

Relaxation Training and Behaviour Therapy

Some patients with chronic anxiety find techniques of relaxation beneficial (Thomas and Abbas 1978). However, these procedures require a considerable degree of cooperation from the patient and many find it difficult to continue their exercises for any length of time.

Various forms of behaviour therapy may be beneficial for those patients with phobias, especially if a phobia is specific to a relatively small number of stimuli such as in an animal phobia. However, behaviour therapy for agoraphobia and other phobic disorders can also be helpful, especially in those patients who are reluctant to take medication. Rohs and Noyes (1978) in their review of available behavioural treatments for a given phobia conclude that methods which incorporate flooding are probably the most effective.

Psychosurgery

Finally, for those individuals who have suffered from very severe, long-standing anxiety and depression which have proved refractory to all other methods of treatment, a psychosurgical procedure should be considered, particularly if there is a strong risk of suicide.

References

CLANCY, J., NOYES, R., HOENK, M.S.W. & SLYMEN, D.J. (1978) Secondary depression in anxiety neurosis. *J. nerv. ment. Dis.*, **166**, 846.

DEROGATIS, L.R., LIPMAN, R.S., COVI, L. & RICKELS, K. (1972) Factorial invariance of symptom dimensions in anxious and depressive neuroses. *Archs gen Psychiat.*, **27**, 659.

DOWNING, R. & RICKELS, K. (1974) Mixed anxiety-depression—Fact or myth? *Archs gen. Psychiat.*, **30**, 312.

GRANVILLE-GROSSMAN, K.L. & TURNER, P. (1966) The effect of propranolol on anxiety. *Lancet*, **i**, 788.

GREENBLATT, D.J. & SHADER, R.I. (1974) *Benzodiazepines in Clinical Practice.* New York: Raven Press.

GURNEY, C., ROTH, M., GARSIDE, R.F., KERR, T.A. & SCHAPIRA, K. (1972) Studies in the classification of affective disorders. The relationship between anxiety states and depressive illnesses-2. *Br. J. Psychiat.*, **121**, 162.

GURNEY, C., ROTH, M., KERR, T.A. & SCHAPIRA, K. (1970) The bearing of treatment on the classification of the affective disorders. *Br. J. Psychiat.*, **117**, 251.

HALLAM, R.S. (1978) Agoraphobia: A critical review of the concept. *Br. J. Psychiat.*, **133**, 314.

JOHNSTONE, E.C., CUNNINGHAM OWENS, D.G., FRITH, C.D., MCPHERSON, K., DOWIE, C., RILEY, G. & GOLD, A. (1980) Neurotic illness and its response to anxiolytic and antidepressant treatment. *Psychol. Med.*, **10**, 321.

LIPSEDGE, M.S., HAJIOFF, J., HUGGINS, P., NAPIER, L., PEARCE, J., PIKE, D.J. & RICH, M. (1973) The management of severe agoraphobia: a comparison of iproniazid and systematic desensitization. *Psychopharmacologia*, **32**, 67.

MARKS, I.M. (1969) *Fears and Phobias.* London: Heinemann Medical.

MOUNTJOY, C.Q., MARSHALL, E.F., CAMPBELL, I.C., GARSIDE, R.F. & ROTH, M. (1980) Prediction of response to treatment with phenelzine in neurotic patients. Progress in Neuro-Psychopharmacology, Vol. 4, p. 303. Oxford: Pergamon Press.

MOUNTJOY, C.Q., ROTH, M., GARSIDE, R.F. & LEITCH, I.M. (1977) A clinical trial of phenelzine in anxiety, depressive and phobic neuroses. *Br. J. Psychiat.*, **131**, 433.

NOYES, R. Jr., CLANCY, J., HOENK, P.R. & SLYMEN, D.J. (1980) The prognosis of anxiety neurosis. *Archs gen. Psychiat.*, **37**, 173.

PARISER, S.F., PINTA, E.R. & JONES, B.A. (1978) Mitral valve prolapse syndrome and anxiety neurosis/panic disorder. *Am. J. Psychiat.*, **135.2**, 246.

PAYKEL, E.S., PARKER, R.R., PENROSE, R.J.J. & RASSABY, E.R. (1979) Depressive classification and prediction of response to phenelzine. *Br. J. Psychiat.*, **134**, 572.

PRUSOFF, B. & KLERMAN, G.L. (1974) Differentiating depressed from anxious neurotic outpatients. *Archs gen. Psychiat.*, **30**, 302.

RAO, V.A.R. & COPPEN, A. (1979) Classification of depression and response to amitriptyline therapy. *Psychol. Med.*, **9**, 321.

RAVARIS, C.L., NIES, A., ROBINSON, D.S., IVES, J.O., LAMBORN, K.R. & KORSON, L. (1976) A multiple-dose, controlled study of phenelzine in depression anxiety states. *Archs gen. Psychiat.*, **33**, 347.

ROBINSON, D.S., NIES, A., RAVARIS, C.L. & LAMBOURN, K.R. (1973) The monoamine oxidase inhibitor, phenelzine, in the treatment of depressive-anxiety states. *Archs gen. Psychiat.*, **29**, 407.

ROHS, R.G. & NOYES, R. Jr. (1978) Agoraphobia: Newer treatment approaches. *J. nerv. ment. Dis.*, **166**, 701.

ROTH, M., GURNEY, C., GARSIDE, R.F. & KERR, T.A. (1972) Studies in the classification of affective disorders. The relationship between anxiety states and depressive illnesses—I. *Br. J. Psychiat.*, **121**, 147.

SARGANT, W. & DALLY, P. (1962) Treatment of anxiety states by antidepressant drugs. *Br. med. J.*, **i**, 6.

SCHAPIRA, K., ROTH, M., KERR, T.A. & GURNEY, C. (1972) The prognosis of affective disorders: the differentiation of anxiety states from depressive illnesses. *Br. J. Psychiat.*, **121**, 175.

THOMAS, D. & ABBAS, K.A. (1978) Comparison of transcendental meditation and progressive relaxation in reducing anxiety. *Br. med. J.*, **ii**, 1749.

TYRER, P. (1974) The benzodiazepine bonanza. *Lancet*, **ii**, 709.

TYRER, P., CANDY, J. & KELLY, D. (1973) A study of the clinical effects of phenelzine and placebo in the treatment of phobic anxiety. *Psychopharmacologia*, **32**, 237.

TYRER, P., RUTHERFORD, D. & HUGGETT, T. (1981) Benzodiazepine withdrawal symptoms and propranolol. *Lancet*, **i**, 520.

17

Management of Obsessive–Compulsive Disorders

J.H. Dowson

INTRODUCTION

Obsessions and compulsions can occur in association with various psychiatric syndromes but, if these phenomena are predominant, a diagnosis of obsessive–compulsive neurosis is usually made.

OBSESSIVE–COMPULSIVE DISORDERS

Obsessions and Compulsions

The following criteria have been used in various definitions of an obsession: a distressing content of consciousness which is intrusive, unwanted or unacceptable; a feeling of subjective compulsion, pressure or inner compelling force; internal resistance; internal attribution; a recognition that it is alien, unrealistic or, on quiet reflection, senseless; mental activity which is groundless, meaningless or relatively incomprehensible; and a difficulty in controlling the recurrence or persistence of the mental event (Schneider 1925; Jaspers 1963; Lewis 1966). However, as most of these attributes are not invariable, it can be argued that the only characteristics of an obsession which can properly be used as defining criteria are an abnormal degree of recurrence or persistence, and internal attribution. (The latter requirement excludes passivity experiences, in which the individual may believe that his mental events, or actions, are influenced by external forces) (Walker 1973; Dowson 1977; Rachman and Hodgson 1980*b*).

Compulsions can be considered as overt behavioural equivalents of obsessions and have been described as repetitive or stereotyped actions which are at least partly irrational (Rachman and Hodgson 1980*l*). Definitions of compulsions have also involved the underlying mental events and, as compulsions almost invariably seem to give expression to underlying obsessions, they can be described as 'purposive', in contrast to behaviour such as tremor or choreiform movements.

Obsessive–Compulsive Neurosis

Definition. Obsessive–compulsive neurosis has been defined as a disorder in which obsessions and compulsions cause distress or impair functioning (Black 1974; Rachman and Hodgson 1980*b*), although most clinicians would not make the diagnosis of obsessive–compulsive neurosis in the presence of psychosis or if the phenomena were judged to be part of another psychiatric disorder, such as anorexia nervosa.

Phenomenology. Obsessions and compulsions are invariably associated with other features such as anxiety, depression, marital and family problems, and social difficulties. These, particularly depression, may be the major determinants of hospital admission.

Obsessions take many forms, including images, urges, doubts, certain phobias, and 'thought-chain' ruminations, in which the patient is involved in inconclusive ruminations, usually about possible future events (Akhtar et al. 1975). The commonest content of an obsession appears to be dirt or contamination, while themes of harm, sex, religion, disgust, aggression, meticulousness and orderliness have often been described (Stern and Cobb 1978; Rachman and Hodgson 1980*s*).

Compulsions involve overt behaviour which is usually repetitive, although it may be merely persistent, when it is not so readily recognized by an observer. Cleaning behaviour, checking and avoidance are the commonest compulsions (Dowson 1977; Stern and Cobb 1978). Checking may involve underlying thoughts of security, safety or accuracy. Avoidance may be active, when additional actions are aimed at avoiding certain stimuli, or passive, when certain actions are omitted. If compulsions are present, most patients show more than one type (Hodgson and Rachman 1977). Obsessional slowness is a special type of compulsive behaviour in which some (but not necessarily all) activities are performed in an extremely slow, meticulous manner (Rachman 1974). Compulsions often have a magical or symbolic quality, for example, a patient repeatedly 'cleaned' herself with a specified handkerchief, and they have been classified as either 'yielding', when they give expression to the underlying urges, or 'controlling', when they are considered by the patient to 'neutralize' or displace an obsession (Akhtar et al. 1975).

An adverse mood state, which may involve depression, anxiety and hostility, is often associated with obsessions and compulsions, but although Walker and Beech (1969) have pointed out that mood may worsen during compulsive rituals, Rachman and Hodgson (1980*p*) have claimed that the performance of compulsions (but not the experience of obsessions alone) is usually accompanied by an improvement in mood, while only a minority of patients experience either no change in mood or an increase in anxiety and discomfort. Checking compulsions are over-represented in the minority group.

A feeling of resistance to carrying out compulsions together with varying degrees of insight are commonly found, although the former characteristic often appears to be variable or absent (Rachman and de Silva 1978; Stern and Cobb 1978). However, some patients show neither resistance nor insight. Patients have different levels of explanation for their symptoms; some statements may be apparently rational, but irrationality will eventually be found by repeatedly asking 'Is there a reason underlying that?' (Rachman and Hodgson 1980*l*). Compulsions can often be suspended by the patient, indicating that a degree of voluntary control is present, and some patients may seek out anxiety-provoking situations which initiate compulsions. Contrasting elements of behaviour may be seen; for example, cleaning compulsions may be combined with dirty personal habits (Beech 1974; Rachman and Hodgson 1980*g*). Compulsions are often mainly confined to one place, while interruption of rituals seldom leads to increased discomfort and often improves the patient's mood state (Stern and Cobb 1978; Rachman and Hodgson 1980*q*).

Natural history. The reported incidence of obsessive–compulsive neurosis in groups of psychiatric patients ranges from 0.1% to 4.6% (Black 1974; Rachman and de Silva 1978). The onset, which is typically in adolescence or in the early twenties, may be acute or insidious, and the course may be static, gradually worsening, fluctuating or phasic with remissions (Beech and Vaughan 1978*b*). It has been claimed that a relatively good outcome is associated with mild symptoms, an absence of compulsions, a short interval between onset and referral, a depressed mood, precipitating factors, and an absence of previous personality disorder. A poor prognosis has been associated with previous obsessional personality (although the evidence is conflicting), childhood onset, pervasive symptoms and lack of insight (Goodwin et al. 1969; Black 1974; Beech and Vaughan 1978*c*; Rachman and Hodgson 1980*c,j*).

Associated psychiatric syndromes. Obsessions and compulsions may be found in conjunction with several psychiatric disorders, in particular with depressive syndromes. A depressive syndrome with 'neurotic' phenomenology often develops in the course of an obsessive–compulsive neurosis, while a primary depressive disorder may be followed by the appearance of obsessions and compulsions, which may sometimes be considered as symptoms of an affective psychosis, if there is evidence to support this diagnosis (Gittelson 1966; Lewis 1966; Kendell and Discipio 1970; Kringlen 1970; Black 1974; Videbech 1975; Welner et al. 1976; Rachman and Hodgson 1980*h*). Rare examples of recurrent 'endogenous obsessive–compulsive neurosis' have been attributed to atypical affective psychoses, and it has been reported that obsessions and compulsions can remit in manic illness, although Lewis (1966) has claimed that they can be secondary to mania (Mayer-Gross et al. 1969).

There are reports of obsessive–compulsive phenomena preceding or accompanying schizophrenic syndromes, but the development of a schizophrenic illness in the course of obsessive–compulsive neurosis is rare, with an incidence of up to 3.3% in various samples (Black 1974).

Several supposed attributes of the obsessional (or anankastic) personality include being methodical, rigid, parsimonious, obstinate and conscientious, in addition to being a chronic worrier (Slade 1974). However, although there appears to be an association between obsessive–compulsive neurosis and obsessional personality, many patients do not have these premorbid personality traits to a marked degree.

Some postencephalitic syndromes, parkinsonism, anorexia nervosa, Lesch –Nyhan syndrome, epilepsy, childhood autism and Gilles de la Tourette syndrome have been reported to be associated with obsessions and compulsions, although such phenomena may not be identical with those in obsessive –compulsive neurosis (O'Regan 1970; Lindley et al. 1977; Marks 1979; Yaryura-Tobias et al. 1980).

It is clear that the occurrence of obsessions and compulsions in various psychiatric syndromes presents considerable problems in the delineation of the syndrome of obsessive–compulsive neurosis and, in addition, the boundaries between obsessive–compulsive neurosis and disorders such as phobic neurosis, anorexia nervosa, obsessional personality disorder and some examples of morbid jealousy or hypochondriasis, can be difficult to determine (Docherty and Ellis 1976; Cobb and Marks 1979).

Aetiology. Many factors, both essential and non-essential, may contribute to the development of the syndrome; some will mainly affect the occurrence and form of the symptoms, while others will merely shape their contents.

There is insufficient evidence to assess the importance of genetic factors, but a specific and/or a non-specific contribution is possible (Black 1974; Welner et al. 1976; McGuffin and Mawson 1980; Rachman and Hodgson 1980*d*; Murray and Reveley 1981). A relationship between the syndrome and blood group A has been reported (Rinieris et al. 1978).

Psychoanalytic theorists have claimed that conflicts in the early years of life may be unresolved due to events such as strict or early toilet training, and that if these conflicts are reactivated by subsequent sexual or aggressive impulses, obsessions and compulsions can be the result; these symptoms have been considered to derive from the psychological defences which operated at the time of the original unresolved conflict (Freud 1966; Schwartz 1977). Although there is insufficient evidence to support this theory (Cawley 1974), Rachman and Hodgson (1980*l,m,n,w*) have claimed that there is evidence of excessive parental control in groups of patients with obsessive–compulsive neurosis, and these authors considered that parental overprotection may contribute to the development of cleaning rituals, while excessive parental criticism may contribute to the development of checking compulsions. There is evidence that there is a significant excess of firstborn male patients with obsessive–compulsive neurosis, and it has been suggested that this may be the result of excessive demands to which a first born child can be subjected (Snowdon 1979). Parental preoccupation with cleanliness, early or excessive punishment of aggression, and a strict religious upbringing have also been suggested as possible aetiological factors (Teasdale 1974).

It is possible that conditioning can play a part in the development or maintenance of the disorder by producing a response of fear to originally neutral stimuli, or by reinforcing compulsions if they lead to a reduction of anxiety (Teasdale 1974). Although some rituals are accompanied by increasing anxiety, in such cases it is possible that compulsions may be reinforced by the fulfilment of a desire to reduce guilt or to provide safety in the long term, even though anxiety and discomfort are increased in the short term (Rachman and Hodgson 1980*t*). Observational learning may also be of aetiological significance, at least for the content of some symptoms, although this is probably not a major factor (Marks et al. 1969). However, social learning which leads to timidity and overdependence may be a non-specific predisposing factor for the development of obsessive–compulsive neurosis (Rachman and Hodgson 1980*l*).

It has been considered that premorbid personality may be an aetiological factor, and Lewis (1936) has described two obsessional personality types which he found to be associated with obsessive–compulsive neurosis. One is obstinate, morose and irritable, while the other is vacillating and submissive. Sandler and Hazari (1960) have also reported that there are two relatively independent groups of traits which appear to be related to those described by Lewis; one group is characterized by being very systematic, methodical and meticulous, while the other includes a marked tendency to worry. Rachman and Hodgson (1980*j*) have claimed that Lewis's former group of traits are associated with cleaning compulsions and the latter traits with checking rituals. However, there have been many reports of between 16% and 36% of patients with obsessive–compulsive neurosis who did not have marked obsessional personality traits (Black 1974). Non-obsessional personality traits have also been studied in relation to obsessive–compulsive neurosis and there is some evidence of an association between obsessive–compulsive neurosis and both neuroticism and introversion (Slade 1974; Blacker and Levitt 1979; Rachman and Hodgson 1980*o*), for which there is evidence of a genetic contribution.

Mood state, involving depression, anxiety and hostility, has been identified as an important determinant of compulsive behaviour, and Beech has suggested that a predisposition to the development of an exaggerated state of arousal in response to adverse stimuli is a major underlying defect in the obsessive–compulsive syndrome (Beech and Vaughan 1978). However, not all patients appear to have an abnormal mood at the onset of their rituals.

Inappropriate displacement activity in animals can follow conflict or frustration (Delius 1970), and although it is not clear whether this behaviour is akin to compulsions, it is generally accepted that certain events can precipitate obsessive–compulsive neurosis. Reported examples include pregnancy, abortion, childbirth, sexual problems, illness or death, increased criticism or responsibility, and thwarted self-assertion (Kringlen 1970).

Several avenues of research have indicated an association between brain dysfunction and obsessive–compulsive neurosis (Ananth 1976; Yaryura-Tobias and Bhagavan 1977; Rinieris et al. 1978; Moskovitz and Lingao 1979; Rachman and Hodgson 1980*i*; Yaryura-Tobias et al. 1980). Many early studies which reported EEG abnormalities are of poor quality, but Flor-Henry et al. (1979) have recently provided EEG evidence of left frontal dysfunction in the syndrome, which has also been associated with diabetes insipidus and a history of obstetric difficulties at birth (Barton 1976; Capstick and Seldrup 1977).

ASSESSMENT OF OBSESSIVE–COMPULSIVE DISORDERS

Obsessive–compulsive neurosis may affect many aspects of the patient's life, so that assessment should not be restricted to the obsessions and compulsions.

Unstructured interviews with the patient and family are, of course, commonly used in clinical practice, while numerous questionnaires, rating scales and check lists have been employed for both the initial assessment and for monitoring response to treatment. These may be self-administered or completed by an assessor (Capstick 1975; Hackman and McLean 1975; Beech and Vaughan 1978*d*; Ananth et al. 1979; Donnelly et al. 1979).

There are five main instruments for the assessment of obsessions and compulsions: the Leyton Obsessional Inventory (Cooper 1970; Murray et al. 1979; Robertson and Mulhall 1979; Snowdon 1980), the Lynfield Obsessional/ Compulsive Questionnaire (Allen and Tune 1975; Allen 1977), the Obsessive–Compulsive Interview Checklist (Philpott 1975), the Obsessive–Compulsive Checklist (Marks 1979), and the Maudsley Obsessional–Compulsive Inventory (Hodgson and Rachman 1977). Other aspects of obsessive–compulsive neurosis such as depression, anxiety, hostility, neuroticism and impaired social adjustment have been evaluated by a wide range of methods, and a common device in clinical practice is to ask the patient to complete a diary at regular intervals.

Other assessment methods include in vivo tests of avoidance behaviour, automatic counting devices operated by the patient, automated monitoring of behaviour, recording of behaviour by an observer for set periods, and physiological measurements of heart rate and skin conductance.

THERAPEUTIC INTERVENTIONS IN OBSESSIVE–COMPULSIVE NEUROSIS

Introduction

Initial assessment and diagnosis may indicate that obsessive–compulsive phenomena are secondary to another psychiatric syndrome which requires specific treatment.

It is probably not appropriate to consider obsessive–compulsive neurosis as a unitary disorder from either the aetiological or the phenomenological viewpoint, so that an eclectic approach to management is needed to produce the optimal combination of treatment methods for each patient (Beech 1978).

Psychotherapy

Psychotherapy can be divided into two main, but overlapping categories: supportive psychotherapy involves such ingredients as interest, concern, empathy, advice, and helping the patient to avoid self-deception, while insight-directed psychotherapy is more intensive (i.e. time consuming) and provides an emphasis on interpretations of behaviour and attitudes, in particular those which are found in the treatment sessions (Cawley 1974).

Supportive psychotherapy may have the aim of symptom relief, or be directed towards problems which are secondary to a particular psychiatric syndrome, and has an important role in the management of obsessive–compulsive neurosis. Also, interviews with the patient's spouse or family are often indicated. Advice can be given regarding potential distractions from obsessions and compulsions; examples include listening to music, mental arithmetic, compiling lists, recalling songs, crosswords, work and social events. Such activities may alleviate or inhibit symptoms, and strategies can be planned which may be especially useful for those patients who recognize episodic build-up of a tendency to engage in their symptoms (Beech 1978). In addition, the patient's life style should be reviewed; it is known that some patients improve when they are in a controlled environment with routine, such as is found in the armed forces, prisons, or hospitals, and symptoms may be exacerbated by work involving excessive pressure or uncertainty (Black 1974). Reassurance that the patient will not commit violent or socially embarrassing acts in response to resisted urges, or will not 'go insane', is usually helpful, albeit for a limited period, so long as the therapist does not repeatedly reinforce a ritual of asking for reassurance (Teasdale 1974; Rachman and Hodgson 1980*a*). Supportive psychotherapy should also be directed towards attitudes to the obsessions and compulsions, problems of living with the symptoms, and marital, social or occupational problems. Various facets of the therapist –patient relationship, such as the therapist's capacity for empathy, and the therapist being seen as assuming responsibility for the patient's actions, may improve the patient's mood, and such a mood change may then improve both personal adjustment and obsessive–compulsive symptoms (Beech and Vaughan 1978*j*).

Insight-directed psychotherapy may sometimes be undertaken when there is evidence of maladaptive psychological defence mechanisms, and an attempt may be made to modify attributes of the patient's personality (see Chapters 8 and 9) (Blacker and Levitt 1979). However, although many claims have been made for the beneficial effects of intensive, insight-directed psychotherapy, this 'procedure' is not standardized, and reports have been uncontrolled, often consisting of a mixture of observation and theory (Cawley 1974; Freud 1966). Although a minority of patients may benefit, there is no convincing evidence to confirm the efficacy of intensive psychotherapy based on psychoanalytic techniques for obsessive–compulsive neurosis (Rachman and Hodgson 1980*j*). However, aggression and insecurity may merit exploration.

Drug Treatments

Many studies have claimed that clomipramine can alleviate obsessive –compulsive neurosis and some apparently dramatic 'cures' are recorded. In the early days of its use for obsessions and compulsions, it was thought that the intravenous administration of this drug enhanced its action (Rack 1977; Ananth et al. 1979), and clomipramine was given by daily infusions in increasing doses up to 375 mg daily, if side effects permitted; however, the value of this procedure has not been confirmed and clomipramine should not be routinely administered intravenously.

A controlled trial which was supported by the Medical Research Council has recently investigated the effects of both oral clomipramine and exposure in vivo (with modelling and self-imposed response prevention), in 40 obsessive– compulsive patients (Rachman et al. 1979; Marks et al. 1980; Stern et al. 1980*a*). Although clomipramine produced a significant improvement in compulsions, mood and social adjustment, this only occurred in those patients who were initially depressed. There was no evidence of a primary antiobsessional effect and no conclusive evidence of an interaction between the drug and the behavioural treatment, which was also shown to be effective. The maximum effect of clomipramine was between 10 and 18 weeks after starting treatment, and the patients often relapsed after stopping the drug. It was concluded that although behaviour therapy is the treatment of choice for compulsions in the absence of depression, clomipramine should be used in combination with behavioural treatment if depression is present, and that the drug may need continuation for at least a year. Clomipramine may be given as a single dose at night, starting with 10 mg which is increased to 225 mg within 2 weeks, unless side effects become intolerable, although in another publication derived from this study, which focussed on plasma levels of clomipramine and desmethylclo- mipramine in relation to clinical response, it was claimed that there may be a therapeutic window for plasma levels of clomipramine and its primary metabo- lite (Stern et al. 1980*a*). In another publication based on the same plasma level data, Stern et al. (1980*b*) claimed that the level of unchanged clomipramine (and not desmethylclomipramine) may be related to the outcome of compulsive rituals, while the level of the metabolite may correlate with the outcome of depression. Although this study did not provide evidence for a specific antiobsessional effect of clomipramine, there are other controlled trials and case reports which have claimed that a dramatic effect on symptoms is not always dependent on the presence of a depressed mood, suggesting that this drug may have a primary action on obsessive–compulsive symptoms (Ananth 1980; Rack 1980). For example, Thorén et al. (1980) reported that clomipramine was superior to placebo and nortriptyline in relieving the severity of obsessive –compulsive phenomena, and that this effect could not be predicted by the presence of secondary depressive symptoms. However, Mawson et al. (1982) found that clomipramine treatment did not have a detectable effect on rituals after a 2-year follow-up period.

Various other drugs have been used for obsessive–compulsive neurosis including other antidepressants such as doxepin, amitriptyline, imipramine and mianserin (Sternberg 1974; Ananth et al. 1975; Väisänen et al. 1977; Snyder 1980a,b). Although, in general, monoamine oxidase inhibitors (MAOIs) have not been considered to be useful, there are some case reports of apparently beneficial effects of these drugs, while the use of a combination of a tricyclic antidepressant with a MAOI has also been advocated (Ananth 1976). Other drugs which have been tried are various benzodiazepines, L-tryptophan, chlorpromazine, perphenazine, amphetamine (associated with abreaction), intravenous acetylcholine, LSD (weekly injections for 57 weeks), and haloperidol (O'Regan 1970; Sternberg 1974; Yaryura-Tobias and Bhagavan 1977). Haloperidol apparently produced good results in two patients, but there is no good evidence that any of these drugs have a specific antiobsessional effect, although anxiolytic and antidepressant drugs may provide relief of an adverse mood state, and may facilitate behavioural treatment.

Electroconvulsive therapy (ECT)

Although ECT may alleviate obsessive–compulsive phenomena which are secondary to a depressive syndrome with an endogenous aetiology, its value in obsessive–compulsive neurosis is, at best, limited and short lived. However, ECT has a place in the management of severe depression which develops in the course of an obsessive–compulsive neurosis, and which does not respond to other methods of treatment (Sternberg 1974).

Behaviour Therapy

In vivo exposure, modelling and response prevention. Mayer et al. (1974) reported a method with these three ingredients, in which the emphasis was on prevention of compulsions. Patients were usually admitted to hospital, where they were continually supervised by a nurse who tried to prevent compulsions by a mixture of persuasion, praise, prompting, diversion and mild physical restraint which was applied with the patient's consent. After the rituals had been controlled under supervision, the patient was exposed, with the help of participant modelling, to a hierarchy of eliciting stimuli, starting with those which produced the least anxiety. When the rituals had been eliminated in the presence of eliciting stimuli, supervision was gradually withdrawn and sessions were organized at the patient's home.

Marks et al. (1975) have described a similar method, for either in- or out-patients, which put more emphasis on exposure and modelling (Rachman and Hodgson 1980*u*). Response prevention was minimally supervised and the patients were simply asked to refrain from, limit, or delay carrying out their compulsions between treatment sessions. The patient was initially told that the treatment involved facing feared situations and putting up with discomfort, but that this would eventually lead to improvement. A hierarchy of eliciting stimuli was constructed but, if possible, treatment began with exposure to the most feared situation. However, if this could not be tolerated, the patient was exposed to items which provoked less anxiety. Treatment sessions consisted of exposure and participant modelling, which involved a demonstration by the therapist, followed by a repetition of the therapist's actions by the patient; sometimes the therapist would manually guide the patient to the feared stimuli. Home treatment was arranged and the patient was asked to record his behaviour between sessions. The patient's family was often encouraged to be involved in treatment.

There are other studies of the relative importance and optimal characteristics of exposure, modelling and response prevention, and there are case reports of the success of exposure alone (Beech and Vaughan 1978*e,j*; Emmelkamp et al. 1980). It appears that the duration of exposure may be more important than the associated level of discomfort, and there is evidence that participant modelling, in which the patient copies the therapist's actions, is superior to passive modelling, in which the patient merely observes the therapist. The results of Rachman et al. (1973) indicated that the therapeutic effects of exposure alone did not differ significantly from those of modelling (which may of course, include exposure), and that their combination produced only slightly better results than either procedure alone. Foa et al. (1980) have investigated the differential effects of exposure and response prevention in patients with washing compulsions. In this study, 'exposure' involved the experience of a discomfort-evoking stimulus for 6 h daily for 2 weeks, but although the patients were allowed to wash, it was found that they voluntarily delayed their compulsions until after each exposure period so that 'response prevention' was also part of this component of the regimen. Response prevention consisted of a continuous period of 2 weeks during which patients were constantly supervised and discouraged from carrying out their rituals; subjects were allowed to avoid 'contaminatory' stimuli. The authors reported that exposure had more ther-apeutic effect on anxiety than on overt compulsive behaviour, while response prevention had relatively more influence on the washing compulsions. It was suggested that for many patients, especially those with long-standing disorders, 'second-order' stimuli, such as mood state, stress, water, and bathrooms can be important determinants of compulsions, in addition to the 'first-order' stimuli, which are believed by the patient to be the source of contamination.

Foa et al. (1980) considered that while their exposure principally reduced the harmful consequences of first-order stimuli, response prevention had significant effects on both first- and second-order stimuli. However, the differential effects which were reported may also have been partly due to the fact that exposure was for limited periods, while response prevention was continuous. These authors claimed that a combination of their exposure and response prevention was more effective than either used singly.

These behavioural techniques represent a considerable advance in the treatment of many patients with obsessive–compulsive neurosis, although their use is not usually appropriate for patients with obsessional slowness or with obsessions alone. Of those patients who are suitable for treatment, about 75% can be expected to improve, although only a minority lose all their symptoms (Rachman and Hodgson 1980v). Problems other than obsessions and compulsions also may improve, with the usual exception of any sexual maladjustment, and there is no evidence of symptom substitution.

A typical arrangement would be to admit the patient to hospital for a minimum of 3 weeks. This would be followed by home treatment and 'booster sessions' for relapse, as required. Marks (1979) reported that the mean number of 90-min treatment sessions was 11, and follow-up studies have indicated that improvement is likely to be maintained for at least 2 years (Marks et al. 1975). Some patients found exposure too distressing and discontinued their treatment, but of those who completed their behaviour therapy the main reason for failure was an inability to comply with instructions to stop or limit compulsions between sessions, and a regimen of continuous supervision might have been more appropriate for these patients (Rachman and Hodgson 1980t). Pervasive checking rituals appeared to be relatively resistant to behavioural treatment, and an early ability to limit rituals between treatment sessions was claimed to be a good prognostic sign.

Thought stopping and related techniques. These procedures helped a minority of patients with obsessions alone, although the effects are unpredictable (Beech and Vaughan 1978h). The patient is seated with his eyes shut and is instructed to induce an obsession, perhaps by describing it aloud. After 15–30 s he signals to the therapist who shouts 'stop' or makes some loud noise. The patient is instructed to keep his mind blank after the 'stop' signal, or to substitute some other mental activity such as imaging pleasant scenery. Tape recordings of sounds such a bird song have been used to assist the substitution process. If this procedure is repeatedly effective, control of the 'stop' signal is passed to the patient who is instructed to gradually reduce the intensity of the signal.

Eventually the patient may simply whisper 'stop' inaudibly. Three studies have compared thought stopping with other behavioural treatments, and several case studies have reported successful results (Stern 1978). These techniques deserve further attention, and it has been suggested that the 'stop' signal should be applied earlier, during the emergence of the obsession.

Satiation. This method has also been applied to obsessions in the absence of compulsions, and can occasionally be helpful (Rachman 1976; Beech and Vaughan 1978g). During the sessions, which may last for up to an hour, or consist of much shorter periods with intervening breaks, the patient is asked to evoke the obsession and describe it aloud. The patient is also instructed to carry out this procedure on his own, spend time repeatedly writing the obsession, and to bring himself into contact with eliciting stimuli. Stern (1978) has reported how two patients with horrific thoughts responded well to this method. A variation of this procedure is the so-called paradoxical intention method, in which an attempt is made to elaborate and exaggerate the obsessional thoughts. This has been described by Solyom et al. (1972).

Prompting, pacing and shaping. These techniques have been successfully applied to the few patients in whom obsessional slowness is the predominant problem (Bilsbury and Morley 1979). In addition to the prompting, pacing and shaping of behaviour, this procedure may involve setting targets, modelling, and organizing treatment in the patient's home. Not all patients with obsessional slowness respond, but significant and rapid improvement has been reported.

Miscellaneous techniques. Self-monitoring, which forms part of many behavioural methods can, by itself, produce improvement (Frederiksen 1975). Various self-administered aversive stimuli, such as an electric shock or snapping an elastic band against the wrist, have been paired with obsessions or compulsions, and the latter method was reported to have helped two patients (Beech and Vaughan 1978i). Attempts have also been made to modify patients' concepts of appropriate behaviour, and various other cognitive manipulations have been suggested, which include the patient imagining himself to be refraining from rituals by acting normally, or associating imagined eliciting stimuli or compulsions with imagined unpleasant experiences (Wisocki 1970; Meyer et al. 1974; Rachman and Hodgson 1980w). A patient with trichotillomania responded dramatically to instructions to repeatedly say, "No, stay where you are" (Taylor 1963).

Adjuncts to behavioural treatment. These include asking the patient to vary the order of a ritual, organizing special distraction tasks and helping the patient to restructure his life after treatment (Beech and Vaughan 1978i). The therapist can arrange to follow up the patient partly by telephone, and relatives may be encouraged to supervise the patient's record of his symptoms. Relaxation training and social skills training may also be helpful (Beech and Vaughan 1978*j*).

Psychosurgery

In England and Wales, 30 psychosurgical operations were performed for obsessive–compulsive neurosis during 1974–76. Unwanted effects such as epilepsy or personality change were infrequent, and it was recently concluded that 'it is reasonable to assume that a maintained remission soon after surgery in patients with severe and hitherto intractable symptoms is largely the result of the operation'. An enquiry sponsored by the US Congress came to the same conclusion (Anon 1980).

Various types of operation have been performed. Lewin advocated bilateral destruction of the anterior cingulate cortex, and Knight has developed a technique (bilateral stereotactic tractotomy) for implanting yttrium in the subcaudate region. This latter procedure was reported to produce improvement in 16 out of 24 patients, although it has been suggested that it should be combined with lesions of the cingulum (Knight 1972; Bridges et al. 1973). Kelly and his colleagues have reported the results of stereotactic limbic leucotomy, which involved bilateral lesions in both the lower medial quadrant of the frontal lobe and the cingulum; 89% of 66 patients had maintained an improvement at a 16-months follow-up (Kelly et al. 1973*a,b*; Mitchell-Heggs et al. 1976). Crow has reported another technique, while other procedures include coagulation of the intralaminar and medial thalamic nuclei (Hassler and Dieckmann 1967; Crow 1973).

Psychosurgery should be considered for patients with chronic (5 years or more), intractable obsessive–compulsive neurosis when it is associated with marked suffering, especially if the risk of suicide seems high. All other treatments should have been tried over a period of at least 2 years and full and effective consent must be obtained (Anon 1980). Postoperative improvement is often gradual, and active postoperative rehabilitation and treatment for at least several months is usually essential. It has been reported that previously ineffective behaviour therapy may produce beneficial results in the postoperative period (Knight 1972). Obsessions and compulsions may be improved, and there may also be a reduction of tension and depression which helps the patient to tolerate any residual symptoms (Sternberg 1974; Rachman and Hodgson 1980*k*).

CONCLUSIONS

The management of obsessive–compulsive neurosis usually involves the coordination of several professional disciplines, and therapeutic interventions may involve psychotherapy, behavioural treatments, drugs and social work. Psychosurgery should be considered for patients with severe intractable symptoms.

The patient may attend as an out-patient or day-patient, and home treatment sessions are often required. Hospital admission may be necessary to carry out intensive behavioural treatment, to manage severe anxiety and depression, or to relieve family distress. If local resources cannot provide the behavioural treatments which are indicated, the patient should be referred to a unit which specializes in these techniques.

References

AKHTAR, S., WIG, N.H., VERMA, V.K., PERSHOD, D. & VERMA, S.K. (1975) A phenomenological analysis of symptoms in obsessive–compulsive neurosis. *Br. J. Psychiat.*, **127**, 342.

ALLEN, J. (1977) The measurement of obsessionality: first validation studies of the Lynfield Obsessional/Compulsive Questionnaires. *J. Int. Med. Res. 5, Suppl., (5)*. 12.

ALLEN, J.J. & TUNE, G.S. (1975) The Lynfield Obsessional/Compulsive Questionnaires. *Scot. med. J.*, **20**, 21.

ANANTH, J. (1976) Treatment of obsessive–compulsive neurosis: pharmacological approach. *Psychosomatics*, **17:4**, 180.

ANANTH, J. (1980) Systematic studies with clomipramine in obsessive neurosis. *Pharm. Med.*, **1:1**, 148.

ANANTH, J., SOLYOM, L., BRYNTWICK, S. & KRISHNAPPA, U. (1979) Clomipramine therapy for obsessive–compulsive neurosis. *Am. J. Psychiat.*, **136:5**, 700.

ANANTH, J., SOLYOM, L., SOLYOM, C. & SOOKMAN, D. (1975) Doxepin in the treatment of obsessive–compulsive neurosis. *Psychosomatics*, **16:4**, 185.

ANON, (1980) Is leucotomy ever justified? *Drug. Ther. Bull.*, **18:15**, 57.

BARTON, R. (1976) Diabetes insipidus and obsessional neurosis. *Am. J. Psychiat.*, **132:2**, 235.

BEECH, H.R. (1974) Approaches to understanding obsessional states. In: *Obsessional States*. Ed. Beech, H.R. London: Methuen.

BEECH, H.R. (1978) Advances in the treatment of obsessional neurosis. *Br. J. hosp. Med.*, **January**, 54.

BEECH, H.R. & VAUGHAN, M. (1978) *Behavioural Treatment of Obsessional States* pp. 3a, 9b, 10–12c, 13–30d, 31–50e, 51–84f, 85–100g, 101–116h, 117–138i, 150–151j. Chichester: John Wiley and Sons.

BILSBURY, C. & MORLEY, S. (1979) Obsessional slowness: a meticulous replication. *Behav. Res. Ther.*, **17**, 405.

BLACK, A. (1974) The natural history of obsessional neurosis. In: *Obsessional States*, ed. Beech, H.R. London: Methuen.

BLACKER, K.H. & LEVITT, M. (1979) The differential diagnosis of obsessive–compulsive symptoms. *Compreh. Psychiat.*, **20:b**, 532.

BRIDGES, P.K., GOKTEPE, E.O. & MARATOS, J. (1973) A comparative review of patients with obsessional neurosis and with depression treated by psychosurgery. *Br. J. Psychiat.*, **123**, 663.

CAPSTICK, N. (1975) The Shapiro cards scale as a method of assessment of obsessional symptoms in clomipramine therapy. *Scot. med. J.*, **20**, 17.

CAPSTICK, N. & SELDRUP, J. (1977) Obsessional states. *Acta psychiat. neurol. scand.*, **56**, 427.

CAWLEY, R. (1974) Psychotherapy and obsessional disorders. In: *Obsessional States*, ed. Beech, H.R. London: Methuen.

COBB, J.P. & MARKS, I.M. (1979) Morbid jealousy featuring as obsessive–compulsive neurosis: treatment by behavioural psychotherapy. *Br. J. Psychiat.*, **134**, 301.

COOPER, J. (1970) The Leyton Obsessional Inventory. *Psychol. Med.*, **1**, 48.

CROW, H.J. (1973) Intracerebral polarization and multifocal leucocoagulation in some psychiatric illness. *Folia psychiat. neurol. neurochir. neerl.*, **76**, 365.

DELIUS, J.D. (1970) Irrelevant behaviour, information processing and arousal homeostasis. *Psychol. Forsch.*, **33**, 165.

DOCHERTY, J.P. & ELLIS, J. (1976) A new concept and finding in morbid jealousy. *Am. J. Psychiat.*, **133:6**, 679.

DONNELLY, E.F., MURPHY, D.L. & WALDMAN, I.N. (1979) Obsessionalism and response to lithium. *Br. med. J.*, **i**, 1627.

DOWSON, J.H. (1977) The phenomenology of severe obsessive–compulsive neurosis. *Br. J. Psychiat.*, **131**, 75.

EMMELKAMP, P.M.G., VAN DER HELM, M. VAN ZANKEN, B.L. & PLOCHG, I. (1980) Treatment of obsessive–compulsive patients: the contribution of self-instructional training to the effectivenss of exposure. *Behav. Res. Ther.*, **18**, 61.

FLOR-HENRY, P., YEUDALL, L.T., KOLES, Z.J. & HOWARTH, B.G. (1979) Neuropsychological and power spectral EEG investigations of the obsessive–compulsive syndrome. *Biol. Psychiat.*, **14**, No. 1, 119.

FOA, E.B., STEKETEE, G. & MILBY, J.B. (1980) Differential effects of exposure and response prevention in obsessive–compulsive washers. *J. consult. clin. Psychol.*, **48:1**, 71.

FREDERIKSEN, L.W. (1975) Treatment of ruminative thinking by self-monitoring. *J. Behav. Ther. Exp. Psychiat.*, **6**, 258.

FREUD, A. (1966) Obsessional neurosis. (Summary of 24th International Psychoanalytic Congress, 1965). *Int. J. Psycho-Analysis*, **47**, 116.

GITTELSON, N. (1966) The effect of obsessions on depressive psychosis. *Br. J. Psychiat.*, **112**, 253.

GOODWIN, D.W., GUZE, S.B. & ROBINS, E. (1969) Follow-up in obsessional neurosis. *Archs gen. Psychiat.*, **20**, 182.

HACKMAN, A. & McLEAN, C. (1975) A comparison of flooding and thought stopping in the treatment of obsessional neurosis. *Behav. Res. Ther.*, **13**, 263.

HASSLER, R. & DIECKMANN, G. (1967) Stereotaxic treatment of compulsive and obsessive symptoms. *Confinia neurol. (Basel)*, **29**, 152.

HODGSON, R.J. & RACHMAN, S. (1977) Obsessional–compulsive complaints. *Behav. Res. Ther.*, **15**, 389.

JASPERS, K. (1963) *General Psychopathology*, p. 134. Chicago: University of Chicago.

KELLY, D., RICHARDSON, A. & MITCHELL-HEGGS, N. (1973a) Stereotactic limbic leucotomy: neurophysiological aspects and operative technique. *Br. J. Psychiat.*, **123**, 133.

KELLY, D., RICHARDSON, A., MITCHELL-HEGGS, N., GREENUP, J., CHEN, C. & HAFNER, R.J. (1973b). Stereotactic limbic leucotomy. *Br. J. Psychiat.*, **123**, 141.

KENDELL, R.E. & DISCIPIO, W.J. (1970) Obsessional symptoms and obsessional personality traits in patients with depressive illnesses. *Psychol. Med.*, **1**, 65.

KNIGHT, G. (1972) Psychosurgery today. *Proc. R. Soc. Med.*, **65**, 1099.

KRINGLEN, E. (1970) Natural history of obsessional neurosis. *Semin. Psychiat.*, **2**, 403.

LEWIS, A.J. (1936) Problems of obsessional illness. *Proc. R. Soc. Med.*, **29**, 325.

LEWIS, A.J. (1966) Obsessional disorder. In: *Price's Textbook of the Practice of Medicine*, ed. Scott, R. 10th ed. London: Oxford University Press.

LINDLEY, P., MARKS, I., PHILPOTT, R. & SNOWDEN, J. (1977) Treatment of obsessive–compulsive neurosis with history of childhood autism. *Br. J. Psychiat.*, **130**, 592.

MARKS, I. (1979) Exposure therapy for phobias and obsessive–compulsive disorders. *Hosp. Practice*, **14(2)**, 101.

MARKS, I.M., CROWE, M., DREWE, E., YOUNG, T. & DEWHURST, W.G. (1969) Obsessional –compulsive neurosis in identical twins. *Br. J. Psychiat.*, **115**, 991.

MARKS, I.M., HODGSON, R. & RACHMAN, S. (1975) Treatment of chronic obsessive–compulsive neurosis by in-vivo exposure. *Br. J. Psychiat.*, **127**, 349.

MARKS, I.M., STERN, R.S., MAWSON, D., COBB, J. & McDONALD, R. (1980) Clomipramine and exposure for obsessive–compulsive rituals. *Br. J. Psychiat.*, **136**, 1.

MAWSON, D., MARKS, I.M. & RAMM, L. (1982) Clomipramine and exposure for chronic obsessive–compulsive rituals. *Br. J. Psychiat.*, **140**, 11.

MAYER, V., LEVY, R. & SCHNURER, A. (1974) The behavioural treatment of obsessive–compulsive disorders. In: *Obsessional States*, ed. Beech, H.R. London: Methuen.

MAYER-GROSS, W., SLATER, E. & ROTH, M. (1969) *Clinical Psychiatry*, 3rd ed. London: Baillière Tindall.

McGUFFIN, P. & MAWSON, D. (1980) Obsessive–compulsive neurosis: two identical twin pairs. *Br. J. Psychiat.*, **137**, 285.

MITCHELL-HEGGS, N., KELLY, D. & RICHARDSON, A. (1976) Stereotactic limbic leucotomy—a follow-up at 16 months. *Br. J. Psychiat.*, **128**, 226.

MOSKOVITZ, R.A. & LINGAO, A. (1979) Binge eating associated with oral contraceptives. *Am. J. Psychiat.*, **136:5**, 721.

MURRAY, R.M., COOPER, J.E. & SMITH, A. (1979) The Leyton Obsessional Inventory: An analysis of the responses of 73 obsessional patients. *Psychol. Med.*, **9**, 305.

MURRAY, R.M. & REVELEY, A. (1981) The genetic contribution to the neuroses. *Br. J. Hosp. Med.*, **Feb.**, 185.

O'REGAN, J.B. (1970) Treatment of obsessive–compulsive neurosis with haloperidol. *Can. med. Ass. J.*, **103**, 167.

PHILPOTT, R. (1975) Recent advances in the behavioural measurement of obsessional illness. *Scot. med. J.*, **20**, 33.

RACHMAN, S. (1974) Primary obsessional slowness. *Behav. Res. Ther.*, **11**, 463.

RACHMAN, S. (1976) The modification of obsessions: a new formulation. *Behav. Res. Ther.*, **14**, 437.

RACHMAN, S., COBB, J., GREY, S., McDONALD, B., MAWSON, D., SARTORY, G. & STERN, R. (1979) The behavioural treatment of obsessional–compulsive disorders, with and without clomipramine. *Behav. Res. Ther.*, **17**, 467.

RACHMAN, S. & DE SILVA, P. (1978) Abnormal and normal obsessions. *Behav. Res. Ther.*, **16**, 233.

RACHMAN, S.J. & HODGSON, R.J. (1980) *Obsessions and Compulsions*. pp. 17a, 21b, 28c, 38–d, 46e, 54f, 65g, 70–74h, 90i, 101j, 102–105k, 110l, 117m, 137n, 162o, 166p, 186q, 192r, 254s, 317t, 362u, 351v, 391–393w. New Jersey: Prentice-Hall, Inc.

RACHMAN, S., MARKS, I. & HODGSON, R. (1973) The treatment of chronic obsessive–compulsive neurosis by modelling and flooding in vivo. *Behav. Res. Ther.*, **11**, 463.

RACK, P.H. (1977) Clinical experience in the treatment of obsessional states. *J. Int. Med. Res.*, **5 Suppl. (5)**, 81.

RACK, P.H. (1980) The chemotherapy of obsessive–compulsive disorders. *Pharm. Med.*, **1:2**, 22.

RINIERIS, P.M., STEFANIS, C.N., RABAVILAS, A.D. & VAIDAKIS, N.M. (1978) Obsessive–Compulsive neurosis, anancastic symptomatology and ABO blood types. *Acta. psychiat. neurol. scand.*, **57**, 377.

ROBERTSON, J.R. & MULHALL, D.J. (1979) The clinical evaluation of obsessionality: a development of the Leyton Obsessional Inventory. *Psychol. Med.*, **9**, 147.

SANDLER, J. & HAZARI, A. (1960) The obsessional: On the psychological classification of obsessional character traits and symptoms. *Br. J. Med. Psychol.*, **33**, 113.

SCHNEIDER, K. (1925) Schwangszustände und Schizophrenie. *Arch. Psychiat. NervKrankh.*, **74**, 93.

SCHWARTZ, J.E. (1977) Obsessional phenomena and the concept of intentionality. *Internat. J. Psychoanal. Psychother.*, **6**, 450.

SLADE, P.D. (1974) Psychometric studies of obsessional illness and obsessional personality. In: *Obsessional States*, ed. Beech, H.R. London: Methuen.

SNOWDON, J. (1979) Family-size and birth-order in obsessional neurosis. *Acta psychiat. neurol. scand.*, **60**, 121.

SNOWDON, J. (1980) A comparison of written and postbox forms of the Leyton Obsessional Inventory. *Psychol. Med.*, **10**, 165.

SNYDER, S. (1980a) Trichotillomania treated with amitriptyline. *J. nerv. ment. Dis.*, **168:8**, 505.

SNYDER, S. (1980b) Amitriptyline therapy of obsessive–compulsive neurosis. *J. Clin. Psychiat.*, **41**, 286.

SOLYOM, L., GARZA-PEREZ, J., LEDWIDGE, B. & SOLYOM, C. (1972) Paradoxical intention in the treatment of obsessive thoughts: a pilot study. *Compreh. Psychiat.*, **13**, 291.

STERN, R.S. (1978) Obsessive thoughts: the problem of therapy. *Br. J. Psychiat.*, **132**, 200.

STERN, R.S. & COBB, J. (1978) Phenomenology of obsessive–compulsive neurosis. *Br. J. Psychiat.*, **132**, 233.

STERN, R.S., MARKS, I.M., MAWSON, D. & LUSCOMBE, D.K. (1980a) Clomipramine and exposure for compulsive rituals. *Br. J. Psychiat.*, **136**, 161.

STERN, R.S., MARKS, I.M., WRIGHT, J. & LUSCOMBE, D.K. (1980b) Clomipramine: plasma levels, side effects and outcome in obsessive–compulsive neurosis. *Post-grad. med. J.*, **56 (Suppl. 1)**, 134.

STERNBERG, M. (1974) Physical treatments in obsessional disorders. In: *Obsessional States*, ed. Beech, H.R. London: Methuen.

TAYLOR, J.G. (1963) A behavioural interpretation of obsessive–compulsive neurosis. *Behav. Res. Ther.*, **1**, 237.

TEASDALE, J.D. (1974) Learning models of obsessional–compulsive disorder. In: *Obsessional States*, ed. Beech, H.R. London: Methuen.

THORÉN, P., ASBERG, M., CRONHOLM, B., JÖRNESTEDT, L. & TRASKMAN, L. (1980) Clomipramine treatment of obsessive–compulsive disorder. *Archs gen. Psychiat.*, **37**, 1281.

VÄISÄNEN, E., RANTA, P., NUMMIKKO-PELKONEN, A. & TIENARI, P. (1977) Mianserin hydrochloride in the treatment of obsessional states. *J. Int. Med. Res.*, **5**, 289.

VIDEBECH, T. (1975) The psychopathology of anancastic endogenous depression. *Acta psychiat. neurol. scand.*, **52**, 336.

WALKER, V.J. (1973) Explanation in obsessional neurosis. *Br. J. Psychiat.*, **123**, 675.

WALKER, V.J. & BEECH, H.R. (1969) Mood state and the ritualistic behaviour of obsessional patients. *Br. J. Psychiat.*, **115**, 1261.

WELNER, A., REICH, T., ROBINS, I., FISHMAN, R. & VAN DOREN, T. (1976) Obsessive–compulsive neurosis. *Compreh. Psychiat.*, **17**, 527.

WISOCKI, P.A. (1970) Treatment of obsessive–compulsive behaviour by covert sensitisation and covert reinforcement: a case report. *J. Behav. Ther. Exp. Psychiat.*, **1**, 233.

YARYURA-TOBIAS, J.A. & BHAGAVAN, H.N. (1977) L-Tryptophan in obsessive–compulsive disorders. *Am. J. Psychiat.*, **134:11**, 1298.

YARYURA-TOBIAS, J.A., NEZIROGLU, F.A. & FULLER, B. (1980) An integral approach in the management of the obsessive–compulsive patient. *Pharm. Med.*, **1:2**, 155.

18

Management of Hysterical, Hypochondriacal and Psychosomatic Disorders

C. de B. White and J.H. Dowson

HYSTERICAL DISORDERS

Definitions

Hysterical disorders encompass a variety of dissociative (mental) and/or conversion (physical) symptoms, a history of chronic multiple complaints (Briquet's syndrome), and hysterical (or histrionic) personality disorder (Lewis 1975; Reed 1975; and Merskey 1978). The American Psychiatric Association in their Diagnostic and Statistical Manual (DSM III) designate hysterical disorders with physical symptoms as 'somatoform disorders' (which also include Briquet's syndrome, psychogenic pain and some forms of hypochondriasis), while those with mental symptoms alone are known as 'dissociative disorders'.

Dissociative phenomena involve varying degrees of loss of the conscious awareness of aspects of mental function which were previously available to awareness, or have the potential to become so available. However, these mental events may still affect behaviour, as can be convincingly demonstrated by implanting a posthypnotic suggestion, in which the hypnotized individual may subsequently carry out an action without realizing that he has been so instructed. Impairment of conscious awareness is not an all-or-nothing phenomenon, and Crown (1978) has pointed out that day-dreaming, the semi-autonomous creative process shown by some authors, the promises of some alcoholics (when they declare they will never drink again), so-called pathological lying, and the Munchausen syndrome, are all associated with varying degrees of dissociation. The most common examples in clinical practice are fugue states, which may involve varying degrees of circumscribed amnesia, and trance states, in which subjects may relive a past experience, or act as if they are in a fantasized situation. 'Double' or 'multiple' personalities appear to be rare variants of hysterical fugue (Cutler and Reed 1975).

Conversion phenomena involve dissociation and are characterized by signs or symptoms of apparent bodily disorder, which result from psychological mechanisms, in the absence of an adequate somatic cause. It is presumed that a conversion symptom usually serves to provide relief from an unpleasant psychological state. Almost any bodily disorder can be mimicked, including fits, paralysis, aphonia, and areas of anaesthesia.

Chronic multiple complaint disorder (Briquet's syndrome) involves the repeated production of a variety of conversion phenomena over a period of years, and ranges from a persistent preoccupation with bodily feelings to a dramatic presentation of many (often bizarre) complaints. The 'gain' involved often appears to be the gratification from creating a drama, gaining concern and attention from others, or the reinforcement of fantasized 'sick roles'. The importance of social sanctions and illness roles in the genesis of hysterical phenomena has been stressed (Hamdi et al. 1981).

A varying number of the constellation of personality traits associated with the term 'hysterical (histrionic) personality disorder' are frequently seen in clinical practice, although the nosological status of this disorder is unclear (Slavney and McHugh 1975; Slavney and Rich 1980). These traits include an excessive dependence on others, a labile mood, an inability to contribute sufficiently to sustain a satisfactory close relationship, and a tendency to attract the attention of others. Individuals with such traits are liable to episodes of self-injury and, possibly, to dissociative and conversion symptoms.

The Management of Hysterical Disorders

Assessment. This involves determining the nature of the phenomena and then exploring possible causal factors, which may include somatic disease, as well as the interaction between the individual and aspects of his environment.

It is usually possible to distinguish dissociative states from cognitive impairment due to an identifiable somatic disorder, but it may be more difficult to separate a conversion phenomenon from its 'genuine' counterpart. However, if a physical symptom is clearly discrepant with known diseases, and/or appears to have been precipitated by marked stress, the presence of a conversion is indicated. Also, if the disorder is improved by suggestion or resolves when the apparent precipitants are relieved, the likelihood of a diagnosis of a hysterical disorder is further increased. Sometimes, the nature of an apparent somatic disorder seems to have a personal significance for the patient—this also suggests the presence of a conversion.

However, when all appropriate investigations have been carried out, the diagnosis may still be in doubt. In such a situation it is vital to keep the issue open by resisting the demands for a definitive opinion; such an approach protects the patient from being dismissed as 'not ill', and reminds the various doctors involved to be vigilant. A diagnostic delay will also provide an opportunity for detailed evaluation of the patient's previous personality, history and current life situation. Further information may help to clarify the diagnosis but, if in doubt, it is wise to assume that the symptoms may be due to, or associated with, somatic disease. At times, patients with undoubted somatic disease develop additional conversion symptoms, so that there is a mixture of 'organic' and hysterical phenomena which present particular diagnostic difficulty. In such cases there is a tendency for the patient to be referred backwards and forwards from general physician to psychiatrist, and it is most important that the various doctors involved devise an integrated management strategy. This may include telling the patient that although part of his problem is due to his disease, some of his symptoms are likely to improve with the help of a psychiatrist.

Even if the nature of the conversion symptom is clear, follow-up studies of patients with hysterical disorder have shown that the proportion who subsequently develop somatic pathology is considerably higher than expected, which indicates that various disease processes (especially cerebral disorder) may be heralded by hysterical conversion (Hafeiz 1980). Any hysterical phenomenon developing in middle age or beyond, in a person who has not been exposed to marked stress and has no psychiatric history, is very often the first sign of serious somatic disease (Slater 1961; Merskey and Buhrich 1975). It should also be remembered that conversion symptoms can occur in conjunction with somatic disease or other psychiatric disorders.

The separation of hysterical phenomena from malingering may be difficult, partly because some malingerers, as well as some individuals with the Munchausen syndrome (in which patients actively feign illness) may show a fluctuating impairment of conscious awareness. However, if an apparently paralysed patient is observed striding away from the clinic, malingering may be inferred. With some individuals, close observation in hospital may elucidate the problem.

Interventions. First, it must be decided if the patient should be admitted to a psychiatric hospital. This is often appropriate, and provides an opportunity for thorough assessment. If the presence of dissociation or conversion is confirmed, the discovery of the apparent precipitating factors may suggest ways in which causal psychological stress can be resolved. For example, a fugue state may have resulted from a domestic argument, when psychotherapeutic help may resolve the crisis. Thus, an attempt must be made to reduce the value of the primary gain associated with the avoidance of psychological discomfort. In addition, the value of any secondary gain (e.g. gratification of a tendency to become overdependent on others by being a patient, or avoidance of becoming involved in legal proceedings resulting from a precipitating incident), must also be kept to a minimum. An extension to this strategy is the provision of alternative gains (i.e. rewards) which can be made contingent on the reduction of symptoms. This could involve withholding approval for home leave from hospital and providing this when the desired behaviour occurs. Of course, the patient's cooperation is needed for this example, but the provision of special attention and praise from hospital staff can also be used as a reward. Various reports have suggested other behavioural approaches in conditions such as dissociative blindness, deafness and anaesthesia (Lehtinen and Puhakka 1976; Bird 1979).

Following, or in parallel with, the reduction of gain, the second basic strategy involves the use of persuasion and suggestion in a variety of settings. In many instances the patient is simply told informally, and as often as possible, that he has the kind of condition that gets better with time and that he has already shown a degree of improvement. This can be coupled with praise; e.g.,'You have obviously been trying to remember'. It is important to avoid giving the patient the impression that you think there is 'really' nothing wrong with him as, in this situation, improvement will (often unconsciously) be associated by the patient with a loss of dignity and self-respect; thus recovery will become less likely. In some cases, formal sessions can be organized when the patient is hypnotized or given an injection of sodium amytal. The latter is preferable to the former as the doctor may lose 'credibility' if an attempt at hypnosis fails. The placebo and pharmacological effects of the barbiturate-induced state makes some patients more susceptible to suggestion.

Psychoanalysis was founded on the demonstration that discussion of emotionally loaded topics could ameliorate conversion disorder, and the third strategy involves inducing abreaction (i.e. the experience and expression of emotions associated with the sources of symptom formation). Abreaction may be encouraged by simply talking to the patient about the relevant events, but drugs such as sodium amytal (sometimes combined with a stimulant such as methedrine), and hypnosis, may be employed to assist this process. Drug-induced abreaction is of particular value when hysterical disorder follows a clear-cut and severe stress, such as an accident or battlefield incident, but it should always be undertaken with care, as patients may show extreme emotional arousal involving violence or self-injury, which may persist for many hours after the treatment session. A tranquillizer may have to be given subsequently, especially if methedrine has been used. In general, abreaction should be avoided when hysterical phenomena occur in the setting of severe personality disorder, when clearly stressful life events are absent, and when underlying conflicts are likely to be insoluble.

A fourth strategy is to embark on an intensive (once- or twice-weekly) series of psychotherapeutic sessions with the aim of making the patient increasingly aware of unconscious conflicts, motives, or memories which have contributed to the development of the hysterical disorder. If these can be uncovered, perhaps by using such techniques as encouraging 'free association', the analysis of transference, and helping the patient to discard certain psychological defence mechanisms which are apparent in the treatment sessions, the patient may be helped to develop new ways of resolving psychological conflicts or other problems, thereby reducing the primary gain. However, long-standing dissociation and conversion is often not helped by this approach, which may make the situation worse by fostering overdependence on the therapist. Thus, intensive psychotherapy should only be considered in carefully selected patients.

Patients with hysterical neurosis should not generally spend more than a few weeks as an in-patient; if, after this period, the condition has not recovered completely, it is often appropriate to continue management on an out-patient basis. Further improvement may occur gradually over months or years.

The Management of Chronic Multiple Complaints Disorder (Briquet's Syndrome)

Patients with this disorder, who may often be identified by the thickness of their medical notes, can provoke strong negative feelings in their doctors. This may lead to three main kinds of inappropriate management: insufficient attention is paid to those symptoms which do result from underlying somatic disease, excessive investigations are carried out, or the doctor displays irritation and anger which may exacerbate the problems of management.

Many of these patients have marked hysterical (histrionic) personality traits. They make considerable demands on their doctor's time and patience, and often display the well-known combination of hostility and excessive dependency. The doctor must monitor his own feelings and should try to ensure that these do not significantly influence the patient's management. The doctor must be firm in setting limits; for example, he must not give way to demands for increasingly frequent or lengthy consultations, or escalating doses of sleeping pills. This may involve receiving complaints and abuse which have to be accepted calmly; the emotional lability of many individuals with hysterical (histrionic) personality disorders often produces a polite, cooperative patient at the following interview. Such patients should not, if possible, be frequently transferred from doctor to doctor, as stable support provides the most useful form of intervention. Long-term containment of the problem is one of the main goals of management, as is the prevention of harm by resisting unnecessary investigations or treatment. New symptoms must be properly evaluated, but without unnecessary reinforcement of the illness role. Regular, firm reassurance is useful, but the patient must not be told that the symptoms are 'only in the mind'. It is often appropriate to say that many people get various aches and pains for which no cause can be found, and that while doctors are not able to cure such symptoms, they are not a serious threat to life or health. Often patients are temporarily satisfied by a demonstration of concern which allows them to feel that their demands are at least recognized. The doctor may, in time, effect a somewhat ritualized compromise between the patient's demands and his own need to use his time cost-effectively. Despite Balint's (1964) suggestion that a more intensive psychotherapeutic approach may help such patients, maladaptive dependency is often the result of such attempts. For certain individuals, behavioural management in hospital may have some value (Dickes 1974).

The Management of Hysterical (Histrionic) Personality Disorder

The principles of not giving way to inappropriate demands, and keeping calm in the face of anger and hostility, have been outlined above. However, a minority of individuals with the most severe forms of personality disorder do not respond to these methods and may repeatedly come to medical attention with self-injury, violence and other antisocial acts. If violence is directed to others, the police, courts, and prisons are often involved, but when episodes of extreme emotional arousal and/or self-injury occur, admission to hospital (sometimes on a compulsory basis) may be necessary. However, compulsory admission must be a last resort, and if such individuals are admitted to hospital, they should normally be discharged within 2 weeks. The structured environment of the hospital, together with psychotherapeutic and social help, may produce a rapid resolution of a crisis and help the patient towards a more stable adjustment. However, such patients must not be encouraged to believe that the hospital will continually absolve them of all responsibility for repeated acts of antisocial behaviour, which often occur in a setting of domestic argument and alcohol abuse, even if this involves self-injury. Ideally, a special setting with experienced staff and a highly structured environment is required for the management of such crises, but this type of facility is rarely available in a psychiatric service.

HYPOCHONDRIACAL DISORDERS

Definitions

Hypochondriasis involves anxious concern about health which is persistently exaggerated and resistant to reassurance (Kenyon 1976). In its most extreme forms this may reach delusional proportions, either as a monosymptomatic 'hypochondriacal psychosis' (Munro 1980) or as a more diffuse conviction of illness. Certain hypochondriacal complaints are not easily classified as part of (i.e. secondary to) another psychiatric disorder, and Pilowsky (1970) concluded that, for this group, hypochondriasis may be usefully regarded as a separate syndrome. However, in other cases, the symptoms are clearly secondary to a depressive syndrome, a schizophrenic illness, an anxiety or phobic state, obsessive–compulsive neurosis, or a personality disorder with obsessional or paranoid traits. Chronic polysymptomatic hypochondriasis overlaps with Briquet's syndrome.

Management

When hypochondriasis is secondary, treatment of the underlying disorder is indicated, although when it develops in the setting of personality disorder, significant change is difficult to achieve.

Some cases of monosymptomatic delusional hypochondriasis have been reported to respond to neuroleptic medication, and pimozide has been advocated. Also, there are anecdotal accounts of improvement following monoamine oxidase inhibitors. However, although relatively pure hypochondriacal syndromes vary in severity, at their most persistent they often fail to respond to all forms of reassurance and intervention, and can end in suicide (Kenyon 1976; Bebbington 1976). Despite this, the adjustment of such patients can usually be stabilized by regular supportive interviews and reassurance, without which deterioration would probably occur. In this situation, perseverance by the psychiatrist is needed in the face of a seemingly intractable problem.

PSYCHOSOMATIC DISORDERS

Definitions

A psychosomatic condition can be defined as a disorder in which conscious (or potentially conscious) mental events are judged to have played a significant role in the aetiology, exacerbation or maintenance of changes in somatic structure or function which are judged to be undesirable. This does not incorporate hysterical conversion, in which somatic function is unimpaired. If the consequences of the mental events are mediated by somatic mechanisms, such as autonomic changes, the condition can be termed a 'direct' psychosomatic disorder while an 'indirect' disorder results from the effects of overt behaviour. Examples of indirect psychosomatic disorders include anorexia nervosa, alcoholism, the effects of smoking, and dermatitis artefacta.

In addition, the term 'psychosomatic medicine' is often used to include the evaluation and management of the psychological concomitants of disease; the psychiatrist's work in this sphere, in the setting of the general hospital, is often called 'liaison psychiatry' (Hackett and Cassem 1978; Connolly 1979; Lloyd 1980; Gomez 1981).

Management

The nature and clinical significance of direct psychosomatic mechanisms is uncertain (Lipowski 1977; Hill 1976; Lloyd 1980). There are many reports which apparently support the claim that significant life events (particularly those which are perceived as stressful) are correlated with the subsequent development of a wide range of diseases, including neoplasia (Rahe 1975;

Holmes and Masuda 1974; Greer and Morris 1975; Hurst et al. 1976; Murphy and Brown 1980). However, it can be difficult to rule out the role of an indirect mechanism (such as smoking) in such studies, and even if a causal association were to be established, the relevance of such findings to clinical practice is uncertain.

Other studies of various forms of neoplastic disease have reported an association between outcome and psychological variables, such as attitude and emotional state (Abse et al. 1974; Crisp 1970; Greer et al. 1979; Rogentine et al. 1979). If such associations prove to be causal, non-specific psychotherapeutic help for some cancer patients might be indicated. However, the potential value of such a general policy is highly speculative.

The likelihood of the clinical importance of direct psychosomatic factors is more generally accepted with regard to coronary artery disease (Connolly 1974), the aftermath of myocardial infarction (Naismith et al. 1979), peptic ulceration, cerebrovascular accident in hypertensive individuals, ulcerative colitis (and certain other bowel disorders), asthma (Cohen 1971), certain skin disorders including eczema and psoriasis (Russel 1967; Surman et al. 1973; Whitlock 1976; Seville 1977), and some forms of epilepsy, in which specific psychological events, boredom, and stress may affect the seizure frequency. However, the importance of a direct psychosomatic mechanism in relation to other causal factors (both essential and non-essential), no doubt varies considerably between the above diseases, and between individuals. In clinical practice, the psychiatrist may be able to contribute to the management of patients with these diseases by various non-intensive psychotherapeutic or pharmacological interventions (Kellner 1975). The uses and limitations of biofeedback, other behavioural techniques, various forms of relaxation therapy, hypnosis and treatment with psychoactive drugs have all been described (Frankel 1975; Waxman 1975; Jacob et al. 1977; Agras et al. 1980; Maher-Loughnan 1980).

Other disorders in which psychosomatic mechanisms have been postulated include hypertension (Heine 1971), Raynaud's disease, vomiting (Hill 1977), constipation, diabetes (Bradley 1979; Wilkinson 1981), diarrhoea, irritable bowel, abdominal pain, regional ileitis (Sheffield and Carney 1976), hyperventilation, dyspnoea (Heim et al. 1972), menstrual disorders (Clare 1979), sexual dysfunctions, infertility (Kipper et al. 1977), migraine, other forms of headache (Martin and Mathews 1978; Nuechterlein and Holroyd 1980), rheumatoid arthritis (Silverman 1975; Gardiner 1980), autoerythrocyte sensitization (Asle et al. 1969), and hyperemesis gravidarum (Wolkind and Zajicek 1978).

Pain may be produced, aggravated, or maintained by psychological mechanisms and by the presence of depression, anxiety or conversion hysteria (Lascelles 1966; Bond 1980). The psychiatrist may help to alleviate pain which is partly or wholly due to psychiatric disorder and may also help to modify secondary psychological effects of chronic pain. Clomipramine and/or chlopromazine are often used in conjunction with analgesics for certain forms of chronic pain and for the terminally ill (Stengel 1965; Merskey 1973; Gomez and Dally 1977; Pilowsky 1976; Lipowski 1977).

Aspects of the management of indirect psychosomatic mechanisms such as those associated with smoking, self-injury, alcoholism and eating disorders (Stunkard 1975; Mitchell 1980) are dealt with in other chapters.

The psychiatrist's work in the general hospital (liaison psychiatry) rarely involves intensive management of direct or indirect psychosomatic mechanisms, and is often concerned with the assessment and management of psychological and social problems, many of which are related to the effects of the patient's disease. The physician or surgeon may find it difficult to evaluate such problems adequately, partly due to lack of time, and partly because some inexperienced hospital doctors require further training in the development of interviewing techniques. The liaison psychiatrist may usefully spend some time providing a regular teaching seminar for junior hospital doctors, in which interviewing technique is demonstrated by the psychiatrist, after a trainee has conducted a preliminary interview. The subsequent discussions provide feedback regarding interviewing skills and also focus on the management in relation to psychological and social factors. Also, there has been an increasing awareness of the psychological problems of hospital staff, particularly in such settings as intensive care or renal dialysis units. The liaison psychiatrist may be able to provide support and advice; this is best done informally, but regular staff meetings, which discuss ward administration, cooperation and morale, may be valuable.

References

ABSE, D.W., WILKINS, M.M., VAN DE CASTLE, R.L. et al. (1974) Personality and behavioural characteristics of lung cancer patients. *J. psychosom. Res.*, **18**, 101.

ASLE, D.P., RATNOFF, O.D. & WASNMAN, M. (1969) Conversion reactions in autoerythrocyte sensitization: their relationship to the production of ecchymoses. *Arch. Gen. Psychiatry*, **20**, 438.

AGRAS, W.S., TAYLOR, C.B., KRAMER, H.C., ALLEN, R.A. & SCHNEIDER, J.A. (1980) Relaxation training. Twenty-four-hour blood pressure reductions. *Arch. Gen. Psychiatry*, **37**, 859.

BALINT, M. (1964) *The Doctor, His Patient and the Illness.* London: Pitman Medical.

BEBBINGTON, P.E. (1976) Monosymptomatic hypochondriasis, abnormal illness behaviour and suicide. *Br. J. Psychiat.*, **128**, 475.

BIRD, J. (1979) The behavioural treatment of hysteria. *Br. J. Psychiat.*, **134**, 129.

BOND, M.R. (1980) New approaches to pain. *Psychol. Med.*, **10**, 195.

BRADLEY, C. (1979) Life events and the control of diabetes mellitus. *J. psychosom. Res.*, **23**, 159.

CLARE, A.W. (1979) The treatment of pre-menstrual symptoms. *Br. J. Psychiat.*, **135**, 576.

COHEN, S.I. (1971) Psychological factors in asthma: a review of their aetiological and therapeutic significance. *Postgrad. med. J.*, **47**, 533.

CONNOLLY, J. (1974) Stress and coronary artery disease. *Br. J. Hosp. Med.*, **11**, 297.

CONNOLLY, J. (1979) Psychiatry in a general hospital. In: *Essentials of Postgraduate Psychiatry*, ed. Hill, P., Murray, R. & Thorley, A., pp. 599–625. London: Academic Press.

CRISP, A.H. (1970) Some psychosomatic aspects of neoplasia. *Br. J. med. Psychol.*, **43**, 313.

CROWN, S. (1978) Disorders of conscious awareness. *Br. J. Hosp. Med.*, **April**, 303.

CUTLER, B. & REED, J. (1975) Multiple personality. *Psychol. Med.*, **5**, 18.

DICKES, R.A. (1974) Brief therapy of conversion reactions: An in-hospital technique. *Am. J. Psychiat.*, **131**, 584.

FRANKEL, F.H. (1975) Hypnosis as a treatment method in psychosomatic medicine. *Int. J. Psychiatry, Med.*, **6**, 75.

GARDINER, B.M. (1980) Psychological aspects of rheumatoid arthritis. *Psychol. Med.*, **10**, 159–163.

GOMEZ, T.J. (1981) Liaison Psychiatry. *Br. J. Hosp. Med.*, **Sept.**, 242.

GOMEZ, T.J. & DALLY, P. (1977) Psychologically mediated abdominal pain in surgical and medical outpatient clinics. *Br. med. J.*, **1**, 1451

GREER, S. & MORRIS, T. (1975) Psychological attributes of women who develop breast cancer: a controlled study. *J. psychosom. Res.*, **19**, 147.

GREER, S., MORRIS, T. & PETTINSALE, K.W. (1979) Psychological response to breast cancer: effect on outcome. *Lancet*, **11**, 785.

HACKETT, T.P. & CASSEM, N.H. (1978) *Handbook of General Hospital Psychiatry*. St. Louis: The C.V. Mosby Company.

HAFEIZ, H.B. (1980) Hysterical conversion: a prognostic study. *Br. J. Psychiat.*, **136**, 548.

HAMDI, T.I., AL-HASANI, L., MAHMOOD, A. & AL-HUSANI, A. (1981) Hysteria: a large series in Iraq. *Br. J. Psychiat.*, **138**, 177.

HEIM, E., BLASER, A. & WAIDELICH, E. (1972) Dyspnea: psychophysiologic relationships. *Psychosom. Med.*, **24**, 405.

HEINE, B. (1971) Psychosomatic aspects of hypertension. *Postgrad. med. J.*, **47**, 451.

HILL, O.W. (1976) *Modern Trends in Psychosomatic Medicine*. London: Butterworths.

HILL, O.W. (1977) Functional vomiting. *Br. med. J.*, **1**, 1491.

HOLMES, T.H. & MASUDA, M. (1974) Life change and illness susceptibilities. In: *Stressful Life Events: Their Nature and Effects*, ed. Dohrenwend, B.S. & Dohrenwend, B.P., pp. 45–72. New York: John Wiley & Sons.

HURST, M.W., JENKINS, C.D. & ROSE, R.M. (1976) The relation of psychological stress to onset of medical illness. *A. Rev. Med.*, **27**, 301.

JACOB, R.G., KRAEMER, H.C. & AGRAS, W.S. (1977) Relaxation therapy in the treatment of hypertension. *Arch. Gen. Psychiatry*, **34**, 1417.

KELLNER, R. (1975) Psychotherapy in psychosomatic disorders. *Arch. Gen. Psychiatry*, **32**, 1021.

KENYON, F.E. (1976) Hypochondriacal states. *Br. J. Psychiat.*, **129**, 1.

KIPPER, D.A., ZIGLER-SHAMI, Z., SEVR, D.M. & INSLER, V. (1977) Psychogenic infertility, neuroticism and the feminine role: a methodological enquiry. *J. psychosom. Res.*, **353**.

LASCELLES, R.G. (1966) Atypical facial pain and depression. *Br. J. Psychiat.*, **112**, 651.

LEHTINEN, V. & PUHAKKA, H. (1976) A psychosomatic approach to the globus hystericus syndrome. *Acta psychiat. neurol. scand.*, **53**, 21.

LEWIS, A. (1975) The survival of hysteria. *Psychol. Med.*, **5**, 9.

LIPOWSKI, Z.J. (1977) Psychosomatic medicine in the seventies: an overview. *Am. J. Psychiat.*, **134**, 233.

LLOYD, G. (1980) Whence and whither 'liason' psychiatry? *Psychol. Med.*, **10**, 11.

MAHER-LOUGHNAN, G.P.(1980) Clinical applications of hypnosis in medicine. *Br. J. Hosp. Med.*, **23**, 447.

MARTIN, P.R. & MATHEWS, A.M. (1978) Tension headaches: Psychophysiological investigation and treatment. *J. psychosom. Res.*, **22**, 389

MERSKEY, H. (1973) The management of patients in pain. *Br. J. Hosp. Med.*, **9**, 574.

MERSKEY, H. (1978) Hysterical phenomena. *Br. J. Hosp. Med.*, **19**, 305.

MERSKEY, H. & BUHRICH, N.A. (1975) Hysteria and organic brain disease. *Br. J. med. Psychol.*, **48**, 359.

MITCHELL, E.M. (1980) Obesity, psychological aspects and management. *Br. J. Hosp. Med.*, **24**, 523.

MUNRO, A. (1980) Monosymptomatic hypochondriacal psychosis. *Br. J. Hosp. Med.*, **24**, 34.

MURPHY, E. & BROWN, G.W. (1980) Life events, psychiatric disturbance and physical illness. *Br. J. Psychiat.*, **136**, 326.

NAISMITH, L.D., ROBINSON, J.F., SHAW, G.B. & McINTYRE, M.M.J. (1979) Psychological rehabilitation after myocardial infarction. *Br. med. J.*, **1**, 439.

NUECHTERLEIN, K.H. & HOLROYD, J.C. (1980) Bio-feedback in the treatment of tension headache. Current status. *Arch. Gen. Psychiatry*, **37**, 866.

PILOWSKY, I. (1970) Primary and secondary hypochondriasis. *Acta. psychiat. neurol. scand.*, **46**, 273.

PILOWSKY, I. (1976) The psychiatrist and the pain clinic. *Am. J. Psychiat.*, **133**, 752.

RAHE, R.H. (1975) Epidemiological studies of life change and illness. *Int. J. Psychiatry Med.*, **6**, 133.

REED, J.L. (1975) The diagnosis of 'hysteria'. *Psychol. Med.*, **5**, 13–17.

ROGENTINE, G.N., VAN KAMMEN, D.P., FOX, B.H., DOCHERTY, J.P., ROSENBLATT, J.E., BOYD, S.C. & BUNNEY, W.E. (1979) Psychological factors in the prognosis of malignant melanoma: a prospective study. *Psychosom. Med.*, **41**, 647.

RUSSEL, B.G. (1967) Emotional factors in skin disease. *Br. J. Hosp. Med.*, **Sept.**, 1117.

SEVILLE, R.H. (1977) Psoriasis and stress. *Br. J. Dermatol.*, **97**, 297.

SHEFFIELD, B.F. & CARNEY, M.W.P. (1976) Crohn's disease: A psychosomatic illness? *Br. J. Psychiat.*, **128**, 446.

SILVERMAN, A.J. (1975) Rheumatoid arthritis. In: *Comprehensive Textbook of Psychiatry*—II, ed. Freedman, A.H., Kaplan, H.I., Sadock, B.J., pp. 1694–1704. Baltimore: The Williams and Wilkins Company.

SLATER, E. (1961) Hysteria 311. *J. ment. Sci.*, **107**, 359.

SLAVNEY, P.R. & McHUGH, P.R. (1975) The hysterical personality. An attempt at validation with the MMPI. *Arch. Gen. Psychiat.*, **32**, 186.

SLAVNEY, P.R. & RICH, G. (1980) Variability of mood under diagnosis of hysterical personality disorder. *Br. J. Psychiat.*, **136**, 402.

STENGEL, E. (1965) Pain and the psychiatrist. *Br. J. Psychiat.*, **111**, 795.

STUNKARD, A.J. (1975) From explanation to action in psychosomatic medicine: the case of obesity. *Psychosom. Med.*, **37**, 195.

SURMAN, O.S., GOTTLIEB, S.K., HACKETT, T.P. & SILVERBERG, E.L. (1973) Hypnosis in the treatment of warts. *Arch. Gen. Psychiat.*, **28**, 439.

WAXMAN, D. (1975) Hypnosis in the psychotherapy of neurotic illness. *Br. J. med. Psychol.*, **48**, 339.

WHITLOCK, F.A. (1976) *Psychophysiological Aspects of Skin Disease.* London: Saunders.

WILKINSON, D.G. (1981) Psychiatric aspects of diabetes mellitus. *Br. J. Psychiat.*, **138**, 1.

WOLKIND, S. & ZAJICEK, E. (1978) Psycho-social correlates of nausea and vomiting in pregnancy. *J. psychosom. Res.*, **22**.

19

Offender Patients

D.J. West

THE OVERLAP BETWEEN CRIMINALITY AND PSYCHIATRIC DISORDER

Whether it is a symptom of their illness, or whether the link arises less directly, patients with psychiatric disorders have a greater than average liability to arrest for criminal offences. Conversely, persons convicted of crime have a raised incidence of psychiatric morbidity. It has even been suggested (Penrose 1943) that institutional populations of prisoners and mental hospital patients are to some extent interchangeable, so that communities with large prison populations have small hospital populations and vice versa.

We are all occasional law-breakers. A surprisingly high proportion of males, especially working-class males, have been convicted of an offence of sufficient seriousness to lead to the opening of a file at Scotland Yard. A recently published calculation (Farrington 1981) based upon the incidence of first convictions in different age groups in England and Wales in 1977, suggests that, on those figures, the chance of a man acquiring a criminal record by the 25th birthday has become more than one in four. From such a large section of the population only a relatively small percentage can be seriously disordered.

Almost any troublesome youngster might attract the catch-all label of behaviour disorder, but in practice even this highly flexible diagnosis is applied to no more than a minority of the vast number of juveniles and adolescents who pass through the courts. A very small percentage have any ascertainable neuropsychiatric condition other than behaviour disorder. The position is different, however, among the minority of persistent and serious offenders who make up the population of the prisons. According to an English survey carried out by Professor John Gunn's research team 'a third of the sentenced prison population in the south eastern region could be regarded as psychiatric cases' (Gunn et al. 1978). About 20% had had psychiatric treatment prior to sentence, most of them as hospital in-patients. Although 'personality disorder' and 'alcoholism' were the commonest conditions, a primary diagnosis of neurosis,

372

affective psychosis or schizophrenia was applied to about 11% of the prisoners. An even higher morbidity rate was reported in a survey in St Louis, Missouri (Guze 1976). Among 232 men imprisoned for felonies, 90% were found to have some psychiatric condition. About 3% were suffering from schizophrenia, grand mal epilepsy or organic brain syndromes, and 12% from anxiety neurosis, but as many as 85% were considered to have one or more of the three commonest disorders, namely sociopathy, alcoholism or drug dependence.

Even more than in other kinds of epidemiological work, surveys of criminal populations are handicapped by variations in standards of assessment, but a few broad generalizations can be made with confidence. First, among the kinds of adult criminals who find their way into prison, a small but significantly raised percentage are diagnosable as psychotic, borderline mentally subnormal, or suffering from organic brain syndrome, and this notwithstanding the existence of a legal system and medical facilities intended to divert such cases into hospital. Second, a surprisingly high proportion of prisoners, and recidivist prisoners especially, are former mental hospital patients. Third, at the most conservative estimates, the incidence of antisocial personality disorder is extraordinarily high among prisoners.

American psychiatrists have taken a particular interest in the criminality of mental hospital inmates, especially since the implementation of more liberal release policies has led to some questioning of the degree of risk to which the community may be exposed from the behaviour of the mentally ill. The arrest rates of a sample of 867 patients passing through the acute wards of Bellevue Hospital, New York City, were compared with that of the population of the catchment area of the hospital (Zitrin et al. 1976). The arrest rates of the patients was higher than that of the general population, both for the period of 2 years preceding their hospital admission, and for the 2-year period of follow-up after release. The difference was particularly evident in regard to some of the more serious crimes of personal violence, such as aggravated assault and rape. An earlier study of mental hospital patients in Maryland had reached similar conclusions, namely that 'for some serious offenses the psychiatric population has a higher arrest rate than the general population' (Rappeport and Lassen 1965). Much larger differences were later found between the preadmission arrest rates of patients in a Californian mental hospital and that of the surrounding population (Sosowsky 1978). It was thought that at least some of the apparent increase in the criminality of mental patients may have been due to a change in policy in California resulting in larger numbers of psychiatrically disordered individuals being allowed to remain free in the community.

The association between liability to ascertainment as a psychiatric case and liability to conviction for crime does not in itself establish a direct causal connection. Both forms of disturbance might arise from similar stresses. Moreover, a certain amount of overlap could arise from overlapping definitions. In different contexts the same behaviour, physical assault for example, may lead to conviction for an offence, to a diagnosis of psychiatric illness, or sometimes to both at once.

REFERRAL FROM THE CRIMINAL JUSTICE SYSTEM

Persons with a criminal background enjoy no special immunity from psychiatric illness, so any population of patients will include a proportion of such individuals. The prevalence of criminality is particularly high among patients admitted to hospital as a result of certain medicosocial emergencies, notably alcoholism, drug-induced illness, attempted suicide or an explosive family crisis. The numerous legal complications with which some of these patients are involved may not always be evident at their first appearance.

Patients referred through the criminal justice system comprise a special category. Their offender status is, as it were, officially recognized, their offending behaviour has been suspected of being a symptom of illness or at any rate associated with a psychiatric condition, and their treatment is a matter of concern to authorities outside the medical services. The legal statutes for treatment or examination are specific in England and Wales.

Mental Health Act, 1959, Section 136. A constable who finds 'in a place to which the public have access a person who appears to him to be suffering from a mental disorder and to be in immediate need of care or control' is empowered to remove that person to a 'place of safety', which normally means to a hospital or police station. The individual may then be compulsorily detained for up to 72 h, after which he must be let go, become a voluntary patient, or be further held 'for observation' or 'for treatment' by the customary procedures for compulsory commitment (sections 25 or 26 of the Mental Health Act).

Some police forces make very little use of this power, preferring, instead, to deal with persons causing a public nuisance by calling in the duty social worker (either before or after the offender has been taken to the police station). Even simpler, the police can, and often do, opt out of the problem by merely issuing a caution, provided they know that there are relatives or others available to look after the situation. Police are fairly experienced in dealing with such matters, so often being the first on the scene when an excited or deluded individual begins to cause trouble.

Magistrates' Courts Act, 1980, Section 30. If the magistrates' court is satisfied that the evidence shows that a person accused of an imprisonable offence 'did the act or made the omission charged but is of the opinion that an inquiry ought to be made into his physical or mental condition before the method of dealing with him is determined' it may adjourn the case and remand the offender, either in custody or on bail, to enable an appropriate examination and report to be made. Examinations in custody are normally carried out by prison medical officers, but for offenders on bail the court clerk or a probation officer arranges an appointment with a psychiatrist, usually on an out-patient basis, and asks for an official report, for which a fee is payable. The courts are allowed to remand on bail for 4 weeks at a time, or in custody for 3 weeks, so the time available for psychiatric enquiries and the submission of a considered opinion is limited. If there is a substantial waiting list for appointments, the prospective offender–patient may have to be allowed to 'jump the queue' on the grounds that a pending criminal conviction is a circumstance of urgency.

Under Section 10 (3) of the same act, the magistrates have a more general power 'for the purpose of enabling inquiries to be made or of determining the most suitable method of dealing with the case', after convicting the accused, to adjourn for a period of 4 weeks at a time (or 3 weeks if the accused is remanded in custody). Inquiries can include requests for psychiatric reports. It is also possible for an offender's own solicitor, either during a remand period, or while awaiting appearance on a summons, to make a private request for a psychiatric examination and opinion, which he may then use at the trial hearing, either as an argument for a medical rather than a penal disposal, or as evidence for psychological factors that reduce the offender's culpability and should mitigate the punishment. The courts can impose lesser penalties, or order conditional or absolute discharge, because of the offender's mental state.

The psychiatric report should not advance explanations for offences not yet proved. This can constitute a considerable impediment to frank reporting on offenders who have not yet been found guilty or pleaded guilty. Privately requested reports do not always have the effect the psychiatrist might wish, for they can be used, or discarded, or quoted in part only, at the discretion of the defending solicitor. Reports requested by the court are seen intact and become a matter of semi-public record. They may be used again, for example, if the offender is imprisoned and subsequently considered for parole, or if he re-appears at a later date on another charge.

Powers of the Criminal Courts Acts, 1973, Section 3. If a court has obtained satisfactory evidence from a duly qualified medical practitioner who is approved by a local authority as having special experience in the diagnosis or treatment of mental disorder (for the purposes of section 28 of the Mental Health Act, 1959) 'that the mental condition of an offender is such as requires and may be susceptible to treatment', then submission to such treatment may be made a requirement of a probation order. The order has to state whether the treatment shall be as a resident patient in a named hospital, or as a non-resident patient under a specified institution or medical practitioner, or as directed by a named practitioner (without specifying whether it need be residential). The duration of the treatment is set either for part or for the whole of the period during which the probation order remains in force (i.e. up to 3 years).

Usually it is the psychiatrist who has been asked to examine and report on the offender and has recommended treatment who offers to carry it out or to arrange for it. The court cannot make the requirement 'unless it is satisfied that arrangements have been made for the treatment intended'. In practice, offenders who have been examined by the prison medical service are less often recommended for an order under this section, perhaps because prison doctors are less likely to be able to arrange for treatment in the community, or perhaps because the kind of offenders who have not been allowed bail are less suitable for this disposal.

At least in principle, this is a voluntary contractual system. The offender has to agree to the probation order and its requirements before the court can put it into force. Once having accepted, he is liable to be brought back to court and charged with breach of probation if he fails to comply with the terms to which he has agreed.

Acceptance of a patient under a psychiatric probation order does not oblige the psychiatrist to continue treatment if that is seen as inappropriate. If, in due course, it appears that the offender is after all not susceptible to treatment, or that no further treatment is required, or that different treatment is needed, or that the psychiatrist is for any reason unable or unwilling to continue, he can notify the probation officer accordingly, who can in turn refer the matter to the court for cancellation or alteration of the treatment requirement. If the psychiatrist who has arranged the treatment wants to transfer the patient elsewhere he can do so by giving notice in writing to the supervisory probation officer.

If the offender fails to cooperate, for instance by walking out of hospital, or by not turning up for out-patient appointments, the psychiatrist is expected to notify the probation officer who can bring the matter before the court in order to have the offender tried for a breach of probation. This can result in a fine, a community service order, or a sentence appropriate to the offence for which the probation order was originally made (Home Office 1978). Refusal to undergo surgical, electrical or other treatment under circumstances considered reasonable by the court does not amount to a breach of probation.

In practice, owing to the reluctance of doctors to give evidence against their own patients, and owing to lack of liaison between doctors and the probation service, prosecutions for breach of a treatment requirement are rare, although failure by patients to comply with their orders is by no means uncommon.

Mental Health Act (1959) Section 60, Hospital Orders. If, after remanding for psychiatric examinations, a crown court, or a magistrates' court dealing with an offence that is imprisonable, receives evidence from two separate reports to the effect that the offender is suffering from 'mental illness, psychopathic disorder, subnormality or severe subnormality' which is 'of a nature or degree which warrants the detention of the patient in hospital for medical treatment' then the court may make a hospital order for compulsory admission for treatment. This is in lieu of any penal sentence that might otherwise have been imposed and, unlike the psychiatric probation order, it effectively brings to an end the court's concern with the case, transferring all responsibility to the medical authorities.

The medical evidence may be presented orally or by written report, but at least one of the doctors must be approved by a local authority as having special experience in mental disorder. They must agree on the category of illness or disorder from which the offender suffers. A copy of each report must be given to the accused's counsel or solicitor or, if he is not represented, the substance of it must be communicated to him. The accused has the right to insist on the doctor's presence in court and also to call evidence in rebuttal of statements in the report.

Since the Mental Health Act was formulated, sensitivity to civil liberties has increased and patients are recommended for compulsory commitment only if there are very clearly justifiable grounds. Hospital orders can be made legally on grounds of psychopathy, regardless of the age of the offender, but in practice this hardly ever happens. It has become customary to recommend hospital orders for the mentally ill only if the patient is floridly psychotic at the time he is examined, obviously requiring residential care, and not ready to accept voluntarily the necessity for admission to hospital. The number of hospital orders made annually has diminished to about 800.

The court cannot make a valid order until 'satisfied that arrangements have been made for the admission of the offender' to a named hospital. The difficulty of finding hospitals willing to accept such cases has increased in recent years. Normally, it is a consultant who offers to have the patient in one of his own beds who provides one of the two reports. Unless a prison medical officer can persuade a Health Service consultant to examine a prisoner and provide for his admission, there is little point in making a hospital order recommendation. This is one reason why numbers have declined and the prison medical service complains of the increasing frequency with which mentally ill offenders who need hospitalization are being received into prisons under sentence.

Like patients committed without reference to the courts, those admitted under a hospital order have the right to appeal to a Mental Health Review Tribunal, which has the power to order them to be released if it appears that continued compulsory detention is not justified on medical grounds. An ordinary commitment to hospital can originate from a petition by the nearest relative, who has the right to ask for the patient's discharge at any time, but this provision does not apply to hospital order cases. However, if a patient under a hospital order absconds from hospital and remains at large for 28 days (or 6 months in the case of a subnormal or psychopathic patient) he becomes free 'by process of law' and cannot thereafter be compulsorily brought back. This provision, which seems to give semi-official support to a flouting of the intentions of the courts, has been criticized by the Home Office (Butler) 'Report on mentally abnormal offenders' (Home Office 1975). In the opinion of that committee, the assumption that a patient capable of remaining at large is not sufficiently incompetent to justify detention 'may have been to some extent justifiable when asylums took considerable precautions against escape, and energetic steps to recapture escapers, but it is much less justifiable in the era of the open door, when hospitals take no trouble to recapture most absconders'.

The responsible medical officer of the hospital can discharge the hospital order at any time. After 1 year authority to detain lapses, unless renewed by the same procedure as for patients committed by civil process under a treatment order. Unlike the probation order, the hospital order does not allow for compulsory after-care. A hospital order patient can be given 'trial leave', but once formally discharged from hospital he is free of any legal obligation to report back.

Restricted patients. Mental Health Act, 1959, Section 65. Where an offender's mental state at the time of examination justifies compulsory hospitalization, but his antecedents and the risk of his committing further offences if set at large make it necessary to protect the public, the crown courts have the power, under section 65 of the Mental Health Act, to add to the hospital order a further order prohibiting the discharge of the patient, prohibiting leave of absence, and prohibiting transfer to another hospital, without the formal consent of the Home Secretary. These restriction orders may be made to apply for a specified period or, more usually, as the ominous legal phrase expresses it, 'without limit of time', so that the patient might never be released. Appeals to a Mental Health Review Tribunal are allowable at specified intervals, but in such cases tribunals can only advise and the Home Secretary is not obliged to act on a recommendation for release. The Home Secretary is empowered, under section 66 (3), to order release of a restricted patient subject to specified conditions, such as regular reporting to a probation officer. So long as the order is not expired or discharged, the patient can be recalled to hospital at any time.

Restriction orders can be made only by the crown courts, but if the necessity arises the magistrates can commit a mentally abnormal offender to the crown court, who may then impose a restriction order or pronounce such other sentence as they see fit. If a restriction order is under consideration, at least one of the two doctors providing the medical recommendations must be present in court to give evidence orally.

The restriction order system gives formal recognition to the reality that a decision to release a criminal patient who may pose a serious danger to the public involves sociopolitical as well as purely medical considerations. In effect, responsibility is divided between the doctors and Home Office officials. It could be argued that continued residence in hospital beyond the period required on mental health grounds is an improper use of medical facilities. It is sometimes suggested that a legal power to refer back to the court should be introduced so that such an offender could be sentenced to imprisonment on the grounds that he has recovered sufficiently to be punished for his crime. This would seem to many people unduly harsh. Hospitals should, perhaps, accept some responsibility for providing asylum for patients who cannot be placed in the community.

Often, the kind of patient who needs a restriction order is suitable only for the special hospitals, where adequate security can be enforced. Admissions to special hospitals are controlled by the Department of Health and are generally provided only for offenders convicted of serious crimes, such as homicide, arson or sexual violence, who are considered to require strict security. Some of the patients who need restriction orders, so that they can be legally detained after their immediate disturbance has subsided, or recalled after discharge if disturbance recurs, can be managed satisfactorily in an ordinary hospital, given sufficient supervision. Others, after a period of treatment in a special hospital, are thought fit enough for transfer to an open hospital as a preliminary to gradual release into the community.

Each year, a handful of offenders committed to crown courts are found to be mentally unfit to stand trial, being too ill to follow the proceedings or instruct counsel in their defence. Legally, under the Criminal Procedure (Insanity) Act, 1964, section 4, the unfitness decision is one for the jury to make after hearing medical evidence. In practice, the provision is used only for offenders who are obviously out of touch with what is happening to them, and it is hardly ever a matter for dispute. Pleas of insanity, on the grounds that the offender did not know what he was doing at the time of the crime, are almost obsolescent. If successful, this plea results in a finding of 'not guilty by reason of insanity' but, like the offender found unfit for trial, the 'insane' criminal is automatically subject to indefinite detention in hospital at the discretion of the Home Secretary, an outcome virtually identical to having a restriction order. A patient who has been found unfit for trial can be prosecuted if he recovers, but this is rarely done. After a long lapse of time the necessary witnesses may be no longer available.

Finally—given the necessary recommendations and the consent of the Home Secretary—offenders in prison found to be mentally disordered, either under sentence or on remand, can be transferred to hospital (Mental Health Act, 1973, sections 72 and 73). This does not happen very often. There were 83 such transfers in 1979, but almost as many, 74, were awaiting transfer or decision. This reflects the difficulty experienced by the prison medical service in finding hospitals willing to take such cases. In making a transfer of a prisoner, the Home Secretary can add a restriction which prevents the responsible medical officer from discharging the patient for the duration of his sentence. If he recovers in the meantime, and no longer requires hospitalization, he may be returned to prison to serve the balance of his sentence.

MAKING APPROPRIATE USE OF LEGAL PROVISIONS

Psychiatric views differ as to the advisability of collaboration with non-medical authorities in the implementation of treatment under compulsion for patients capable of making choices for themselves. Among both psychotherapists and behaviour therapists there are some who consider absolutely voluntary cooperation to be either an essential prerequisite of effective therapy or an ethically imperative condition before any intervention should be attempted. If that is the psychiatrist's honest opinion, then he should express it frankly when called upon to make a report for the court on an offender who stands in need of treatment. The practitioner can explain that he is willing to provide treatment on a strictly informal basis, but not to have a patient attend under any kind of legal requirement or constraint. The court can then decide whether it is prepared to deal with the offender in such a way (by conditional discharge, deferred or suspended sentence, or fine) that he remains free to take up the psychiatrist's offer of treatment. Some courts are reluctant to accept advice along these lines, either because they do not expect the offender to cooperate if left to his own devices, or because they want to know what happens to the offender and be able to take some action if things go wrong.

In common with many psychiatrists who have had experience of dealing with offender patients I take the view that a formal order can be helpful. The crisis of criminal prosecution, coupled with the threat of a punitive sentence, serves to bring home to some disordered individuals the necessity for making a change in their lives. At that point they begin to admit and to discuss their problems in a way that they may never have done before. Once the immediate stress is over, and a definite sentence has been passed, many offenders who previously complained of a multiplicity of symptoms or problems, recover magically and deny any wish for further help. One may know these bland denials to be a defence against facing up to unpleasant realities, and believe that further trouble is almost inevitable, but nothing can be done unless the offender has formally agreed on the need for change and entered into a contract which he cannot easily refute. Another advantage of a formal requirement in a probation order is that it can help to sustain a wavering resolution to cooperate long enough for a constructive therapeutic relationship to develop that would not otherwise have been established.

Some psychiatrists are reluctant to share responsibility, or to divulge information about their confidential interchanges with patients, and for this reason do not like to have a probation officer in any way involved with treatment. A contrary, and probably more realistic view, is that offender patients frequently have continuing social problems, and that it is therefore beneficial to have available a social worker experienced in such matters, whose duty it is to explore the home circumstances and maintain supervisory contact with the offender and his family, especially after discharge from residential treatment.

The 1973 statute lays down in section 3(4) that during residential treatment the probation officer 'shall carry out the supervision to such extent only as may be necessary for the purpose of discharge or amendment of the order'. This provision has been criticized, for instance by the Butler committee and by Lewis

(1980), a probation officer who carried out a survey of the roles and expectations of psychiatrists and probation officers. If the system is to work satisfactorily doctors and probation officers need to collaborate from the outset. For instance, at the stage when a report is being prepared and recommendations formulated, consultation is necessary to obtain from the probation officer particulars of home background and social history (since the courts often order a social inquiry report from the probation service at the same time as they request a medical report). This helps in making an informed decision as to whether the treatment should be as an in-patient or an out-patient, and to clarify the goals of treatment and how the probation officer can assist. On some matters that may be highly relevant to treatment, such as settling accommodation difficulties, monitoring drinking problems, or assistance with socio-legal issues like eviction orders or separation orders, the probation officer is better placed than the psychiatrist to provide help. Experience suggests that lack of adequate liaison between psychiatrist and probation officers is often an important contributing factor when treatment plans fail through patients drifting away, not turning up for appointments or committing further offences.

Published surveys show that the practice of remanding for a psychiatric report varies considerably from one locality to another (Binns et al. 1969; Bowden 1978; Gibbens et al. 1977; Prins 1976). The availability of forensic psychiatric facilities and the attitudes of the magistrates greatly influence how many medical remands are requested, and how many are remands in custody rather than on bail. Only a small proportion of offenders are remanded and an even smaller proportion (about 0.5% of all defendants found guilty in adult courts of non-motoring offences) receive any formal treatment order. Except for juveniles, who are remanded to specialized assessment centres outside the jurisdiction of the prison department, those remanded in custody are less likely to receive a positive recommendation. Among the reports prepared on adults remanded in custody for psychiatric investigations, of which there were 8494 in 1979, under 10% include a positive recommendation for a treatment order, and the vast majority of the recommendations that are made are for hospital orders rather than treatment on probation. As Bowden found, prison medical officers 'are essentially recommending for treatment only those individuals who are suffering from acute psychiatric illness'. Other things being equal, a bad criminal history, as reflected in the number of previous convictions and length of previous imprisonments, or the presence of 'psychopathy' or alcohol problems, reduced significantly the likelihood of receiving a positive recommendation. The more difficult, obstreperous or dangerous an offender appears to be, the less likely he is to receive a treatment recommendation for the obvious reason that hospitals will not accept such cases.

When recommendations for supportive treatment in the community (hostel placements, out-patient psychotherapy and so forth) are made, it is usually in respect of individuals examined by Health Service consultants while on bail.

Among the offences which lead to a psychiatric remand, sexual offences, especially offences of a deviant kind such as indecent exposure or child molestation, alcohol-related offences, drug offences, public disorderliness or vagrancy and personal violence, are all over-represented in comparison with what would be expected in an unselected population of convicted persons. This reflects the kinds of behaviour which magistrates believe may be related to psychiatric disorder and may be modifiable through medical treatment. In many cases, in relation to drugs and alcohol for example, the courts are more optimistic in their evaluation of the feasibility of treatment than are the reporting doctors. Remands in custody of acutely disordered individuals may seem inappropriate, but often the courts resort to this as the quickest and easiest way to obtain swift care and safe keeping.

The commonest forensic task that the hospital psychiatrist may be called upon to perform is the preparation of a report on a patient referred by the courts for an assessment. The style and substance is important, since these reports greatly influence court decisions and can have devastating consequences for the individual in question. The likelihood that the court will act upon whatever recommendation may be made depends in part upon the clarity with which the proposals are formulated and the manner in which reasons for them are set out (Scott 1953). Since the bench is made up of lay persons, technical jargon has to be avoided or paraphrased. For instance 'involuntary blinking' is preferable to 'blepharospasms', 'anxiety in sexual situations', though less specific, may convey more than 'castration complex' and 'socially withdrawn' may be more understandable than 'schizoid personality'. Stock labels, such as 'immature' and 'unstable', that carry no precise information, should be either avoided or amplified by practical examples of the kinds of behaviour or attitude that justify the epithet.

Courts do not often explain exactly what they want from the psychiatrist, so it is best to assume that they are interested in a general assessment of background, present state, amenability and prospects of effective help for the offender. Brief statements such as 'this man is not suffering from mental illness within the meaning of the Mental Health Act', with no comment as to what can or cannot be done for him, are irritatingly inadequate. On the other hand, long personal histories with numerous details about family relationships, although relevant to psychotherapy, are not only unnecessary but positively undesirable if they involve the public revelation of sensitive and confidential material. In the case of juveniles, especially, one needs to consider carefully before releasing information that may prejudice an already delicate relationship with the parents. Furthermore, the wording with which unpleasant comments are expressed can make a difference. For example, Scott suggests substituting for 'This boy is illegitimate and has always been rejected by his mother' the phrase 'His mother's anomalous situation at the time of his conception appears to have affected her feelings towards him ever since'. It is advisable, if confidential matters, such as a previous suicide attempt, or an extramarital affair, need to be mentioned, to point them out to the offender and obtain his specific agreement to include them.

Reports requested by the courts are privileged, in that they cannot be used as grounds for actionable defamation. Nevertheless, since the document may be seen by many people and may be preserved and cited on subsequent occasions, it is only right to be scrupulously fair in avoiding speculative suggestions of a pejorative kind and limiting statements to matters that can be reliably substantiated. Sometimes it is as well to make clear the origin of the information by prefacing statements with such phrases as, 'His wife states that...' or, 'According to the records of his previous hospital admission...'. This precaution works both ways, for one may also say, 'He asserts that...', instead of appearing to accept automatically the offender's version of events.

Needless to say the court is interested in the prognosis, not only as regards psychiatric symptoms, but also as regards risk of reoffending. Sometimes it is justifiable to say that a certain course of action or treatment is likely to reduce the risk of reoffending. The courts are obliged to make definite decisions between a restricted range of choices, and consequently welcome a clear-cut recommendation. If no treatment or advice on psychiatric grounds can be given, perhaps because the patient appears unwilling or unamenable, or the necessary facilities are not available, or there is nothing that requires treatment, this should be fully explained. It is not the psychiatrist's business, however, to tell the court what penal sentence should be given. Some such phrase as, 'There are no psychiatric grounds for modifying any decision the court may wish to make', goes far enough. The psychiatrist can, of course, point out, even if treatment is not on offer, that the individual is anxious to cooperate with a probation officer, or that imprisonment might exacerbate the individual's problems. Such statements should not be made too lightly, but only if the doctor is confident that they are fully justifiable.

VARIETIES OF DISORDER

Offenders referred to a psychiatrist may be suffering from anything or nothing. A few are plainly psychotic, some appear to have nothing the matter save for a wish to avoid the penal consequences of their offences, most fall somewhere in between. The commonest situations in which psychotics are involved are not dramatic outbursts of violence but rather petty offences of larceny arising out of the vagrant way of life of the chronic or 'burnt out' schizophrenic, who may have no relatives able or willing to look after him and no inclinations or ability to undertake a normal job. Paranoid schizophrenics with persecutory delusions are more likely to be a nuisance than a danger, constantly complaining to police about neighbours or, as in one memorable case, travelling on a train without a ticket in an effort to reach Sandringham to appeal to the Queen. The acutely ill schizophrenic who will not cooperate voluntarily, for whom a compulsory order is clearly justifiable, poses less of a problem of management than the moderately disturbed psychotic who retains clear volition, but persists in an unsatisfactory mode of life and declines treatment or advice. Particularly difficult are the cases of morbidly jealous husbands, whose preoccupations and suspicions are held with delusional intensity and unreason, who nevertheless retain clear and rational thinking on other topics. Some of these individuals ultimately deteriorate, show clear signs of thought disorder, and can be confidently diagnosed as paranoid schizophrenics, but the ones who remain monosymptomatic, but totally lacking in insight, are virtually impossible to control and their wives, if they remain together, run a considerable risk (Mowat 1966).

Serious violence, usually against members of the patient's family, is liable to occur in states of acute, psychotic excitement, agitation or severe depression. In the case of depressives, attacks by women on their children, or husbands on their wives, are sometimes part of an attempt at extended suicide, meant to ensure that all die together. When their immediate disturbance is brought under control with medication, they often become quite easy to manage in hospital, in spite of the fact that they have committed horrendous crimes when acutely ill.

Sex offenders, especially those involved in activities of a deviant nature (such as child molestation, indecent exposure, homosexual indecency, larceny of women's underwear, etc.) are frequently referred for treatment. Some of these offenders are incapable of ordinary heterosexual life, being entirely fixated upon some inappropriate sexual interest or ritual. Others have strong inclinations towards opposite-sexed adults, but take to deviant acts because their social ineptitude, or severe repressions, prevent them from finding a partner. This is often the situation with mentally subnormal patients who have got into trouble for minor indecencies. Some of these offenders, homosexuals and paedophiles for example, are content with their particular sexual preferences, have no wish to change, and appear before the psychiatrist only because ordered to do so by the courts. Assessment of such cases calls for considerable experience, and treatment may involve specialist psychological techniques such as 'orgasmic reconditioning', as well as group psychotherapy or social skills training. Ideally there should be specialist units for the assessment and treatment of these offenders, on the lines of the facilities available in part of the United States (West 1980), but in the UK there are very few psychiatrists who specialize in these matters, and many men who want and need special help do not receive treatment. The courts tend to reflect the public's concern over sexual offences, even those which cause no harm and little shock to the victim. One of the services psychiatrists can perform in this regard is to reassure, whenever possible, that there is no evidence that the offender is physically dangerous. It is not generally appreciated that the risk of reconviction for further sex crime of a man found guilty for the first time is quite low.

Many offenders have no particular psychiatric disorder to treat other than persistent antisocial behaviour, which the usual deterrents appear powerless to alter. Others, who do have a psychiatric complaint, also have an underlying antisocial personality, which hampers treatment. Antisocial personality is by far the most prevalent feature of offender patients, and it makes for endless problems of management and great difficulty in fitting into the kind of psychiatric regime that suits the majority of patients. The concept of antisocial personality has been criticized as ill defined, relative to the cultural standards of the diagnostician, of questionable aetiology, possibly more of a situational reaction than a pathological state, and not sufficiently consistent to deserve the term 'syndrome'. Whatever the scientific (or unscientific) status of the concept, from the clinicians' point of view the phenomena not only exist, but obtrude all too frequently and unpleasantly. Roth (1972) has no doubt of the existence of the syndrome. It 'has a characteristic sex distribution, age at onset, family history of similar symptoms and disorders, and family constellations and influences that show a considerable measure of consistency in their course and outcome'.

Typically, the history of the antisocial personality clearly reveals a socially deprived home background in which parental care was erratic, intermittent or neglectful. The disturbance may be obvious even during preschool years, with temper tantrums, wandering from home, stubbornness and backwardness. Later on, troublesomeness in the classroom, truancy, quarrelsomeness, resistance to discipline, poor scholastic performance, alienation from the more conventional members of the peer group and delinquent behaviour mark the youngster as a social deviant. Wayward traits continue in youth, with drinking problems, sexual promiscuity, drug abuse, neglect of work, no interest in job training, involvement in gang fights and a generally impulsive, hedonistic style of life unrestrained by normal social rules. If these characteristics persist, they lead to an erratic work record, welfare dependency, continued criminality, neglect of family responsibilities and consequent breakdown of marriages or cohabitations. Accident proneness, drunken violence, homelessness and attempted suicide are frequent features. The long-term prognosis for children referred to a psychiatric clinic with severe behaviour disorder is poor. As was shown in a 30-year follow-up in St Louis (Robins 1966) the incidence of social and psychiatric disorders of all kinds in later life, including psychotic illness, suicide, violent and sometimes lethal confrontations with police, alcoholism, drug problems, chronic unemployment, social alienation and criminal life style, was significantly raised among those who had been antisocial as children.

Many young delinquents display some of these features in youth, but settle down in their early twenties, taking family and work responsibilities more seriously, and becoming much like their peers who have never been delinquents (Osborn and West 1980). On the other hand, the more extreme cases, especially those from the very worst kinds of background, remain unsocialized much longer, perhaps permanently, and are liable to that malignant progression of social pathology described by Robins. The antisociality syndrome is sometimes accompanied by a variety of non-specific electroencephalographic abnormalities, suggestive of some organic brain damage, or at least of delayed maturation (Syndulko 1978). Recent research on disturbance of brain laterality in psychopathic disorders are also strongly suggestive of an organic factor (Yeudall and Wardell 1978). In the majority of cases, however, the most obvious feature is a history of social deprivation. This might account for the defective social learning, the failure to internalize acceptable moral rules, and the formation of what psychologists might call an instinct-driven character with very weak super-ego. A psychophysiological characteristic, under-reactivity of the autonomic nervous system, resulting in slowness of 'conditioned avoidance learning' and consequent resistance to punishment, has also been suggested as an explanation for the failure of the usual socialization processes to take effect (Hare 1980).

There seems little doubt that the antisociality syndrome, like other psychiatric syndromes, is the outcome of a complex interaction between social, psychological and organic constitutional factors. Aetiological research in this case has contributed little to effective treatment. Fortunately, very few examples of the antisociality syndrome are so severe that the individual is completely impervious to environmental pressures. Some highly impulsive characters react well to a controlled, authoritarian regime which rewards acceptable behaviour while reacting to deviant acts with swift and certain reprisals. Some of the more inadequate, dependent types improve in a supportive and undemanding situation in which decisions are made for them and rewards are not conditional upon much constructive activity on their part. Others, again, are capable of fitting into a tolerant but stimulating therapeutic community in which peer influences and group discussions challenge their attitudes and habits and help them to achieve greater insight into and more control over their destructive impulses (Whiteley 1968). These kinds of milieu therapy require special facilities and units separate from the ordinary patient population. If the system of 'regional secure units', proposed by the Butler Report, ever becomes fully operational (Bluglass 1978), it may be possible to cater more readily for the special needs of offender patients. In a controlled setting, disgruntled attitudes, hostility to authority and disregard of other patients' needs and rights make useful occasions for 'reality confrontations'. In an ordinary ward the same phenomena can be totally disruptive.

THE 1982 LEGISLATION

The Mental Health (Amendment) Bill (1982) proposes to change some of the arrangements described. For example, courts will be specifically empowered to remand to hospital rather than to prison for medical assessment, and to make interim orders of up to three months detention in hospital for assessment before finally deciding on a hospital order. Mental Health Review Tribunals will be empowered to direct, not merely to advise on, the discharge of patients on restriction orders. Sexual deviancy or drug dependence will no longer in themselves suffice to permit detention as a 'psychopath'. The circumstances in which detained patients may be given treatment without their consent are also to be restricted.

CONCLUDING THOUGHTS

Offender patients are unpopular, more particularly perhaps among nurses who have to bear the brunt of any unpleasant behaviour. Well-publicized complaints against mental hospital nurses, arising out of their handling of obstreperous patients, are not calculated to improve the offender–patient's chances of admission. Nevertheless, although there is every justification for caution and discrimination, a policy of near-total rejection is both misguided and inhumane. These patients can be very rewarding, the long-term prognosis is better than for many of the psychogeriatric disorders which form an increasing part of the mental hospital work load, and treatments that succeed in reducing risk of reoffending are of great value to the community as well as to the individual patient and his family. No one wants a return to the prison-like atmosphere of the totally closed hospital, but the total abolition of locked wards has possibly gone too far. In many cases, as Bluglass (1978) points out, the greatest need is not for secure accommodation, but for 'a recognition that more intensive care and a carefully constructed daily programme is indicated for these patients'.

Bluglass also points out that for some uncontrollable, asocial personalities, and particularly perhaps for some partially recovered chronic schizophrenics, long-term hospital care may still be necessary. This goes against the modern trend, but the fact remains that lack of basic life supports in the community, and unsuitability for most hostel placements, leaves behind a residue of patients who need hospital asylum. It is some of these currently rejected patients who make up the disgracefully large number of former mental hospital patients languishing unnecessarily in expensive secure accommodation in prison.

The social problems of the antisocial personality can only be permanently solved in community living. Many of the less serious offender patients are best dealt with outside hospital, but for those who have to spend some of their treatment period in residence the most important phase comes when they have to return to their usual environment and try to withstand all the stresses that may involve. For this reason the built-in after-care provided by a probation order is, as was previously mentioned, decidedly advantageous.

References

BINNS, J.K., CARLISLE, J.M., NIMMO, D.H., PARK, R.H. & TODD, N.A. (1969) Remanded in custody for psychiatric examination. *Br. J. Psychiat.*, **115**, 1133.

BLUGLASS, ROBERT (1978) Regional secure units and interim security for psychiatric patients. *Br. med. J.*, **25 February**, 489.

BOWDEN, P. (1978) Men remanded into custody for medical reports. *Br. J. Psychiat.*, **132**, 320.

FARRINGTON, D.P. (1981) A note on the prevalence of convictions. *Br. J. Crim.* **21**.

GIBBENS, T.C.N., SOOTHILL, K.L. & POPE, P.J. (1977) *Medical Remands in the Criminal Courts*. London: Oxford University Press.

GUNN, J., ROBERTSON, G., DELL, S. & WAY, C. (1978) *Psychiatric Aspects of Imprisonment*. London: Academic Press.

GUZE, S.B. (1976) *Criminality and Psychiatric Disorders*. New York: Oxford University Press.

HARE, ROBERT D. (1980) Psychopathy. In: *Handbook of Biological Psychiatry, Part II*. Ed. Van Praag, H.M. New York: Marcel Dekker.

HOME OFFICE (1975) *Report of The (Butler) Committee on Mentally Abnormal Offenders*, Command 6244. London: H.M.S.O.

HOME OFFICE (1978) *The Sentence of the Courts*, 3rd ed. London: H.M.S.O.

LEWIS, P. (1980) *Psychiatric Probation Orders*. Cambridge: Institute of Criminology.

MOWAT, R.R. (1966) *Morbid Jealousy and Murder*. London: Tavistock.

OSBORN, S.G. & WEST, D.J. (1980) Do delinquents really reform? *J. Adolescence*, **3**, 99.

PENROSE, L.S. (1943) A note on the statistical relationship between mental deficiency and crime in the United States. *Am. J. ment. Defic.*, **47**, 462.

PRINS, H.A. (1976) Remands for psychiatric reports. *Med. Sci. Law*, **14**, 129.

RAPPEPORT, J.R. & LASSEN, G. (1965) Dangerousness—arrest rate comparisons of discharged psychiatric patients and the general population. *Am. J. Psychiat.*, **121**, 776.

ROBINS, L. (1966) *Deviant Children Grown Up*. Baltimore: Williams and Wilkinson.

ROTH, MARTIN (1972) Human Violence as Viewed from the Psychiatric Clinic. *Am. J. Psychiat.*, **128**, 1043.

SCOTT, P.D. (1953) Psychiatric reports for magistrates' courts. *Br. J. Delinq.* **4**, 1.

SOSOWSKY, L. (1978) Crime and violence among mental patients reconsidered in view of the new legal relationship between the state and the mentally ill. *Am. J. Psychiat.*, **135**, 33.

SYNDULKO, K. (1978) Electrocortical investigations of sociopathy. In: *Psychopathic Behaviour*, ed. Hare, R.D. & Schalling, D. New York: Wiley.

WEST, D.J. (1980) (ed.) *Sex Offenders in the Criminal Justice System*. (Cropwood Conference Series No. 12). Cambridge: Institute of Criminology.

WHITELEY, J.S. (1968) The response of psychopaths to a therapeutic community. *Br. J. Psychiat.*, **114**, 517.

YEUDALL, L.T. & WARDELL, D., (1978) Neurophysiological correlates of criminal psychopathy. In: *Human Aggression and Dangerousness*, ed. Beliveau, L., Canepa, G. & Szabo, D. Montreal: Pinel Inst.

ZITRIN, A., HARDESTY, A.S., BURDOCK, E.I. & DROSSMAN, A.K. (1976) Crime and violence among mental patients. *Am. J. of Psychiat.*, **133**, 142.

20

Management of Alcoholism and Drug Addiction

F. Arroyave and G.E. Berrios

ALCOHOLISM

Introduction

The term 'alcoholism' refers to several patterns of alcohol abuse and can be defined as an absent or impaired ability to control alcohol consumption (Arroyave and McKeown 1979), or as repeated consumption of alcohol leading to dependence, physical disease, or other types of harm (Paton and Saunders 1981). Thus alcoholism can refer to the behaviour of those who are particularly sensitive to the harmful effects of alcohol, and induce somatic damage by drinking socially acceptable amounts of alcohol; of those who drink relatively heavily without loss of performance until alcohol-related disease develops; of those whose regular drinking is associated with social and physical problems; and of those who develop a severe withdrawal syndrome if alcohol is stopped.

Although this group of disorders has been considered by some as a disease which results from brain dysfunction (Jellinek 1960; Keller 1976), it has been pointed out that the attitudes arising from this hypothesis may encourage people to avoid responsibility for their drinking. On the other hand it has been claimed that the consideration of drinking problems as an 'illness' provides the alcoholic with a sense of dignity (Gitlow 1980).

The disease concept of alcoholism has led to the identification of a genetic factor, although it is difficult to determine what is inherited; loss of control, tolerance and mood response to alcohol have been considered in this context (Partanen 1966; Goodwin 1979). However, interactions of the individual with environmental variables are crucial to the development of the disorder (Winokur et al. 1970; El-Guebaly and Offord 1977), and epidemiological analysis has shown that increases in per capita consumption of alcohol are associated with increases in rates of alcohol-related problems such as liver cirrhosis, and mortality and hospital admissions of persons diagnosed as alcoholics (Cartwright and Shaw 1978).

Jariwalla et al. (1979) have recently shown that 27% of a series of acute medical admissions were related to alcohol, and Holt et al. (1980) reported that 40% of those attending a Casualty Department had consumed alcohol before the emergency. Lee (1979) found that cerebrovascular accidents in non-hypertensive males under 50 had alcoholism as the only common denominator.

Physical dependence. This involves an increased tolerance to the pharmacological effects of alcohol, a tendency to develop withdrawal phenomena on cessation of drinking, and the subjective awareness of a desire to drink (Arroyave and McKeown 1979).

Psychological dependence. This can be defined as a subjective desire to drink alcohol accompanied by a fear that lack of alcohol will lead to intellectual or emotional dysfunction.

Tolerance. This refers to the increased capacity of the individual to resist the effects of alcohol intake on the CNS. This may be due to accelerated hepatic alcohol metabolism (as a result of induction of microsomal enzymes) or to hyposensitivity of CNS receptors.

Impaired control. This involves an impaired ability to stop drinking, either in the case of the regular heavy drinker, or in the so-called bout drinker once he has restarted (Keller 1972).

Controlled drinking. This has also been termed 'normal' or 'social' drinking, and has been defined as the drinking of self-monitored amounts of alcohol in non-clinical settings to an extent that does not interfere with intellectual, affective, physical, or social functioning. The individual retains the ability to stop at will, or whenever external circumstances render it appropriate (Arroyave and McKeown 1979). It can also be defined in terms of a recommended upper limit of alcohol; the Royal College of Psychiatrists (1979) have suggested a maximum of four pints of beer a day, or its equivalent. This involves 60–80 g alcohol daily, and a pint of beer is roughly equivalent to a single measure of spirits, one small glass of sherry, or one glass of wine. Paton and Saunders (1981) considered that 60 g of alcohol daily for men, and 30 g daily for women, is a relatively safe upper limit, but they pointed out that this may be too high in some individuals and that there may be no absolutely safe limits (Lebachs 1975).

The goal of controlled drinking in the management of alcoholism can be criticized on a number of grounds. For example, the routine ingestion of a relatively small amount of alcohol may be harmful in the long term, and the effects of a given intake depend on constitution, pattern of drinking, diet, body weight, hepatic function, tolerance and the presence of a psychiatric illness. Also, it has been recently shown that liver disease can result from lower levels of alcohol consumption than previously reported, and that a regular intake of above three pints of beer a day (or its equivalent) can produce biochemical changes in liver function tests within 6 weeks. Saunders et al. (1981) have reported that alcohol may have a differential and more marked effect upon the liver in females, in that they tend to develop alcoholic hepatitis after a shorter period of excessive drinking and at a lower daily alcohol intake. This may reflect some difference in the immune reactivity between the sexes and it has been suggested that greater emphasis should be placed on designing specific abstinence programmes for female patients and on earlier detection of liver disease. In addition, it is possible that relatively small quantities of alcohol may continue to have harmful effects on pre-existing alcohol-induced cerebral damage or cirrhosis of the liver.

The rationale of controlled drinking is based on the belief that this goal is more readily attainable by most alcoholics and there are several studies which have claimed satisfactory results from treatment programmes with the goal of controlled drinking (Armor et al. 1976; Schuckit 1980; Smith 1981a). However, some clinicians still consider that this approach is experimental. It has recently been stated that there is probably a place and a need for controlled drinking in routine clinical practice (Heather and Robertson 1981).

Interventions Directed Towards Abstinence

Introduction. It has been concluded that the majority of alcohol-related problems remain resistant to any attempts at treatment, and that individuals improve only as a result of certain life events (Anon 1981; Smith 1981a). Also, in relation to large groups of alcoholic individuals, the value of any kind of treatment (except, perhaps, the newer forms of behaviour therapy) has been questioned (Smith 1981a), although it should be remembered that the assessment of outcome is beset with methodological difficulties. However, Smith (1981a) has reviewed several studies which indicated that relatively intensive in-patient treatment was not superior to out-patient treatment, and although data on heterogeneous groups may obscure the effects of certain treatments on individual patients, it was suggested that the limited resources that are available should be invested in relatively simple treatment programmes, and that organizations such as Alcoholics Anonymous may play a valuable role. The problem of providing appropriate facilities for the habitual drunken offender is still unsolved (Smith 1981b). Even though detoxification centres do not appear to modify drinking behaviour to a significant extent, many of these individuals require some kind of provision for their basic care, other than the hospital and prison services (Arroyave et al. 1980).

There has been an increasing emphasis on the early detection of various forms of alcoholism, particularly in women, by general medical practitioners, and by the recognition of 'problem drinkers' at work (Paton and Saunders 1981; Smith 1981c). The general practitioner should be on the look-out for the physical stigmata of alcoholism, and blood tests may show a macrocytosis or elevation of the MCV without anaemia. γ-Glutamyl transpeptidase, glutamate dehydrogenase and aspartate transaminase may be raised, while a low albumin or increased alkaline phosphatase also indicates liver disorder. Advice is more likely to be therapeutic at an early stage, and the patient can be asked to abstain from alcohol, at least until the blood tests return to normal. If abstinence is an unrealistic goal, a limit for the daily alcohol intake can be negotiated (Anon 1981).

Disulfiram (Antabuse). It has been claimed that alcoholics can be deterred from drinking by the severe physiological effects that characterize the disulfiram −ethanol reaction, which are due to accumulation of acetyldehyde together with a relative deficiency of noradrenaline, mainly in myocardial tissue and arterioles (Morgan and Cagan 1974). The reaction starts between 10 and 25 min after ingestion of alcohol, and is characterized by palpitations, profuse sweating, skin flushing, nausea (which is sometimes followed by vomiting), 'splitting' headache and general malaise. A severe reaction could include a fall in blood pressure followed by cardiovascular shock. This might prove fatal.

Disulfiram should not be prescribed without first inducing a 'controlled' disulfiram reaction in hospital; this ensures that the patient becomes acquainted with the symptoms and risks involved, and provides the physician with the opportunity of assessing the individual's response to disulfiram. The selected patient is given disulfiram (400 mg daily by mouth), for at least 4 days, during which alcohol abstinence is essential, followed by 600 mg on the day of the controlled reaction. An hour after the dose, 50 ml ethanol is given, and the patient is observed closely. Blood pressure and pulse should be recorded at 10-min intervals, and subjective signs of distress noted. If no reaction occurs, administration of the same quantity of ethanol is repeated at 15-min intervals up to a maximum of 150–200 ml. In the case of hypotensive shock, 10 mg of intravenous noradrenaline may be indicated, and the administration of alcohol is discontinued. It is believed that this induced reaction can reinforce the deterrent effect of the drug.

The daily maintenance dose is 200 mg. Side effects include a disagreeable taste in the mouth, persistent headache, nausea, fatigue or impotence, which may require its substitution by calcium carbamide (Abstem) at a daily dose of 100 mg. Occasionally psychotic states (Reisberg 1978; Major et al. 1979) and neurological syndromes involving the basal ganglia (Rainey 1977) have been described associated with disulfiram. Both disulfiram and calcium carbamide can be taken for an indefinite period.

Abdominal wall implants have been tried in subjects who, although accepting the deterrent effect of the drug, lack the determination or motivation to take it by mouth (Wilson 1975). Since implants, however, do not frequently produce the plasma levels required for a reaction to take place, it must be postulated that the symptoms reported after the ingestion of alcohol may sometimes be of psychological origin.

The use of disulfiram should be considered for:

(1) The patient who believes that without it he will be unable to abstain, and who has the wish to use it.

(2) Clinical situations where the potential for psychotherapeutic intervention is limited, for example, when the patient has a low intelligence.

(3) The patient who has difficulties in relating to professional helpers. By requiring regular hospital attendance, prescription of the drug may create the possibility of developing a relationship.

(4) Individuals who have a history of law-breaking related to alcoholism.

However, even in these cases disulfiram should constitute only one element of a wider treatment plan.

Behavioural techniques. Behavioural approaches to the treatment of alcoholism are based on classic or instrumental learning principles (Sobell and Sobell 1973), and may have controlled drinking as the goal (Hamburg 1975; Lloyd and Salzberg 1975; Sobell and Sobell 1976). It should be noted that the methodological aspects of the work reported by the Sobells (1973, 1976) have recently come under severe criticism (Pendery et al. 1982).

The most common behavioural technique is aversive therapy, which involves establishing an association between the drinking of alcohol (or the thought of it) and an unpleasant stimulus, such as nausea and vomiting resulting from the administration of apomorphine. However, this procedure carries some risk (e.g. inhalation of vomit), and therapeutic results are modest and transitory. Injections of succinylcholine have also been tried as an aversive stimulus and the ensuing apnoea paired with the drinking or the smell of alcohol. Other aversive stimuli have included electric shocks. In general, the more unpleasant aversive techniques are rarely recommended as they tend to damage the development of a therapeutic relationship which is vital in the treatment of an alcoholic. However, behavioural strategies which have been claimed to be of value include filming the patient when intoxicated and subsequently showing him the film, and electric shock coupled with inappropriate drinking behaviour (e.g. drinking too fast), as well as identifying environmental situations which lead to excessive alcoholic intake, prior to working out strategies for their modification or avoidance.

Informal psychotherapy. This refers to organized situations where the patient may derive help and understanding from friends, relatives, spouse or strangers, who may sometimes share the same problem. Alcoholics Anonymous or similar self-help groups provide regular meetings and may offer emergency visits during a crisis. In general, group members are not expected to 'put up with everything', as this is often counter-productive, and are encouraged to set limits to any disruptive behaviour of the alcoholic by, if necessary, excluding the individual.

Alcoholics Anonymous (AA) has proved successful in the treatment of some patients but assessment of this organization is difficult as anonymity is given to those who attend.

Formal psychotherapy. This type of intervention is offered by specially trained practitioners in specific settings (see Chapter 8), although there is reasonable evidence to suggest that the most relevant outcome variable is not the theoretical framework in which the therapist operates, but the personality of the therapist. Also, it has been claimed that 'alcoholics may be effectively treated in long-term interactional group therapy and that, hour for hour, the group therapist achieves as much therapeutic change as in groups of non-alcoholic neurotic patients' (Brown and Yalom 1977).

The value of group psychotherapy in the treatment of alcoholism is difficult to assess, partly because most published studies have considered their patient sample as homogeneous. However, Finney and Moos (1979) identified eight subgroups of alcoholics and correlated these with treatment programmes and outcome, and Willems et al. (1973) attempted to categorize alcoholics into four subgroups in terms of their awareness of illness. These consisted of:

(1) Those with full awareness of their disorder. (Individuals in this category often recover without specialized help.)

(2) Individuals who are aware that 'there is something wrong',but who do not know what, and 'are unaware of the criteria for, and the implications of, the diagnosis'. (This is the group which is most likely to benefit from admission to a specialized unit.)

(3) Those who are unaware that there is anything wrong and/or who reject the diagnosis of alcoholism, but have the capacity to gain insight.

(4) Individuals who lack the capacity to develop insight.

The Oxford Regional Alcoholism Unit does not use stringent admission criteria and only demands a willingness to attend. The initial stage of management is a 2-week in-patient programme which begins with 'detoxification'. This is the beginning of treatment as well as the process of 'sobering up', and has three aspects: 'drying out', which involves the management of any symptoms of physical withdrawal (this may also take place in a general medical ward); medical, psychological and social assessment; and the development of a relationship between patient and staff. Thereafter, in 30 h of group psychotherapy, the patient is confronted with the realities of his situation and with his psychological defence mechanisms (Arroyave et al. 1980).

Treatment of Alcohol-Induced Syndromes

Withdrawal symptoms. There is marked individual variation in the manifestation of symptoms, which usually begin between 4 and 12 h after the last drink, although onset may be delayed for up to 24 h. Of over 3000 patients who have been admitted to the Oxford Regional Alcoholism Unit, about a third exhibited sweating, tremor, agitation and restlessness, while anxiety and bewilderment were the predominant mood states. These symptoms often respond well to sympathetic care and a supportive environment, and drugs are not usually required. Disorders of sleep and hypnagogic perceptual disturbances may also occur and, in severe cases, confusion, auditory and visual hallucinations can be accompanied by fever which may be due to a concomitant infection. Grand mal fits ('rum fits') may appear after between 6 and 72 h of abstinence. Alcohol consumption may also precipitate or increase the frequency of epileptic seizures.

Medication should not be given as a matter of routine and its need is assessed on a day-to-day basis. Chlormethiazole can be prescribed in doses of 500–2000 mg every 6–8 h for the first few days, and then in a progressively reducing dose (Arroyave et al. 1980). This drug can induce psychological and physical dependence and should not be given for longer than 8 days. Chlordiazepoxide is also useful in doses ranging between 30 and 60 mg every 6–8 h. 'Parentrovite' injections should be given as a matter of routine, as alcoholic patients often malabsorb due to gastrointestinal disorders. If grand mal fits are likely (for example, if there is a previous history of this complication) phenytoin 300 mg daily can be prescribed, and should be continued until at least 2 weeks after recovery from withdrawal symptoms. The Oxford Unit does not advocate the use of alcohol for the management of withdrawal.

Delirium tremens. If this complication develops, its onset is most likely to occur after about 3 days of abstinence from alcohol (Hemmingsen et al. 1979). It usually lasts 1–3 days. Untreated delirium tremens still carries a significant mortality due to hyperthermia, dehydration, hypotension and coma. Onset is often at night with fear, hyperactivity, clouding of consciousness and visual, auditory and tactile hallucinations. The patient may experience visual hallu-cinations involving small objects, animals or people (Lilliputian hallucina-tions), or may feel and see insects crawling on his skin. Also, he may hear accusatory and abusive voices. Delirium tremens constitutes a severe medical emergency whose aetiology is not yet clear (Salum 1975; Victor and Wolfe 1973).

Treatment of the disorder should always take place in hospital. Indiscrimin-ate rehydration is hazardous as rebound hyperhydration may easily occur (Balsano and Reynolds 1970). Thiamine (usually in combination with other vitamins) should be given in daily doses of 50–100 mg parenterally, and sedation with intravenous benzodiazepines, (e.g. diazepam 10 mg 4-hourly), is usually required. The likelihood of fits is reduced by giving phenytoin 100 mg three times daily. In cases of severe excitation haloperidol 10 mg hourly (intramuscularly) may be given until control has been achieved. This regimen is then reviewed. Not uncommonly, the delirious state is compounded by other conditions such as head injury, infections, cardiac failure, circulatory collapse, hypoglycaemia, hepatic failure or Wernicke's encephalopathy with nystagmus and other eye signs.

Alcoholic hallucinosis. ICD-9 describes alcoholic hallucinosis as a 'psychosis usually of less than six months duration with slight or no clouding of consciousness and much anxious restlessness in which auditory hallucinations, mostly of voices uttering insults and threats, predominate' (W.H.O. 1978). However, Cutting (1978) has argued that this definition does not distinguish the disorder from auditory hallucinations occurring in other disorders, and that only a small number of patients diagnosed as having alcoholic hallucinosis retain a similar syndrome when they are followed up. The clinical implications of this debate are uncertain, and the interactions between schizophrenic symptoms and alcohol abuse is a complex one (Freed 1975).

The management of alcoholic hallucinosis involves the treatment of the symptoms and of the underlying condition. Alcohol must be withdrawn from the patient and neuroleptics are prescribed, e.g. chlorpromazine 100 mg three times daily. Such measures are usually followed by marked diminution in the intensity of the hallucinations within a few days. Any physical disorder must be corrected, and a course of Parentrovite may be indicated. If the hallucinatory syndrome is persistent and threatens the life of the patient (e.g. by commanding him to commit suicide), then ECT may be given with good results. Patients suffering from this syndrome often live on their own and have no social support. In such cases, determined efforts should be made to modify the alcohol addiction and to provide help with social disability.

So-called pathological intoxication (mania a potu) is a rare phenomenon, and probably refers to excited states of varied aetiology in which alcohol is only one factor (Coid 1979).

Korsakoff's psychosis. Wernicke (1881) described a neurological syndrome characterized by confusion, ataxia and oculomotor palsies, while Korsakoff (1887) reported a symptom complex associated with alcoholism which involved anterograde and retrograde amnesia, polyneuritis and a tendency to confabulate. In the so-called Korsakoff's psychosis, the characteristic memory impairment is associated with bilateral structural damage which involves the mamillary bodies and/or other brain structures (Victor et al. 1971). This results from vascular pathology, and is associated with thiamine deficiency. About 25% of Korsakoff patients may recover after the first episode, and in a series of 11 collected by the first author, four patients showed steady progress during periods of sobriety ranging from 6 months to 3 years. Another patient made an almost complete recovery over a period of 2 years.

Thiamine hydrochloride, e.g. 500 mg (as part of Parentrovite) intramuscularly or intravenously should usually be given daily for a week, and thereafter until a normal diet is resumed. If a degree of impairment is permanent, rehabilitation may be required, and some patients can be trained to make better use of their remaining memory function, for example, by using lists and a diary.

Alcoholic dementia. Prolonged and heavy alcoholic intake may lead to chronic cognitive impairment, and this effect seems more marked in females. It has been claimed that alcoholism is associated with cerebral atrophy as shown by air encephalography (Brewer and Perrett 1970), CAT scan (Ron 1977), or psychometric testing (Carlsson et al. 1979), but the aetiology and severity of the cognitive impairment is not yet clear (Tarter 1975).

MANAGEMENT OF ABUSE OF DRUGS OTHER THAN ALCOHOL

ICD-9 defines drug (or polydrug) addiction (304) as:

A state, psychic and sometimes also physical, resulting from taking a drug, characterized by behavioural and other responses that always include a compulsion to take a drug on a continuous or periodic basis in order to experience its psychic effects, and sometimes to avoid the discomfort of its absence. Tolerance may or may not be present. A person may be dependent on more than one drug. (W.H.O. 1978)

The following are indexed: morphine type (304.0): barbiturate type (304.1): cocaine (304.2); cannabis (304.3); amphetamine type (304.4); hallucinogens (304.5); other (e.g. glue) (304.6); combinations of morphine type drug with any other (304.7); combinations excluding morphine type drug (304.8); and unspecified (304.9). Non-dependent abuse of drugs (305) is defined as:

Cases where a person, for whom no other diagnosis is possible, has come under medical care because of the maladaptive effect of a drug on which he is not dependent, and that he has taken on his own initiative to the detriment of his health or social functioning. (W.H.O. 1978)

It can be argued that the W.H.O. definition of drug addiction (304) should be modified to take into account the setting in which the drug (or drugs) is abused and the quantity consumed, and it should also be noted that a distinction between therapeutic and intoxicating drugs is not always easy to make.

This section offers guidelines for the treatment of abuse of drugs by the general psychiatrist. However, complex cases should often be referred to a specialist unit.

General Principles

A physiological approach to drug addictive behaviour has been supported by studies of animal pharmacology of drug addiction, which shows a number of behavioural patterns closely resembling human addiction (Woods 1978). Thus, an identifiable form of individual psychopathology may not be necessary for the development of some aspects of drug addiction. However the role of psychological, social and cultural factors cannot be denied.

Concepts such as tolerance and physical dependence, on which a physiological approach is based, are far from simple. First of all, the early appearance of tolerance does not necessarily entail physical dependence. For example, a number of drugs (e.g. anticholinergics) produce tolerance without physical dependence, while others (e.g. chlorpromazine) may develop physical dependence without tolerance. Furthermore neither of these two concepts is necessarily associated with abuse of drugs.

Three types of tolerance must be recognized: pharmacokinetic, pharmacodynamic and behavioural. The first refers to a change in drug availability mainly resulting from increased metabolism (Curry 1980); the second to adaptive change in receptor sensitivity which leads to a reduced response in the presence of the same concentration of the drug (Collier 1966); and the third to changes in the behavioural response to a given dose of drug. Behavioural tolerance involves the reduced expression of the behavioural effects of the drug and may develop when these have too high a 'cost' for the individual. Thus, regular drug abusers tend to produce less behavioural effects (to the same plasma level) in structured situations (e.g. the work place) than in an evening drug-taking session.

Tolerance is, therefore, not a homogeneous state, and a form of tolerance 'learning' has been described, in which retaking the drug after a period of abstinence can lead to a relatively rapid development of tolerance.

Physical dependence is recognized clinically by the appearance of a withdrawal syndrome on acute discontinuation of the drug. However, the detection of physical effects of withdrawal depends upon the rate of removal of the drug from the site of action, and on the sensitivity of techniques used; for example the EEG may identify changes which are not apparent on a clinical examination. It has been suggested that the presence and severity of a withdrawal syndrome may be associated with factors such as the previous development of receptor hypersensitivity, a compensatory proliferation of receptors, the functional utilization of redundant nervous pathways, or the inhibition of enzymes involved in the production of various neurotransmitters (Fishman 1978). Cross-dependence must be mentioned in this context, as a number of treatment programmes have been developed on the basis that one drug may suppress the manifestations of a withdrawal syndrome produced by another. Cross-dependence may be partial, such as between alcohol and barbiturates, or complete, as between methadone and morphine.

Learning is also an important factor in the persistence of drug addictive behaviour as this is often maintained by such consequences as the production of pleasurable effects, or the termination of unpleasant symptoms, including a chronic disillusionment with life. During the early stages of drug-taking, side effects may be outweighed by social reinforcers such as the need to gain membership of a drug-taking subculture, or the 'status' which the drug taking may confer. Learning principles can also be used to understand the various behaviours and rituals which often surround the drug-taking behaviour. The setting, time of the day, type of syringe, group membership, attire and other external cues are often associated with drug abuse and, on occasions, the mere presence of these cues can produce pleasurable effects or at least alleviate the pharmacological side effects. Knowledge of these associations is important to the development of treatment programmes.

However, pharmacological factors, learning, and social factors cannot completely explain the development of drug addiction. For a long time, clinicians have suspected that certain personality factors increase its likelihood, and it is said that individuals with sociopathic personality traits, who may be impulsive and unable to tolerate frustration, are particularly prone to develop dependence on drugs.

Barbiturate Addiction (304.1)

About ten barbiturates are available and are mainly used as short-term anaesthetics or antiepileptics. Oral barbiturates have both hypnotic and sedative actions and are still occasionally indicated for patients who have developed moderate dependence but have no tendency to escalate the dose. Intravenous use leads to early physical dependence (see Chapter 1).

The persistent reporting of severe withdrawal symptoms (Wikler 1968), seizures (Gardner 1967) and successful suicide or accidental overdosage due to barbiturates (Stevens 1978) gave rise to a drive to curb their use during the early 1970s. Thus, in the period 1970–75, the number of prescriptions for barbiturate hypnotics fell from 13 104 to 7331 in England and Wales (Williams 1980). Withdrawal from barbiturates was a common cause of confusional states in general hospitals (Gault 1976) and occasionally of seizures (Essig 1967). Withdrawal symptoms may commence 16–48 h after ceasing drug intake and include anxiety, apprehension, emotional lability, perspiration, muscular twitching, restlessness, tremor, hyper-reflexia, tachycardia, nausea, vomiting, lacrimation and, in severe cases, confusion, slurred speech, ataxia, hallucinations, fits and occasionally death. The EEG may show predominant frontocentral β-activity and, in cases of impending seizure, diffuse slowing, recurrent spikes and high-voltage paroxysmal discharge (Wulff 1959).

Treatment. Physical and psychiatric assessment should be carried out before gradual withdrawal is commenced. The following points must be kept in mind:

(1) Withdrawal from barbiturate abuse in doses above 600 mg daily should be carried out in hospital.

(2) Intravenous abusers must always be managed in hospital.

(3) The dose should be progressively decreased by 100 mg every 1 or 2 days.

(4) Small doses of benzodiazines are useful to reduce anxiety. Phenothiazines should not be used as they may induce seizures. Placebos are rarely indicated.

(5) Supportive or other forms of psychotherapy should be provided to maintain recovery.

Benzodiazepine Abuse

Benzodiazepines are used to relieve anxiety, to facilitate sleep and as muscle relaxants and anticonvulsants. In large doses they may produce respiratory depression and coma, but an overdose with the drug alone is rarely fatal. Benzodiazepines produce psychological, and occasionally physical, dependence characterized by a withdrawal syndrome consisting of anxiety, dysphoria, malaise, depersonalization and perceptual changes such as hyperacusis and unsteadiness (Pettursson and Lader 1981): see Chapter 1.

Treatment consists in progressive dose reduction and supportive follow up. Benzodiazepines should not be routinely prescribed for a period in excess of 8 weeks.

Benzodiazepines may be useful in the treatment of alcohol withdrawal, but they should not generally be prescribed for alcoholics outside this specific treatment situation.

Methaqualone

This drug, developed as an antimalarial, has anxiolytic, anticonvulsant, local anaesthetic, antihistaminic and hypnotic properties. It accumulates after repeated usage and may produce psychological and physical dependence. In the drug-taking subculture it is mixed with alcohol as it is claimed to produce a pleasant sensation (Editorial 1973). The mixture, however, may be lethal (Ostrenga 1973), as alcohol seems to reduce the excretion of the drug (Whitehouse et al. 1977). It is marketed in a combination with diphenhydramine as 'Mandrax'. Withdrawal symptoms are similar to those of alcohol. Treatment is by progressive reduction of the drug and supportive psychotherapy.

Amphetamines and Amphetamine-like Drugs

These stimulant drugs exert their action on the cerebral cortex and the reticular activating system. Their short-term effects are euphoria, a sense of well-being, excitement, restlessness, tachycardia, sleeplessness and, occasional-ly, nausea and anorexia. In the long term they may produce a severe psychosis and stereotyped motor behaviour (Connell 1958; Kiloh and Brandon 1962; Rylander 1972; Janowski and Risch 1979). Such a psychosis may be difficult to differentiate from a schizophrenic illness and usually responds to neuroleptics.

Psychological dependence is a major problem, while tolerance develops rapidly and it is not uncommon to find subjects taking up to 500 mg daily. The main withdrawal symptoms are dysphoria, depression and fatigue, and the treatment of severe amphetamine addiction should be carried out in hospital. The drug should be withdrawn abruptly and no medication is required. Moral support and special attention to the mood disorder that often develops in the wake of withdrawal are important. The clinical indications for amphetamines (or related drugs) are rare and its usage in depressive illness is controversial.

Hallucinogens (Fuxe et al. 1976)

D-Lysergic acid diethylamide (LSD) is a potent hallucinogenic agent and may produce acute toxic states as well as prolonged psychotic reactions (Bowers 1977). LSD may produce other distortions of perception such as illusions, and can also affect thought processes, leading to impaired train of thought, as well as to emotional changes. These may include euphoria, anxiety and terror.

The treatment depends on the effect of 'the trip'. Observation in a safe environment is often sufficient; sometimes benzodiazepines are necessary to relieve anxiety, and neuroleptics may be indicated to control the psychotic symptoms. 'Flashbacks' (i.e. the recurrence of psychotic symptoms without the subject having taken the drug) occur occasionally. The aetiology of these phenomena is unknown, but see Alarcon et al. (1982).

Opioid Substances

Stimson (1973) distinguished four types of addicts attending the London clinics, showing that any stereotyping or generalization about the opioid substance addict is inappropriate. Although the so-called British System (i.e. the free prescribing for registered users), afforded some protection to addicts, there is still a high risk of physical disease and accidental death (Sapira 1968; Thornton and Thornton 1974). Also, the association of this kind of drug addiction with depression and other psychiatric syndromes is high. Less clear is the association between crime and drug taking, as opioids reduce aggression and sexual drive. Nonetheless, burglary and assault in males, and prostitution in females, may be undertaken as a means of obtaining supplies of drugs.

The prognosis of opioid substance addicts is not good. Stimson et al. (1978), in a follow-up study of young heroin addicts attending London clinics, found that, 7 years later, 48% were still using drugs (43% being registered), 12% were dead, while only 32% were abstinent.

Heroin and morphine are the commonest substances abused. The former has greater lipid solubility and crosses the blood–brain barrier without difficulty; hence it is preferred by addicts, who can distinguish it from morphine when given intravenously.

In spite of regular intravenous administration, some pharmacological effects (e.g. miosis) do not show tolerance and hence can be used as indicators of recent usage. The withdrawal state is usually stereotyped, and presents 8–12 h after the last dose with sweating, yawning, rhinorrhea and lacrimation; after 12–14 h drowsiness and hypersomnia develop. After sleeping for a few hours, the addict may then feel worse and exhibit tremor, marked irritability, an excited state, confusion, anorexia and midriasis; after about 72 h the full-blown syndrome may start, which can involve insomnia, sneezing, total anorexia, nausea, vomiting, intestinal spasm, diarrhoea, increased pulse and blood pressure, prominent goose-flesh (cold turkey), changes in temperature, and violent muscle spasms, (i.e. 'kicking the habit'). Ejaculation in males and orgasm in women may occasionally occur.

The combination of these symptoms leads to medical complications such as dehydration, ketosis, disturbed electrolytic balance and, occasionally, cardiovascular collapse.

Treatment . Withdrawal should take place in hospital or in a specialized unit where personality, degree of dependence and motivation can be properly assessed.

The need for methadone to treat the withdrawal symptoms should be regularly assessed, but methadone should not routinely be prescribed. A suitable regimen for relatively less severe withdrawal syndromes may be methadone 60–80 mg daily, orally or intramuscularly, which is reduced over a period of about 8 days by increments of 10 mg daily. Clonidine also reduces opiate withdrawal symptoms (Gold 1978).

In relatively severe cases of heroin addiction, methadone should still be the drug of choice, and the daily (oral) dose is calculated on the basis of 1 mg methadone = 1 mg heroin. The dose regimen must be discussed with the patient, and should involve gradual discontinuation over 2–3 weeks. No other drugs are needed during detoxification except moderate doses of benzodiazepines for anxiety and insomnia.

In the long term, the only realistic goal is total abstinence together with personality growth and maturation. To achieve this, a number of treatments has been tried, such as the 'therapeutic community' approach, which demands total abstinence and a long-term in-patient stay of perhaps 18–24 months. No data are available for either the numbers of those who stay for the whole treatment or for those who remain abstinent for at least 5 years.

Long-term 'maintenance' on methadone is unsatisfactory as it is just another way of delaying the decision to give up opioids and to face personal conflicts and difficulties. However, long-term prescription of a modest dose of methadone may be the appropriate management for a small number of individuals who are otherwise unable to cope. In such cases, the clinician may be able to 'use' methadone replacement as a compromise during which a therapeutic relationship can be developed. The goal of abstinence can then be pursued with more chance of success.

A therapeutic relationship is crucial to management and is often difficult to achieve. Patients dependent on opioids usually place strong pressure on the clinician, who should be particularly aware of his own ways of dealing with patients' inappropriate demands.

References

ALARCON, R.D. et al. (1982) Flashback phenomena. *J. nerv. ment. Dis.*, **170**, 217.

ANON (1981) What GPs can do for problem drinkers. *Drug. Ther. Bull.*, **19:23**, 89.

ARMOR, D.J., POLICH, J.M. & STAMBUL, H.B. (1976) *Alcoholism and Treatment.* Santa Monica, California: Rand Corporation.

ARROYAVE, F. & MCKEOWN, S. (1979) Controlled drinking—a perspective. *Br. J. hosp. Med.*, **22**, 604.

ARROYAVE, F., MCKEOWN, S. & COOPER, S. (1980) Detoxification—an approach to developing a comprehensive alcoholism service. *Br. J. Addiction*, **75**, 187.

BALSANO, N.A. & REYNOLDS, B.M. (1970) Fluid restriction in the management of acute alcoholic withdrawal. *Surgery*, **68**, 283.

BOWERS, M.B. (1977) Psychoses precipitated by psychotomimetic drugs. *Archs gen. Psychiat.*, **34**, 832.

BREWER, C. & PERRETT, L. (1971) Brain damage due to alcohol consumption: an air-encephalographic, psychometric and E.E.G. study. *Br. J. Addiction*, **66**, 170.

BROWN, S. & YALOM, I.D. (1977) Interactional group therapy with alcoholics. *J. Stud. Alcohol*, **38**, 426.

CARLSSON, C. et al. (1979) Clinical, psychometric and radiological signs of brain damage in chronic alcoholism. *Acta Neurol. Scand.*, **60**, 85.

CARTWRIGHT, A.K.J. & SHAW, S.J. (1978) Trends in the epidemiology of alcoholism. *Psychol. Med.*, **8**, 1.

COID, J. (1979) Mania a potu: a critical review of pathological intoxication. *Psychol. Med.*, **9**, 707.

COLLIER, H.O.J. (1966) Tolerance, physical dependence and receptors. *Adv. Drug. Res.*, **3**, 171.

CONNELL, P.H. (1958) *Amphetamine Psychosis*, Maudsley Monograph No. 5. Chapman and Hall, London: Oxford University Press.

CURRY, S.H. (1980) *Drug Disposition and Pharmacokinetics.* Oxford: Blackwell Scientific Publication.

CUTTING, J. (1978) A reappraisal of alcoholic psychoses. *Psychol. Med.*, **8**, 285.

EDITORIAL (1973) Mixing mandrax and alcohol. *Br. med. J.*, **ii**, 45.

EL GUEBALY, N. & OFFORD, D.R. (1977) The offspring of alcoholics: a critical review. *Am. J. Psychiat.*, **134**, 357.

ESSIG, C.F. (1967) Clinical and experimental aspects of barbiturate withdrawal convulsions. *Epilepsy*, **8**, 21.

FINNEY, J.W. & MOOS, R.H. (1979) Treatment and outcome for empirical subtypes of alcoholic patients. *J. consult. clin. Psychol.*, **47**, 25.

FISHMAN, J. (ed.) (1978) *The Bases of Addiction.* Berlin: Abakon.

FREED, E.X. (1975) Alcoholism and schizophrenia. *J. Stud. Alcohol*, **36**, 853.

FUXE, K. et al. (1976) On the biochemistry and pharmacology of hallucinogens. In: *Schizophrenia Today*, ed. Kemali, D. et al. Oxford: Pergamon Press.

GARDNER, A.J. (1967) Withdrawal fits in barbiturate addicts. *Lancet*, **ii**, 337.

GAULT, F.P. (1976) A review of recent literature in barbiturate addiction and withdrawal. *Bol. Stud. Med. Biol.*, **29**, 75.

GITLOW, S.E. (1980) *Alcoholism. A Practical Treatment Guide.* Ed. Gitlow, S.E. & Peyser, H.S. New York: Grune & Stratton.

GOLD, M.E. (1978) Clonidine blocks acute opiate-withdrawal symptoms. *Lancet,* **ii,** 599.

GOODWIN, D.W. (1979) Alcoholism and heredity. *Archs gen. Psychiat.,* **36,** 57.

HAMBURG, S. (1975) Behavior therapy in alcoholics. A critical review of broad spectrum approaches. *J. Stud. Alcohol.,* **36:1,** 69.

HEATHER, N. & ROBERTSON, I. (1981) *Controlled Drinking.* London: Methuen.

HEMMINGSEN, R. et al. (1979) Delirium tremens and related clinical states. *Acta psychiat. scand.,* **59,** 337.

HOLT, S. et al. (1980) Alcohol and the emergency service patient. *Br. med. J.,* **281,** 638.

JANOWSKI, D.S. & RISCH, C. (1979) Amphetamine psychosis and psychotic symptoms. *Psychopharmacology,* **65,** 73.

JARIWALLA, A.G., ADAMS, P.H. & HORE (1979) Alcohol and acute general medical admissions to hospital. *Health Trends,* **II,** 95.

JELLINEK, E.M. (1960) *The Disease Concept of Alcoholism.* New Haven: Hill House Press.

KELLER, M. (1972) On the loss-of-control phenomenon in alcoholism. *Br. J. Addiction,* **67,** 153.

KELLER, M. (1976) The disease concept of alcoholism revisited. *J. Stud. Alc.,* **37,** 1694.

KILOH, L.G. & BRANDON, S. (1962) Habituation and addiction to Amphetamines. *Br. med. J.,* **ii,** 40.

KORSAKOFF, S.S. (1887) (Quoted in Victor et al. 1971, q.v.)

LEBACHS, W. (1975) Cirrhosis in the alcoholic and its relation to the volume of alcohol abuse. *Ann. N.Y. Acad. Sci.,* **252,** 85.

LEE, K. (1979) Alcoholism and cerebrovascular thrombosis in the young. *Acta neurol. scand.,* **59,** 270.

LLOYD, R.W. & SALZBERG, H.C. (1975) Controlled social drinking: an alternative to abstinence as a treatment goal for some alcohol abusers. *Psychol. Bull.,* **82,** 817.

MAJOR, L.F. et al. (1979) The role of plasma amine oxidase, platelet monoamine oxidase and red cell catechol-*o*-methyl transferase in severe behavioural reactions to Disulfiram. *Am. J. Psychiat.,* **136,** 679.

MORGAN, R. & CAGAN, E.J. (1974) Acute alcoholic intoxication, the disulfiram reaction and methyl alcohol intoxication. In: *Biology of Alcoholism,* vol. 3, ed. Kissin, B., & Begleiter, H. New York: Plenum Press.

OSTRENGA, J.A. (1973) Methaqualone. *Clin. Toxicol.,* **6,** 607.

PARTANEN, J. et al. (1966) *Inheritance of drinking behaviour: a Study on Intelligence, Personality and Use of Alcohol of adult twins,* pp. 14–159. Helsinki: Finnish Foundation for Alcohol Studies.

PATON, A. & SAUNDERS, J.B. (1981) ABC of alcohol. *Br. med. J.,* 283, 1248 and 1458.

PENDERY, M.L. et al. (1982) Controlled drinking by alcoholics. *Science,* **217,** 169.

PETTURSSON, H. & LADER, M.H. (1981) Benzodiazepine dependence. *Br. J. Addiction,* **76,** 133.

RAINEY, J.M. (1977) Disulfiram toxicity and carbon disulfide poisoning. *Am. J. Psychiat.,* **134,** 371.

REISBERG, B. (1978) Catatonia associated with disulfiram therapy. *J. ner. ment. Dis.,* **166,** 607.

RON, M.A. (1977) Brain damage in chronic alcoholism. *Psychol. Med.,* **7,** 103.

ROYAL COLLEGE OF PSYCHIATRISTS (1979) *Report of a Special Committee on Alcohol and Alcoholism.* London: Tavistock.

RYLANDER, G. (1972) Psychoses and the punding and choreiform syndromes in addiction to central stimulant drugs. *Psychiat. Neurol. Neurochir.,* **75,** 203.

SALUM, I. (1975) Treatment of delirium tremens. *Br. J. Addiction,* **70,** (Conference Suppl.) 75.

SAPIRA, J.D. (1968) The Narcotic addict as a medical patient. *Am. J. Med.,* **45,** 555.

SAUNDERS, J.B. et al. (1981) Do women develop alcoholic liver disease more readily than men? *Br. med. J.,* **i,** 1140.

SCHUCKIT, M. (1980) Alcoholism Treatment in Transition. In: *Alcoholism. New Knowledge and New Responses,* ed. Edwards, G., and Grant, M. London: Croom Helm.

SMITH, R. (1981*a*) Treating alcohol problems: making ends meet. *Br. med. J.,* **283,** 1043.

SMITH, R. (1981*b*) The habitual drunken offender: everybody's fool, nobody's friend. *Br. med. J.,* **283,** 1251.

SMITH, R. (1981*c*) Alcohol and work: a promising approach. *Br. med. J.,* **283,** 1108.

SOBELL, M.B. & SOBELL, L.C. (1973) Individualized behaviour therapy for alcoholics. *Behav. Ther.,* **4,** 49.

SOBELL, M.B. & SOBELL, L.C. (1976) Second year treatment outcome of alcoholics treated by individualized behaviour therapy results. *Behav. Res. Ther.,* **14,** 195.

STEVENS, B.C. (1978) Deaths of drug addicts in London during 1970–74. *Med. Sci. Law*, **18**, 128.

STIMSON, G.V. (1973) *Heroin and Behaviour: Diversity Amongst Addicts Attending London Clinics*. New York: John Wiley.

STIMSON, G.V. et al. (1978) Seven years follow up of heroin addicts: drug use and outcome. *Br. med. J.*, **i**, 1190.

TARTER, R.E. (1975) Psychological deficit in chronic alcoholics: a review. *Int. J. Addiction*, **10**, 327.

THORNTON, W.E. & THORNTON, B.P.(1974) Narcotic poisoning. *Am. J. Psychiat.*, **131**, 867.

VICTOR, M. et al. (1971) *The Wernicke-Korsakoff Syndrome Vol. 7 Contemporary Neurology Series*. Philadelphia: F.A. Davis.

VICTOR, M. & WOLFE, S.M. (1973) Causation and treatment of the alcohol withdrawal syndrome. In: *Alcoholism*, ed. Bourne, P.G. & Fox, R. London: Academic Press.

WERNICKE, C. (1881) *Lehrbuch der Gehirnkrankheiten Vol. 2*, pp. 229–242. Kassel: Fischer.

WHITEHOUSE, L.W. et al. (1977) Effect of ethanol on the pharmacokinetics of 2-14-c Methaqualone. *Life Sci.*, **20**, 1871.

WIKLER, A. (1968) Diagnosis and treatment of drug dependence of the barbiturate type. *Am. J. Psychiat.*, **125**, 758.

WILLEMS, P.J., LETEMENDIA, F.J. & ARROYAVE, F. (1973) A categorization for the assessment of prognosis and outcome in the treatment of alcoholism. *Br. J. Psychiat.*, **122**, 649.

WILLIAMS, P. (1980) Recent trends in the prescribing of psychotropic drugs. *Health Trends*, **12**, 6.

WILSON, A. (1975) Disulfiram implantation in alcoholism treatment: a review. *J. Stud. Alcohol.* **36**, 555.

WINOKUR, G. et al. (1970) Alcoholism III: diagnosis and familial psychiatric illness in 259 alcoholic probands. *Archs gen. Psychiat.*, **23**, 104.

WOODS, J.H. (1978) Behavioural pharmacology of drug self-administration. In: *Psychopharmacology: A Generation of Progress*, ed. Lipton, M.A. et al., p. 595. New York: Raven Press.

WORLD HEALTH ORGANIZATION (1978) *Mental Disorders: Glossary and Guide to Their Classification in Accordance with ICD-9*.

WULFF, M.H. (1959) The barbiturate withdrawal syndrome: a clinical and E.E.G. study. *Electroenceph. Clin. Neurophysiol.*, (Suppl. 14).

21

Management of Eating Disorders

N.J.R. Evans

ANOREXIA NERVOSA

Description

Anorexia nervosa is regarded as a distinct syndrome by most authorities. It consists of a triad of persistent refusal to eat leading to emaciation, an endocrine disorder manifested typically as amenorrhoea in females, and a psychopathological syndrome (considered as characteristic by some) which involves an abnormal attitude to the patient's own body weight, size and shape. The latter has been conceptualized as a phobia of body weight and regarded as the central feature (Crisp 1967). The case reports of Gull (1874), who proposed the name of 'anorexia nervosa' are still pertinent, while detailed information relating to signs and symptoms, background factors, cause, treatment and outcome is available in several British series (Kay and Leigh 1954; Morgan and Russell 1975; Dally and Gomez 1979; Crisp et al. 1980). Theander's (1970) study reported a Swedish series, and an American view was given by Bruch (1974a).

The syndrome is uncommon in males so that when it does occur, the diagnosis may be missed. Besides the triad already mentioned, other common psychological features include an overconscientious personality, rather poor sexual adjustment and a depressive syndrome which may lead to suicide. Also, there seems to be a high incidence of stealing, which is unexpected if the background and personality of many of these patients is taken into consideration. The behaviour employed to keep weight down may involve severe dieting and various methods of concealing or disposing of food, self-induced vomiting, purging, and taking excessive exercise. It has been claimed that there is a subgroup (Beumont et al. 1976) in which episodic overeating and vomiting, named by Russell (1979) 'bulimia nervosa', is correlated with a later onset, better sexual development, but a more prolonged and stormy course. However, this may simply be an outcome variant. Physical complications of the starvation include endocrine abnormalities, while cardiac dysfunction, and the electrolyte disturbances in vomiters and purgers, may constitute an immediate threat to life. Anorexia nervosa should be differentiated from loss of appetite, poor eating and weight loss arising in the course of a physical illness or of a psychiatric disorder such as a severe depressive syndrome.

The aetiology of anorexia nervosa is not known, and there is no specific remedy. It has long been held to have a psychological origin, and recent reviews of the endocrine abnormalities did not challenge this view (Beumont 1979; Isaacs 1979), although rare cases of hypothalamic tumours associated with the syndrome have been reported (Lewin et al. 1972; BMJ 1973). However, it is known that amenorrhoea can develop in response to psychological stress, and may present, in anorexia nervosa, before significant weight loss has developed. Some of the features of anorexia may seem understandable in terms of the adolescent's struggle for independence, as a reaction against emotional conflicts within a family, as a response to the fashionable demands for slimness or a retreat from sexuality, but such understandability need not constitute a causal explanation. Although certain characteristics of modern society have been considered to be causal, the syndrome has been clearly described as early as the seventeenth century. However, its incidence appears to be increasing (Kendell et al. 1973; Crisp et al. 1976). While it is possible to adopt a theoretical view of both essential and non-essential causal factors on which to base treatment, a purely eclectic approach appears justifiable in the light of present knowledge.

Management

It can be seen that there are likely to be many physical and psychological features which require intervention, and the practice of such authors as Crisp (1965) and Russell (1970) has been generally accepted in the UK, where there is broad agreement over the strategy to be adopted. Previously, there was a trend for more intensive medical measures, exemplified by Dally and Sargant (1960), which developed partly because the treatments became available, but also because, as Kay and Leigh (1954) put it, 'the time-honoured treatment, by persuasion and meticulous supervision of the patient's diet, practised so successfully by earlier physicians, has in recent years been found less satisfactory'.

The Initial Interview

Management begins with a careful interview with the patient, and then with other informants, usually the parents, in order to collect enough information to make the individual formulation on which the details of management will depend. This may be difficult because the patient is commonly unwilling and claims that nothing is wrong. A young patient may defend herself with the brittle obstinacy of immaturity, while the visit to the psychiatrist is often the last resort, following months or years of strife at home. In spite of this, it may be possible to gain her confidence at this crucial stage, and every effort should be made to do so. Both the patient and the doctor may find advantages in making a 'contract' in which she agrees to put on weight and the doctor promises to do his utmost to help with the emotional problems as they arise.

Treatment has two aims; the restoration of normal weight and eating, and the amelioration of mental symptoms and environmental disturbance. The first may be urgent while the second may need long-term intervention.

Out-Patient or In-Patient Treatment?

A decision has to be made as to whether in-patient admission is required. As the disorder has a spectrum of severity, straightforward discussion and advice may be sufficient for mild or early cases but, as a rule, the disorders reaching psychiatrists are relatively severe, and textbooks often recommend admission (Slater and Roth 1969). However, some of the reported series show that admission is not, by any means, inevitable; nine of Kanis's (1974) series of 24 were treated as out-patients, and so were 31 out of Crisp's (1980) series of 102.

Admission may prove valuable by removing the patient from an environment which is invariably an emotional battlefield, and many patients accept the suggestion with relief. If admission is indicated, it is often prudent to arrange this immediately, in case the patient should change her mind on returning home. The possible indications for admission include degree of emaciation, other physical consequences, suicidal intent and unsatisfactory home circumstances.

If the patient is not gravely ill, the case for a trial of out-patient management is made more reasonable if she is older and more mature, or is living in surroundings which are not highly charged with emotion, which is usually away from the parental home. Many (but certainly not all) patients are unreliable and uncooperative, and it is sensible to persuade the patient to agree to be admitted to hospital if, after a stated period of a few weeks, a predetermined weight gain has not been achieved.

Compulsion

Compulsory admission and treatment under Section 26 of the UK Mental Health Act of an unwilling patient at grave risk of her (or his) life seems fully justifiable and may be the only possible course of action. However, this is rarely necessary.

Psychiatric or Medical Ward

A patient who is at risk of her life and requires intensive intravenous therapy and frequent monitoring to restore electrolyte balance may need general hospital facilities, as may a patient who steadfastly refuses to go into a psychiatric ward but who agrees to enter a medical ward. An immature teenager may be at an awkward age for the available psychiatric facilities, if this involves a choice between an adult psychiatric ward with highly disturbed and disturbing patients and an adolescent unit with minimal provision for medical care. In this situation a medical ward is a more satisfactory option, and a large general hospital may have part of a ward which usually accommodates a certain number of these patients, if referrals are sufficiently frequent. The essential requirement is that the staff of whatever ward it may be are skilled and experienced in handling these often difficult patients, who may be manipulative and resourceful in deception. However, a general medical ward may not be able to provide 'special nursing' in the midst of the unpredictable and urgent requirements of the other patients.

Physical Investigation

Many authors refer to investigations, for example, Crisp (1965) advocated 2 weeks of psychiatric observation and physical investigation, but there are no detailed suggestions. The extent of the investigations will naturally depend on the history and examination, but as misdiagnosed cases seem to be rare, the main aim will not be towards unearthing a latent physical disorder, but rather establishing the extent and effects of starvation. The results may have direct practical implications for salt and water replacement.

In-Patient Regimen

The patients who are admitted to hospital will be mainly those whose weight loss is severe, whose effective food intake is very small and who have a variety of other problems; the regimens which are usually described are appropriate for such cases. It is a mistaken kindness to refrain from an attempt to exert firm control, as by the time of admission there are likely to have been many failures and it is important for the patient's morale that further interventions succeed from the outset. Curiously, many patients are amenable to firm instructions and encouragement despite much uncooperative behaviour.

A target weight is fixed and the patient is encouraged to stay in hospital at least until it is attained and, initially, the patient may be confined to bed. The target weight should be in the 'normal' range, taking into account age, height and 'frame'; an appropriate weight can be determined by consulting tables. This procedure may be perceived as unreasonable, but if the patient's stated premorbid weight is selected as a target, this may have been low or even excessive, and the information may be unreliable. The patient should be weighed at irregular intervals, approximately twice weekly, and the time of weighing should be varied as some patients might drink excessive amounts of fluid beforehand if they knew when the weighing was due to take place.

The 'diet' is normal amounts of ordinary food; high-calorie preparations are normally unnecessary and do not rehearse conditions in everyday life. Some patients have food 'fads' and compromises over content may have to be made, but it will be necessary to include high-carbohydrate foods such as bread, potatoes and rice; patients with anorexia are often extremely averse to these substances, probably because they are generally considered 'fattening'. The total daily intake should be between 3000 and 5000 calories in order to achieve a satisfactory weight gain of 1–2 kg per week. It is prudent to increase the food intake gradually over a week or two, explaining that the increases will then stop. The patient should be encouraged to eat everything that is given to her, and arguments over, for instance, the precise number of potatoes, are not entered into; it will soon be apparent to her that she is not presented with any surprises. It is the general experience that most anorexic patients can be encouraged and persuaded, by skilled and patient nursing, to eat what is required, and that nasogastric tube feeding is seldom needed. The nurse remains with her throughout each meal and tries to ensure that all is eaten, no matter how long it takes. In this way there is little chance for the patient to conceal the food and dispose of it later, and control is strengthened if the patient is initially put to bed; certainly she should be persuaded not to take excessive exercise.

Perhaps the most difficult practical problem is the control of regurgitation or vomiting, especially if it is claimed to be involuntary. Some patients eat their meals readily but secretly induce vomiting soon after; in such cases, careful supervision between meals is necessary if the patient is not gaining weight, despite adequate food intake. The advice of Dally and Gomez (1979) to let the patient know that anything vomited will have to be eaten again may not be generally accepted and, in any case, cannot be enforced.

The patient may need to be in hospital for periods up to 2 or 3 months, during which the framework of this management is filled in with other treatment, which can be considered under the broad headings of psychotherapy, behaviour therapy and medical treatment. The scheme described by Silverman (1974) illustrates the combination of a strict regimen for the control of eating with provision of four weekly sessions of psychotherapy.

Psychotherapy

Insofar as most anorexic patients have manifest neurotic symptoms, prominent mental conflicts and disturbed relationships with other people, they may be considered eligible for whatever psychotherapy is available. However, the degree of malnutrition is associated with the severity of some of the psychological components of the syndrome, so that successful refeeding may render the patient more susceptible to psychotherapeutic measures.

Intensive psychotherapy based on psychoanalytic principles or on the theory that anorexia nervosa stems from oral impregnation fantasies (Waller et al.

1940) has not been successful and, after reviewing much psychoanalytic literature, Bemis (1978) found that psychoanalytically based treatment 'has proven singularly ineffectual'. Other conceptual frameworks for intensive psychotherapy which aim at fundamental reconstruction of the personality have been evolved by, for example, Selvini (1965) and Bruch (1974a), who have claimed that successful outcome can be the result of intensive psychotherapy. However, the problem of the lack of controls on such studies makes it impossible to answer such simple questions as whether there is any correlation between outcome and time invested in psychotherapy.

Group psychotherapy does not appear to have been advocated as a specific treatment for anorexia nervosa, but some patients may benefit. A good many, however, are particularly reserved and find any public disclosure painful, and it is unwise to exert pressure for such patients to participate in group therapy for such reasons as 'ward policy'.

'Family therapy' encompasses a wide range of interventions, from the normal medical practice of doing what one can to support the family with an ill member, to a sociological reconsideration of who should be the patient (Laing 1960), or making family interviews the focus of treatment (Howells 1976). A thorough assessment of current family relationships should be made. This may involve the patient's parents and siblings, or, if the patient has married and left the parental home, the relationship with the spouse may be particularly relevant. The value of attempting to modify family relationships varies, and this should not routinely form the focus of treatment; but, if obvious problems are present, an attempt to resolve current difficulties is often indicated. However, even if part of the family may seem to have contributed to the development of the syndrome, there is a danger of putting the 'blame' on the family on the basis of unproven hypotheses regarding the aetiology of this disorder. Medical approval should not be given to theories of the causes of an anorexia nervosa if they are liable to produce guilt and distress in the patient's family.

Behaviour Therapy

The abnormal fears, perceptions and eating behaviour in anorexia nervosa are a challenge to behaviour therapists. Three important questions are: Does a behavioural programme facilitate feeding? Does it have a long-lasting effect on eating behaviour? and Does it influence other aspects of the psychopathology? It is relatively easy to undertake behavioural treatment programmes on one or two patients, and reports abound, but it is difficult to assemble a group of comparable subjects, and the organization of a prospective controlled trial requires a formidable effort. Consequently, answers to these questions are not easy to find.

The routine refeeding regimen has characteristics which can easily be structured into an operant conditioning programme: thus, if there are initial restrictions such as being confined to bed, or having limited activities, these are lifted in a series of steps which are made contingent on achieving desired results, such as eating meals or putting on weight. In theory, reinforcements should be early rather than delayed, so that desired eating behaviour would seem suitable for reward but, in practice, weekly weight gain is usually the target for reinforcement. This is a better indication of progress, as it is much less vulnerable to dispute and subterfuge. Bhanji and Thompson (1974), who followed up 11 patients for unusually long periods (the average was 34 months), described a regimen in which rewards were contingent on eating a certain number of meals within specified times, while Blinder et al. (1970) gave permission to carry out physical activity which was contingent on a daily weight gain. Halmi et al. (1975) used a variety of privileges which had to be earned by weight gain, which was monitored every 5 days (their eight patients were not given other treatment, unlike some of those in Bhanji and Thompson's study). Other studies have been reviewed by Bemis (1978). In a rare controlled study (Eckert et al. 1979), 81 patients were randomly assigned to operant conditioning or ward milieu treatment, and there was no significant difference in immediate outcome between the groups. Most authorities seem to agree that achieving a normal weight is relatively easy in comparison with maintaining the improvement and modifying the psychological component of the syndrome. Unfortunately, lack of long-term follow-up studies, and the errors inherent in comparing groups selected from different sources, prevent any definite inference that behavioural treatment influences the outcome. But many clinicians believe that careful analysis of behaviour, and the use of behavioural principles in designing each treatment programme, does contribute to the practical management of these patients, particularly if they are in-patients.

It should also be mentioned that it is important to obtain full consent from the patient for programmes involving deprivation (Bruch 1974b).

Medical Treatment

A drug may be used to alleviate anxiety, especially in connection with meals, and a safe tranquillizer such as a benzodiazepine is suitable. Sedation with a major tranquillizer may be necessary in the rare instance when a patient is compulsorily detained in hospital because her life is in imminent danger, but the routine use of relatively high doses of chlorpromazine is unnecessary as this seems to have no specific effect on weight gain, and side effects are to be expected. However, many clinicians still advocate a modest dose of chlorpromazine (i.e. up to 100 mg daily) which may assist weight gain. The 'modified insulin' regimen, described by Dally and Sargant (1960), has not been shown to have a specific effect on eating or weight gain, and seems to have fallen into disuse.

If a patient is depressed, or becomes depressed during admission, then antidepressant treatment should be considered. The routine use of a tricyclic in all patients depends on various hypothesis (Lopez Ibor 1972; Mills 1976), but there is some evidence that neurotic depressive syndromes, even without an underlying manic–depressive psychosis, may benefit from tricyclics, although in general the results are, at best, modest. If the depression is coloured with obsessive–compulsive features, clomipramine may be of special value. If depressive symptoms are prominent, a trial with a tricyclic or other antidepressant may be indicated, but their routine use is not recommended.

The occasional patient who proves completely resistant to treatment, whose life is in constant danger, and particularly if she has a range of other severe neurotic symptoms, may be considered for psychosurgery. Crisp and Kalucy (1973) presented four of their patients (out of a series of 250) who had had a leucotomy, and discussed possible psychological as well as physical reasons for the results. These authors concluded that 'leucotomy has a small but definite place in the treatment of patients with intractable anorexia nervosa'.

Space does not allow a consideration of all the treatments which have been tried and abandoned, but it is worth mentioning that appetite stimulants, such as cyproheptadine hydrochloride, which has some appetite stimulating properties in the organically ill, do not work in anorexia nervosa; steroids and other hormones have not helped, but some patients whose menses do not return when they reach normal weight may be reassured by the induction of ovulation with clomiphene (Marshall and Russell Fraser 1971). This is said to be useful if the patient wishes to conceive, but one would be cautious in encouraging the responsibility of parenthood soon after a major psychological disturbance. Various agents which have actions on the hypothalamus are of theoretical interest in anorexia, but bromocriptine has not been found to assist weight gain (Harrower 1977, 1978).

Long-Term Support

Reports of outcome after long-term out-patient treatment tend to be uncontrolled because it is virtually impossible from an ethical viewpoint to allocate patients known to be suffering from a chronic condition to a 'no treatment' group. It is to be assumed that there may be benefit in continuing to see some of these patients for out-patient psychotherapy, usually for years, but it is not known if this prevents relapse. Correlations of clinical and family factors with outcome have not yielded practical implications for treatment.

Summary

Hsu (1980) reviewed the long-term outcome of 16 studies and concluded that 'the effects of treatment cannot be gauged at present'. However, it is clear that in the short- and medium-term, a great deal can be done to improve the symptoms of anorexia nervosa, and to alleviate concomitant neurotic symptoms and social or family difficulties. Occasionally, admission to hospital to encourage weight gain is a life-saving procedure, but there is a wide range of severity for this syndrome; many patients never present to the medical services while, for others, short-term problem-orientated out-patient psychotherapy is all that is indicated.

OBESITY AND OVEREATING

Introduction

Obesity has to be defined arbitrarily, either as a certain degree of excessive body weight, or of excessive body fat. Reference tables of sex, height, 'frame' and weight give 'ideal' weights from the point of view of life expectancy: those of the Metropolitan Life Insurance Company of New York are frequently used. Skinfold thickness measurement gives an indication of the quantity of body fat; its relation to other measures was examined by Womersley and Durnin (1977).

The superficial cause of obesity is an excess of energy intake over energy expenditure. Definable organic disorders which predispose to a disturbance of this balance, such as hypothyroidism or hypothalamic lesions, are relatively uncommon (Bray and Gallagher 1975), but it is an everyday observation that some healthy people eat well, exercise little and remain thin, while others, equally healthy, eat sparingly and have a constant tendency to get fat. The source of these variations remains elusive, but a promising field for investigation is non-shivering thermogenesis by brown adipose tissue, recently reviewed by Jung and James (1980). There is an association between obesity and lower social class, which may be mediated by a cheap, easily prepared diet which is heavy with sugar, starch and fat, but some evidence suggests that the eating habits of many obese individuals are not significantly different from those of the non-obese (Ries 1973; Adams et al. 1978; Leon and Roth 1977). In addition, it has been well established that there are wide variations in individual energy expenditure (Edholm et al. 1955). The whole subject of energy balance, and the weaknesses of theories of its regulation, has been discussed by Garrow (1978).

In rough proportion to the degree of obesity are the associated disadvantages, both social and medical, which include increased morbidity from various diseases including diabetes, cardiovascular disorders, gall-bladder disease and osteoarthritis. In addition, obesity is associated with increased risks in surgery and childbirth.

The majority of severely obese patients show no psychiatric aetiology and, in contrast to anorexia nervosa, there is no special psychopathology. Although the non-random selection of subjects has produced some series with a high prevalence of mental disturbance, there are surveys conducted in general practice (Silverstone 1968) or in the general population (Crisp and McGuinness 1976), which find no such excess. On the other hand, there are many patients, whether obese or not, who have a neurotic pattern of overeating, sometimes followed by vomiting, which briefly assuages unpleasant feelings. This behaviour is commonly described by patients as 'compulsive', though it is usually different from obsessive–compulsive symptoms in that the behaviour provides gratification. It has been considered to be a correlate of excessive emotional dependence on others (Russell 1976), anxiety or depressive neurosis or even, on occasions, as a result of a sensitivity to an anticonvulsant (Green and Rao 1974). Also, bulimia and periods of obesity are sometimes encountered in anorexia nervosa.

Management

The energy balance must be altered in order to lose weight at an acceptable rate, but even the 0.5–1 kg per week which most authorities recognize as a desired result appears painfully slow to many patients. The time required for losing 10–20 kilograms, which is a common target, is many months of sustained effort. The patient must be aware of the expected rate of weight loss, and be prepared to make a permanent change in dietary habits. Increasing energy output by taking more exercise often has many indirect benefits, but this usually has only a small effect on weight. Increasing energy output by accelerating metabolism with drugs, notably thyroid hormones, has fallen into disrepute, except in the investigation of starvation-induced metabolic changes (Moore et al. 1980); there remains an unconfirmed suspicion that some appetite-suppressant drugs may also have a peripheral metabolic action.

Diet

There is no consensus on the best way to bring about a reduction in energy intake, and common sense asserts that different people with different personalities, habits and circumstances will find some methods more successful than others. Although most patients who seek medical advice about obesity will have tried dieting on their own, and perhaps have joined a 'slimmers' organisation, it does not follow that further dieting with medical supervision is hopeless. But it must be admitted that, in the long term, only a small number of patients maintain large losses (Binnie 1977; Craddock 1977). Craddock's monograph (1973) gave a collection of diets and much practical advice. No single diet will be universally helpful, but it is likely that many patients are confused by a wide choice. It is the responsibility of the doctor to assess each patient before making definite recommendations; some may succeed with the Marriott (1949) type of diet (i.e. 'eat as much as you want of everything except...'), as some individuals can lose weight by altering the pattern of eating, without resort to a relatively low calorie intake; but, for most people, a strict diet entails a daily intake of about 1000 calories.

Drugs

Amphetamine and phenmetrazine should not be prescribed for obesity because of the danger of addiction. Anorectic drugs such as phentermine, mazindol, diethylpropion and fenfluramine can assist adherence to a diet, but such drugs must always be part of a management plan which includes dietary advice. Diethylpropion hydrochloride is probably the least harmful of the stimulant drugs, although it is used illicitly for its psychotropic effects, while tense patients may prefer fenfluramine, which has some depressant properties and does not stimulate the CNS in therapeutic doses. The stimulant drugs should not be given to those with a history of drug abuse or with evident sociopathic personality traits. Bulk-forming substances such as methylcellulose are free of serious side effects, but do not seem to be effective in suppressing appetite.

Psychotherapy and Behaviour Therapy

The value of enthusiasm and effort on the part of the doctor are difficult to measure, but it is generally believed that most patients respond best to personal supervision by the same person or team of people, seen at every attendance. The psychiatrist may also be able to provide a programme of behaviour modification to reinforce dieting advice and change eating habits. There has been much research in this field which has involved investigation of stimuli which provoke eating, and experimental treatments (Foreyt 1977). Stunkard et al. (1980) examined the effects of fenfluramine, a highly structured regimen of behaviour therapy (which included self-monitoring, stimulus control, slowing of eating and cognitive restructuring), or both treatments combined. Although fenfluramine, alone or in combination with behaviour therapy, produced significantly greater initial weight loss compared with behaviour therapy alone, the group treated with behaviour therapy had a significantly lower mean weight than those of the other groups at the end of a 1-year follow-up period. Thus it appeared that fenfluramine compromised the long-term effects of behaviour therapy, and that behaviour therapy alone was the best treatment for maintained weight reduction.

The Role of the Psychiatrist

Most psychiatrists seldom treat obesity but they may have a special role in trying to modify the behaviour of some patients who overeat in association with neurotic symptoms such as anxiety. Standard methods of intervention which are used include pharmacological treatment, psychotherapy and, perhaps, behaviour modification. Beyond this, and in the particular cases of the extremely obese and those who cannot keep to a diet, referral for more drastic but often successful treatment may be indicated, if the potential benefits to the patient outweigh the discomfort and risks of the procedures involved. These include admission to hospital for starvation (Munro et al. 1970), jaw-wiring (Garrow and Gardiner 1981) and major surgery such as gastric bypass (Mason et al. 1978) and jejunoileal bypass (Baddeley 1979). The report by Quaade (1974) of hypothalamic psychosurgery attracted unfavourable comment and this treatment does not seem to be in current use.

PICA

Pica is the eating of, or desire to eat, substances which are not normally considered edible. Earth and clay are often chosen, while eating coal has also been described. Pica can arise in association with deficiencies of trace elements such as iron or zinc, and it is possible that a similar mechanism is responsible for the occurrence of apparently related phenomena (craving for particular foods) in pregnancy. Cooper's study (1957) concluded that there was a nutritional basis for the pica which was reported in almost a quarter of 784 children seen by a Mothers' Advisory Service. The treatment of a proven deficiency is, of course, replacement, once a remediable cause has been excluded.

Pica from ignorance is normal in infants and in adults of severely subnormal intelligence. Precautions to exclude potentially poisonous objects from the environment, especially those covered with lead-containing paint, are a normal part of the care of both groups. Severely demented patients may show similar behaviour which may have the same explanation, although it has been said to be equivalent to the excessive eating component of the Kluver–Bucy syndrome produced in monkeys by removal of both temporal lobes.

Secondary pica may appear in psychosis, as a result of delusional thinking, in hysteria, in the Ganser syndrome, and in feigned madness. The treatment is that of the underlying disorder.

SECONDARY EATING DISORDERS

Disturbances of appetite and eating are common in patients with psychiatric illness, when it is important to treat the primary disorder. This is of particular relevance in the elderly, whose physiology may be more easily disturbed and who are likely to become trapped in a vicious circle of poor food intake and declining health, leading to cognitive impairment. Other relatively rare disorders include water intoxication, and aerophagy.

Nowadays, the vague label of 'nervous dyspepsia', a relic of the period when medical dictionaries such as Quain's carried complex classifications of 'gastric neuroses', tends to be subsumed under the broad heading of anxiety, and treated as such.

References

ADAMS, N., FERGUSON, J., STUNKARD, A.J. & AGRAS, W.S. (1978) The eating behaviour of obese and nonobese women. *Behav. Res. Ther.*, **16**, 225.

BADDELEY, R.M. (1979) The management of gross refractory obesity by jejuno-ileal bypass. *Br. J. Surg.*, **66**, 525.

BEMIS, K. (1978) Current approaches to the etiology and treatment of anorexia nervosa. *Psychol. Bull.*, **85**, 593.

BEUMONT, P.J.V. (1979) The endocrinology of anorexia nervosa. In: *Recent Advances in Clinical Psychiatry*, Vol. 3, ed. Granville-Grossman, K. London: Churchill Livingstone.

BEUMONT, P.J.V., GEORGE, G.C.W. & SMART, D.E. (1976) 'Dieters' and 'vomiters and purgers' in anorexia nervosa. *Psychol. Med.*, **6**, 617.

BHANJI, S. & THOMPSON, J. (1974) Operant conditioning in the treatment of anorexia nervosa. A review and retrospective study of 11 cases. *Br. J. Psychiat.*, **124**, 166.

BINNIE, C.C. (1977) Obesity in general practice. Ten year follow-up of obesity. *Jl. R. Coll. gen. Practit.*, **27**, 492.

BLINDER, B.J., FREEMAN, D.J. & STUNKARD, A.J. (1970) Effectiveness of activity as a reinforcer of weight gain. *Am. J. Psychiat.*, **126**, 1093.

BRAY, G.A. & GALLAGHER, T.F. (1975) Manifestation of hypothalamic obesity in man. *Medicine* (Baltimore), **54**, 301.

B.M.J. (1973) Clinicopathological conference: A case of anorexia. *Br. med. J.*, **ii**, 158.

BRUCH, H. (1974a) *Eating Disorders. Obesity, Anorexia Nervosa and the Person Within*. London: Routledge Kegan Paul.

BRUCH, H. (1974b) Perils of behaviour modification in the treatment of anorexia nervosa. *J. Am. med. Ass.*, **230**, 1419.

COOPER, M. (1957) *Pica*. Springfield, Illinois: Charles C. Thomas.

CRADDOCK, D. (1973) *Obesity and Its Management*, 2nd ed. London: Churchill Livingstone.

CRADDOCK, D. (1977) The free diet: 150 cases personally followed-up after 10 to 18 years. *Int. J. Obes.*, **1**, 127.

CRISP, A.H. (1965) A treatment regime for anorexia nervosa. *Br. J. Psychiat.*, **112**, 505.

CRISP, A.H. (1967) Anorexia nervosa. *Hosp. Med.* **(May)**, 713.

CRISP, A.H., HSU, L.K.G., HARDING, B. & HARTSHORN, J. (1980) Clinical features of anorexia nervosa. *J. psychosom. Res.*, **24**, 179

CRISP, A.H. & KALUCY, R.S. (1973) The effect of leucotomy on intractable adolescent weight phobia (primary anorexia nervosa). *J. postgrad. Med.*, **49**, 883.

CRISP, A.H. & McGUINNESS, B. (1976) Jolly fat: relation between obesity and psychoneurosis in general population. *Br. med. J.*, **i**, 7.

CRISP, A.H., PALMER, R.L. & KALUCY, R.S. (1976) How common is anorexia nervosa? *Br. J. Psychiat.*, **128**, 549.

DALLY, P. & GOMEZ, J. (1979) *Anorexia Nervosa*. London: Heinemann.

DALLY, P.J. & SARGANT, W. (1960) A new treatment of anorexia nervosa. *Br. med. J.*, **i**, 1770.

ECKERT, E.D., GOLDBERG, S.C., HALMI, K.A., CASPER, R.C. & DAVIS, J.M. (1979) Behaviour therapy in anorexia nervosa. *Br. J. Psychiat.*, **134**, 55.

EDHOLM, O.G., FLETCHER, J.G., WIDDOWSON, E.M. & McCANCE, R.A. (1955) The energy expenditure and food intake of individual men. *Br. J. Nutr.*, **9**, 286.

FOREYT, J.P. (1977) *Behavioural Treatments of Obesity*. Oxford: Pergamon Press.

GARROW, J.S. (1978) *Energy Balance and Obesity in Man*. Amsterdam: Elsevier.

GARROW, J.S. & GARDINER, G.T. (1981) Maintenance of weight loss in obese patients after jaw wiring. *Br. med. J.*, **i**, 858.

GREEN, R.S. & RAO, J.H. (1974) Treatment of compulsive eating disturbances with anticonvulsant medication. *Am. J. Psychiat.*, **131**, 428.

GULL, W.W. (1874) Anorexia nervosa (apepsia hysterica, anorexia hysterica). *Trans. clin. Soc. Lond.*, **7**, 22.

HALMI, K.A., POWERS, P. & CUNNINGHAM, S. (1975) Treatment of anorexia nervosa with behaviour modification. *Archs gen. Psychiat.*, **32**, 93.

HARROWER, A.D.B. (1978) Bromocriptine in anorexia nervosa. *Hosp. Med.*, **(Dec)**, 672.

HARROWER, A.D.B., YAP, P.L., NAIRN, I.M., WALTON, H.J., STRONG, J.A. & CRAIG, A. (1977) Growth hormone, insulin and prolactin secretion in anorexia nervosa and obesity during bromocriptine treatment. *Br. med. J.*, **ii**, 156.

HOWELLS, J.G. (1976) *Principles of Family Psychiatry*. London: Pitman Medical.

HSU, K.G. (1980) Outcome of anorexia nervosa. A review of the literature (1954 to 1978). *Arch. gen. Psychiat.*, **37**, 1041.

ISAACS, A.J. (1979) Endocrinological section. In: *Anorexia Nervosa*, ed. Dally, P. & Gomez, J. London: Heinemann.

JUNG, R.T. & JAMES, W.P.T. (1980) Is obesity metabolic? *Br. J. hosp. Med.*, **(Dec)**, 503.

KANIS, J., BROWN, P., KIRKPATRICK, K., HIBBERT, D.J., HORN, D.B., NAIRN, I.M., SHIRLING, D., STRONG, J.A. & WALTON, H.J. (1974) Anorexia nervosa: A clinical psychiatric and laboratory study. *Quart. J. Med.*, **43**, 321.

KAY, D.W.K. & LEIGH, D. (1954) The natural history, treatment and prognosis of anorexia nervosa, based on a study of 38 patients. *J. ment. Sci.*, **100**, 411.

KENDELL, R.E., HALL, D.J., HAILEY, A. & BABIGIAN, H.M. (1973) The epidemiology of anorexia nervosa. *Psychol. Med.*, **3**, 200.

LAING, R.D. (1960) *The Divided Self*. London: Tavistock.

LEON, G.R. & ROTH, L. (1977) Obesity: psychological causes, correlations and speculations. *Psychol. Bull.*, **84**, 117.

LEWIN, K., MATTINGLEY, D. & MILLIS, R.R. (1972) Anorexia Nervosa associated with hypothalamic tumour. *Br. med. J.*, **ii**, 629.

LOPEZ IBOR, J.J. (1972) Masked depressions. *Br. J. Psychiat.*, **120**, 245.

MARRIOTT, H.L. (1949) A simple weight reducing diet. *Br. med. J.*, **ii**, 18.

MARSHALL, J.C. & RUSSELL FRASER, T. (1971) Amenorrhoea in anorexia nervosa: assessment and treatment with clomiphene citrate. *Br. med. J.*, **iv**, 590.

MASON, E.E., PRINTEN, K.J., BLOMMERS, J.J. & SCOTT, D.H. (1978) Gastric bypass for obesity after ten years' experience. *Int. J. Obes.*, **2**, 197.

MILLS, I.H. (1976) The disease of failure of coping. *Practitioner*, **217**, 529.

MOORE, G., GRANT, A.M., HOWARD, A.N. & MILLS, I.H. (1980) Treatment of obesity with triiodothyronine and a very low calorie liquid formula diet. *Lancet*, **i**, 223.

MORGAN, H.G. & RUSSELL, G.F.M. (1975) Value of family background and clinical features as predictors of long-term outcome in anorexia nervosa: four year follow-up study of 41 patients. *Psychol. Med.*, **5**, 355.

MUNRO, J.F., MacCUISH, A.C., GOODALL, J.A.D., FRASER, J. & DUNCAN, L.J.P. (1970) Further experience with prolonged therapeutic starvation in gross refractory obesity. *Br. med. J.*, **iv**, 712.

QUAADE, F. (1974) Stereotaxy for obesity. *Lancet*, **i**, 267.

RIES, W. (1973) Feeding behaviour in the obese. *Proc. Nutr. Soc.*, **32**, 187.

RUSSELL, G. (1979) Bulimia nervosa: An ominous variant of anorexia nervosa. *Psychol. Med.*, **9**, 429.

RUSSELL, G.F.M. (1970) Anorexia nervosa: its identity as an illness and its treatment. In: *Modern Trends in Psychological Medicine*. 2, ed. Price, J.H. London: Butterworths.

RUSSELL, M.A.H. (1976) What is dependence? In: *Drugs and Dependence*. ed. Edmunds, G., Russell, M.A.H., Hawks, D. & MacCafferty, M. London: Saxon House/Lexington Books.

SELVINI, M.P. (1965) Interpretation of mental anorexia. In: *Anorexia Nervosa*. ed. Meyer, J.E. & Feldman, H. Stuttgart: Thieme.

SILVERMAN, J.A. (1974) Anorexia nervosa. Clinical observation on a successful treatment plan. *J. Pediat.*, **84**, 68.

SILVERSTONE, J.T. (1968) Psychological aspects of obesity. *Proc. R. Soc. Med.*, **61**, 371.

SLATER, E. & ROTH, M. (1969) *Clinical Psychiatry*. 3rd ed., p. 125. London: Baillière Tindall.

STUNKARD, A.J., CRAIGHEAD, L.W. & O'BRIEN, R. (1980) Controlled trial of behaviour therapy, pharmacotherapy and their combination in the treatment of obesity. *Lancet*, **ii**, 1045.

THEANDER, S. (1970) Anorexia nervosa—A psychiatric investigation of 94 female patients. *Acta. psychiat. scand. Suppl.*, 214.

WALLER, J.V., KAUFMAN, M.R. & DEUTSCH, F. (1940) Anorexia nervosa—a psychosomatic entity. *Psychosom. Med.*, **2**, 3.

WOMERSLEY, J. & DURNIN, J.V.G.A. (1977) A comparison of the skinfold method with extent of 'overweight' and various weight–height relationships in the assessment of obesity. *Br. J. Nutr.*, **38**, 271.

22

Management of Disorders of Sexual Function

J.H. Dowson

INTRODUCTION

This chapter will consider the management of individuals who complain of inadequate sexual performance within a heterosexual relationship (Haslam 1974); problems associated with so-called sexual deviations are dealt with elsewhere.

There are many interacting determinants of sexual function, including genetic endowment, somatic disease, events which condition behaviour, personality, sexual technique and a variety of psychological factors. The latter may involve conscious or unconscious effects of remote events, as well as the current social environment—in particular the relationship with the sexual partner.

The first step in management is to obtain a detailed sexual, personal, medical, and psychiatric history. Any current medication should be reviewed and the patient is then physically examined. At this stage, any fundamental ignorance of sexual technique or the range of commonly practised sexual behaviour should be corrected, and the patient can be reassured that many people with sexual difficulties can be helped. It is important to stress that an inability to achieve simultaneous orgasm should not be equated with 'failure'.

In some sexual dysfunctions further physical investigations may be required, as may treatment for underlying somatic disorders. Some dysfunctions respond to specific advice aimed at modifying the couple's sexual behaviour, and relatively short-term psychotherapeutic intervention may be directed at all aspects of the couple's relationship, as well as at individual problems such as anxiety, fear of sexual failure, guilt, or psychological defence mechanisms which prevent the individual from experiencing sexual pleasure (see glossary, Chapter 9). Often, the couple's difficulties are compounded by poor communication, when frank discussion of sexual behaviour is encouraged. In rare cases, it may be appropriate for one partner (or possibly both) to receive relatively long-term psychotherapy, especially if probable unconscious factors are considered to be

421

relevant; however, this component of management is not readily available, and the results are uncertain.

Other forms of intervention include certain forms of behaviour therapy, including biofeedback (Editorial 1973; Nemetz et al. 1978; Wright et al. 1977), surgically implanted prostheses for erectile impotence, and various mechanical devices which either support the flaccid penis, exert pressure on male genitalia, or provide genital stimulation in either sex.

Although treatment of sexual dysfunction resulting from a somatic cause, and advice on technique or mechanical aids, can be offered to all who may benefit, a series of interviews with both partners are not usually indicated if one or both partners is uncooperative or regularly involved in other sexual relationships.

Advice for physically disabled people can be obtained from the SPOD or Disabled Living Foundation (see references), while Burnfield (1979) has discussed problems associated with multiple sclerosis.

TAKING THE HISTORY

A sexual, personal and medical (including psychiatric) history must be obtained, together with information regarding recent and current medical or surgical treatment. However, as patients are invariably anxious and embarrassed, the establishment of a rapport must often take precedence over fact-gathering, especially in the initial interview.

A sexual history should include details of attitudes to sex in the parental home and the way in which sexual information was first obtained, together with previous heterosexual and homosexual experience. Any traumatic sexual incidents should be identified. Enquiries should be made about sexual fantasies and the frequency of masturbation. The nature of many aspects of the couple's relationship needs to be explored, and patterns of behaviour are noted. Details of contraceptive practice are often relevant, together with each partner's attitude to future pregnancies. Female patients should be asked if they have ever had a termination of pregnancy, and the circumstances and emotions surrounding this should be explored. Enquiry should also be made regarding possible alcohol abuse. In addition, the couple should be asked if they have ever separated, or, with married couples, if solicitors have ever been consulted with a view to divorce.

THE PHYSICAL EXAMINATION

This may reveal anatomical abnormality or a disease process which is known to cause sexual dysfunction. Relevant somatic diseases are considered under the various categories of disorder.

SEXUAL DYSFUNCTION IN THE MALE

In order to complete the sexual act to the mutual satisfaction of both partners, the male must be able to develop a penile erection of sufficient firmness to penetrate the vagina, must maintain the erection for the time necessary to allow his partner to come to orgasm, and himself experience orgasm, with the discharge of seminal fluid. Problems occur at various stages of this complex process.

Impotence

Definition. Impotence is defined as an inability to produce or sustain an erection which is sufficient to allow vaginal penetration. The term 'primary' impotence implies that all previous attempts at intercourse have been unsuccessful, while the impotence is 'secondary' if successful intercourse has previously occurred. Libido may be impaired, and loss of libido is one of the factors which can lead to impotence. It should be noted that ejaculation can sometimes occur from a flaccid penis.

Aetiology. Impotence may result from congenital abnormalities such as absence or fibrosis of the corpora cavernosa, chromosomal disorders (Johnson 1975), or spinal cord lesions. Traumatic causes include injury (to the penis, pelvis or spinal cord) and surgery, including sympathectomy, cystectomy, abdominoperineal resection and suprapubic prostatectomy. Impotence may result from vascular disorders such as priapism, atherosclerosis (including the Leyriche syndrome) and varicocoele, while neurological causes may involve spinal cord lesions and peripheral neuropathies. Impotence is a common complication of hypertension, renal failure and diabetes mellitus. In the latter disorder, the onset of impotence does not always correlate with the duration or severity of the disease and may be due to autonomic neuropathy. Impotence may also be associated with haemochromatosis, adrenal or thyroid disorders, primary or secondary hypogonadism with low androgen levels, feminizing interstitial tumour, the effects of alcohol and certain drugs, and hypothalamic/pituitary disorders such as hyperprolactinaemia.

Hyperprolactinaemia has been reported in association with impotence, gynaecomastia, galactorrhoea and impaired sperm counts. (The administration of dopamine agonists to reduce serum prolactin may improve potency in such individuals.) A degree of hyperprolactinaemia may result from treatment with phenothiazines, haloperidol, metoclopramide or methyldopa. Chronic alcoholism can induce impotence, sterility, gynaecomastia and changes in body hair, even when liver function is within normal limits, while a variety of liver disorders may also lead to impotence. Hypothyroidism is a rare cause of hypogonadism and impotence, and if testicular biopsy demonstrates testicular damage, reversal of thyroid deficiency may not improve potency. Also, hyper-thyroidism can cause impotence.

Drugs which may cause impotence include some antihypertensive drugs (especially bethanidine), steroids, spironolactone, androgen antagonists, oestrogens, phenothiazines (especially thioridazine), haloperidol, tricyclic antidepressants, monoamine oxidase inhibitors, disopyramide and opiates.

It has been reported that ageing produces a fall in plasma testosterone and impaired spermatogenesis after the age of 60. It is possible that impotence in such individuals may respond to hormonal replacement therapy but this is controversial.

Impotence is often associated with anxiety, hostility, disgust, personality factors, ignorance, misinformation, and the functional psychoses. Although anxiety is often secondary, it has been suggested that it can often be of aetiological significance. Stress, fatigue, 'performance anxiety' and unconscious conflicts can also be relevant. Ansari (1975) highlighted anxiety in sexual situations, and the sexual response and personality of the partner, as aetiological factors. Kaplan (1974) has pointed out that a woman can engage in unwelcome intercourse more easily than a man, who may develop a 'vicious circle' of increasing anxiety when the female partner makes sexual demands which he feels unable to supply.

Management. After a detailed assessment and examination, any relevant somatic disorder should be identified. The history may suggest the presence of 'organic' aetiology when impotence tends to be associated with loss of morning erections and libido, in contrast with the usual presentation of psychogenic impotence. Examination should pay particular attention to evidence of gonadal failure, postural hypotension (which may indicate autonomic neuropathy), gynaecomastia, galactorrhoea, and signs of hepatic cirrhosis. It has been suggested that routine investigations should include measurement of luteinizing hormone, follicle-stimulating hormone, testosterone, prolactin, thyroid-stimulating hormone and triiodothyronine, liver function tests and a 2 h postprandial blood sugar. [Most cases of hyperprolactinaemia have low testosterone levels (Editorial 1978; Davies and Mountjoy 1981).] Other investigations which may be indicated include radiology, full blood count, erythrocyte sedimentation rate, fasting blood sugar, chromosomal analysis, Valsalva manoeuvre, bladder function studies and studies of penile vascular supply.

If the patient is taking drugs (or alcohol) which could influence potency, these should be withdrawn, if this is possible. Alternatively, they may be replaced by other drugs which are less likely to produce impotence.

If impotence is due to reduced testosterone, replacement treatment may involve sublingual testosterone or injections of testosterone esters. Although there is no clear evidence that hormonal treatment is indicated without evidence of androgen deficiency, its use in 'normal' older men has yet to be evaluated. The dopamine agonist drug bromocriptine may be therapeutic in the rare case of impotence resulting from hyperprolactinaemia. This may be combined with irradiation of the pituitary. It should be remembered that stress can induce mild prolactin elevation, and consecutive samples taken within 30 min of the insertion of an indwelling intravenous catheter may aid diagnosis (Davies and Mountjoy 1981). Luteinizing-hormone-releasing-hormone (LH-RH) has also been used in an attempt to treat hypogonadism of hypothalamic origin (Editorial 1978).

The sexual problems of individuals with chronic neurological deficits have been considered by Silver (1975); the maintenance of manually stimulated erection may be assisted by plastic rings which encircle either the penis, or both scrotum and penis (Rhodes 1975).

Variants of the techniques of Masters and Johnson (1970, 1976) have been reported to benefit many individuals with impotence, although there is a wide range of reported failure rates which may reflect variation in the selection criteria for the samples studied (Ansari 1976; Bancroft and Coles 1976; Editorial 1976). Masters and Johnson advocated an intensive 2-week period of treatment in which the couple are seen regularly by male and female co-therapists. At first, the couple is advised to avoid intercourse and to engage in daily periods of 'sensate focus' exercises, in which each partner takes it in turn to caress the other in a manner designed to produce pleasure in a 'no-demand' situation. Also, verbal 'feedback' is encouraged. This strategy usually removes 'performance anxiety' in which both partners may worry that an attempt at intercourse will be unsuccessful. This is eventually followed by 'genital focus' exercises, when the stimulation is directed to the genital and perineal area. In addition, other therapists have advocated the development of erotic fantasies, which may both increase arousal and displace the patient's anxiety-provoking preoccupation with the monitoring of his own performance. A degree of 'selfishness' is also encouraged; some impotent men neglect their own needs for arousal because they concentrate exclusively on the needs of their partner. Eventually, the therapists suggest that intercourse is resumed, but this should be done gradually; thus the couple may, at first, be told to achieve penetration, but to avoid orgasm. The use of the 'female superior position', in which the male lies on his back and the female is astride him, is often of use for this as well as for other sexual problems (Kaplan 1974).

In some patients, the 'stop-start' procedure, which was advocated primarily for the treatment of premature ejaculation by Dr James Semans in 1956, can be helpful for erectile impotence, if an erection has been produced by the 'genital focus' exercises. In this procedure, the female stimulates her partner's penis manually until he gives the signal that orgasm is imminent; she then discontinues but subsequently resumes until the male's previous sensations recur. This process is repeated several times and may give some men confidence that a 'lost' erection can be regained, thus reducing fear of failure.

Various techniques of behaviour therapy involving desensitization and positive conditioning have been reported (Bancroft 1975; Glick 1975; Reynolds 1977), but an approach based on the principles of Masters and Johnson, together with short-term psychotherapy (which may involve both individual and joint interviews), should be the first line of management for psychogenic impotence. The psychotherapeutic input may include education and an attempt to modify many aspects of the couple's relationship. Benzodiazepines may help to reduce performance anxiety, while successful treatment of a depressive syndrome may alleviate impotence which is secondary to such a disorder. Sexual aids such as rings and penile splints have been reviewed by Rhodes (1975). One type of ring encircles both penis and scrotum, and can be worn much of the day. A variant of this incorporates electro-galvanic plates which produce an electric current that is said to have beneficial effects. Although Cooper (1974) found no significant difference between an electric and non-electric ring, there was a tendency for the electric ring to be associated with a greater degree of improvement.

Surgical implantation of different forms of penile prostheses (for example, tubes of silicone implanted inside the corpora) is another potetial form of management (Editorial 1977, 1979; Pryor 1979). This should be seriously considered for relatively young men with erectile failure due to an irreversible somatic disorder, but an appliance which splints the penis should be tried initially.

The literature on the various treatment methods for this disorder (and for premature ejaculation) has recently been reviewed by Kilmann and Auerbach (1979).

Premature Ejaculation

Definition. This occurs when the male is unable to exert a degree of voluntary control on the timing of ejaculation, which occurs soon after attaining erection, either before penetration or soon afterwards. Premature ejaculation has been reported to be the most prevalent of the male dysfunctions in clinical practice.

Aetiology. Somatic causes include spinal cord pathology, due to such diseases as multiple sclerosis and prostatitis. Psychogenic factors are often relevant and are invariably associated with anxiety.

Management. For some individuals, improvement follows the lowering of performance anxiety by a series of interviews with the couple, although the male partner may also be seen individually. The use of a condom may also be beneficial. Prescription of a monoamine oxidase inhibitor will usually bring symptomatic relief, presumably due to reduced sympathetic activity, but a relapse tends to occur when the drug is discontinued. Clomipramine has also been advocated for this disorder (Goodman 1977).

The stop-start technique which is outlined above was specifically developed by Semans for the management of premature ejaculation, and excellent results have been reported from this simple procedure, which is easily explained to the couple.

Masters and Johnson introduced a variant which is known as the 'squeeze technique': the man lies on his back and his partner manually stimulates his penis until he signals that orgasm is imminent. She then squeezes the shaft of his penis, just below the glans, to induce a partial loss of erection. Stimulation is then restarted and the procedure is repeated on several occasions. If the simpler Semans technique is ineffective, this method may be of value to those men who find it difficult to prevent ejaculation resulting from the premonitory sensations of orgasm, even when the stimulation has been discontinued.

After this exercise has been successfully practised on a number of occasions (e.g. 6–12), the couple can be advised to attempt intercourse, perhaps in the female-superior position. At first, withdrawal should take place when male orgasm is imminent, and the level of arousal is allowed to subside. Further application of the squeeze method may be necessary. After this procedure has been repeated, orgasm is then permitted. Subsequently, the cessation of pelvic movements by both partners is substituted for withdrawal, and the male is encouraged to monitor his own sensations of impending orgasm, so that he can achieve the maximum degree of voluntary control.

Retarded Ejaculation (Ejaculatory Incompetence)

Definition. This disorder consists of an inability to ejaculate, even though erection and penetration have been achieved. Intercourse is usually prolonged and unsatisfactory, and the female partner may be concerned about being unable to become pregnant.

Aetiology. A disorder which impairs erectile potency will usually impair ejaculation, while a 'dry ejaculation', in which the seminal fluid is directed into the bladder, can be caused by thioridazine, other phenothiazines, some antihypertensive drugs and neurological disease. It appears that various psychogenic factors leading to anxiety are often relevant.

Management. As in every case of sexual dysfunction, probable somatic causes are considered, and an attempt is made to identify ignorance of sexual matters, specific conflicts and fears, and difficulties in the couple's relationship. Psychological management may involve reducing performance anxiety, encouraging the provision of erotic stimuli, and, in some individuals, a psychotherapeutic attempt to reduce a tendency to be excessively controlled with regard to expression of emotion. Some patients can learn to distract themselves from this tendency by developing erotic fantasy.

The patient and his partner may benefit from instructions which are based on

Masters' and Johnson's methods. They are advised not to attempt intercourse initially and to carry out sensate focus exercises. The female is then instructed to develop a technique for stimulating her partner's penis to produce ejaculation, which may be assisted by the male's concentration on erotic fantasy, or a battery-operated vibrator (Geboes et al. 1975). After extravaginal ejaculation has been regularly achieved, intercourse can be attempted after the female has manually stimulated her partner to a stage when the orgasm is close. At this point, penetration should occur. The female (or male) can provide additional manual stimulation of the penis during intercourse or, if necessary, the penis is withdrawn for additional stimulation if ejaculation does not occur within a reasonable time.

DYSFUNCTION IN THE FEMALE

The female equivalents of impotence and ejaculatory incompetence are lack of libido and orgasmic dysfunction, respectively. The third type of female dysfunction which will be considered is vaginismus. In general, female sexual disorder is less vulnerable to somatic changes than male function, although stress, fatigue and illness can all have adverse effects. In some women, lack of libido and impaired orgasm may be related to hormonal contraceptives.

Lack of Libido

Definition. This term refers to impaired (or lack of) sexual interest and drive, together with a lack of psychological and physical response to sexual stimulation. However, it should be noted that some women can experience orgasm in the absence of vaginal lubrication and vascular engorgement of the genitalia.

Aetiology. This disorder can be primary, when sexual interest has always been deficient, or develop after a period of 'normality'. Aetiological factors include ignorance of sexual 'norms' and technique, ill-health, stress, intrapsychic conflicts or difficulties in the relationship with the partner.

Management. Assessment and physical examination is followed by the appropriate medical and psychotherapeutic interventions. It should be remembered that lack of libido may be due to a depressive syndrome of endogenous aetiology, or be associated with breast feeding. Other causes include tiredness due to the strain of looking after young children, impaired self-image with regard to femininity (perhaps due to hirsuties or operations such as mastectomy), fear of pregnancy, and chronic marital tension or resentment.

It is important to determine whether the male partner is aware of the circumstances which produce female sexual arousal, as management involves the encouragement of adequate psychological and physical stimulation. Initially, the couple can be advised to avoid intercourse and to concentrate on sensate and genital focus exercises, which include stimulation of nipples, clitoris and the vaginal entrance. A battery operated vibrator may be helpful. In due course, instructions are given to attempt intercourse after an initial period of mutual stimulation, but not to attempt orgasm. Such non-demand intercourse is designed to lower anxiety. The female-superior and side-to-side positions have been recommended for this and other disorders (Kaplan 1974). If non-orgasmic intercourse is successfully achieved, intercourse with both female and male orgasm (but not necessarily simultaneously) can then be attempted.

Behavioural techniques have been used for this disorder (Glick 1975) and, in a controlled study, Carney et al. (1978) reported that treatment with testosterone had therapeutic effects; but it is not known if the routine use of this latter regimen is appropriate or safe.

Orgasmic Dysfunction

Definition. This condition involves an impaired (or lack of) ability to experience orgasm during sexual intercourse. It should be noted that many women with this complaint have satisfactory libido and are able to come to orgasm by masturbation, or as a result of manual stimulation by their partner. Also, the preliminary physical responses to erotic stimuli (i.e. vaginal lubrication and vascular engorgement of the genitalia), are often unimpaired. Orgasm can be described as a progressive physical and psychological sexual excitement culminating in a pleasurable peak, which may be accompanied by a transient reduction of self-control.

Aetiology. Orgasmic dysfunction may be primary or secondary. It has been stated that clitoral adhesions can (very rarely) be responsible, but this is controversial. Another suggested aetiological factor is impaired tone of the pelvic musculature, in particular of the pubococcygeal muscle. Other possible causes include ill-health, the effects of certain drugs (including hormonal contraceptives), and faulty sexual technique. Relevant psychogenic factors include a fear of 'letting go', which may result from obsessional personality traits or a fear of being overheard or interrupted, perhaps by older children. Sometimes the woman is afraid of her partner's reaction to possible uncontrollable utterances during orgasm. As with other forms of sexual dysfunction, difficulties in the couple's relationship are common causes, particularly if resentment or anxiety is involved.

Management. Any medical interventions are usually combined with specific advice and psychotherapeutic help. The principles of management are to enhance sexual stimulation, to reduce anxiety, and to encourage the 'over-controlled' or 'detached' person to develop erotic fantasy.

Particular attention must be paid to giving the couple specific advice on sexual technique. A variable period of 'foreplay' (of up to, and sometimes beyond, half an hour) is often necessary if the female is to achieve orgasm. The man may kiss and caress his partner in a way which includes contact with the so-called 'erogenous zones' consisting of the clitoris, other parts of the genital and perineal area, and the breasts, particularly the nipples. Stimulation of certain parts of the vaginal entrance is particularly liable to induce sexual arousal (Kaplan 1974). General advice can be given, or the particular behavioural approach of Masters and Johnson (1970), involving sensate and genital focus exercises, can be employed. Other behavioural approaches have been described (Munjack et al. 1976). Cunnilingus, involving mouth and tongue genital contact may also be employed, provided it is not distasteful to either partner. After a degree of physical arousal has been obtained in the female, which has included the secretion of the vaginal lubricant, penetration follows. Further mutual genital stimulation is provided by movement of the penis within the vagina which results from pelvic movements of both partners. Such movements may continue for a variable time, during which each partner may continue to kiss and caress the other. Although mutual orgasm is usually the goal of intercourse, some couples find this difficult to achieve; in such cases they may try and take turns as to who should initially experience orgasm. Sometimes it is necessary for the male partner to induce his partner's orgasm by manual stimulation after he has experienced orgasm during intercourse.

It may be possible for the couple to delay the man's orgasm by stopping pelvic movements, or by withdrawal, in an effort to arrive at orgasm simultaneously.

Psychological factors such as a 'romantic atmosphere', a pleasant and undisturbed environment, verbal communication with compliments, and the development of erotic fantasy are also important.

It may be necessary for the foreplay to involve self-stimulation, or the use of a battery operated vibrator by the woman or her partner. Programmes for masturbation training have been reported to be useful in some cases. However, long-term over-reliance on mechanical aids should not be encouraged. Sometimes a woman requires privacy to develop a degree of self-stimulated arousal before joining her partner. In some cases, orgasm can be induced by the process of manual clitoral stimulation during intercourse by the male partner. This is easily achieved in the female-superior position.

Certain exercises designed to improve the tone of pelvic musculature have been claimed to be beneficial, together with advice to regularly contract the abdominal, perineal and vaginal musculature during intercourse.

Vaginismus

Definition. This refers to involuntary sustained contraction of the muscles surrounding the entrance to the vagina, which is sufficient to result in incomplete or total failure of penetration. This is often accompanied by a phobic avoidance of attempts at intercourse.

Aetiology. Rarely this is associated with a rigid or imperforate hymen, hymenal tags, senile vaginitis or painful pelvic disease (Munsick 1980). Psychogenic factors of particular relevance may include lack of information on sexual matters, sexual guilt, a negative attitude to intercourse—perhaps engendered by the woman's mother, hostility to her partner, fear of pregnancy and previous unsuccessful or traumatic sexual encounters.

Management. As part of initial assessment, physical examination should be carried out with particular care. The patient is often young, with little or no sexual experience. It is not uncommon for such individuals to have received hurried vaginal examinations which may have reinforced the problem and the first attempt at examination should often just involve an inspection of the external genitalia and the placing of the examiner's (or patient's) finger on the vaginal orifice. The patient can be asked to use her own hand to explore the opening, and this may provide sufficient information to exclude a relevant physical cause. However, if a full vaginal examination is necessary, this may be attempted in gradual stages, at subsequent visits. In such cases the patient may find it reassuring to be asked to manoeuvre herself so that the doctor's finger, which is held still, enters the vagina. It may sometimes be appropriate to examine the male partner's genitalia, if the nature of the problem is in doubt.

As for other disorders, a combination of relevant medical treatment, practical advice and psychotherapy is usually indicated. Kaplan (1974) has described detailed instructions for the couple to carry out in privacy. The first step involves the patient and her partner identifying the vaginal orifice with the aid of a mirror. Then she is told to gently insert her own finger, or her partner's finger, into her vagina, and keep it there until discomfort subsides. Throughout this and subsequent procedures the woman is in control of events and, at her own pace, in a series of sessions, the finger is repeatedly inserted and eventually moved back and forth. When this has been achieved without vaginismus, two fingers can be inserted and eventually moved and rotated. This graded sequence of stimuli can be carried out by the patient alone, or in the presence of her partner. Graduated plastic or glass dilators may be helpful in some cases. Also, advice to practise contraction and relaxation of the perineal and vaginal musculature may help the patient to produce relaxation when necessary.

In addition, the couple can be instructed to engage in sensate and genital focus exercises in the knowledge that intercourse will not be attempted until regular self-insertion of two fingers, or of a dilator of the appropriate size, can be achieved without discomfort. The female-superior position is often useful when the couple are ready to attempt penetration. This may prevent the woman feeling trapped beneath her partner and allows her to exert more control over the process of intercourse. Initially, the woman parts the labia with one hand and lowers herself onto the penis which is guided by her other hand. Penetration should be accomplished in stages, so that just the tip of the penis is inserted at the first attempt at intercourse. After full penetration is obtained, pelvic movements should be initially avoided, and the male must be ready to withdraw at his partner's signal. The encouragement of sexual fantasy may also help to distract the patient from anxiety-provoking thoughts. Behavioural strategies involving desensitization in fantasy have also been reported, and for those patients in whom traumatic sexual experience seem to be relevant, abreaction interviews after diazepam have been reported to be helpful (Mikhail 1976).

An important advantage of the various forms of in vivo desensitization which can be carried out at home is that these procedures can be easily instituted in a relatively short time. The range of treatments has been reviewed by Fertel (1977).

JOINT INTERVIEWS

Irrespective of the nature of the presenting problem, management of sexual dysfunction usually includes a series of joint interviews (i.e. with both partners), although sometimes simple explanation and practical instruction are all that are required. However, even a relatively limited number of joint interviews must not be undertaken unless specific goals have been formulated which are likely to be achieved by a directive approach in the time available (Crowe 1978). Bancroft and Coles (1976) report that those who do well with a modified Masters and Johnson technique do so with relatively few sessions. In many psychiatric services it is not possible to offer more than about four to six joint interviews, which are partly concerned with the modification of various maladaptive aspects of the couple's relationship (Berman and Lief 1975; Dominian 1979), and partly with giving instruction for the practice of a specific programme of sexual behaviour. When the therapist's time is particularly limited, a well-motivated couple can be asked to obtain and read the relevant section of a textbook such as *The New Sex Therapy* by Kaplan (Baillière Tindall 1974). However, it has been shown that some follow-up interviews are necessary (Zeiss 1978). Despite the claims for the benefits of the directive behavioural methods pioneered by Masters and Johnson, residual difficulties and relapse are not uncommon (Levay and Kagle 1977; Meyer et al. 1975). Evidence for their efficacy is derived from highly selected populations (Wright et al. 1977).

References

ANSARI, J.M.A. (1975) A study of 65 impotent males. *Br. J. Psychiat.*, **127**, 337.
ANSARI, J.M.A. (1976) Impotence: prognosis. (A controlled study). *Br. J. Psychiat.*, **128**, 194.
BANCROFT, J. (1975) The behavioural approach to marital problems. *Br. J. med. Psychol.*, **48**, 147.
BANCROFT, J. & COLES, L. (1976) Three years' experience in a sexual problems clinic. *Br. med. J.*, **1**, 1575.

BERMAN, E.M. & LIEF, H.I. (1975) Marital therapy from a psychiatric perspective: an overview. *Am. J. Psychiat.*, **132:6**, 583.

BURNFIELD, P. (1979) Sexual problems and multiple sclerosis. *Br. J. Sexual Med.*, **33**.

CARNEY, A., BANCROFT, J. & MATHEWS, A. (1978) Combination of hormonal and psychological treatment for female sexual unresponsiveness: a comparative study. *Br. J. Psychiat.*, **132**, 339.

COOPER, A.J. (1974) A blind evaluation for a penile ring. *Br. J. Psychiat.*, **124**, 402.

CROWE, M.J. (1978) Conjoint marital therapy: a controlled outcome study. *Psychol. Med.*, **8**, 623.

DAVIES, T.F. & MOUNTJOY, C.Q. (1981) Unpublished data—personal communication.

DISABLED LIVING FOUNDATION, 346 Kensington High Street, London W14 8NS, UK.

DOMINIAN, J. (1979) Management: basic counselling. *Br. med. J.*, **ii**, 915. Choice of partner. *Br. med. J.*, **ii**, 594. First phase of marriage. *Br. med. J.*, **ii**, 654. Second phase of marriage. *Br. med. J.*, **ii**, 720. Third phase of marriage. *Br. med. J.*, **ii**, 781. Management: Sexual counselling. *Br. med. J.*, **ii**, 1053.

EDITORIAL. (1973) Behaviour therapy for sex problems. *Lancet*, **i**, 1295.

EDITORIAL. (1976) Treatment of erectile impotence. *Br. med. J.*, **i**, 1298.

EDITORIAL, (1977) Prostheses for impotence. *Br. med. J.*, **i**, 404.

EDITORIAL, (1978) Endocrine basis for sexual dysfunction in men. *Br. med. J.*,**ii**, 1516.

EDITORIAL, (1979) Penile prostheses in erectile impotence. *Br. med. J.*, **ii**, 816.

FERTEL, N.S. (1977) Vaginismus: a review. *J. Sexual Marital Ther.*, **3:2**, 113.

GEBOES, K., STEENO, O. & DE MOOR, P. (1975) Primary anejaculation: diagnosis and therapy. *Fertil. Steril.*, **26:10**, 1018.

GLICK, B.S. (1975) Desensitization therapy in impotence and frigidity: review of the literature and report of a case. *Am. J. Psychiat.*, **132:2**, 169.

GOODMAN, R.E. (1977) The management of premature ejaculation. *J. Int. Med. Res.*, **5, (Suppl. (1)**, 78.

HASLAM, M.T. (1974) Psycho-sexual disorders and their treatment: Part I. *Curr. Med. Res. Opin.*, **2:8**, 488.

JOHNSON, J. (1975) Impotence. *Br. J. Psychiat.*, **Special Publication, No. 9**, 206.

KAPLAN, H.S. (1974) *The New Sex Therapy*. London: Baillière Tindall.

KILMANN, P.R. & AUERBACH, R. (1979) Treatments of premature ejaculation and psychogenic impotence: A critical review of the literature. *Archiv. Sexual Behav.*, **8:1**, 81.

LEVAY, A.N. & KAGLE, A. (1977) A study of treatment needs following sex therapy. *Am. J. Psychiat.*, **134:9**, 970.

MASTERS, W.H. & JOHNSON, V.E. (1970) *Human Sexual Inadequacy*. London: J. & A. Churchill.

MASTERS, W.H. & JOHNSON, V.E. (1976) Principles of the new sex therapy. *Am. J. Psychiatry*, **133:5**, 548.

MEYER, J.K., SCHMIDT, C.W., LUCAS, M.J. & SMITH, E. (1975) Short-term treatment of sexual problems: Interim report. *Am. J. Psychiat.*, **132:2**, 172.

MIKHAIL, A.R. (1976) Treatment of vaginismus by i.v. diazepam abreaction interview. *Acta psychiat. scand.*, **53**, 328.

MUNJACK, D., CRISTOL, A. & GOLDSTEIN, A. et al. (1976) Behavioural treatment of orgasmic dysfunction: a controlled study. *Br. J. Psychiat.*, **129**, 497.

MUNSICK, R.A. (1980) Introital operations for dyspareunia. *Chin. Obstet. Gynecol.*, **23:1**, 243.

NEMETZ, G.H., CRAIG, K.D. & REITH, G. (1978) Treatment of female sexual dysfunction through symbolic modeling. *J. Cons. Chin. Psychol.*, **46:1**, 62.

PRYOR, J.P. (1979) The surgery of erectile impotence. *Br. J. Sex. Med.*, **July**, 24.

REYNOLDS, B.S. (1977) Psychological treatment models and outcome results for erectile dysfunction: A critical review. *Psychol. Bull.*, **84:6**, 1218.

RHODES, P. (1975) Sex aids. *Br. Med. J.*, **11**, 93.

SILVER, J.R. (1975) Sexual problems in disorders of the nervous system. *Br. med. J.*, **iii**, 480.

SPOD (Sexual and Personal Relationships of Disabled People), 25 Mortimer Street, London W1 N8AB, UK.

WRIGHT, J., PERREAULT, R. & MATHIEU, M. (1977) The treatment of sexual dysfunction: a review. *Arch. gen. Psychiat.*, **34**, 881.

ZEISS, R.A. (1978) Self-directed treatment for premature ejaculation. *J. Cons. Clin. Psychol.*, **46:6**, 1234.

23

Management of Sexual Deviations

W.M. Braude

INTRODUCTION

There is no clear demarcation between normal and abnormal sexual behaviour as many of the sexual deviations (e.g. fetishism, sadomasochism and voyeurism) differ only quantitatively from normal sexual behaviour. To a large extent, sexual deviation, like behavioural deviation in general, is determined by the mores and practices of society. This inevitably raises ethical dilemmas for the psychiatrist receiving a request for the treatment of such a problem.

The sexual deviations are a heterogeneous group of conditions which show considerable overlap (Wilson 1981). Thus, any attempt at classification is

Table 23.1. Classification of the sexual deviations

Deviations of sexual-object preference
Homosexuality
Paedophilia
Fetishism and transvestism
Bestiality
Necrophilia
Deviations of mode of sexual behaviour
Sadomasochism
Voyeurism
Fetishism
Transvestism
Exhibitionism
Frotteurism
Abnormality of gender identity
Transsexualism

unlikely to be either exhaustive or exclusive. The sexual deviations are listed in Table 23.1 and may involve an abnormality of sexual-object preference, mode of sexual behaviour, or gender identity. The individual sexual deviations should be regarded as possible symptoms and not as definitive syndromes. They are not singularly predictive of treatment response or prognosis.

Deviations of Sexual-Object Preference

Homosexuality. This refers to a strong preferential erotic attraction to members of the same sex. Western society has adopted an increasingly tolerant attitude to homosexuality, and only a small minority of practising homosexuals are in contact with psychiatric services or in conflict with the law.

Siegelman (1972*a,b*) has shown that a sample of homosexuals and lesbians who were not attending a psychiatric clinic were as well adjusted as normal controls on certain questionnaire measures. Furthermore, it is rare for a homosexual who is attending a psychiatric clinic to be motivated to change his choice of sexual partner preference (Marks 1978). Thus, homosexuality per se should not be regarded as a clinical problem.

Paedophilia. This refers to an erotic desire for sexual contact with pre- or early-pubertal children of either sex. Paedophiliac offences incur strong censure from society and heavy legal penalties.

Deviations of Mode of Sexual Behaviour

These conditions encompass a range of behaviour, which in milder and less exclusive forms, may often be incorporated into sexual practices in which the 'object' is still an individual of the opposite sex.

Fetishism. This may be defined as the obligatory use of an inanimate object (most commonly aspects of female clothing) in order to attain sexual arousal. This deviation may be described as an abnormality of sexual object preference or mode of sexual behaviour, depending on its predominant manifestations.

Transvestism. This refers to the wearing of clothes of the opposite sex (usually female) as a source of sexual arousal.

Sadism and masochism. These terms refer to conditions in which sexual excitement and release depend on inflicting or suffering pain, respectively.

Exhibitionism. This describes intentional yet inappropriate genital display, almost invariably by a man to adults or children of the opposite sex (Rooth 1980). For most (especially first time offenders) this is a temporary phase of deviant sexual activity (Rooth 1980).

Abnormalities of Gender Identity

Transsexualism. This is a disorder of gender identity. Transsexuals are individuals with a firm conviction of belonging to the opposite sex, despite normal genitalia. They have a strong desire to physically resemble the opposite sex and may seek hormonal 'treatment' or surgery to attain this end (Wålinder 1968).

ASSESSMENT

Management is tailored to the characteristics of the individual so that a wide range of factors have to be evaluated before treatment is considered.

The Deviation

The characteristics of the sexual deviation to be identified include its type, duration, frequency of expression, exclusiveness, intensity, recent life event contingencies, legal consequences, relevant positive and negative reinforcing factors, and social effects. Depending on these features, approach to treatment will vary widely. Homosexuality, for example, may vary from being a transient practice, such as a substitutive form of sexual behaviour in single-sex prisons, to an established exclusive form of sexual preference which is independent of environmental factors. Also, a single episode of exhibitionism occurring in the context of obvious stress carries a good prognosis, whereas exhibitionism may be an established recurrent form of behaviour.

Because of the overlap between normal and abnormal sexual behaviour, it is useful to evaluate the context of the so-called deviation. It must be determined whether the deviant behaviour is an obligatory component of sexual arousal, and whether it has become an exclusive form of sexual behaviour. If it is an occasional feature of normal sexual behaviour, it may be possible to identify precipitating factors. If the individual is married, the effects of the deviation on the relationship with the spouse must be considered in detail.

Sexual Arousability

This refers to the capacity to respond to sexual stimulation with increased sexual arousal (Bancroft 1974). In the male, penile erection is the most specific physiological expression of sexual arousal, which can be measured by penile plethysmography. This technique may be used to measure the erectile response to specific stimuli, although failure to respond is not necessarily evidence for low arousability (Bancroft 1971). Despite this and other limitations, this technique may aid diagnosis and the monitoring of change during treatment.

Sexual Performance

Impairment of sexual performance (sexual dysfunction) may be an important concomitant of any deviation. For example, exhibitionism, episodic homosexual soliciting, or excessive sadism may occur, albeit rarely, in response to impotence. In such cases, appropriate treatment may involve treatment of the underlying sexual dysfunction.

Personality and Social Factors

Bancroft (1974) considered that three aspects of the assessment of personality were especially important in this context. These are gender and sexual identity, social skills, and 'ego syntonicity'.

The likelihood of assisting an individual to change his or her sexual behaviour is considerably diminished if it is congruent with an established gender or sexual identity. Thus, if the transsexual is established in the identity of his/her opposite sex, or if the homosexual is established in a homosexual social milieu, the prospect of change is unlikely.

A lack of social skills may prevent normal sexual adjustment. Gosselin and Wilson (1980) found a significant number of fetishists, sadomasochists and transvestites to be shy and introverted while Rooth (1971) describes a similar personality profile for some exhibitionists.

The term 'ego syntonicity' refers to the extent to which the individual accepts deviant tendencies as being an integral part of his/her make-up. Conversely, the term 'ego alien' refers to the degree of the individual's distaste for, and alienation from, the sexual deviance (Bancroft 1974). Clearly, this latter group are most likely to seek help aimed at reducing or eliminating the relevant aspect of their sexual interest.

A further important aspect of personality assessment involves the evaluation of sociopathic tendencies. In some individuals the sexual deviation is found in the context of impulsive, poorly controlled antisocial behaviour, when any proposed intervention must try to help the individual to consider the consequences of his/her behaviour, and to develop strategies (e.g. including avoidance) for their control. It is not appropriate to focus exclusively on the sexual manifestations.

Motivation and External Pressures

As many patients are coerced into 'treatment' by external pressures, such as courts, parents, spouse and the attitudes of society, it is important to determine whether the individual wishes to change. Many treatment techniques are doomed to failure if the individual is not fully cooperative.

Psychiatric Illness

All sexual deviations may occasionally be symptoms of an underlying psychiatric disorder. Schizophrenia and especially mania may be associated with increased libido (Slater and Roth 1969), which may exacerbate a tendency to engage in deviant behaviour, while the disinhibition of many manic patients may lead to the expression of deviation for the first time. A depressive syndrome occurring in association with sexual deviance is a more complex clinical problem as cause and effect may be difficult to unravel. Bancroft (1974) has commented that behavioural techniques are unlikely to be successful in a depressed patient. Sexual deviations may rarely be manifestations of temporal lobe epilepsy (Hunter et al. 1963; Taylor 1969), frontal lobe lesions (Lishman 1978), or dementia (Slater and Roth 1969).

TREATMENT TECHNIQUES

Introduction

Once the assessment is complete, the following decisions must be made: 'Should the patient be treated?' 'What should be treated?' and 'How should the patient be treated?'

At times, severely antisocial deviance may result in imprisonment or, when appropriate, detention in a psychiatric hospital, or special hospital, under the provisions of the Mental Health Act. However, with regard to the treatment techniques for the modification of sexual behaviour, the individual must give informed consent and be motivated to achieve the specified goals. Furthermore, the psychiatrist must be convinced that a successful treatment outcome is likely to result in a more successful social or personal adaptation.

The goals of treatment should be formulated for each individual, and may involve modification of sexual behaviour, treatment of a causal or concomitant psychiatric disorder, or the provision of psychotherapeutic support and advice.

There are two broad approaches to 'treatment'. Firstly, the target symptom (the sexual deviance) may be reduced by aversive, self-regulatory or pharmacological methods, which may be combined with behavioural techniques which encourage the development of 'normal' sexual behaviour. Secondly, relatively intensive psychotherapeutic treatment may occasionally be appropriate.

Techniques Designed to Abolish or Reduce Deviant Sexual Behaviour

Aversion therapy. This involves the pairing of an unpleasant stimulus with relevant cues associated with deviant sexual acts, which may involve fantasies, photographs or real life situations. The timing of the aversive stimulus may vary from the moment of contact with the deviant sexual cue to the presence of sexual arousal (e.g. erection) (Marks 1978). Various aversive stimuli have included electric shock, chemical agents (e.g. apomorphine to induce nausea and vomiting) and unpleasant smells. However, chemical aversion has now fallen into disfavour because it is more cumbersome, less precise, and potentially more dangerous than electric aversion (Marks 1978). Another form of aversion treatment is called 'covert sensitization', which utilizes the individual's imagination of unpleasant stimuli instead of an external unpleasant agent (Cautela 1967; Barlow et al. 1969). The imagined unpleasant situation is paired with the deviant behaviour. However, its efficacy is, as yet, unproven (Marks 1981). Yet another technique is known as 'shame aversion' in which the individual performs the deviant act in front of people; the associated embarrassment is the aversive stimulus (Serber 1970). 'Aversion relief' (Thorpe et al. 1964) is another therapeutic ingredient which may be used in conjunction with aversion therapy; the individual is given a stimulus (which would 'normally' be expected to induce sexual arousal) at the termination of an aversive procedure. Thus, the relief and pleasure at the termination of the aversive stimulus is paired with any non-deviant arousal which is produced.

Self-regulatory methods. These involve encouraging the individual to control deviant fantasies and actions by preventing their occurrence (Rooth and Marks 1974). Firstly, the precise conditions under which self-control is deficient are identified, and then strategies for blocking the progression of recurring antecedent events are considered. For example, an exhibitionist may be trained to distract himself from a situation in which he is most likely to be tempted to expose himself. The distraction may involve 'thought stopping', leaving or avoiding the tempting situation, executing alternative behaviour, or introducing an aversive stimulus. An aversive form of self-regulation involves the patient producing self-inflicted pain by stretching and then releasing an elastic band around the wrist. This may help to prevent the progression of events which habitually lead to the deviant act.

Pharmacological agents. Certain drugs lead to a reduction of the sexual drive without modifying the choice of sexual object or the mode of sexual behaviour (Barnes et al. 1979). Oestrogens, progesterones, antiandrogens (e.g. cyproterone acetate) and neuroleptics, have all been used as antilibidinal agents.

Oestrogens rapidly reduce male sexual drive, but their use has been limited by unwanted side effects, in particular nausea, vomiting, feminization with gynaecomastia, and testicular atrophy, which is usually reversible (Scott 1964; Field and Williams 1968). Also, there has been a report of carcinoma of the breast apparently resulting from oestrogen treatment (Symmers 1968). If oestrogen treatment is considered appropriate, Wakeling (1977) recommended stilboestrol 5 mg daily until sexual activity is diminished, followed by a maintenance dose of 1 mg daily. Progesterones are now seldom used in clinical practice (Wakeling 1977).

Phenothiazines and butyrophenones (in particular benperidol) have also been used as antilibidinal agents. Scott (1964) has suggested that neuroleptics may help those individuals who commit sexual offences which are associated with generalized frustration rather than primary sexual arousal; the behaviour of some paedophiles and exhibitionists often appears to be related to maladaptive interpersonal relations with consequent stress and frustration. Benperidol, a butyrophenone, has been claimed to have specific antilibidinal properties (Field 1973; Wakeling 1977), and Tennant et al. (1974), in a double-blind controlled study, compared benperidol, chlorpromazine and placebo in 12 patients with deviant sexual behaviour. No difference between treatments was found with regard to a reduction in sexual activity or arousal in response to erotic stimuli, but benperidol was superior to the other treatments in reducing frequency of sexual thoughts. This suggests that benperidol reduces the level of sexual interest and thus the subsequent seeking out of deviant stimuli, but that arousability is not affected when the patient is confronted with an effective sexual stimulus. The use of benperidol is limited by a high incidence of extrapyramidal side effects (Wakeling 1977).

Cyproterone acetate, an antiandrogen, has also been used to control antisocial sexual behaviour (Cooper et al. 1972). It exerts a competitive blocking effect on androgens at target organ receptor sites, blocks gonadal androgen synthesis, and has progestational activity (Editorial 1976). It is usually prescribed at a dose of 100 mg a day, up to a maximum of about 200 mg per day. Feminizing side effects are reported, although less commonly than with oestrogens. Dose-dependent reduction and inhibition of spermatogenesis has been reported, although this is usually reversible by withdrawing treatment (Wakeling 1977). Bancroft et al. (1974) found no difference in efficacy between cyproterone acetate and ethinyl oestradiol.

Bancroft (1975) suggested that the antilibidinal drugs exert their effect by decreasing sexual interest but not the erectile response to erotic stimuli. Thus, in theory, such treatment may help people to control antisocial sexual behaviour while not inhibiting normal physiological responses to their current marital or other sexual relationships. Antilibidinal drugs should only be prescribed with the full written consent of the patient. Wakeling (1977) recommends that their use should be limited to situations where 'extreme measures' are needed to prevent such consequences as a prison sentence, dismissal from a job, or a marital breakdown.

If the deviant behaviour is related to generalized anxiety, it may be appropriate to prescribe an anxiolytic. However, Rooth (1980) has warned that as benzodiazepines may produce a degree of disinhibition, antidepressants with sedative effects may be preferable in such circumstances.

Techniques for Encouraging 'Normal' Sexual Behaviour

A range of behavioural techniques have been used to encourage 'normal' sexual functioning.

Masturbatory training is a form of conditioning in which masturbatory fantasies are systematically associated with non-deviant fantasies.

'Social skills training' may help an individual obtain a partner, and would be indicated if poor social competence has encouraged a drift into sexually deviant behaviour which is associated with ambivalence.

Training in sexual techniques may likewise be appropriate for those whose sexual deviance seems to be related to sexual dysfunction.

Psychotherapeutic Techniques

Supportive psychotherapy is an important adjunct to all the above forms of therapy. Rooth (1980) highlighted the importance of confronting denial of the deviance, while relatively intensive psychotherapy may sometimes be useful in those who are considered suitable (Bloch 1979).

Group psychotherapy has been attempted for some sexual offenders with evidence of poor impulse control and social incompetence (Rooth 1980). These groups are usually homogeneous for the sexual deviation and provide opportunities for gaining support, confidence, social skills and limited insight. For non-offenders, membership of a psychotherapy group which contains individuals with a variety of neurotic and personality problems may be indicated.

THE MANAGEMENT OF TRANSSEXUALISM

The individual is normally assessed in respect of the intensity, duration and consistency of his or her conviction of mistaken gender identity. It is particularly important to evaluate the consistency of the various manifestations of this belief in all aspects of sexual and social life. Transsexuals should be distinguished from transvestites and homosexuals, in particular from sexually passive effeminate male homosexuals who occasionally 'cross-dress'. However, unlike transsexuals, transvestites and homosexuals do not show distaste for their genitalia and, within the context of their deviance, are more likely to engage in sexual activity (Meyer et al. 1971; Finney 1975). Sociopathic personality disorder, psychosis, temporal lobe epilepsy and Klinefelter's syndrome have been reported in association with transsexualism, but the significance of these observations is unclear (Money and Pollitt 1964).

Schapira et al. (1979) outlined three stages in the management of transsexualism, if the clinician considers that the individual should be helped to live as a member of his/her opposite gender. Stage one consists of assisting the person to develop modes of behaviour and social skills which are appropriate to the opposite gender role. The second stage involves hormone therapy, for which written consent should be obtained. Oestrogens are prescribed for males and induce mild gynaecomastia, deposition of fat around the hips and thighs, and a reduction in sexual drive. However, the feminizing effects are limited. The oestrogens used include stilboestrol 0.25–0.5 mg daily, and injectable oestradiol valerate 5–20 mg twice weekly. Androgens may be prescribed for females and are usually administered by monthly intramuscular injections of 250 mg testosterone oenanthate. This may increase body weight, encourage the growth of facial hair, lower the pitch of the voice, and suppress menstruation. The third stage involves 'sex-change' surgery which has aroused understandable controversy, as it produces irreversible changes to normal sexual characteristics of an individual. However, such surgery has been justified on the grounds that some transsexuals suffer greatly from their condition (Schapira et al. 1979) and are refractory to conventional psychiatric treatments (Bancroft 1974; Marks 1978), and that surgery in appropriate cases may result in a favourable social and sexual adjustment (Money and Gaskin 1970; Randell 1971; Laub and Fisk 1974). Laub and Fisk (1974) have applied stringent criteria for the selection of individuals for surgery in their clinic at Stanford, California. These include:

(1) The individual is aged between 21 and 58 years.

(2) There has been a significant degree of endocrine feminization or masculinization, with 1–3 years in which the person has been totally 'cross-living' in the gender of choice, with satisfactory social and psychological adjustment.

(3) The individual must not be married as a person of his/her anatomical gender.

(4) There must be an absence of psychosis, psychopathy or criminality.

(5) The individual must be free from any life-limiting medical disease.

By these criteria, less than 10% of individuals who requested surgery were considered suitable.

The surgery is extensive, and complications are common. Feminizing surgery has included excision of the body of the penis, shortening the urethral tube, and the creation of a simulated vaginal cavity. Complications such as infections and fistulae are common. Other cosmetic procedures may include breast augmentation, rhinoplasty, thyroid cartilage reduction and blepharoplasty. Masculinizing surgery has involved mastectomy, hysterectomy and the construction of a simulated penis, which may incorporate a rigid prosthesis. It is estimated that up to 25% of such procedures have postoperative complications (Laub and Fisk 1974).

The management of transsexualism, therefore, presents considerable clinical and ethical problems. Decisions which may lead to irreversible, mutilating and frequently complicated surgery, must be made at specialized centres.

References

BANCROFT, J.H.J. (1971) The application of psychophysiological measures to the assessment and modification of sexual behaviour. *Behav. Res. Ther.*, **9**, 119.

BANCROFT, J.H.J. (1974) *Deviant Sexual Behaviour.* Oxford: Clarendon Press.

BANCROFT, J.H.J. (1975) The control of deviant sexual behaviour by drugs. *J. Int. Med. Res.*, **3**, suppl. 4, 20.

BANCROFT, J.H.J., TENNANT, G., LOURAS, K. & CASS, J. (1974) The control of deviant sexual behaviour by drugs. I: Behavioural changes following oestrogen and antiandrogens. *Br. J. Psychiat.*, **125**, 310.

BARLOW, D.H., LEITENBERG, H. & AGRAS, W.S. (1969) The experimental control of sexual deviation through manipulation of the noxious scene in covert desensitisation. *J. abnorm. Psychol.*, **74**, 596.

BARNES, T.R.E., BAMBER, R.W.K. & WATSON, J.P. (1979) Psychotropic drugs and sexual behaviour. *Br. J. hosp. Med.*, 594.

BLOCH, S. (1979) Review article: assessment of patients for psychotherapy. *Br. J. Psychiat.*, **135**, 193.

CAUTELA, J.R. (1967) Covert sensitization. *Psychol. Rep.*, **20**, 459.

COOPER, A.J., ISMAIL, A.A.A., PHANJOO, A.L. & LOVE, D.L. (1972) Antiandrogen (cyproterone acetate) therapy in deviant hypersexuality. *Br. J. Psychiat.*, **120**, 59.

EDITORIAL (1976) Cyproterone acetate. *Lancet*, **i**, 1003.

FIELD, L.M. (1973) Benperidol in the treatment of sexual offenders. *Med. Sci. Law*, **13**, 195.

FIELD, L.M. & WILLIAMS, M. (1968) The hormonal treatment of sexual offenders. *Medicine Sci. Law*, **10**, 27.

FINNEY, J.C. (1975) A study of transsexuals seeking gender reassignment. *Am. J. Psychiat.*, **132**, (9), 962.

GOSSELIN, C.C. & WILSON, G.P. (1980) *Sexual Variations: Fetishism, Sadomasochism and Transvestism*. London: Faber and Faber.

HUNTER, R., LOGUE, V. & McMENEMY, W.H. (1963) Temporal lobe epilepsy supervening on long standing transvestism and fetishism. *Epilepsia*, **4**, 60.

LAUB, D.R. & FISK, N. (1974) A rehabilitation programme for gender dysphoria syndrome by surgical sex change. *Plast. reconstr. Surg.*, **53**, 388.

LISHMAN, W.A. (1978) *Organic Psychiatry. The psychological consequences of cerebral disorder*, pp. 227. Oxford: Blackwell.

MARKS, I. (1978) Behavioural psychotherapy of adult neurosis. In: *Handbook of Psychotherapy and Behavioural Change. An empirical analysis*, ed. Garfield, S.L. & Bergin, A.E., Ch. 13, p. 525. New York: John Wiley & Sons.

MARKS, I. (1981) Review of behavioural psychiatry, II: Sexual disorders. *Am. J. Psychiat.*, **138**, 6, 755.

MEYER, J.K., KNORR, N.J. & BLUMER, D. (1971) Characterisation of a self designated transsexual population. *Archs Sex. Behav.*, **1**, (3), 219.

MONEY, J. & GASKIN, R.J. (1970) Sex reassignment. *Int. J. Psychiat*, **9**, 249.

MONEY, J. & POLLITT, E. (1964) Cytogenetic and psychosexual ambiguity; Klinefelter's Syndrome and transvestism compared. *Arch. gen. Psychiat.*, **11**, 589.

RANDELL, J. (1971) Indications for sex reassignment surgery. *Archs Sex. Behav.*, **1**, (2), 153.

ROOTH, G. (1971) Indecent exposure and exhibitionism. *Br. J. hosp. Med.*, **5**, 521.

ROOTH, G. (1980) Exhibitionism: an eclectic approach to its management. *Br. J.H. Med.*, (*April*) 366.

ROOTH, G. & MARKS, I.M. (1974) Aversion, self regulation and relaxation in the treatment of exhibitionism. *Archs Sex. Behav.*, **3**, 227.

SCHAPIRA, K., DAVISON, K. & BRIERLY, H. (1979) The assessment and management of transsexual problems. *Br. J. hosp. Med.*, 63

SCOTT, D.D. (1964) Definition, classification, prognosis and treatment. In: *Pathology and Treatment of Sexual Disorders*, ed. Rosen, J., ch. 4, pp. 87–119. London and New York: Oxford University Press.

SERBER, M. (1970) Shame aversion therapy. *Behav. Ther. Exper. Psychiat.*, **1**, 219.

SIEGELMAN, M. (1972a) Adjustment of male homosexuals and heterosexuals. *Archs. Sex. Behav.*, **2**, 9.

SIEGELMAN, M. (1972b) Adjustment of homosexual and heterosexual women. *Br. J. Psychiat.*, **120**, 477.

SLATER, E. & ROTH, M. (1969) *Clinical Psychiatry*. 3rd ed. London: Baillière Tindall.

SYMMERS, W. ST. C. (1968) Carcinoma of breast in transsexual individuals after surgical and hormonal interference with primary and secondary sex characteristics. *Br. med. J.*, **11**, 83.

TAYLOR, D.C. (1969) Sexual behaviour and temporal lobe epilepsy. *Arch. Neurol.*, **21**, 510.

TENNANT, F., BANCROFT, J. & CASS, J. (1974) The control of deviant sexual behaviour by drugs: a double blind controlled study of benperidol, chlorpromazine and placebo. *Archs. Sex. Behav.*, **3**, 261.

THORPE, J.G., SCHMIDT, E., BROWN, P. & CASTELL, D. (1964) Aversion—relief therapy: a new method for general application. *Behav. Res. Ther.*, **2**, 71.

444   TREATMENT AND MANAGEMENT IN ADULT PSYCHIATRY

WAKELING, A. (1977) *Antilibido Agents in Psychopharmacology*, Series vol. 2. *Psychotherapeutic Drugs* Part II, *Applications*, ed. Usdin, E. & Forrest, I.S. New York: Marcel Dekker.

WÅLINDER, J. (1968) Transsexualism: definition, prevalence and sex distribution. *Acta psychiat. scand.*, Suppl., **203**, 255.

WILSON, G.D. (1981) Sexual deviations. *Br. J. hosp. Med.*, 8.

24

Management of Psychiatric Disorders in Old Age

Peter Brook

DEMENTIA

Introduction

No apology is needed for devoting the longest section of this chapter to the management of chronic disorders due to structural brain changes which are present in 8–10% of people over 65, while in those over 80 the proportion with clinically significant dementia increases to 22% (Kay et al. 1970). The disorder usually involves either Alzheimer (senile) or multi-infarct (arteriosclerotic) dementia, and about half of these individuals are severely affected. Although 80% of all elderly dements in the UK are outside institutions, thus creating a burden on relatives, the rest make a heavy demand on geriatric facilities (Sainsbury and Grad de Alarcon 1973).

In a community study of the elderly, 61% of those with significant dementia had been admitted to an institution, in contrast to 19% of those without psychiatric disorder and 25% of those with other psychiatric syndromes. In addition, the demented group spent longer in institutions (on average 12 weeks) despite their higher mortality, compared with 0.9 weeks for a comparable group of elderly physically infirm (Kay et al. 1970).

The incidence of dementia is associated with growing life expectancy. In this century there has been a three-fold increase in the proportion of people over 65, the present figure being 14%, while the number of individuals over 75 will have increased by a third at the end of the century (DHSS 1978).

Organization of a Psychogeriatric Service

A clear definition of the aims of the service should be formulated. Requests for assessment should receive prompt attention, close collaboration should be established with other disciplines, and in-patient beds should be available (Arie 1970; Jolley and Arie 1978; Hemsi 1980). The service should also include beds in a geriatric unit so that patients with physical illness and psychiatric disorder can be managed by a psychiatrist and geriatrician in collaboration (Arie and Dunn 1973). Good working relationships with others involved in the care of the elderly are essential and are forged by personal contacts.

Assessment

If possible a patient should not be admitted to a psychogeriatric unit without having been assessed by a home visit which can be supplemented in the out-patient clinic or day hospital (Arie 1973*a*). It should rarely be necessary to admit an elderly patient to hospital merely for assessment. Because the cause of mental disorder in the elderly is often multifactorial, assessment needs to be undertaken by a team which includes doctors (a specialist and general practitioner), nurses (the district nurse or health visitor) and a social worker. The initial assessment team should not exceed three members as a larger number could alarm the confused individual.

Occupational therapists may advise on aids in the home, and in the hospital they have a valuable role in the assessment of the patient's capacity to undertake the tasks of daily living, together with his disabilities. The assessment should include:

(1) A careful history of the onset and progression of symptoms, together with factors which might have exacerbated or improved the patient's condition.

(2) A list of current problems and a detailed description of the patient's current behaviour, for example, how he spends the day and how much he can do for himself.

(3) An assessment of the social situation, including the state of home, the patient's position and the extent of support from relatives and friends. It is important to contact those who have been involved in providing support.

(4) Information about background and past personality. This may explain the family's attitude towards the patient.

(5) A full physical assessment. Reversible causes for dementia in the elderly are uncommon but physical illness where present may further impair brain function.

(6) Chest and skull X-rays, blood electrolytes, erythrocyte sedimentation rate, full blood count, liver, kidney and thyroid function tests, serum vitamin B_{12} and folate, Venereal Disease Research Laboratory (VDRL) test, microscopy and culture of a midstream specimen of urine, and electroencephalogram. Further investigations may be needed especially for the younger patient with dementia, for those with a rapidly progressive dementia, for those with atypical clinical features, and when there is the possibility that the disorder is a so-called pseudodementia due to a primary depression. These special investigations may include lumbar puncture, computerized axial tomography, positron emission tomography (if available) or isotope scan.

Psychometry is rarely of value in the differential diagnosis of pseudodementia or in the detection of early dementia, although it has recently been claimed that the 'Kendrick battery' comprising an object learning test and a digit copying test might discriminate between elderly normals, depressives and dements (Gibson and Moyes 1979). Psychological tests are also of value in identifying assets or deficits, particularly in patients with a multi-infarct dementia, and monitoring changes in the severity of the disorder (Whitehead 1976). Validated tests of speech and parietal lobe function which are easy to administer can be of help in establishing the diagnosis of dementia and in the identification of those with a poor life expectancy (Hare 1978).

Treatable Causes of Dementia

Effective treatment of any concomitant reversible disorder may reduce disability and avoid institutionalization. Examples of conditions which cause demential states include chronic subdural haematomata, poorly controlled epileptic seizures, uraemia, liver disorder, hypothyroidism, chronic barbiturate intoxication, anaemia (which may be due to inadequate diet or silent bleeding), congestive cardiac failure, chronic pulmonary disease, deficiency of vitamins such as thiamine, nicotinic acid, B_{12} and folic acid and normal pressure hydrocephalus (Lishman 1978). Episodes of acute confusion, or a sudden exacerbation of pre-existing dementia, should always lead to a search for a superimposed pathological process which may respond to treatment.

Drug Treatment for Dementia

Drugs to improve cognition. Yesavage et al. (1979) in a review of the effect of so-called vasodilator drugs concluded that there was some evidence in favour of the clinical usefulness of dihydroergotoxine and naftidrofuryloxalate. However, it is the experience of the author that these drugs have, at best, modest practical value, especially in the severely demented. Dihydroergotoxine may improve mood (Drug and Therapeutics Bulletin 1975) and it has been claimed that other drugs such as piracetam and meclofenoxate can have some therapeutic value (see Chapter 4).

Major tranquillizers. Thioridazine is valuable for controlling sleep disturbance (Linnoila and Viukari 1976), aggression or restlessness and is relatively free from side effects, although drowsiness and ataxia may develop; the dose should not exceed 300 mg daily. Haloperidol (usually up to 10 mg daily), is also of value in the management of behavioural disorder, and doses up to 60 mg daily may rapidly reduce agitation (Silverman 1977). Small doses of fluphenazine decanoate such as 12.5 mg every 4 weeks may also be of value when there is poor compliance.

Hypnotics. Chlormethiazole is effective as a night- or day-time tranquillizer, is not cumulative, and is relatively free from side effects (Witts et al. 1979). However, it may produce nasal irritation and reduce mucosal secretions with a consequent risk of respiratory tract infections. In certain patients, especially those with a history of alcoholism, prolonged use can lead to dependence, but this is not usually a problem with elderly demented patients. The use of barbiturates should generally be avoided, and benzodiazepines are usually contraindicated because of the risk of confusion, loss of strength and incoordination (Linnoila and Viukari 1976; Committee on the Review of Medicines 1980). In addition it should not be forgotten that ageing is associated with a decreasing need for sleep, and that a degree of fragmentation of sleep may need to be accepted. Simple measures such as talking to the patient for an hour or two in the early part of the night may be preferable to medication.

Review of medication. Old people are frequently on a number of different medications which may reflect multiple pathology of old age or an accumulation without adequate review (Law and Chalmers 1976). Drugs may produce more problems than they solve, because of side effects or intermittent compliance, and a thorough review of medication should be undertaken at the first assessment. Old people, even if they are not significantly demented, often make mistakes with their medication so that the number of drugs should be kept to the minimum, and the dose regimen should be as simple as possible. Typewritten instructions may be provided, but relatives, or others, should be asked to supervise the medication whenever possible (Drug and Therapeutics Bulletin 1980).

Psychological Treatments

These have been reviewed by Miller (1977). The two main approaches consist of attempting to alter the individual, or of adapting the environment, and are usually combined. Although ability to learn new information is always impaired in the demented individual, there is often a significant residual capacity which enables some demented patients to be taught to improve their level of self-care. In practical terms, patients sometimes show a cognitive improvement as a result of being exposed to situations involving mental stimulation which, if done in a formal way, is known as 'reality orientation'. Miller (1977) described this therapy as 'relearning and then continually using essential information relating to his orientation for time, place and person; knowing the names and uses of commonly encountered objects and environmental features is usually included in this.' Reality orientation training may take place in a special room but should always include constant informal reinforcement in the setting of the ward or home. As would be expected, patients with mild to moderate dementia respond best, while patients who are severely affected show little improvement (Brook et al. 1975). Behaviour modification techniques may also improve specific problems such as incontinence, restlessness or aggression, while techniques to modify the environment can include the provision of special equipment to enable the patient to manipulate objects such as kettles more easily, and special notices which ensure that the lavatories are easily identifiable.

Conclusion

Arie (1973b) has outlined the three main needs of old people with dementia; first, security, because their capacity to function outstrips their ability to adapt; second, stimulation, because of the withdrawal and apathy which are frequently found; and third, patience in those who provide care and support. Although it may be more convenient for a nurse to dress a patient who could manage without help, albeit slowly, this may produce an unnecessarily high degree of dependence.

Management

Home or institution? The first question to be resolved is whether the patient should be managed at home or in an institution. The former is usually preferable because of the risk of increased confusion by a transfer of the patient to a strange environment; being in an institution may rapidly remove whatever residual skills are left and produce apathy. Admission of an elderly patient to hospital, particularly if unplanned, is often followed by great difficulties in organizing discharge, so that when admission to hospital takes place it should be for clearly defined reasons. It is often valuable to set out the proposed length of admission in a written form, which should be given to the relatives before admission. It should always be made clear that admission may itself produce further impairment, which is usually temporary but can sometimes be permanent. The reasons for a short admission may include an attempt to modify specific behavioural problems (such as wandering at night), special investigations when these are not feasible on an out-patient basis, and to give relatives a period of relief. However, permanent admission may be required either because of lack of community-based support, or because of the severity of the presenting problems. Permanent admission often occurs when a demented old person lives on his own or when it is no longer economical to provide the necessary degree of community support, especially when this is limited and would be better deployed in helping those who have the most potential to remain in their own homes (Bergmann et al. 1978). Patients with a mild or moderate degree of dementia, who do not require specialist nursing, are usually suitable for an old people's home run by the local Social Services Department while, if there is significant physical illness, it is more appropriate to admit a patient to a geriatric hospital (DHSS 1972). If permanent institutional care is needed, it is usually more desirable to admit the patient to an old people's home than to hospital, as the former provides a more homely and pleasant environment. In the UK, Local Government Authorities provide some specialist homes (and parts of ordinary homes) which have been designed for the elderly mentally infirm, and these 'EMI Units' are reserved for the more severely demented who do not present with severe behavioural problems. One local government authority in the UK has proposed that its EMI homes will generally accept wandering and restlessness, urinary incontinence, deterioration in personal habits, and even a degree of aggression or antisocial behaviour, but not faecal incontinence or persistent aggressive or antisocial acts. The possibilities of using private or voluntary residential or nursing homes should be kept in mind. In the UK a list of such places will be kept by the local Social Services Department.

Day hospitals and day centres. Day hospitals are provided by the UK National Health Service; they should provide full facilities for treatment and assessment with a bathroom, a daily living activity area, chiropody, physiotherapy, recreation and occupational therapy. Day Centres (usually administered by Local Government) normally provide recreation, occupational therapy, and perhaps a sheltered workshop; both types should be able to offer meals. Arie (1979) has pointed out that most of those attending day hospitals are being given long-term care and fall into one of three groups; first, the mildly to moderately demented, who need little more than general supervision and tolerance of odd behaviour; second, those individuals with other chronic psychiatric disorders who are often socially isolated, but who can be kept going with support; and third, the group who attend for relatively short periods for investigation or assessment, or who have had a spell as an in-patient when day-centre attendance can offer a bridge between hospital and home. Ideally the day hospital or centre should have its own transport service but in practice this has to be provided by the local ambulance service, or by arrangement with local taxi firms. Because of transport problems it is usually only feasible to take patients from within a 10-mile radius.

The day hospital provides opportunities for close assessment and treatment without the disruptive effect of leaving home, while the day centre offers stimulation, companionship and a mid-day meal, as well as providing relief for a patient's relative who may be given the opportunity to go out to work (Bergmann et al. 1978).

Domiciliary support services. The extent of these varies, and will depend on local circumstances. Arie (1973*b*) lists the following in the UK:

(1) Support and surveillance from social workers, health visitors or district nurses; it is important for one of these to be responsible for coordination of the various professional disciplines.

(2) Home helps and 'meals on wheels' operated by the local Social Services Department.

(3) Aids such as Zimmer frames, commodes and disposable sheets. In a few areas a local domiciliary occupational therapy service is available to advise on appropriate modification to the home and to facilitate such tasks as getting on and off the lavatory or up and down stairs.

(4) Chiropody services, which are in short supply. Attention to the feet is an important unmet need in the elderly (Hunt 1980).

(5) Local organizations which provide 'good neighbour' surveillance or 'granny sitters'.

(6) Relatives may be eligible for an 'attendance allowance'.

Support for relatives. Arie (1973*b*) has emphasized that it is not the immediate burden of caring for an elderly relative which often makes the relatives despair, but the prospect of carrying on indefinitely, sometimes without even the expectation of a holiday or without some recognition by others of the size of their burden. All possible measures to support the relatives should be arranged, including the patient's attendance at a day centre, and a short 'holiday relief' admission either to a local authority home or to hospital. In addition, relatives need to feel that they are being listened to and that it is recognized that their task is valuable as well as arduous. It has been shown that relatives can benefit greatly not only from specific advice, but also from the opportunity to express feeling of anger or resentment together with the realization that the problems which they felt were unique were, in fact, quite common (Fuller et al. 1979).

Specific Management Problems

Sanford (1975) conducted a survey to discover which behavioural problems in the elderly were the most frequent and poorly tolerated; major problems arising from dementia included the following:

Sleep disturbance. This was one of the most common problems reported and one of the least well tolerated. When the disturbance occurs early in the night, a short-acting hypnotic such as chlormethiazole is usually appropriate, and when broken sleep or early waking is a problem, thioridazine may be indicated. Sometimes a combination of both will be needed.

Urinary incontinence. It must be emphasized that this common problem often responds to treatment or appropriate management. The first step is to establish whether there is any specific cause, such as urinary tract infection, chronic constipation or vaginitis, and to treat these disorders appropriately. When restricted mobility is a major determinant of incontinence then either the patient should be moved nearer the lavatory, or a bottle or commode must be provided, particularly when incontinence is a problem at night. If the old person is incontinent because of failure to find or identify the lavatory, such expedients as labelling the lavatory door may be tried. Regular 'toiletting' by the nurse or relatives often reduces urinary incontinence to an acceptable level, while nocturnal incontinence can be made more manageable by the use of absorbent or disposable sheets. Either an indwelling catheter or 'Paul's tubing' can be used for the occasional patient who has constant urinary dribbling. However the introduction of a catheter almost always produces a urinary infection. Emepronium bromide at a dose of 200 mg three times daily is claimed to reduce the frequency of urinary incontinence in demented patients by increasing bladder capacity and decreasing voiding pressure, but in the author's experience it is rarely effective in dementia.

Faecal incontinence. This may sometimes be due to faecal impaction associated with diarrhoea, and in this situation the problem can be resolved by relief of the constipation. Thereafter, regular bowel movements may be encouraged by advising the patient to take daily bran. Even when faecal incontinence is a product of the mental state, it is sometimes possible to reduce the problem by arranging for the district nurse to give regular 'high' enemas and arrange for special laundry services. However, faecal incontinence has a poor prognosis in terms of the old person remaining at home.

Irresponsible and dangerous behaviour. Common-sense measures such as turning the gas tap off at the mains, locking doors to prevent wandering outside, and placing electric fires on the wall above the patient's reach, may minimize danger. However, if the patient cannot be left alone when a caring relative is out working or shopping, attendance at a day centre may be indicated.

Personal conflicts. Dementia may exacerbate previous personality traits and thus exacerbate conflicts within the household. Support and counselling may help the relatives but often the only effective management is to reduce the amount of contact by means of day centre attendance and relief admissions. A disparity between a patient's behaviour at home and in hospital, which has been described as the 'Jekyll and Hyde syndrome' (Boyd and Woodman 1978), usually indicates considerable domestic tensions and is often only alleviated by separation. This may be partial or temporary, but sometimes repeated aggressive behaviour may be so severe that only permanent separation will suffice.

Restlessness . This often takes the form of exploring activity when the patient moves from one room to another or wanders outside. It is sometimes possible to reduce this behaviour by ensuring that the patient has sufficient exercise outdoors, but otherwise tranquillizers such as thioridazine or chlormethiazole are often necessary.

Aggression. An attempt should be made to establish the circumstances in which aggressive outbursts take place; sometimes quite simple measures such as using a quiet, tactful approach with clear explanations may be effective, but medication may be necessary. Haloperidol is often effective or, where compliance is a problem, depot injections of fluphenazine or flupenthixol may be tried. However, sometimes relatives use the term 'aggression' to describe verbal abuse, when counselling and explanation is often more appropriate than drugs. Persistent aggressive outbursts have a bad prognosis in terms of the patient remaining at home and the other side of the coin is that fractious old people may themselves be assaulted by their exasperated relatives. If all other measures fail, then this problem may also require admission to an institution.

Inability to communicate. Demented patients often show considerable disorganization of speech, or they may be deaf and unable to manipulate their hearing aids. This problem is frequent and is not well tolerated by many relatives.

Psychogeriatric emergencies. One of the commonest precipitants of a crisis situation is when the spouse, who has been supporting the patient and has often concealed the extent of the disability, dies or is taken into hospital. An emergency also may arise from homelessness due to accidental fire raising, a declaration from the family that they cannot or will not cope any longer, and episodes of agitation or hypochondriasis in the elderly person living alone. In addition, sudden behavioural disturbances are frequently caused by concomitant illness.

ACUTE CONFUSIONAL STATES

Introduction

The elderly are particularly prone to develop acute or subacute confusional states which may be precipitated by relatively trivial causes, such as constipation or removal to strange surroundings, if there is a pre-existing degree of dementia (Bergmann 1974). A reliable history is important for the diagnosis, as a sudden deterioration in a patient who is known to be demented should always suggest an acute confusional state. This should be particularly borne in mind if there is evidence of clouding of consciousness, worsening of symptoms towards the evening, or the appearance of hallucinations. An acute confusional state may need to be distinguished from a paranoid state in which the patient does not show significant impairment of orientation and consciousness.

Aetiology

The common causes of acute confusional states have been described by Lishman (1978) and include subdural haematoma (which may follow a quite trivial head injury), infections of the chest and urinary tract, cerebrovascular disorders, electrolyte disturbance (often caused by excessive use of diuretics) hypoglycaemia, alcohol withdrawal, drug toxicity, anoxia (e.g. due to 'silent bleeding' or a coronary infarction) and hypothermia. In addition, reduction of visual cues may contribute to an increase in confusion after retiring to bed, or after awakening in the dark, which may be relieved by providing some light in the patient's room throughout the night.

Treatment and Management

The first step is to establish the cause and institute treatment where appropriate. Correction of dehydration and the restoration of normal electrolyte levels is often necessary and if nutrition has been poor, injections of high potency vitamins (Parentrovite) for 7–10 days may be prescribed. If sleep pattern is disturbed, tranquillizers should be kept to the minimum during the day, and chlormethiazole or thioridazine (or both in combination) can be given in the early evening. During the day medication should only be given if the patient is very restless or aggressive. Thioridazine or haloperidol should generally be tried first but sometimes chlormethiazole is effective. The use of paraldehyde is not recommended. For severely disturbed behaviour intravenous or intramuscular haloperidol 5–10 mg combined with procyclidine 5–10 mg can be given and repeated hourly intramuscularly, until the severely disturbed behaviour is controlled. Thereafter, a twice-daily regimen of oral haloperidol (perhaps adding the syrup to the patient's food and drink) is often appropriate. The appropriate daily dose usually varies between 2 and 30 mg, but in rare cases up to 60 mg may be required. Regular monitoring of the dose and route of administration is necessary until the patient is maintained on a regular dose, or the need for medication has passed. If possible the anticholinergic drug should be gradually discontinued. Haloperidol does not usually produce drowsiness or hypotension, so that it is particularly valuable for day-time control of agitation and restlessness.

All staff and relatives should be aware that such patients need constant reassurance and explanation as to where they are and what is happening. Unpleasant or painful procedures such as intramuscular injections should be avoided if at all possible, so that the risk of intensifying aggression, confusion and restlessness is minimized.

NEUROSES AND PERSONALITY DISORDERS

Prevalence

Community surveys have shown a prevalence of clinically significant neurosis and/or personality disorders about 12.5% in those over the age of 65 (Kay et al. 1964a, 1964b) while Bergmann (1971) found that 11% of a sample of 300 individuals over the age of 65 and living outside hospital appeared to have clinically significant neurotic disorder which began over the age of 60.

Aetiological factors

It might be expected that the social stresses which are common in old age, such as bereavement and financial difficulties, are associated with the appearance of neurotic symptoms but investigation has not confirmed this association (Bergmann 1978). Life-threatening illnesses, especially affecting the heart are, however, likely to produce neurotic symptoms. The contribution of genetic factors to the neuroses has recently been reviewed: the importance of these seems to be less in the elderly than in younger age groups (Reveley and Murray 1980).

Treatment and Management

After a thorough assessment, explanation and reassurance may be therapeutic in itself. As in younger patients, management usually consists of a combination of psychotherapeutic, pharmacological and social interventions such as arranging attendance at a day centre. If benzodiazepines are used they should be given intermittently in small doses, because they may induce drowsiness, ataxia and eventual dependence.

It is important to treat concomitant illness as effectively as possible and the psychiatrist can sometimes help the patient to come to terms with feelings of guilt, anger, hostility and helplessness which may follow the restriction of activities due to ageing or disease (Bergmann 1978).

MANIC–DEPRESSIVE PSYCHOSIS

'Endogenous' Depression

Although in the elderly this syndrome may be readily recognized by such features as depressive delusions, sleep disturbance, characteristic diurnal variation, psychomotor retardation or agitation, the presentation may resemble a dementing process (Slater and Roth 1969). This has been called 'pseudodementia' and the patient can show what appears to be considerable cognitive impairment (Kiloh 1961; Post 1965; Roth and Myers 1969), resulting from a combination of psychomotor retardation and withdrawal (Lishman 1978). A feature of the history which may suggest the correct diagnosis is a relatively acute onset with no previous cognitive impairment. In addition, patients with pseudodementia may appear depressed and show a cognitive performance which is inconsistent with that of most demented patients. Thus, pseudodemented patients do not usually show the evasions, confabulations and excuses of demented individuals. The recognition of pseudodementia is, of course, vital, as a good response to tricyclic antidepressants or ECT is to be expected, and the diagnosis can be obscured by a demonstration by CT scan of enlarged cerebral ventricles, which is not always associated with a clinically significant degree of cognitive impairment (Jacoby and Levy 1980).

Treatment and management. A combination of the following treatment methods is often required (Bergmann 1973):

(1) *Drug therapy.* For most patients a tricyclic antidepressant or allied drug is the treatment of first choice. Tricyclic drugs have varying cardiac toxicity (George 1978) and it has been claimed that doxepin is the safest in this respect. Some of the more recently developed antidepressants such as mianserin may also be relatively safe for use with elderly patients (Silverstone 1978), but even with these drugs the minimum dose should be used initially. All the above can be given as a single daily dose in the evening, which improves compliance, reduces side effects, and may improve impaired sleep.

(2) *Electroconvulsive therapy (ECT).* As in younger patients, this is a highly effective treatment for certain patients with depressive syndromes of 'endogenous' aetiology which can often be identified by the presence of endogenous clinical features. ECT should be considered when the patient has failed to respond to antidepressant drugs, when there is a serious risk of suicide, or when failure to eat or drink adequately is producing a serious threat to the patient's life (Slater and Roth 1969; Royal College of Psychiatrists 1977).

(3) *Social and psychotherapeutic measures.*

(4) *Treatment of underlying physical disease.* Depression of endogenous aetiology may be precipitated by physical disease which may require appropriate treatment.

Mania

Paranoid symptoms and irritability are often predominant, while a patient may occasionally present with a confusional state associated with exhaustion and dehydration. General nursing care is important and, as with younger patients, the drug of first choice is haloperidol. Lithium carbonate may be used for treatment and prophylaxis, but it must be remembered that the elderly are relatively sensitive to the side effects of lithium, require relatively low doses for a therapeutic response, and are more likely to be suffering from renal disease (Post 1978; Srinivasan and Hullin 1980).

PARANOID STATES

Introduction

The prevalence of paranoid states in a population over 65 years of age was estimated to be only 1% (Kay 1964a) if elderly patients with long-standing schizophrenia are excluded. Post (1967) has suggested that these patients can be divided into three groups, the first of which consists of those with auditory hallucinations accompanied by relatively circumscribed persecutory delusions. Patients with less predominant (or absent) auditory hallucinations and a more extensive delusional system form the second group, while the third group includes patients who have Schneiderian 'first rank' schizophrenic symptoms (Schneider 1959). Kay et al. (1976) showed that paranoid states in their sample had a significant association with low social class, few or no surviving children, living alone, social deafness and a schizoid premorbid personality.

Treatment and Management

Many of these patients make a satisfactory response to phenothiazine therapy which must often be maintained for the rest of the patient's life (Post 1967). The drugs of first choice are either trifluroperazine, in a dose range of 5–15 mg a day or thioridazine up to 300 mg a day. Trifluroperazine has the advantage of producing relatively little drowsiness or ataxia, but extrapyramidal side effects may require the concurrent use of antiparkinsonian drugs, although a reduction of the dose of phenothiazine is preferable. Thioridazine is less likely to produce parkinsonian side effects but as this drug often produces drowsiness and ataxia it is usually best to prescribe the largest part of the dose towards the end of the day. Patients frequently discontinue oral drugs once they are discharged from hospital and a depot injection may be indicated. Fluphenazine or flupenthixol can be given; the dose of the former is usually about 12.5 mg, while that of the latter is about 20 mg, both at intervals of 3–4 weeks. A test dose of about 6 mg fluphenazine and 10 mg flupenthixol should always be given. The final dose will be determined by the patient's response and the presence of adverse reactions including tardive dyskinesia, the development of which becomes more likely with increasing age.

References (Those particularly recommended are marked with an asterisk)

ARIE, T. (1970) The first year of the Goodmayes Psychiatric Service for Old People. *Lancet*, **ii**, 1179.

*ARIE, T. (1973*a*) Dementia in the elderly: diagnosis and assessment. *Br. med. J.*, **iv**, 540.

*ARIE, T. (1973*b*) Dementia in the elderly: management. *Br. med. J.*, **iv**,602.

ARIE, T. (1979) Day care in geriatric psychiatry 87–91. *Age Ageing, 8* (Suppl. *Geriatric Medicine*, ed. Ferguson Anderson, W. and Dall, J.L.C.).

ARIE, T. & DUNN, T. (1973) A "Do-it-Yourself" psychiatric–joint patient unit. *Lancet*, **ii**, 1313.

*BERGMANN, K. (1971) The neuroses of old age. In: *Recent Development in Psychogeriatrics*, ed. Kay, D.W.K. & Walk, A. *Brit. J. Psychiat. Special Publication No. 6.*

BERGMANN, K. (1973) Operational research to assess the effects of early ascertainment in treatment of psychiatric disorder in the elderly. *Gerontopsychiatrie*, 3. Dusseldorf: Janssen.

*BERGMANN, K. (1974) Psychogeriatrics. *Medicine*, **9**, 643.

*BERGMANN, K. (1978) Neurosis and personality disorder in old age. In: *Studies in Geriatric Psychiatry*. ed. Isaacs, A.D. & Post, F. Chichester: John Wiley.

BERGMANN, K., FOSTER, E.M., JUSTICE, A.W. & MATTHEWS, V. (1978) Management of the demented elderly patient in the community. *Br. J. Psychiat.*, **132**, 441.

BOYD, R.V. & WOODMAN, J.A. (1978) The Jekyll & Hyde syndrome. *Lancet*, **2**, 671.

BROOK, P., DEGUN, G. & MATHER, M. (1975) Reality orientation. *Br. J. Psychiat.*, **127**, 42.

COMMITTEE ON THE REVIEW OF MEDICINES (1980) Systematic review of the Benzodiazepines. *Br. med. J.*, **280**, 910.

DEPARTMENT OF HEALTH AND SOCIAL SECURITY (1972) *Services for Mental Illness Related to Old Age.* London: D.H.S.S.

DEPARTMENT OF HEALTH & SOCIAL SECURITY (1978) *A Happier Old Age.* London: H.M.S.O.

DRUG & THERAPEUTICS BULLETIN(1975) *Drugs for Dementia*, **83**, 85.

FULLER, J., WARD, E., EVANS, A., MASSAM, K. & GARDNER, A. (1979) Dementia: supportive groups for relatives. *Br. med. J.*, **1**, 1684.

GEORGE, C.F. (1978) Adverse effects of psychotropic drugs. *Prescribers J.*, **18**, 75.

GIBSON, A.J. & MOYES, I.C.A. (1979) The Revised Kendrick Battery: clinical studies. *Br. J. soc. clin. Psychol.*, **18**, 329.

HARE, M. (1978) Clinical Check List for the Diagnosis of Dementia. *Br. med. J.*, **2**, 266.

HEMSI, L. (1980) Psychogeriatric care in the community. *Health Trends*, **12**, 25.

HUNT, A. (1980) *The Elderly at Home.* London: H.M.S.O.

JACOBY, R.J. & LEVY, R. (1980) Computed tomography in the elderly. 3. Affective disorder. *Br. J. Psychiat.*, **136**, 270.

*JOLLEY, D. & ARIE, T. (1978) Organisation of psychogeriatric services. *Br. J. Psychiat.*, **132**, 1.

KAY, D.K.W., BEAMISH, P. & ROTH, M. (1964a) Old age mental disorders in Newcastle upon Tyne. Part 2. A study of prevalence. *Br. J. Psychiat.*, **110**, 146.

KAY, D.K.W., BEAMISH, P. & ROTH, M. (1964b) Old age mental disorders in Newcastle upon Tyne. Part II. A study of possible social and medical causes. *Br. J. Psychiat.*, **110**, 668.

KAY, D.K.W., BERGMANN, K., FOSTER, E.M., MCKECHNIE, A.A. & ROTH, M. (1970) Mental illness and hospital usage in the elderly: A random sample followed up. *Compreh. Psychiat.*, **211**, 26.

KAY, D.K.W., COOPER, A.F., GARSIDE, O.F. & ROTH, M. (1976) The differentiation of paranoid from affective psychoses patients premorbid characteristics. *Br. J. Psychiat.*, **129**, 207.

KILOH, L.G. (1961) Pseudo-dementia. *Acta psychiat. scand.*, **37**, 385.

LAW, R. & CHALMERS, C. (1976) Medicines and elderly people: a general practice survey. *Br. med. J.*, **1**, 565.

LINNOILA, M. & VIUKARI, M. (1976) Efficacy and side effects of nitrazepam and thioridazine as sleeping aids in psychogeriatric in-patients. *Br. J. Psychiat.*, **128**, 566.

*LISHMAN, W.A. (1978) The Psychological Consequences of Cerebral Disorder. In: *Organic Psychiatry*. Oxford: Blackwell Scientific Publications.

*MILLER, E. (1977) The Management of Dementia: A review of some possibilities. *Br. J. soc. clin. Psychol.*, **16**, 77.

*POST, F. (1965) *The Clinical Psychiatry of Late Life.* Oxford: Pergamon.

POST, F. (1967) The schizophrenic reaction—type in late life. *Proc. roy. Soc. Med.*, **60**, 249.

*POST, F. (1978) The functional psychoses. In: *Studies in Geriatric Psychiatry.* ed. Isaacs, A.D. & Post, F. Chichester: John Wiley.

REVELEY, A. & MURRAY, R.M. (1980) The genetic contribution to the functional psychoses. *Br. J. Hosp. Med.*, **24**, 166.

ROTH, M. & MYERS, D.H. (1969) The diagnosis of dementia. *Br. J. Hosp. Med.*, **2**, 705.

ROYAL COLLEGE OF PSYCHIATRISTS (1977) Memorandum on the use of electroconvulsive therapy. *Br. J. Psychiat.*, **131**, 261.

SAINSBURY, P. & GRAD DE ALARCON, J. (1973) Evaluating a service in Sussex. In: *Roots of Evaluation*, ed. Wing, J.K. & HAFNER, H. London: Oxford University Press.

SANFORD, J.R.D. (1975) Tolerance of debility in elderly dependants by supporters at home: its significance for hospital practice. *Br. med. J.*, **3**, 471–473.

SCHNEIDER, K. (1959) *Clinical Psychopathology.* London: Grune & Stratton.

SILVERMAN, G. (1977) Management of the elderly agitated demented patient. *Br. med. J.*, **2**, 318.

SILVERSTONE, T. (1978) New antidepressants. *Prescribers J.*, **18**, 133.

*SLATER, E. & ROTH, M. (1969) *Mayer-Gross, Slater & Roth's Clinical Psychiatry*, 3rd ed. London: Baillière Tindall & Cassell.

SRINIVASAN, D.P. & HULLIN, R.P. (1980) Current concepts of lithium therapy. *Br. J. Hosp. Med.*, 466.

WHITEHEAD, A. (1976) Prediction of outcome in elderly psychiatric patients. *Psychol. Med.*, **6**, 469.
WITTS, D.J., BOWHAY, A.A., GARLAND, M., McCLEAN, A.M. & EXTON-SMITH, A.M. (1979) Studies of chlormethiazole in the elderly: pharmacokinetic effects. *Age Ageing*, **8**, 271.
YESAVAGE, J.A., TINKLENBERG, J.R., HOLLISTER, L.E. & BERGER, P.A. (1979) Vasodilators in senile dementia. *Archs gen. Psychiat.*, **36**, 220.

25

Management of Sleep Disorders

G.E. Berrios

NEUROPHYSIOLOGY OF SLEEP

The discovery of electroencephalography (EEG) and description of the ascending reticular activating system by Moruzzi and Magoun (1949) helped to ascertain that sleep does not consist of a discontinuation of wakefulness but is an active and orderly intertwining of two different processes: slow-wave sleep (SWS) (delta wave, non-rapid eye movement, synchronized) and desynchronized sleep (paradoxical, activated, REM, fast wave) (Fig. 25.1).

These two processes, or types of sleep are distinguished on the basis of electroencephalographic, electromyographic and electro-oculographic analyses. SWS is subdivided into four stages: I and II, light sleep, and III and IV, deep sleep. The subject sinks gradually from light to deep sleep and, during the first half of the night, spends longer in SWS than in REM sleep. Short periods of REM sleep appear about 90 min after sleep onset and become longer towards the second half of the night (Fig. 25.2). REM sleep is characterized by:

Maximal muscular relaxation
An EEG pattern resembling awake patterns
Increased pulse, blood pressure and respiration rate
Dreaming
Penile tumescence.

The presence or absence of the last can be used to make a differential diagnosis between organic and psychogenic impotence (Kaya 1979).

Speculation as to the relative importance to life of SWS or REM sleep abated in the 1970s as it became clear that a sharp distinction between the two was difficult to make during experimental work. For example, mentation and even dreaming of a kind occur during SWS (Niedermeyer and Lentz 1976); REM sleep may be reduced in the blind; and SWS takes priority over REM sleep during 'recuperation' after total sleep deprivation (Horne 1976). There is some

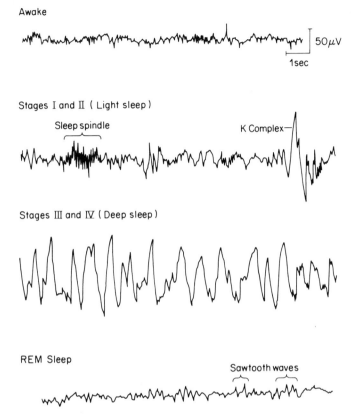

Figure 25.1. Electroencephalographic recording of sleep stages.

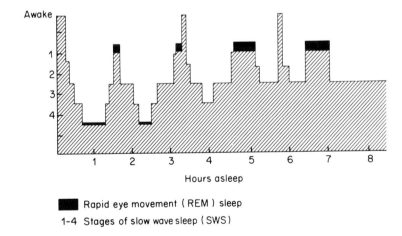

Figure 25.2. Stages of sleep in an eight-hour night.

	Total sleep time	Number of awakenings	Sleep latency	REM	SWS
Benzodiazepines	↑	↓	↓	→	↓
Barbiturates	↑	↓	↓	↓	↓
Phenothiazines	↑	→	↓	→	↑
Tricyclic antidepressants	→	↓	→	↓	↑
MAO Inhibitors	→	→	→	↓	→
Amphetamines	↓	↑	↑	↓	↓
Lithium	↑		→	↓	↑
Alcohol	↓	↑	↓	↓	↓

Sleep latency : Time it takes to fall asleep   ↑ (increase)

REM : Rapid eye movement sleep   → (does not affect)

SWS : Slow wave sleep   ↓ (decrease)

Table 25.1. Effect of certain drugs on common sleep parameters

evidence, on the other hand, that REM facilitates retention of learning (McGrath and Cohen 1978; Webb 1981).

Useful sleep parameters for the clinician are latency (time to get to sleep); total sleep time; total and relative duration of SWS and REM sleep; and number of awakenings. The effect of a number of classes of psychotropic drugs on these parameters can be seen in Table 25.1.

NEUROCHEMISTRY OF SLEEP

Two models have controlled thinking on sleep: Jouvet's during the 1960s and Hobson's in the 1970s. Jouvet's two-stage model (1967, 1977) included the activity of the serotonergic neurones of the Raphe complex, and the noradrenergic neurones of the locus coeruleus. It was suggested that SWS is induced by activity in the rostral Raphe complex, while REM sleep results from activity of the locus coeruleus. The postulated first, or serotonergic, stage gives rise to clinical predictions; for example, that increased 5-HT availability should induce sleep, and clinical trials with L-tryptophan were a consequence of Jouvet's paradigm. The noradrenergic stage has not generated useful hypotheses.

Hobson (1975) put forward a new model involving three neuronal groups—the gigantocellular tegmental field, locus coeruleus and Raphe complex—and three neurotransmitters: acetylcholine, noradrenaline, and serotonin respectively. It was hypothesized that, during wakefulness and SWS, the activity of the gigantocellular tegmental field is under tonic inhibition by the locus coeruleus, which comes under the inhibitory influence of the Raphe complex during stage IV. It was further suggested that the reduction in the inhibitory drive of the locus coeruleus leads to a gradual release of the gigantocellular tegmental field, whereupon this structure stimulates the oculomotor nuclei [producing rapid eye movements (Pink et al. 1977)], the midbrain reticular formation (activating the ECG), and the lateral geniculate nucleus (producing the imagery of dreaming). Hobson's model is complex and tentative. Neither of these models includes dopamine (DA), although there is some evidence that this neurotransmitter is involved in the maintenance of waking behaviour.

ONTOGENY, PHYLOGENY AND GENETICS OF SLEEP

The full-term human neonate sleeps for about 17 h of each day, of which 50% is spent in REM sleep. This is reduced at 6 months of age to 30%, and at age 10 years to 18.5% (Roffwarg et al. 1966). This proportion remains constant until old age, when stages I and II increase at the expense of III and IV, latency before getting to sleep lengthens, awakenings become more frequent, and total sleep time shortens. These objective changes substantiate self-reports by the elderly of broken sleep, difficulties in getting to sleep, and superficial sleep.

REM sleep is non-existent in reptiles; in birds it takes only 0.5% of total sleep time; in ruminants about 6.6; in rodents 15; and in carnivores 20 (Jouvet 1967). In some species it seems that the proportion of REM sleep is inversely related to predatory danger; in others percentage of SWS is inversely proportional to body size (Allison and Cichetti 1976).

The extent to which EEG sleep pattern is determined by inheritance is not clear. EEGs are relatively 'alike' in monozygotic twins for any state of consciousness (Vogel 1970). Total sleep time and organization of sleep stages are also concordant in monozygotic twins (Zung and Wilson 1967), and some sleep disorders seem to have genetic bases. For example, concordance for sleep walking is higher in monozygotic (42%) than in dizygotic twins (7%) (Bakwin 1970). Difficulties in falling to sleep (Abe 1976) and narcolepsy (Kessler 1976) show similar characteristics.

NEUROENDOCRINOLOGY OF SLEEP

In young subjects (not in the elderly) plasma growth hormone (GH) levels peak towards the end of the second hour of sleep and subside by the end of the fourth (Takahashi et al. 1968). However, it is not clear whether this is associated with REM sleep or SWS (Martin 1976). GH secretion may be influenced negatively by tricyclic antidepressants, phenothiazines, benzodiazepines and by Cushing's disease (Martin et al. 1977).

Prolactin is secreted in surges during sleep, and the highest peak occurs towards the end of the night; no specific association with a sleep stage has been established (Sassin et al. 1972). Prolactin secretion is increased by stress but its relationship to night terrors and nightmares is unknown. Adrenocorticotrophic hormone, follicle-stimulating hormone and antidiuretic hormone secretion have no clear pattern during sleep. It has been claimed that melatonin can induce sleep in humans (Hansen et al. 1979), but the mediating mechanisms are unknown.

PATHOLOGY OF SLEEP

The definition of each sleep disorder must ideally include subjective data and objective measurements (e.g. EEG or behavioural). A current classification recognizes four subgroups: primary and secondary sleep disorders, disorders modified by sleep, and parasomnias (Kales and Kales 1974).

Primary and Secondary Sleep Disorders

Primary insomnia. This may be defined as a 'chronic inability to obtain the amount of sleep necessary for efficient daytime functioning', caused by pathology or disturbance of the sleep centres. However, before a diagnosis of insomnia is made, it should be recognized that beliefs as to what constitutes a 'good night's sleep' show considerable variation, and that some complaints of insomnia may not reflect a sleep disorder. Although it has been established that about 13% of the population suffer from 'insomnia', in only one-fifth or fewer of these individuals can the disorder be said to be of 'primary' aetiology (Hauri 1977). In a survey of 1645 adults (age 16 or over), 4% reported frequent trouble in getting to sleep or staying asleep, and 10% used sleeping pills episodically (Karacan et al. 1973). In the UK, 3.8% of patients attending a general practice population presented with insomnia (Clift 1975) and in another survey 15% of male and 25% of female attenders to a general practice had some form of sleep disturbance although this was not necessarily the presenting complaint (Shepherd et al. 1966).

The objective reporting and the polygraphic data may be discrepant (Shimuzu et al. 1970), although subjective sleep disturbance is often accompanied by alterations in the EEG record (Velok et al. 1968), such as atypical wave forms, lack of sleep spindles or intrusions of α-bursts (Phillips 1975). In general, insomnias seem to have longer latency, less total sleep time and less proportion of deep sleep (Frankel et al. 1976).

'Primary' insomnia is not homogeneous, and a number of subgroups can be distinguished. Some of these are identified on a behavioural basis; for example, 'overaroused' and 'underaroused' insomniacs (Peña 1978). The former exhibit higher muscle tension, pulse and core temperature than controls, engage in more worrying and respond well to the 'sleep hygiene' measures of keeping regular sleep hours; sleeping as much as is needed to feel refreshed; taking daily exercise; having a light bedtime snack; avoiding alcohol (as its withdrawal fragments sleep); refraining from drinking coffee, tea, or chocolate in the evening; ensuring a low noise level in the bedroom; and avoiding 'trying hard' to go to sleep by undertaking other activities or practising relaxation exercises. On the other hand, underaroused insomniacs are not anxious or tense, and sleep better in moderately noisy environments (e.g. with background music) or after minor stimulation (e.g. after a cup of coffee). Since the main difficulty with this group is initiating rather than maintaining sleep, it is advisable that the increased sensory input is present only at the beginning of their sleep (e.g. by using an automatic clock-radio which switches itself off). Weitzman et al. (1981) have recently described another subgroup of primary insomniacs as suffering from 'delayed sleep phase insomnia' involving a chronic inability to fall asleep at the desired clock time to meet their required work schedules. (Typically, these patients cannot fall asleep until 2–6 a.m.) However, when not required to maintain a strict timetable, these subjects will sleep without difficulty and, after a sleep period of normal length, will awaken spontaneously feeling refreshed. These patients report that they can function at their best during late evening and are often referred to as 'night people'. If allowed to keep their irregular hours, their sleep EEG recordings are normal. The authors considered that these subjects suffer from an inability to coordinate their sleep pattern to a 24-h cycle as, if left to their own devices, they often fell asleep later at each successive night. No adequate treatment has yet been described for this condition.

Secondary insomnia. This can be defined as a disturbance of sleep function (expressed both in reporting of sleep dissatisfaction and objective disruption of sleep pattern) resulting from overt somatic disease, disorder of brain function, drug-induced states, increasing age, psychological conflict, and stressful life events. Many chronic insomniacs are described as tense, complaining, histrionic, oversensitive and unable to relax (Coursey et al. 1975), and chronic psychiatric disorder is a common cause of disturbed sleep. Delirium and many forms of brain pathology, such as Alzheimer's dementia, Huntington's chorea and Parkinson's disease, severely disrupt the quality, duration and rhythm of sleep, and such patients are often hypersomniac during the day and insomniac at night (Tamura and Karacan 1981). In the case of Parkinson's disease, treatment with L-DOPA may improve an associated sleep disorder. Acute psychiatric disorders, without exception, are accompanied by some form of sleep disturbance (Oswald 1975; Jovanovic 1976). In acute schizophrenia an REM-rebound failure after deprivation has been repeatedly reported, and the duration of REM sleep and SWS are markedly reduced in many patients with acute psychosis (Zarcone 1979).

It has been claimed that hallucinations and delusions in schizophrenics are produced by the intrusion of dreaming activity during awareness; this has been referred to as the 'REM-phasic-events intrusion' hypothesis.

Various forms of depression have been associated with marked sleep difficulties (Hawkins 1979). Also, anxiety states, bereavement reactions, and a general increase in tension and worry have been traditionally related to difficulties in getting to sleep (Lester et al. 1967).

Although there is no doubt that sleep is often disturbed in depressive syndromes (involving increased latency, light sleep, reduced total sleep time or increased number of wakenings), correlations of EEG tracings and clinical diagnosis have failed to demonstrate a clear association with early- or late-onset insomnia, or with presumed neurotic and psychotic aetiology. Endogenous depression, however, is characterized by a shorter than normal latency of the first REM period and by a higher density of eye-movements (McCarley 1982).

Tricyclic antidepressants and ECT temporarily suppress REM sleep, which led to the hypothesis that REM deprivation (by other means) may also improve depression. Early experimental work showed that transient mood elevation takes place after one night of sleep deprivation (Hawkins 1979). Longer periods of REM deprivation (21 days) are occasionally effective in endogenous depression; it is too early and the results are too unreliable to introduce this technique into clinical practice.

Alcoholism also produces severe disruption of sleep. A single dose of ethanol reduces latency, but increases wakefulness in the middle of the night, thereby fragmenting sleep (Pokorny 1978). Under the influence of alcohol, REM sleep is severely suppressed and fragmented, while nightmares, multiple awakenings and abnormal visual and auditory experiences may occur during withdrawal. After 'drying-out', subjects may continue exhibiting fragmented sleep and reduced SWS for up to 6 months.

Physical disease is often associated with sleep disorder (Tamura and Karacan 1981). The mechanisms involved may be metabolic disturbances affecting sleep centres, pain, respiratory difficulties, side effects of medication, changes in diuresis, cough, temporary movement limitations which preclude normal bodily shifting during sleep, worry, or other psychological factors.

Old age seems to be associated with a number of changes in the sleep pattern. Nocturnal wakening periods increase from under 5% of total sleep time (at age 20) to over 20% at age 85 (Feinberg et al. 1967). The factors that determine when these changes will result in subjective dissatisfaction are not clear, but premorbid personality, and quality of life and occupation, are probably important. Early dementia may also play a role, as it enhances the disruptive effect of ageing upon sleep.

External factors such as periodic changes in work shifts, marked variation in environmental noise or room temperature, erratic taking of alcohol, and cerebral stimulants, may all disrupt sleep and engender maladaptive habits of the kind that will perpetuate secondary insomnia.

Rebound insomnia may occur when sleeping pills (e.g. triazolam or nitrazepam) are withdrawn (Kales et al. 1979).

Since secondary insomnia is far more common than a primary disorder, it is important to take a detailed medical and psychiatric history, together with a complete description of the insomnia, its triggers and associations (Regestein 1976; Ware 1979). Occasionally EEG analysis of the sleep disturbances will have to be carried out.

The treatment of insomnia. Barbiturates should never be prescribed for sleep disorders, except in the rare case of the patient who is well stabilized on a small dose of barbiturate (e.g. amylobarbitone, 60 mg nocte) and otherwise has no psychiatric pathology. Phenothiazines are needed only in exceptional circumstances, e.g. insomnia in the setting of extreme emotional arousal; in general, they should be avoided as they may produce 'hangover', deficits in perceptual-motor skills and, most importantly, tardive dyskinesia (TD) with chronic use. Although duration of treatment and dose are related to the production of TD, even short treatments or small doses may precipitate the condition; older age groups are particularly vulnerable.

Benzodiazepines are the most popular 'sleeping tablets'. Of all hypnotics this group is the least likely to produce 'unphysiological' sleep involving disruption of sleep stages. Benzodiazepines increase total sleep time, reduce the number of awakenings and shorten latency. Tolerance may develop, but more gradually than with other sleeping tablets; self-poisoning is less dangerous, and habituation less severe. Benzodiazepines which have short half-life (e.g. triazolam), or constitute terminal metabolites (e.g. temazepam), have less tendency to accumulate in plasma, produce less morning hangover and do not significantly suppress REM sleep. On the other hand nitrazepam, diazepam and medazepam tend to accumulate, producing diurnal sedation.

In general, benzodiazepines should not be prescribed before a complete assessment of the type of insomnia has been made. Not all primary insomnias respond well to benzodiazepines; for example, underaroused and delayed-sleep-phase insomniacs do not benefit. Secondary insomnias should, at first, be treated by reassurance and an attempt must be made to modify their cause. Occasionally, in temporary difficulties such as bereavement, short-term administration of benzodiazepines may be indicated; patients should always be started on a relatively low dose and prescriptions never issued for longer than 2 weeks at a time. If the temporary insomnia does not respond to average doses of benzodiazepines, and there is no evidence of malabsorption (e.g. due to concomitant intake of antacids), or reduced bioavailability as shown by plasma levels, then it is unlikely that higher doses will achieve adequate results. In these cases, alternative management of the insomnia (e.g. by encouraging relaxation techniques—see below) will have to be offered.

The clinical indication for a benzodiazepine must be reviewed every 2 weeks, and the total period of prescription should seldom exceed 8 weeks. During this time, the cause of a secondary insomnia should have been modified (if possible) or, if the insomnia is primary, the type, intensity and complications of the disorder should have been identified. In general, it is easier not to start a patient on a hypnotic drug than to discontinue it once he has become accustomed to its use. For example, patients admitted to hospital for medical or surgical treatment should not be prescribed a sleeping drug unless there is a clear indication, as some patients will continue to request their prescription after leaving hospital.

These recommendations are particularly valid for the elderly. Most available benzodiazepines produce marked muscle relaxation, and this may cause lethargy, unsteadiness and tendency to fall. Cognitive impairment (e.g. memory defect and tendency to confusion) is also a common hazard in the aged, so that doses should be kept to a minimum and prescribed for short periods. When chronic management is needed, more 'physiological' measures such as reduction of daytime naps, or a hot drink before going to bed, may be more appropriate. There is some evidence that snacks such as bran, which are rich in hemi-cellulose, can induce restless sleep and awakening, while milk and other cereal, such as cornflakes, and preparations such as Ovaltine or Horlicks seem to be associated with shorter latency and less disturbed sleep. The mechanisms responsible for this effect are not clear but it may involve the presence of precursor amino acids (e.g. L-tryptophan) or the production by the intestine of hormonal polypeptides (e.g. cholecystokinin).

There is rarely an indication for sleeping tablets such as glutethimide, methaqualone or chloral hydrate.

L-Tryptophan (a precursor of serotonin) has been found to shorten latency and increase SWS. This effect, however, is not consistent. L-Tryptophan is safe, and induces 'physiological' sleep (Hartmann 1977). Aspirin, which increases blood free tryptophan, has also been tried but with indifferent success (Hauri and Silverfarb 1978).

Biofeedback techniques using frontalis electromyography can be tried in cases of hyperarousal insomnia or of insomnia associated with chronic anxiety states and tension headaches. These techniques, however, are no panacea for all forms of insomnia (Hauri 1981). Simple relaxation exercises are not specific but may be of benefit in a number of cases.

Narcolepsy. This is a syndrome of unknown aetiology characterized by short diurnal periods of irresistible need to sleep, and disturbed nocturnal sleep, together with cataplexy, sleep paralysis and hypnagogic hallucinations (Guilleminault et al. 1976). Cataplexy refers to a transient loss of muscle tone associated with sudden emotions, while sleep paralysis is an inability to move after awakening. The narcolepsy and hypnagogic hallucinations are due to intrusions of REM sleep into consciousness (Guilleminault et al. 1973a; Guilleminault 1976; Kales et al. 1982a).

The prevalence of narcolepsy is about 0.5 per thousand and the age on onset is between 10 and 20 years. The most common combination of symptoms is narcolepsy with cataplexy (34%), while narcolepsy alone occurs in 25%. Narcolepsy, cataplexy and hypnagogic hallucinations coexist in 14.5%, and the full tetrad in 11.6%. Secondary narcolepsy may follow head trauma, encephalitis and midline cerebral tumours. There is some evidence in favour of a genetic basis in the primary form of this condition.

Narcolepsy occasionally gives rise to fugue states or 'automatic behaviour', and it has been claimed that some unexplained car accidents may result from the undiagnosed condition (Daly and Yoss 1974). Depression, psychoses, obesity, and hyperphagia have been mentioned as infrequent associations (Kales et al. 1982b).

The narcoleptic attack itself can be adequately managed with amphetamines or methylphenidate. A dose of 10 mg four times daily generally controls the periods of irresistible sleep. Occasionally, however, higher doses are required, and some patients may require up to 100 mg daily. In these cases measurement of the extent to which amphetamines prevent midriasis in standard darkened conditions can indicate optimal dosage (Daly and Yoss 1974).

Psychotic episodes have been described in association with narcolepsy, and it has been suggested that amphetamines may be implicated (Zarcone and Fuchs 1976). However, similar complications were described before this drug began to be used, which suggests that other unknown mechanisms may be involved. The other symptoms of the narcoleptic tetrad do not respond to amphetamines. Tricyclic antidepressants (e.g. imipramine and clomipramine) and monoamine oxidase inhibitors have been tried empirically with indifferent success (Wyatt et al. 1971; Shapiro 1975). Since these other symptoms do not usually produce significant handicap, reassurance is often sufficient.

Hypersomnias. Excessive day-time sleepiness (EDS, drowsiness) is the clinical expression of two different processes: the intrusion of light sleep into consciousness, and insufficient wakefulness (Guilleminault and Dement 1977). The former is due to increased activity of sleep mechanisms while the latter results from reduced arousal involving an impaired inability to 'switch on' to regain full awareness. Hypersomnias can be primary or secondary. The latter may result from brain trauma, tumour, vascular accident, encephalitis, basal tuberculous meningitis, hepatic, renal or respiratory failure, and endocrinological disease. It may also be secondary to other primary sleep disorders such as the sleep apnoea syndrome (Parkes 1981).

Primary hypersomnias, on the other hand, result from pathology intrinsic to the sleep mechanisms. Clinically they do not consist of irresistible urges to sleep, but present with states of variable drowsiness which can be temporarily overcome by physical exercise, intense stimulation or distraction. Electroencephalographically they do not consist of intrusions of REM sleep (like narcolepsy), but the expression of a tendency to sleep is characterized by occasional sleep spindles and 'K' complexes. Sleep spindles are short bursts of fast activity (in the 12–14 Hz range) which characterize light sleep. 'K' complexes consist of generalized bursts of one or two high-voltage slow waves which can also be found during light narcosis which has been induced by a barbiturate.

Short- or long-period hypersomnias can be distinguished by the duration of the episodes. Amongst the former, the most common is the 'sleep drunkenness syndrome', in which patients complain of not being completely awake until 3 or 4 h after getting up; irritability, neurotic depression and headaches are common psychological complications. The 'sleep hygiene' measures outlined above, and minor cerebral stimulants such as pemoline and fencamfamin, are usually sufficient to control this disorder in which hypoarousal seems to be the main causal factor. Patients suffering from sleep drunkenness syndrome often feel that they have 'not had enough sleep' and deliberately increase their total sleep time; however, this only worsens the condition. The main treatment in these cases is to persuade them to shorten the time they spend asleep.

Long-period hypersomnias are very uncommon in clinical practice. An example is the Kleine–Levin syndrome which is characterised by hypersomnia, bulimia (excessive eating), irritability, obesity and sometimes psychiatric disorder (depression, depersonalization, hallucinations and memory disturbance).

Sleep apnoea syndrome. This refers to disruptions of sleep related to respiratory dysfunction: about 10% of the population may suffer from this disorder. Medical and psychiatric complications are not uncommon. This condition is considered as present if: 'during seven hours of nocturnal sleep, at least 30 apnoeic episodes (cessation of air exchange at the nose and mouth lasting at least 10 seconds) are observed in both REM and non-REM sleep'. This definition is a statistical concept, as normal sleepers also experience apnoeic episodes. Useful clinical pointers to the presence of the condition are: loud snoring (with snorting); abnormal motor activity (gross movement of extremities, sleep walking); excessive daytime sleepiness; insomnia; microsleeps (periods of sleep lasting seconds) and enuresis. If the subject is awake at night he tends to exhibit some of the following: automatic behaviour, amnesia, temporal disorientation, poor judgment and hypnagogic hallucinations. Diurnal behaviour in these cases is characterized by irritability, headache and 'neurotic' behaviour, which are relatively pronounced in the morning, together with decreased sexual drive and potency. It has been claimed that hypertension and sinus tachycardia are associated with this disorder (Guilleminault and Dement 1978).

The two types of sleep apnoea syndrome comprise a 'central type' (which may be due to hyposensitivity of the respiratory centre to P_{CO_2}), and an 'upper airway obstructive type', which includes the so-called pickwickian syndrome. Mixed cases are not uncommon (Derman and Karacan 1979). Treatment is difficult and in severe cases there has been resort to chronic tracheostomy. Obstructive apnoeas occasionally respond to dieting (patients are often obese), or theophylline in doses of up to 100 mg nocte (Shkurovick 1976). Protriptyline (Clark et al. 1979), pemoline (Schmidt and Clark 1977) and thioridazine have also been tried with some success.

It is clinically important to recognize these cases as a number of them exhibit psychiatric complications such as 'neurotic' behaviour and irritability. These may be mistakenly treated by psychotherapy or psychopharmacology.

Disorders Modified by Sleep

Anginal pain (Nowlin et al. 1965) and cardiac arrhythmias (Rosenblatt et al. 1973) occur more frequently during REM sleep, and death from myocardial infarction occurs more frequently during sleep. The fact that these deaths peak between 5 and 6 A.M. may indicate that REM sleep is implicated. Asthma attacks may be relatively frequent during sleep but no clear association has been established with any sleep stage (Williams and Karacan 1978). It has been claimed that duodenal ulcer patients who are woken by pain have increased acid secretions during REM sleep (Armstrong et al. 1965), but this finding has recently been challenged (Orr et al. 1974). Nocturnal grand mal seizures occur more often during SWS (Sato et al. 1973). Migraine seems to be associated with REM sleep (Dexter and Weitzman 1970), and this may explain the common clinical finding that affected patients may awake in the morning (i.e. soon after the last REM episode) with a severe headache.

In theory, sleep patterns could be temporarily altered in order to minimize the severity of a condition. For example, an attempt could be made to reduce the proportion of REM sleep for a brief period following a coronary thrombosis, when the patient is particularly at risk for a further episode. However, evidence at this stage does not warrant such a drastic measure.

Parasomnias

Sleep walking (somnambulism), sleep talking (somniloquy), nightmares, night terrors, enuresis, teeth grinding (bruxism) and rhythmic movements are occasionally found clustering together in the same individual or in families. Sleep walking is more common in children, and may be precipitated by lifting the child to its feet during SWS. Since sleep walking occurs only during SWS it cannot be said, as has been suggested by some psychodynamic therapists, that this involves the acting out of a dream. When a somnambulic patient is woken he often feels confused and disorientated. Very seldom, somnambulism is secondary to an organic disorder such as temporal lobe epilepsy.

A genetic factor seems to link sleep walking, sleep talking and enuresis, and young patients tend to grow out of these. A group of sleep walkers, however, continue this behaviour into adulthood. It has been claimed that these subjects have higher levels of psychopathology and of aggression (Kales et al. 1980), but there is no evidence that sleep walking results from the acting out of psychological conflict. Thus, psychotherapy does not seem to be indicated. Benzodiazepines do not alter the condition and therefore should not be prescribed. Sleep walkers rarely get themselves into trouble and are not able to embark on complex behaviours; there is no contraindication to awakening them or redirecting them back to bed. Potential hazards should be removed, and it may be appropriate to secure the bedroom door.

Sleep talking, defined as the 'utterance of speech and other psychologically meaningful sound during sleep and without simultaneous awareness of the event' (Arkin 1966) is commoner in males and occurs during SWS. It may also be related to post-traumatic states, toxic states, helminthiasis and seizural phenomena (Arkin 1966).

There is some confusion in the literature between nightmares, night terrors and dream-anxiety attacks. According to Kramer (1979), nightmares and night terrors should be grouped together as they occur during stages III and IV. They are commoner in males, are associated with enuresis and high arousal, and can only occasionally be recalled. These two parasomnias must be distinguished from 'dream-anxiety attacks', which consist of vivid and frightening dreams with full recollection, which occur in relation to REM sleep and hence are more frequent during the latter part of the night. Autonomic activation in dream-anxiety attacks is less marked than in nightmares or night terrors, but the recall rate is much higher. Benzodiazepines may occasionally help both syndromes (Fisher et al. 1973).

Enuresis in general is a behavioural phenomenon (a 'final common pathway') which is not infrequent in children; 10% of 7 year olds and 3% of 12 year olds still wet their beds. It is associated with psychological, developmental and genetic factors and in only a small proportion of individuals can enuresis be considered as a sleep disorder. Although bed wetting may occur during any sleep stage it is frequently initiated during SWS, so that drugs that reduce stage IV are assumed to reduce the number of enuretic episodes. Imipramine in small doses ($\pm$ 25 mg nocte) has been tried with success, although relapse may occur on sudden withdrawal. It is not clear whether positive results are due to a specific modification of sleep patterns or to a postulated anaesthetic effect of the tricyclic on the bladder. Short-term administration of imipramine (i.e. for intermittent periods of up to 3 months at a time) is more successful than a continuous regimen.

Bruxism (teeth grinding) occurs in stages I and II and may lead to damage to the teeth (Reding et al. 1968). It is commoner in children and tends to run in families. There is no evidence of major individual psychopathology associated with this parasomnia. No treatment is available other than teeth protectors prescribed by dentists, which are worn during sleep. The incidence and aetiology of this disorder is known.

Rhythmic movements may be exhibited by children during sleep. The aetiology is unknown as is their relationship to similar movements which occur during wakefulness. 'Hypnic jerks' or 'startle movements' are normal, and occur as adult subjects fall to sleep, while 'twitching' episodes (nocturnal myoclonus) occur during sleep (Coleman et al. 1980). These are not related to epilepsy and may result from a dysfunction of sleep mechanisms which relate to inhibition of motor behaviour (Guilleminault et al. 1973a). In severe cases, diazepam and GABA analogues have been tried with limited success.

References

ABE, K. (1976) Psychopharmacogenetics, physiological genetics and sleep behaviour. In: Human Behaviour Genetics, ed. Kaplan, A.R. Springfield: Charles Thomas.

ALLISON, T. & CICHETTI, D.V. (1976) Sleep in mammals: ecological and constitutional correlates. Science, 194, 732.

ARKIN, A.M. (1966) Sleep-talking: A review. J. nerv. ment. Dis., 143, 101.

ARMSTRONG, R.H. et al. (1965) Dreams and gastric secretion in duodenal ulcer patients. Nerv. Phys., 14, 241.

BAKWIN, H. (1970) Sleep walking in twins. Lancet, ii, 446.

CLARK, R.W. et al. (1979) Sleep Apnea: treatment with protriptyline. Neurology, 29, 1287.

CLIFT, A.D. (1975) Sleep disturbance in general practice. In: Sleep Disturbance and Hypnotic Drug Dependence. Excerpta Medica. New York: American Elsevier.

COLEMAN, R.M. et al. (1980) Periodic movements in sleep (nocturnal myoclonus): relation to sleep disorders. Annal. Neurol., 8, 416.

COURSEY, R.D. et al. (1975) Personality measures and evoked responses in chronic insomniacs. J. abnorm. Psychol., 84, 239.

DALY, D.D. & YOSS, R.E. (1974) Narcolepsy. In: Handbook of Clinical Neurology, Vol. 15. The Epilepsies. eds. Vinkin, P. & Bruyn, W.G. Amsterdam: North Holland.

DERMAN, S. & KARACAN, I. (1979) Sleep induced respiratory disorders. Psychiat. Ann., 9, 41.

DEXTER, J.D. & WEITZMAN, E.D. (1970) The relationship of nocturnal headaches to sleep stage patterns. Neurol., 20, 513.

FISHER, C. et al. (1973) A psychophysiological study of nightmares and night terrors. *Arch. gen. Psychiat.*, **28**, 252.

FRANKEL, B.L. et al. (1976) Recorded and reported sleep in chronic primary insomnia. *Arch. gen. Psychiat.*, **33**, 615.

GUILLEMINAULT, C. et al. (1973a) Nocturnal myoclonus and phasic events. In: *Sleep Research, Vol. 2*, ed. Chase, M.H. et al. Los Angeles: Brain Information Service.

GUILLEMINAULT, C. et al. (1973b) Continuous polygraphic recording in narcoleptic patients. *Sleep Res.*, **2**, 152.

GUILLEMINAULT, C. (1976) Cataplexy. In: *Advances in sleep research, Vol. 3*, ed. Weitzman, E.D. New York: Spectrum Publications.

GUILLEMINAULT, C. et al. (eds) (1976) Narcolepsy. In: *Advances in sleep research, Vol. 3*, ed. Weitzman, E.D. New York: Spectrum Publications.

GUILLEMINAULT, C. & DEMENT, W.C. (1977) 235 cases of excessive daytime sleepiness. *J. neurol. Sci.*, **31**, 13.

GUILLEMINAULT, C. & DEMENT, W.C. (1978) Sleep apnea syndromes and related sleep disorders. In: *Sleep Disorders*, eds. Williams, R.L. and Karacan, I. New York: Wiley Medical.

HANSEN, T. et al. (1979) Melatonin and sleep in man. In: *Sleep Research*, eds. Priest, R.G. et al. Lancaster: MTP Press.

HARTMANN, E. (1972) L-Tryptophan: a rational hypnotic with clinical potential. *Am. J. Psychiat.*, **134**, 366.

HAURI, P. (1977) *The Sleep Disorders*. Michigan: The Upjohn Company.

HAURI, P. (1981) Treating psychophysiologic insomnia with biofeedback. *Arch. gen. Psychiat.*, **38**, 752.

HAURI, P.J. & SILBERFARB, P.M. (1978) Effect of aspirin on the sleep of insomniacs. (*Paper presented at the 18th meeting of the association for the psychophysiological study of sleep*). California: Stanford University.

HAWKINS, D.R. (1979) Sleep and depression. *Psychiatric Annals*, **9**, 391.

HOBSON, J.A. et al. (1975) Sleep cycle oscillation: Reciprocal discharge by two brain stem neuronal groups. *Science*, **189**, 55.

HORNE, J.A. (1976) Hail slow wave sleep: Goodbye REM. *Bull. Br. psychol. Soc.*, **29**, 74.

JOUVET, M. (1967) Neurophysiology of the states of sleep. In: *The neurosciences*. eds. Quarton, G.C. et al. *Vol. I*, pp. 529–544. Rockfeller University Press.

JOUVET, M. (1977) Neuropharmacology of the sleep-walking cycle. In: *Handbook of Psychopharmacology. Vol. 8*. ed. Iversen, L. et al. New York: Plenum Press.

JOVANOVIC, U.J. (1976) Sleep disturbances in neuropsychiatric patients. *Waking sleeping*, **1**, 67.

KALES, A. & KALES, J.D. (1974) Sleep disorders. *New Engl. J. Med.*, 487.

KALES, A. et al. (1979) Rebound insomnia. A potential hazard following withdrawal of certain benzodiazepines. *J.A.M.A.*, **241**, 1692.

KALES, A., CADIEUX, R.J. & SOLDATES, C.R. et al. (1982a) Narcolepsy–cataplexy: I. *Archs Neurol. (Chicago)*, **39**, 164.

KALES, A., SOLDATES, C.R., BIXLER, E.O. et al. (1982b) Narcolepsy–cataplexy: II. *Archs Neurol. (Chicago)*, **39**, 169.

KALES, J.D. et al. (1980) Night Terrors. *Arch. Gen. Psychiat.*, **37**, 1413.

KARACAN, I. et al. (1973) Prevalence of sleep disturbance in the general population. *Sleep Research*, **2**, 158.

KAYA, N. (1979) Nocturnal penile tumescence and its role in impotence. *Psychiat. Annals*, **2**, 426.

KESSLER, S. (1976) Genetic factors in narcolepsy. In: *Advances in sleep research. Vol. 3*, ed. Weitzman, E. New York: Spectrum Publications.

KRAMER, M. (1979) Dream disturbances. *Psychiatric annals*, **9**, 50.

LESTER, B.K. et al. (1969) A clinical syndrome and EEG sleep changes associated with aminoacid deprivation. *Amer. J. Psychiat.*, **126**, 185.

MARTIN, J.B. (1976) Brain regulation of growth hormone secretion. In: *Frontiers in neuroendocrinology, Vol. 4*, eds. Martini, L. and Ganong, W.F. New York: Raven Press.

MARTIN, J.B. et al. (1977) *Clinical neuroendocrinology*. New York: Davis.

McCARLEY, R.W. (1982) REM sleep and depression. *Am. J. Psychiat.*, **139**, 565.

McGRATH, M.J. & COHEN, D.B. (1978) R.E.M. sleep facilitation of adaptive waking behaviour. *Psychol. Bull.*, **85**, 24.

NIEDERMEYER, E. & LENTZ, W.J. (1976) Dreaming in non-R.E.M. sleep. *Waking sleeping*, **1**, 49.

NOWLIN, J.B. et al. (1965) The association of nocturnal angina with dreaming. *Ann. intern. Med.*, **63**, 1040.

ORR, et al. (1974) Gastric secretion and sleep patterns in ulcer patients and normals. *Sleep Res.*, **3**, 34.

OSWALD, I. (1975) Sleep research and mental illness. *Psychol. Med.*, **5**, 1.

PARKES, J.D. (1981) Day-time drowsiness. *Lancet*, **ii**, 1213.

PEÑA, DE LA, A. (1978) Towards a psychophysiologic conceptualization of insomnia. In: *Sleep disorders*, eds. Williams, R. & Karacan, I. New York: Wiley Medical.

PHILLIPS, R.L. et al. (1975) A study of short arousal in insomniacs and normals. In: *Sleep research*, *Vol. 4*, eds. Chase. M.H. et al. UCLA Brain information center.

PINK, R.T. et al. (1977) Eye Movement-Associated discharge in brain stem neurons during desynchronized sleep. *Brain research*, **121**, 59.

POKORNY, A.D. (1978) Sleep disturbances, alcohol, and alcoholism: A review. In: *Sleep disorders*, eds. Williams, R.L. and Karacan, I. New York: Wiley Medical.

REDING, G.R. et al. (1968) Nocturnal teeth-grinding: All night psychophysiological studies. *J. dent. Res.*, **47**, 786.

REGESTEIN, Q.R. (1976) Treating Insomnia. *Compreh. Psychiatry*, **17**, 517.

ROFFWARG, H.P. et al. (1966) Ontogenic development of the human sleep dream cycle. *Science*, **152**, 604.

ROSENBLATT, G. et al. (1973) Cardiac irritability during sleep and dreaming. *J. psychosom. Res.*, **17**, 129.

SASSIN, J.F. et al. (1972) Human Prolactin: 24 hour pattern with increased release during sleep. *Science*, **177**, 1205.

SATO, S. et al. (1973) The effect of sleep on spikewave discharge in absence of seizures. *Neurology*, **23**, 1335.

SCHMIDT, H. & CLARK, R.W. (1977) Hypersomnia, narcolepsy-cataplexy syndrome and sleep apnea: treatment with protiptyline and pemoline. *Sleep Res.*, **6**, 179.

SHAPIRO, W.R. (1975) Treatment of cataplexy with clomipramine. *Arch. Neurol.*, **32**, 653.

SHEPHERD, M. et al. (1966) *Psychiatric illness in General Practice*. Oxford: Oxford University Press.

SHIMIZU, K. et al. (1970) All night E.E.G. study of insomnia. *Clin. Electroencephal.*, **I**, 21.

SHKUROVICH, Z.M. et al. (1976) The effects of theophylline on the sleep apnea syndrome. *Sleep Res.*, **5**, 188.

TAKAHASHI, Y. et al. (1968) Growth Hormone secretion during sleep. *J. clin. Invest.*, **47**, 2079.

TAMURA, K. & KARACAN, I. (1981) Sleep in neurological disease. *Psychiat. Annals*, **11**, 429.

VELOK, G. et al. (1968) Données polygraphiques sur les insomnies. *Rev. Neurol.*, **119**, 270.

VOGEL, F. (1970) The genetic basis of the normal human E.E.G. *Humangenetik*, **10**, 91.

WARE , J.C. (1979) The symptom of insomnia: causes and cures. *Psychiatric Annals*, **9**, 27.

WEBB, W.B. (1981) Some theories about sleep and their clinical implications. *Psychiat. Annals*, **11**, 415.

WEITZMAN, E.D. et al. (1981) Delayed Sleep phase syndrome. *Arch. gen. Psychiat.*, **38**, 737.

WILLIAMS, R.L. & KARACAN, I. (eds.) (1978) *Sleep Disorders. Diagnosis and Treatment*. New York: John Wiley.

WYATT, R.J. et al. (1971) Treatment of intractable narcolepsy with a monoamine oxidase inhibitor. *New Engl. J. Med.*, **285**, 987.

ZARCONE, V.P. (1979) Sleep and schizophrenia. *Psychiat. Annals.*, **9**, 402.

ZARCONE, V.P. & FUCHS, H.E. (1976) Psychiatric disorders and narcolepsy. In: *Advances in sleep research, Vol. 3*, ed. Weitzman, E.D. New York: Spectrum Publications.

ZUNG, W.W.K. & WILSON, W.P. (1967) Sleep and dream patterns in twins. In: *Recent advances in biological psychiatry. Vol. 9*, ed. Wrotis, J. New York: Plenum Press.

26

Psychiatric Emergencies

G.E. Berrios

INTRODUCTION

The concept of psychiatric emergency is difficult to define but epidemiologic-al analysis (which is essential for the organization of services) requires that one be produced. A common definition states that psychiatric emergencies are situations in which the life of a patient (or of someone else) is in jeopardy on account of his/her abnormal behaviour or psychological state.

This approach appeared in British psychiatry almost a century ago when Newington (1892) defined a psychiatric emergency as 'strong suicidal attempts or desires, refusal of food to a dangerous point, liability to self-injury from violence...the likelihood of harm arising to the patient by his being left his own master, or the possibility of it occurring to others'.

Although consonant with the concept of emergency in general medicine, this definition excludes the less dramatic psychiatric emergencies which are routine-ly encountered in the casualty room or domiciliary visit. These are characte-rized by a disturbance of psychological or social functioning producing personal or social distress but life is rarely threatened (Resnik and Ruben 1975; Soreff 1981).

The concept of 'crisis' has been introduced to incorporate these less serious events, which have been defined as temporary disturbances of the equilibrium between subject and environment that may result from a transient reduction in the individual's coping ability, or from an inordinate increase in external stress (Darbonne 1968; Brandon 1970). Coping mechanisms can be defined in terms of physiological or psychological theory, while stress is classified as social, psychological or physical in origin. For example, severe illness reduces the ability of the subject to cope with normal stress. Similarly, bereavement, or the convergence of several stressful events, can overcome the healthiest of subjects. Concepts of crisis are advantageous in that they encourage a close analysis of the context in which the psychiatric emergency is taking place and thus improve management. On the other hand they are vague and tend to

476

Table 26.1. Five hospital surveys of the characteristics and composition of the 'psychiatric emergencies' population, showing marked variation in some of the parameters

	Reverzy (1978) (Paris)	Ungerleider (1960) (USA)	Mountney et al. (1969) UK (social work sample)	Blaise et al. (1969) (Canada)	Berrios (1980) (Leeds, UK)
Neuroses	3%	40%	15%	13.4%	15%
Psychoses	36.8%	20%	40%	14.6%	17%
Personality disorders	12.3%	17%	22%	15.6%	39%
Others	47.9%	23%	23%	56.4%	29%
Most frequent time of arrival	8p.m.–8a.m.	During the day	?	?	4 p.m.–12 midnight
Age group most represented	10–40	30–39	40–49	30–39	25–35
Self-referral	?	27%	20%	22%	26%
Brought in by relatives	?	50%	?	34%	7%
Admitted	64%	49%	32%	40.1%	39%

engender unrealistic aspirations for the 'primary prevention' of psychiatric morbidity by social interventions.

EPIDEMIOLOGY

Epidemiological information concerning psychiatric emergencies in a given area may not be generally applicable as it is determined by the characteristics of the sample under study, which in turn depend on definitions, socioeconomic parameters of the parent population, the resources of the psychiatric services, and the efficiency of other social agencies acting as filter (or buffers) between the community and the hospital casualty department (Goldberg and Huxley 1980). Such filters include the police, social services and voluntary organizations. Most statistical information originates from casualty department surveys, and refers to the diagnostic composition of the 'psychiatric emergencies' population, the percentage of 'repeaters' or chronic attenders, the presenting complaints, the involvement of other social agencies, the most frequent time of arrival, and the source of referral. Data of this kind are necessary for the organization of psychiatric emergency services but, due to the variations in published studies (Table 26.1), it is advisable that each hospital surveys its own population of attenders.

Table 26.2. Presenting problems of 'psychiatric emergencies' (Detre and Jarecki 1971)

Drunk, fighting with police.
Confusion.
Nervous, delusional, voices.
'I felt tired and sad all the time.'
'My husband is no good.'
Swallowed a number of Seconal capsules.
'Detectives are tailing me and have put waves over my head.'
Has been drinking heavily.
Pain in the head, nervous and mixed up.
'I am nervous, and I'm afraid; sometimes I don't know where I am or who I am.'
Dizziness, 'stomach pain'.
Drinking, nervous, seeing ants.
Can't stop drinking, depressed, suicide 'gesture'.
'Forgetful, losing my sight, nervous.'
Lightheaded, nervous.
'I can no longer go on. I'm depressed and nervous.'
'Can't manage her any more.'
Depression.
Repeated attempted suicide today.
Tantrums, breaking furniture, threatening grandmother.
Attacks of weakness, nervousness, chest pain.
Depression, attempted to gas himself.
'I can't breathe and my heart skips.'
'I want a rest.'
'I am going to kill myself.'
Hearing voices, suspicious.
Threatened to 'kill myself'.
Pain in heart.

In general, only about 25% of patients' presenting problems refer to 'psychiatric conditions' in the conventional sense (Table 26.2) (Detre and Jarecki 1971). The remaining 75% reflect the increasing social demands which are placed upon psychiatric services. Personal sorrows and family conflicts, which are not due to psychiatric disorder, are often brought to the casualty department when 'treatment' is demanded.

Thus, casualty departments are asked to cater for many who are not 'ill' in the conventional sense, and who demand emotional support of the kind which perfunctory physical examination and hurried discharge cannot satisfy. Indeed, this 'medical' way of dealing with crises may be counterproductive in that it enlarges the population of repeaters.

However, stress-related emotional arousal and antisocial behaviour with a 'social' presentation may not infrequently conceal psychopathology of organic origin; thus a number of studies have shown a high level of undiagnosed physical illness in psychiatric emergency populations. For example, Eastwood et al. (1970) detected unknown serious organic disease in 16% of their sample of 100 consecutive attenders.

CLASSIFICATION

Psychiatric emergencies may be variously classified; for example, by whether the source of referral was self, doctor, relatives or other agencies. Ideally, psychiatric emergencies should be categorized by psychiatric diagnosis, but this is not practical as there is often insufficient information available to those working in a busy general hospital casualty department. However, behaviour patterns such as excitement, stupor, panic attacks, fugue states and destructive behaviour (to self or others) can be recognized on the basis of current behaviour without historical or contextual information (Berrios 1979). The recognition of a behavioural syndrome narrows the number of aetiological possibilities and predicts management (Gerson and Bassuk 1980).

PSYCHIATRIC EMERGENCIES INVOLVING KNOWN ('ORGANIC') DISORDERS OF BRAIN STRUCTURE OR FUNCTION

The primary psychological effect of acute organic brain disorder is 'clouding of the sensorium' (see Chapter 13); in addition, phenomena such as hallucinations, paranoid ideation and emotional changes are often present. This stereotyped and non-specific response is described under a variety of names including acute confusional state, delirium, exogenous reaction type, and acute brain syndrome (Lipowski 1980; Berrios 1981a).

Delirium may become a psychiatric emergency if its real nature is not suspected or if it is accompanied by disruptive behaviour. The degree of emergency is mostly determined by the intensity of the behavioural disruption, which usually involves increased or disordered motor activity and/or lack of cooperation.

It has become clear relatively recently that clouding (i.e. disorientation) may be absent in certain acute organic states, for example, in the so-called transitional syndromes (Wieck 1961). DSM III (1980) has also recognized such states. In these cases other signs suggest the organic aetiology of the psychiatric emergency: a history of abrupt personality change, good premorbid social functioning, the presence of adequate family support, fluctuation in behaviour and mental state (e.g. worsening in the evenings), irritability, inability to recover from stress, lowered adaptive capacity, and aggressive or violent behaviour in situations of ordinary stress (i.e. catastrophic reactions).

Minor trauma or stress (whether physical or psychological) may precipitate delirium in patients who are particularly vulnerable, such as the dementing elderly or the physically infirm. Withdrawal from alcohol or drugs is a common cause in all age groups. Cerebrovascular accident without major peripheral neurological signs but with dysphasia may occasionally be referred to mental hospitals as a case of 'schizophrenia'. Drug-induced confusion is not uncommon, and must always be suspected in the elderly, in patients receiving polypharmacy, or in the very young. Analysis of the type and quality of visual hallucinations often assists diagnosis in these states (Berrios and Brook 1982).

Although every effort must be made to treat the underlying disorder, symptomatic management is often the immediate consideration (Varsamis 1978). Sedation must be withheld for as long as possible as it may mask or distort neurological signs such as pupillary size and reaction, reflexes, and the level of arousal. Nursing care should, therefore, be the first line of treatment. The confused patient responds well to being cared for in a well-lit single room. His bladder and bowels should receive regular and anticipatory attention to prevent incontinence, which makes patients embarrassed and restless. He should be reassured during his lucid intervals that his abnormal experiences are transient and the result of illness. This should be done, if possible, by the same nurse who should speak clearly and avoid using phrases that may be misinterpreted. One of the main aims of management is to increase patterned input which helps the patient to regain his hold on reality. Once a relationship between nurse and patient has been established, the latter's defensive excitement and aggression will diminish.

However, this may fail, and the patient's agitated behaviour and lack of insight will continue to disrupt ward functioning or interfere with treatment. For example, the patient may refuse food, become aggressive, suicidal or paranoid, or may pull out an intravenous tube. In such situations, sedation must be used. Barbiturates increase confusion by reducing the level of arousal.

Benzodiazepines do likewise but may be useful in post-ictal confusions or status epilepticus. Phenothiazines or butyrophenones are therefore the drugs of choice. Hypotension, hypothermia, marked sedation and lowering of seizure threshold can complicate treatment with chlorpromazine, and thioridazine or haloperidol are safer tranquillizers. Once the decision has been taken to medicate, adequate doses should be prescribed. Dystonic or pseudoparkinsonian side effects may be controlled with procyclidine 10 mg *i.v.*, but antiparkinsonian drugs should not be prescribed routinely as they may produce cognitive and perceptual disorder.

It is a sound policy habitually to use one or two neuroleptics so that their side effects in relation to dose can be accurately predicted. Paraldehyde or chloral hydrate should not be prescribed except in the rare cases when there are persistent idiosyncratic responses to neuroleptics.

If the patient is so restless that there is danger of injury by falling out of bed, he should be nursed on a mattress on the floor. Extreme measures of this kind should be reviewed every 6 h, and the reasons for such nursing procedures should be periodically explained to the patient. When there are clear clinical indications for restraining the patient physically (to prevent violent behaviour or to administer sedation) this must be carried out only when a sufficient number of helpers have been recruited and in a concerted effort; a useful method is to hold the patient by the main joints, thus avoiding undue damage or pain; in case of drastic emergency and if not enough members of staff are present, the patient can be rolled up in a sheet or blanket until help is at hand. Once tranquillizing medication is started, it should be given regularly around the clock (unless asleep at night), as 'when required' medication produces erratic plasma levels and inadequate behavioural control. The oral route should be used as soon as convenient. If the patient demands discharge or tries to leave, the pertinent sections of the Mental Health Act 1959 (Sections 25, 29 or 30) may be used to keep him in the general hospital, with a view to transferring him to a psychiatric unit when appropriate. However, only an abnormal mental state warrants such action, and the Mental Health Act may *not* be used for the compulsory treatment of physical illness alone.

THE RANGE OF PSYCHIATRIC EMERGENCIES IN THE GENERAL HOSPITAL WARD

Medical or surgical patients may develop psychiatric disturbance that demands rapid control. Causes may be either physical or psychological, and occasionally may result from specific interactions with ward staff or family (Pfeffer 1981). It would be nonsensical to explore staff conflicts or emotions every time that a neurosurgical or 'coronary' patient exhibits acute behavioural disturbance, but if no satisfactory physiological explanation is forthcoming, possible contributory factors must be looked for in the social context. For example, it is not uncommon for self-poisoning patients to be nursed in an 'off-hand' manner which may, in a patient who is still affected by drugs or in the grip of the conflict that originated an overdose, precipitate aggressive behaviour or 'acting out'. Ward staff can be insightless and oblivious to the fact that overt or covert rejection of the patient may engender aggression, and the patient's reaction may be considered as further evidence that self-injury patients suffer from 'personality disorders' and deserve neither understanding nor sympathy.

Neurology, neurosurgery, endocrinology, oncology and surgery contribute the most referrals for psychiatric opinion and assistance (Hackett and Cassem 1978). For example, at a given moment up to 30% of acute neurosurgical patients may be in a confusional state. Endocrinological emergencies may also be accompanied by anxiety, depression, cognitive impairment and, occasionally, psychotic states. Similar symptoms or frank delirium may follow withdrawal from drugs (opiates, alcohol, barbiturates or benzodiazepines) and may occasionally be accompanied by fits and autonomic nervous system overactivity. In these cases the electroencephalogram can be of diagnostic use, as it may show an inordinate increase of fast activity.

Patients in intensive care units may exhibit delirium resulting not only from their primary pathology but from sensory and sleep deprivation (Nadelson 1976). Open heart and eye surgery, prolonged immobility (e.g. due to orthopaedic procedures, or skin grafting) seem to be particularly implicated in this mechanism. Severe burns may also give rise to delirium and psychoses, either associated with an electrolytic disturbance or as a psychological response to the stress. Anticholinergic substances (Johnson et al. 1981), digitalis, tricyclic antidepressants, phenothiazines, oral antidiabetic agents, anaesthetics and many other drugs can also produce confusional states, especially among the very young or the very old.

Physical illness may also be accompanied by psychiatric disorder which is reactive, and not the direct result of disordered brain function. Mastectomy, hysterectomy, termination of pregnancy, vasectomy and mutilating surgery are some of the procedures which may give rise to severe anxiety and depression, to short-lived psychotic episodes, and, occasionally, to suicidal behaviour. Management of these 'psychological' reactions demands both psychiatric skills and compassion.

Excitement (Daumezon et al. 1961)

This is characterized by motor hyperactivity accompanied by disturbance of thought, perception, mood and insight. Motor hyperactivity expresses itself in behaviours such as restlessness, inability to remain seated, frequent pacing up and down the room, hand wringing, mannerisms, aimless exploratory behaviour, overtalkativeness, frequent change of activity, irritability and aggression against objects or people. Restless delirium with disorientation is an example of 'excitement' due to organic brain pathology, while 'functional' excitement occurs in clear consciousness and includes some catatonic states (which can be due to a rare form of schizophrenia), manic excitement (due to the manic phase of bipolar psychosis or less commonly, to physical disease), paranoid excitement, disturbed behaviour in the setting of an hysterical personality disorder and, rarely, a pathological or idiosyncratic response to drugs and alcohol (Coid 1979).

Catatonic excitement is rare, dramatic, short-lived, and unmotivated. The patient is severely ill and occasionally the condition is serious enough to threaten life. Insight is always lost and patients need restraint and sedation, as they are capable of committing serious crimes or acts involving self-injury.

In manic excitement the behaviour is, on the other hand, meaningful; it usually has a gradual onset and may be accompanied by contagious jollity, pressure of speech, flight of ideas, grandiosity and, occasionally, by clouding (Bond 1980). This state may be punctuated by dysphoria, irritability and aggression, and the premorbid personality exerts a pathoplastic or 'modulating' effect. Mixed states are not uncommon with patients exhibiting both hyperactivity and depressive thought content or angry despondency. Manic excitements secondary to physical disease (Bonhoeffer 1909) or to drugs (Krauthammer and Klerman 1978) have also been described. Manic states which appear to have been precipitated by severe grief have been described as 'funeral manias'.

Schizophrenic and other psychoses may produce excited states during which patients exhibit severe disorganization of behaviour and either extreme anger or terror. Fluctuations in the nature of the emotional state are not uncommon and these may be accompanied by 'flight or fight', as delusional beliefs and persecutory ideas are acted upon.

Non-psychotic excitement, perhaps involving hysterical dissociation in the setting of hysterical (or sociopathic) personality disorder, is the commonest type of excitement in clinical practice, and results from deficient behavioural control and episodic disorganization of emotional and cognitive behaviour (Monroe 1970). Secondary gain may sooner or later develop, as behaviour of this kind can be very effective in controlling others; this reinforcing mechanism tends to perpetuate its maladaptive nature. Personality disorders of the explosive or aggressive type may respond to stress with sudden irritability, disorganization of behaviour, terror or aggression. Alcohol or drugs may precipitate this behaviour, particularly in those subjects with marked sociopathic traits who are prone to build up 'psychopathic' tension. The resulting antisocial behaviour, although short lived, can have serious consequences.

Catatonic excitement may respond to phenothiazines and butyrophenones but often ECT is required. Manic excitement can usually be adequately controlled by intramuscular haloperidol; initially several hourly doses of 10–20 mg may be needed, and when sufficient improvement has taken place to resolve the crisis, this can be followed by a regimen which does not usually exceed 80 mg per day. Its long half-life (36 h) allows for twice-daily oral doses. If an initial hourly regimen is indicated, the dose should be under regular review. Haloperidol has negligible hypotensive effects even at high doses (Oldham 1976) and there seems to be some advantage in the intramuscular route during the initial stage of treatment, as a considerable fraction of oral haloperidol is trapped in the enterohepatic circulation (Forsman 1976). ECT is indicated in cases of manic excitement when the patient is nearing exhaustion and is not responsive to drugs. Schizophrenic excitements respond well to neuroleptics and ECT is rarely needed. Excitements in the setting of a hysterical sociopathic personality disorder may require benzodiazepines, but they may resolve without drugs if the subject is removed from the stressful situation. Supportive psychotherapy or social intervention may have a role in situations where life events are precipitating the condition.

Stupor

Stupor is a symptom complex which can follow neurological or psychiatric disease (Berrios 1981). Neurological stupors result from brain stem failure and are defined in terms of unresponsiveness from which the subject can be aroused only by painful stimuli. Psychiatric stupors, on the other hand, refer to states of mutism, reduced motor behaviour and fluctuating consciousness. These two types of stupor probably result from different pathological mechanisms. A number of stupor-like states with uncertain physiopathology have been described: akinetic mutism resulting from midline lesions (Cairns et al. 1941), parkinsonian 'crises', apallic syndromes (Dalle Ore et al. 1977), organic cataleptic states and narcolepsy (Daly and Yoss 1974). It is not yet clear whether the central failure in all forms of stupor involves the level of arousal, or whether each pathological condition causes a different disturbance, and stupor is a 'final common pathway' (Berrios 1981).

Stupor of acute onset should always be investigated neurologically even if there is past history of mental illness; in psychiatric hospital samples, about 20% of stupors can be 'organic', i.e. associated with identifiable pathology (Joyston-Bechal 1966). In another study of patients in neurological units only four out of 386 patients had 'psychogenic' unresponsiveness as a final diagnosis (Plum and Posner 1972). A 'functional' aetiology (i.e. with no identifiable pathology) should only be assumed if tests for cerebral hemisphere and brain stem function are found to be normal; for example, caloric tests should normally produce nystagmus and not tonic deviation of the eyes. Further clinical evidence of aetiology can be obtained from the fact that, after the patient's eyes have been opened by the doctor, a slow, steady closure occurs in organic stupor, while in functional stupor the eyes are often closed more quickly. In addition, after the eyes have been opened, the patient with organic stupor often exhibits slow, rolling eye movements which cannot easily be mimicked. In functional stupors superficial abdominal reflexes are present, plantar reflexes are either absent or flexor, and the EEG is that of an awake patient. Occasionally, however, it is difficult to distinguish psychogenic unresponsiveness (for example, some cases of catatonic unresponsiveness), from a disease process involving identifiable pathology (Plum and Posner 1972).

The most common forms of functional stupor are catatonic, depressive and hysterical. Catatonic stupor usually occurs in young patients, and may be accompanied by waxy flexibility or posturing. It is often preceded by a short period of mood change, thought disorder, or some other features of the schizophrenias. Patients occasionally exhibit a greasy complexion and look empty and remote. Depressive stupors occur more often in the middle-aged or elderly and are not accompanied by bizarre posturing. Patients appear sad and can be mute, although some patients incessantly repeat a few words and wring their hands in desperation. Hysterical stupors are rare, occur in the younger age group, and may fluctuate in intensity from an unresponsive state that mimics coma to a less pronounced alteration of consciousness. Such patients often have a history of previous hysterical conversions or dissociations. Slow intravenous injection of amylobarbitone ($\pm$ 200 mg) may be of help with diagnosis as this procedure may induce verbal production which is incompatible with certain neurological disorders. Catatonic stupors may be suspended for brief periods during which the patient is able to describe his experiences, in contrast to depressive stupors (Stevens and Derbyshire 1958). Patients with hysterical stupors can show extreme forms of regressive and disorganized behaviour (including double incontinence), while those with organic stupors often fall asleep after small doses of sedative drugs, probably due to a low brain 'reserve'. Organic confusions, on the other hand, may sometimes improve after injection of amylobarbitone (Ward et al. 1978).

Functional stupors can compromise life by interfering with eating, drinking or excretion and should be dealt with energetically. Those due to psychotic illness respond well to ECT, while hysterical stupors often respond temporarily and unpredictably to most treatments. As hysterical stupors involve a compromise between intrapsychic conflict and environmental stress, determined efforts should be made to identify precipitating factors and secondary gain, as patients abandon the symptom only after they have been provided with alternative means of coping. Since current or future organic pathology is not uncommon in association with hysterical conversion, the appropriate physical investigations should be carried out (Slater 1965). In a recent study, only 19% of patients exhibiting conversions had 'hysterical personality' as is generally described (Merskey and Trimble 1979).

Panic Attacks (Grunhaus et al. 1981)

These are characterized by a sudden increase in subjective anxiety and/or signs of autonomic overstimulation. Patients may experience fear of death, or feelings of impending disaster involving self or others. Panic attacks are short lived (i.e. involving minutes rather than hours) and stereotyped (Lader and Marks 1971). Panic attacks are common amongst patients suffering from agoraphobic syndromes, anxiety states and obsessive–compulsive disorders.

Occasionally, panic attacks may accompany temporal lobe epilepsy (when they may be followed by a degree of confusion), thyrotoxicosis, phaeochromocytoma (when they are accompanied by hypertension), hypoglycaemic states, carcinoid syndrome (when they are usually accompanied by signs of cardiac disorder, diarrhoea, and a characteristic colour of the face), acute schizophrenic illness, hyperdynamic β-adrenergic states (cardiac awareness, rest tachycardia, circulatory hyperkinesis) (Frohlich 1966), and acute intermittent porphyria.

Management of the panic attack is symptomatic but must take aetiology into account. Panic attacks often settle down in the casualty room but this does not mean that they are unimportant.

Panic attacks can be prolonged by hyperventilation, as the ensuing dizziness, tiredness, paraesthesiae and tetanic response may feed the patient's fears (Lum 1981). If clinical assessment and medical investigations prove negative, and the panic attack persists, a benzodiazepine such as diazepam 10 mg *i.m.* may be administered. Subsequently, a complete psychiatric examination must always be carried out. Symptomatic or even aetiological control of the panic attack may be insufficient in those patients whose symptoms have been overlearned as maladaptive responses. In such cases behavioural and/or psychotherapeutic treatment is indicated.

Phentolamine (Regitine) 10–15 mg *i.v.* is indicated in case of phaeochromocytoma, while hyperdynamic β-adrenergic states and the somatic accompaniments of anxiety respond well to β-blockers (such as propranolol 20–40 mg three times daily) (Tyrer 1976). The latter drug can aggravate asthma, when cardioselective β-blockers such as practolol should be used. The psychiatric component of acute intermittent porphyria may be treated with promazine 100 mg three times daily and a hallucinatory state with propranolol 100 mg four times daily (Goldberg 1968).

Hysterical Fugues (Bergeron 1956; Kirshner 1973)

Individuals, particularly in the younger age group, may occasionally be found wandering in a bewildered and amnestic state which is called a 'hysterical fugue' (see Chapter 18) (Akhtar and Brenner 1979). Almost invariably a fugue is accompanied by a degree of memory failure, which has been called 'motivated' (Talland 1968) or 'psychogenic' loss of memory (Stengel 1966). On examination it is often found that there is a selective loss of those memories which are related to the personal life of the subject; on the other hand 'relational' information, such as language, is not usually affected. The 'personal' memory loss is often total and this (when occurring in a young adult) should alert the psychiatrist to the possibility that the amnesia is not organic in origin. In addition, the pattern of organic amnesia is rather different, in that overlearned material, such as name and address and the identity of close relatives, is particularly resistant to erasure even in cases of advanced dementia. In middle-aged people with no past history of hysterical symptoms, a fugue should not be considered as the most likely primary diagnosis, and the transient global amnesia syndrome (TGA) should be considered. TGA is believed to result from hippocampal circulatory impairment or seizural discharge leading to a temporary inability to register or retrieve information. It lasts less than 24 h, and since patients preserve insight they can be anxious and perplexed; they may occasionally show transient motor or sensory signs (Fisher and Adams 1964).

Narcolepsy may also produce a state of altered consciousness accompanied by a patchy failure to recollect; this may occasionally resemble a hysterical fugue (Daly and Yoss 1974). Petit mal status, dysphasia following a cerebro-vascular accident, and fluctuating stupor (either organic or functional) may superficially resemble a fugue state as patients often answer 'I do not know' to most questions.

Once organic causes have been ruled out, the 'motive' for the hysterical fugue must be identified. Although patients rarely get into serious trouble during the fugue state, admission to hospital is advisable. Persistent accusations of malingering, or the provision of psychodynamic interpretations are all counter-productive in the immediate management of these states. It is important to reassure the patient that his memory loss is genuine, but that the cause of it is not serious and that the memory is likely to return in a few days or weeks. Barbiturate abreactions, hypnosis or intensive psychotherapy usually make no difference to outcome, but abreaction may be attempted when the fugue follows a clear-cut traumatic life event. However, it has been claimed that amylobarbi-tone injection does not improve the chance of obtaining new information (Dysken et al. 1979). It is always important to allow the patient to improve without loss of dignity. Hysterical 'memory loss' is not valid as a defence in Court (Gibbens and Williams 1966).

Destructive Behaviour (Salamon 1976)

This may involve destructive behaviour towards self, others or objects in the environment. Aggression may appear at the height of a crisis, or covert emotion may persist and lead to premeditated destruction. An individual who, during a crisis, breaks the television set (which is not an uncommon cause of psychiatric emergencies), slashes his wrist or attacks another person without apparent motive, is likely to be brought to the casualty room. Details of the incident must be carefully recorded together with its circumstances, and enquiries must be made regarding premorbid personality and factors such as alcohol, drugs or previous mental illness (Fottrell 1981). It is important to determine whether violence is alien to the aggressor (in which case organic or serious psychotic causes must be considered), or constitutes a feature of his social environment or personality.

The presence of severe sociopathic personality disorder of the aggressive type is indicated by such factors as a history of frequent quarrels with family members, association with those who are themselves violent, interest in weapons, excessive use of alcohol and drugs, and fantasies or day-dreaming which involves violence. Subjects with particularly aggressive tendencies have often shown specific childhood behaviour such as pyromania, cruelty to animals, temper tantrums, hyperactivity, stuttering, breath-holding episodes, enuresis, impulsiveness, theft, recklessness and sexual perversion (Sutterfield 1978).

Aggressive behaviour is often specific to certain situations so that once the person is brought to the hospital, there may be no evidence of behavioural disorder during examination; the individual may be contrite, subdued or fearful of the consequences of his actions. In the rare cases in which violent behaviour continues in hospital, it serves no good purpose (as in the case of an excited patient armed with a knife) to be heroic. Doctors are not trained to cope with this kind of situation and the sensible course of action is to contact the police—even if, in the end, psychiatric admission is the outcome.

In the case of an assault resulting from alcoholic intoxication, it is advisable not to interview the patient alone; he should be approached in a firm but reassuring manner, and the doctor must not display hostility or impatience. It is wise not to sedate unless it is strictly necessary. When consciousness is impaired, medication must be withheld until the aetiology of the organic syndrome has been identified. In the alcoholic, intoxication may complicate relatively small amounts of alcohol and subdural haematoma is not an uncommon complication. Benzodiazepines, phenothiazines and butyrophenones are the drugs of choice in severe behaviour disruption due to alcoholic intoxication.

Destructive Acts Against Self

Suicidal and parasuicidal behaviour constitute common psychiatric emergencies (OHE 1981). The term 'suicidal behaviour' implies clear suicidal intention and, when this is present, the patient survives only by chance (McCulloch and Phillips 1972). On the other hand, 'parasuicide' describes self-injury when the motives are mixed or unclear; this often incorporates a 'cry for help' but it should not be dismissed as being only a method for the manipulation of the social environment (Kreitman 1970). Parasuicide is usually part of a repertoire of maladaptive behaviour and about 20% of those who have had more than one episode of self-injury (i.e. repeaters) try again within a year; some repeaters will eventually kill themselves. Suicide is the third most common cause of death in the 15–45 age group and is responsible for one-third of deaths amongst university students (Davidson 1975; Monk 1975).

Parasuicide is often motivated by anger or the need to control others, but the separation of 'genuine' suicidal behaviour from parasuicide is often far from clear. Thus, between the serious suicidal attempt of an elderly widower with chronic physical disease, and the teenager who takes an overdose over a failed love affair, there extends a range of states where intentionality (whether conscious or unconscious) shows considerable variation. Thus, parasuicidal behaviour needs to be taken seriously even if there is no evidence of clear suicidal intent.

Non-accidental poisoning is the most common form of parasuicidal behaviour and is responsible for about 15% of general hospital admissions in the UK (Mathew 1975). Thus the medical and psychiatric management of these states has developed into a specialized skill (Goulding 1972; Lawson 1976; Meredith and Vale 1981).

Attempts have been made to construct scales that measure risk and identify repeaters, so that this group can be provided with follow-up support (McCulloch and Phillips 1972). The Suicide Act of 1961 enjoined psychiatrists to carry out routine assessments when self-injury occurs, and the 1968 Hill Report recommended close liaison between psychiatric and general hospital units. However, these recommendations, which were unsupported by hard data, were never fully implemented. In the middle 1960s Stengel had already advised that psychiatrists should act mainly in a consultative capacity, for there has never been clear evidence to demonstrate that the assessment and management carried out by psychiatrists is any more effective than that by other hospital doctors. Recent work has shown that there seems to be no difference between the effects of assessment by psychiatrists or non-psychiatrists, which suggests that a cost-effective role for the psychiatrist is to provide training for junior general hospital doctors (Gardner 1978). In fact, general practitioners already carry out a great deal of the assessment work and only one self-injury patient in five is referred to a hospital.

Table 26.3 lists the items whose presence leads to an assessment of high suicidal risk. However, these items are based on statistical findings, and do not necessarily have accumulative value. They must be considered in conjunction with other information obtained during interview and modified by the clinical experience of the examiner (Gardner et al. 1981). The central objective of assessing immediate and future suicide risk after self-injury is not so much that of separating a failed genuine suicidal attempt from parasuicidal individuals, but to organize the appropriate management for each patient (Hawton and Catalan 1981). Clearly genuine suicidal attempts are usually admitted to a psychiatric unit, as about 90% may be suffering from a form of mental illness (Sainsbury 1974). Although the parasuicidal population is admitted to a

Table 26.3. Items associated with suicidal risk

1.	Age: Over 50*	12.	Ideas of unworthiness or fantasies* of being reunited with departed relative
2.	Sex: Male		
3.	Social class I or V	13.	Recent bereavement
4.	Status incongruity	14.	Ongoing psychiatric treatment
5.	Social drifting and geographical escaping		
		15.	Violence in relationship with key relatives
6.	Mental illness*		
7.	Depressive illness*	16.	Positive family history of successful suicide
8.	Previous suicidal attempt	17.	Careful planning of act*
9.	Terminal or serious physical illness	18.	Hostile-passive-dependent relationship with doctor
10	Alcoholism*	19.	Bizarre forms of suicide* (throat slashing, hanging, gassing, jumping out of windows)
11.	Drug addiction*		

*Starred items are particularly important

psychiatric hospital less often, ideally all should be offered some form of help which may range from a few supportive interviews to an offer of intensive psychotherapy. The role of social workers, nurse therapists and psychologists is important in this context.

SOCIAL PSYCHIATRIC EMERGENCY

These are behavioural disorders associated with psychological dysfunction resulting primarily from social or family conflict. In the absence of specialized 'crisis intervention' services, these difficulties are usually dealt with as psychiatric emergencies, and may provide 30–40% of the total of psychiatric emergencies in some areas (Berrios 1979). Inadequate cooperation between psychiatrists, other doctors and community agencies may contribute to the number of social psychiatric emergencies. For example, if a general practitioner is not prepared to make a detailed assessment of a behavioural disorder which is causing social problems, he may recommend that the person is brought to the casualty department of the general hospital.

It is essential for the doctor to identify the social precipitants of these emergencies, which may become clear when relatives or friends accompanying the 'patient' are interviewed. The casualty doctor may be in an ideal position to obtain the essential information, as people often talk more readily in an emotionally charged situation, or when threatened by a crisis; by the next morning those concerned may be unapproachable.

Ideally, the increasing frequency of social emergencies requires an improvement of the psychiatric services and the creation of specialized facilities (such as 'flying squads', and 'walk in' clinics), away from the hospital (Cooper 1979). Adequate links between the hospital services and other social agencies must be established. In practice, the provision of such services is difficult, so that casualty departments will continue to cope with their share of social problems, especially if they serve areas of social deprivation.

References

AKHTAR, S. & BRENNER, I.J. (1979) Differential diagnosis of fugue-like states. *J. Clin. Psychiat.*, **40**, 381.

BERGERON, M. (1956) Fugues. Encycl. méd. chir. (Paris). Psychiatrie, Fasc. 37140 E10.

BERRIOS, G.E. (1980) Community psychiatry and the crisis intervention team. *Progr. Psychopharmacol.*, **4**, 83.

BERRIOS, G.E. (1981*a*) Delirium and confusion in the 19th century: a conceptual history. *Br. J. Psychiat.*, **139**, 439.

BERRIOS, G.E. (1981*b*) Stupor revisited. *Compreh. Psychiat.*, **22**, 466.

BERRIOS, G.E. & BROOK, P. (1982) The Charles Bonnet syndrome and the problem of visual perceptual disorder in the elderly. *Age & Ageing*, **11**, 17.

BLAIS, A. & GEORGES, J. (1969) Psychiatric emergencies in a general hospital out-patients department. *Can. psychiat. Ass. J.*, **14**, 123.

BOND, T.C. (1980) Recognition of acute delirious mania. *Arch. gen. Psychiat.*, **37**, 553.

BONHOEFFER, K. (1909) Zur Frage der exogenen Psychosen. *Zentbl. Nervenheilk.*, **32**, 499.

BRANDON, S. (1970) Crisis theory and possibilities of therapeutic intervention. *Br. J. Psychiat.*, **117**, 627.

CAIRNS, H. et al. (1941) Akinetic mutism with an epidermoid cyst of the 3rd ventricle. *Brain*, **64**, 273.

COID, J. (1979) Mania a Potu. A critical review of pathological intoxication. *Psychol. Med.*, **9**, 709.

COOPER, J.E. (1979) *Crisis Admission Units and Emergency Psychiatric Services*. Copenhagen: World Health Organisation.

DALLE ORE, G. et al. (Eds) (1977) *The Apallic Syndrome*. Berlin: Springer.

DALY, D.D. & YOSS, R.E. (1974) Narcolepsy. In: *Handbook of Clinical Neurology. Vol. 16*, eds. Vinken & Bruyn. Amsterdam.

DARBONNE, A. (1968) Crisis: A review of theory, practice and research. *Int. J. Psychiat.*, **6**, 371.

DAUMEZON, G., TOSQUELLES, F. & AUDISIO, M. (1961) Conduites d'agitation. Encycl. méd. chir. (Paris) Psychiatrie, Fasc. 37140 A10.

DAVIDSON, K. (1975) Management of patients at risk of suicide. *Medicine*, 2nd Series, p. 166.

DETRE, T.P. & JARECKI, H.G. (1971) *Modern Psychiatric Treatment*. New York: Lippincott.

D.S.M. III (1980) *Diagnostic and Statistical Manual of Mental Disorder*, 3rd ed. American Psychiatric Association.

DYSKEN, M.W., KOOSER, J.A., HARASZTI, J.S. & DAVIS, J.M. (1979) Clinical usefulness of sodium amobarbital interviewing. *Arch. gen. Psych.*, **36**, 789.

EASTWOOD, M.R. et al. (1970) The physical status of psychiatric emergencies. *Br. J. Psychiat.*, **116**, 545.

FISHER, C.M. & ADAMS, R.D. (1964) Transient Global Amnesia. *Acta psychiat. neurol. scand.*, **40**, (Suppl. 9).

FORSMAN, A.D. (1976) Individual variability in response to Haloperidol. *Proc. roy. Soc. Med.*, **69**, (Suppl.) 9.

FOTTRELL, E. (1981) Violent behaviour by psychiatric patients. *Brit. J. Hosp. Med.*, **25**, 28.

FROHLICK, E.D. et al. (1966) Hyperdynamic beta adrenergic circulatory state. *Arch. intern. Med.*, **117**, 614.

GARDNER, R. et al. (1978) Consultation-liaison scheme for self poisoned patients in a general hospital. *Br. med. J.*, **ii**, 1342.

GARDNER, R., MEREDITH, T.J. & VALE, J.A. (1981) Prevention of Poisoning. In: *Poisoning, Diagnosis and Treatment*. eds. Vale, J.A. and Meredith, T.J. pp. 78–83, London: Update Books.

GERSON, S. & BASSUK, E. (1980) Psychiatric emergencies: an overview. *Am. J. Psychiat.*, **137**, 1.

GIBBENS, T.C.N. & WILLIAMS, J.E.H. (1966) Medico legal aspects of amnesia. In: *Amnesia*. eds. Whitty, C. and Zangwill, O. London: Butterworths.

GOLDBERG, A. (1968) Diagnosis and treatment of the porphyrias. *Proc. roy. Soc. Med.*, **61**, 193.

GOLDBERG, D. & HUXLEY, P. (1980) *Mental Illness in the Community*. London: Tavistock.

GOULDING, R. (1972) Drug Overdose. *Br. J. Hosp. Med.*, **9**, 293.

GRUNHAUS, L., GLOGER, S. & WEISSTUB, E. (1981) Panic attacks. *J. nerv. ment. Dis.*, **169**, 608.

HACKETT, T.P. & CASSEM, N.H. (eds) (1978) *Handbook of General Hospital Psychiatry*. Saint Louis: Mosby.

HAWTON, K. & CATALAN, J. (1981) Psychiatric management of attempted suicide patients. *Br. J. Hosp. Med.*, **25**, 365.

JOHNSON, A.N., HOLLISTER, L.O. & BERGER, P.A. (1981) The anticholinergic intoxication syndrome. Diagnosis and treatment. *J. Clin. Psychiat.*, **42**, 313–317.

JOYSTON-BECHAL, M.P. (1966) The clinical features and outcome of stupor. *Br. J. Psychiat.*, **112**, 967.

KIRSHNER, L.A. (1973) Dissociative reactions. *Acta psychiat. scand.*, **49**, 698.

KRAUTHAMMER, C. & KLERMAN, G.L. (1978) Secondary mania. *Arch. gen. Psychiat.*, **35**, 1333.

KREITMAN, N. et al. (1970) Attempted suicide as language: an empirical study. *Br. J. Psychiat.*, **116**, 465.

LADER, M. & MARKS, I. (1971) *Clinical Anxiety*. London: Heinemann.

LAWSON, A.A.H. (1976) Intensive therapy of acute poisoning. *Br. J. Hosp. Med.*, **16**, 333.

LIPOWSKI, Z.J. (1980) *Delirium, Acute Brain Failure in Man*. Illinois: Charles C. Thomas.

LUM, L.C. (1981) Hyperventilation and anxiety state. *J. Royal Soc. Med.*, **74**, 1.

McCULLOCH, J.W. & PHILLIP, A.E. (1972) *Suicidal Behaviour*. Oxford: Pergamon Press.

MATHEWS, H.J.S. (1975) *Management of Self Poisoning*. Medicine (2nd Series) p. 214.

MEREDITH, T.J. & VALE, J.A. (1981) Poisoning due to hypnotics, sedatives, tranquillisers and anticonvulsants. In: *Poisoning, Diagnosis and Treatment*, eds. Vale, J.A. & Meredith, T.J. pp. 84–89. London: Update Books.

MERSKEY, H. & TRIMBLE, M. (1979) Personality, sexual adjustment and brain lesions in patients with conversion symptoms. *Am. J. Psychiat.*, **136**, 179.

MONK, M. (1975) Epidemiology. In: *A Handbook for the Study of Suicide*, ed. Perlin, S. New York: Oxford Univ. Press.

MONROE, R.R. (1970) *Episodic Behavioural Disorder*. Boston: Harvard Univ. Press.

MOUNTNEY, G. et al. (1969) Psychiatric emergencies in an urban borough. *Br. med. J.*, **i**, 498.

NADELSON, T. (1976) The psychiatrist in the surgical intensive care unit. I. Post operative delirium. *Arch. Surg.*, **111**, 113.

NEWINGTON, H.H. (1892) Certificates. In: *Dictionary of Psychological Medicine*, ed. Tuke, D.H. Vol. I. London: Churchill.

OFFICE HEALTH ECONOMICS (1981) *Suicide and Deliberate Self-Harm*. London: White Crescent Press.

OLDHAM, A.J.P. (1976) The rapid control of the acute patient by Haloperidol. *Proc. roy. Soc. ed.*, **69** (Suppl. 1), 23.

PFEFFER, J.M. (1981) Management of the acutely disturbed patient on the general ward. *Br. J. Hosp. Med.*, **26**, 73.

PLUM, F. & POSNER, J.B. (1972) *The Diagnosis of Stupor and Coma*, 2nd ed. Philadelphia: Davies.

RESNIK, H.L.P. & RUBEN, T. (eds) (1975) *Emergency Psychiatric Care*. Maryland: Charles Press.

REVERZY, J.F. (1978) Les urgences à l'infirmerie psychiatrique de la préfecture de police de Paris. *L'Evolution Psychiatrique*, **43**, 197.

SAINSBURY, P. (1974) Suicide. *Medicine*, (1st Series), No. 30, pp. 1772.

SALAMON, I. (1976) Violent and aggressive behaviour. In: *Psychiatric Emergencies*, ed. R.A. Glick et al., pp. 109–119. New York: Grune & Stratton.

SLATER, E. (1965) Diagnosis of hysteria. *Br. med. J.*, **i**, 1395.

SOREFF, S.M. (1981) *Management of the Psychiatric Emergency*. New York: John Wiley.

STENGEL, E. (1966) Psychogenic memory loss. In: *Amnesia*, eds. Whittey, C. & Zangwill, O. London: Butterworths.

STEVENS, J.M. & DERBYSHIRE, A.J. (1958) Shifts along the alert-response continuum during remission of catatonic "stupor" with amobarbital. *Psychosom. Med.*, **20**, 99.

SUTTERFIELD, J.H. (1978) The hyperactive child syndrome: a precursor of adult psychopathy? In: *Psychopathic Behaviour*. eds. Hare, R.D. & Schalling, D. pp. 329–346. New York: John Wiley.

TALLAND, C.A. (1968) *Disorders of Memory*. Harmondsworth: Penguin Books.

TYRER, P. (1976) *The Role of Bodily Feelings in Anxiety*. Maudsley Monograph No. 23. Oxford: Oxford University Press.

UNGERLEIDER, J.T. (1960) The psychiatric emergency: analysis of six months' experience of a university hospital's consultation service. *Arch. gen. Psychiat.*, **3**, 593.

VARSAMIS, J. (1978) Clinical management of delirium. *Psychiat. Clin. North America*, **1**, 71.

WARD, N.G., ROWLETT, D.B. & BURKE, P. (1978) Sodium amylobarbitone in the differential diagnosis of confusion. *Am. J. Psychiat.*, **135**, 75.

WHITELEY, J.S. & DENISON, D.M. (1963) The psychiatric casualty. *Br. J. Psychiat.*, **109**, 488.

WIECK, H.H. (1961) Zur klinischen Stellung des Durchgangs-Syndroms. *Schweiz. Arch. Neurol. Psychiat.*, **88**, 409.

Index